Diagnostic Sonography Handbook

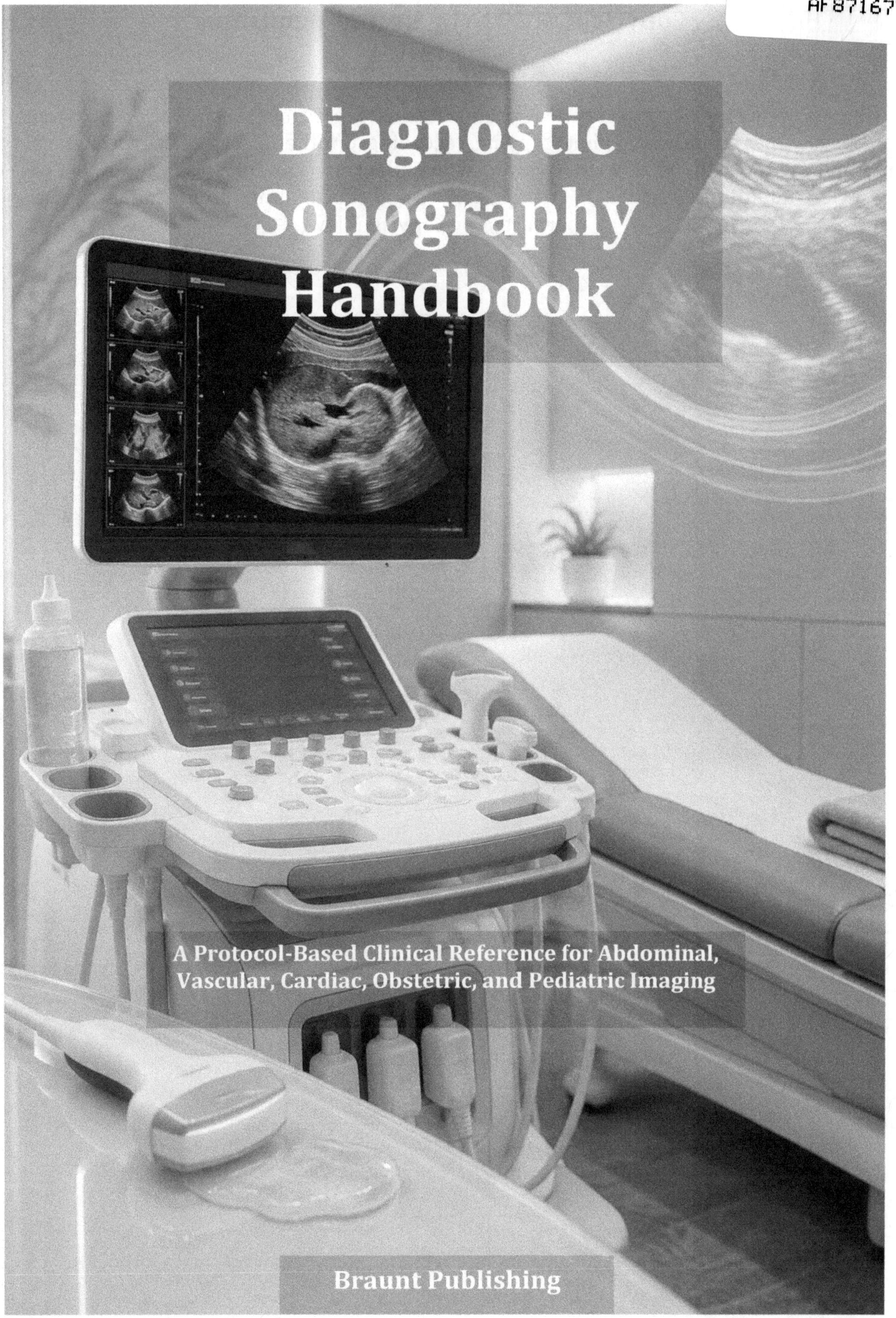

A Protocol-Based Clinical Reference for Abdominal, Vascular, Cardiac, Obstetric, and Pediatric Imaging

Braunt Publishing

DISCLAIMER

This book is intended as an educational reference for qualified sonographers, credentialing candidates, and clinicians training in diagnostic ultrasound. It is not a substitute for formal training, supervised practice, institutional protocol, manufacturer instructions, or clinical judgement.

Medicine changes. Measurement thresholds, classification systems, screening criteria, and management recommendations are revised, and they differ between professional societies and between jurisdictions. Values marked in the text as requiring verification must be confirmed against the current source in force where you practise before being applied to a patient. Where this book and a current practice parameter, guideline, or local policy differ, that document governs.

Ultrasound is operator-dependent. No text can confer competence at a technique the reader has not performed. The dynamic assessments described here in particular are learned at the machine under supervision, and descriptions in prose are not sufficient preparation for performing them.

Nothing in this book establishes a legal standard of care. The authors, contributors, and publisher accept no liability for any loss, injury, or damage arising from the use or misuse of the information it contains. Responsibility for diagnosis, interpretation, and patient management rests with the practising clinician.

Where drugs, contrast agents, devices, or invasive procedures are mentioned, the reader must consult the current product information and applicable licensing status. Some applications described are off-label in some jurisdictions.

This book contains no patient-identifiable information. All illustrations are schematic. Any clinical images are reproduced with appropriate consent and licensing, and are examples rather than diagnostic standards.

Table of Contents

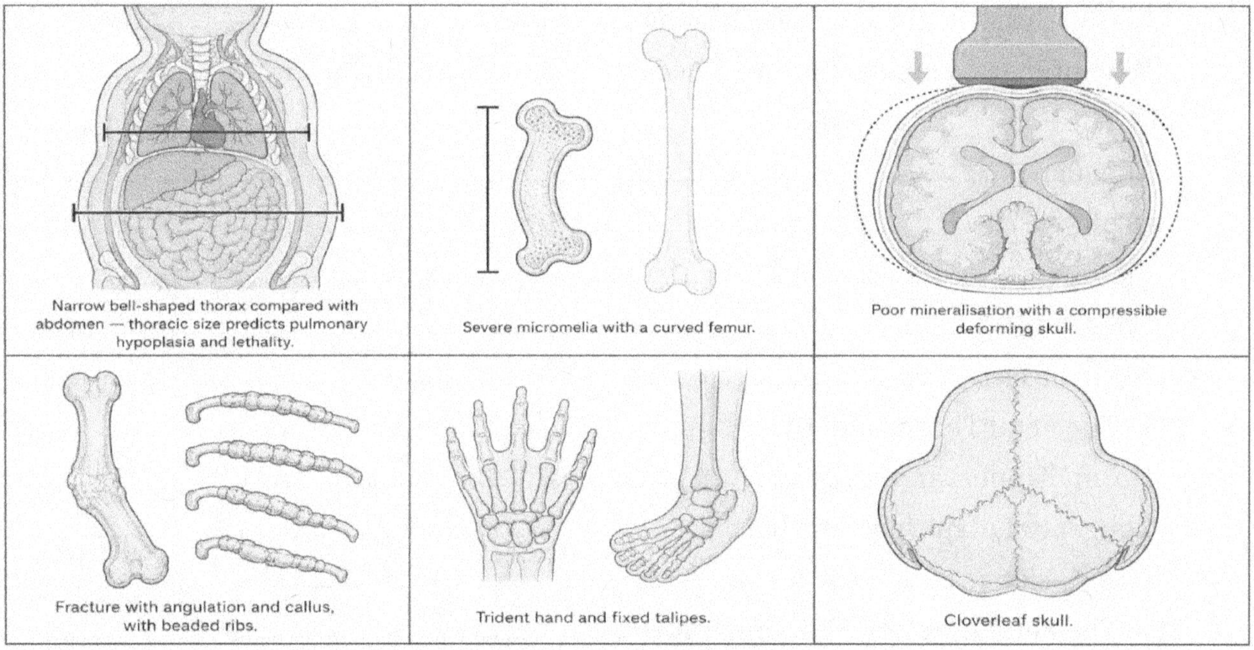

The thorax predicts survival, not the femur.

INTRODUCTION

This is a working reference for people who scan. It is organised around what you do at the machine — the question you have been asked, the window you will use, the measurement that carries the answer, and the finding that changes what happens next — rather than around a taxonomy of disease.

Twenty chapters cover the full scope of general diagnostic sonography: physics and instrumentation, the abdomen, superficial structures and musculoskeletal, neonatal and paediatric imaging, cardiac, vascular, gynaecology, and obstetrics. Each is built to be read once for understanding and returned to for a specific answer.

The book assumes prior anatomy and prior physics. It does not re-teach cross-sectional anatomy, and it does not derive the wave equation. It is written for readers who already know those things and need to know what to do with them.

Sonography students and registry candidates preparing for credentialing examinations; radiology and emergency medicine trainees; and clinicians in any specialty who are credentialing in point-of-care ultrasound and want to understand what the formal examination would have shown them.

It is also written to be useful to a qualified sonographer moving between specialties — the vascular sonographer taking on obstetrics, the abdominal sonographer starting echocardiography — because those transitions are where the most avoidable errors occur. Several of the conventions in this book reverse between chapters, and the text says so explicitly where they do.

One fact governs everything in these pages, and it is stated at the beginning of Chapter 1 because the rest of the book follows from it.

Ultrasound is operator-dependent in acquisition as well as interpretation. Every other cross-sectional modality produces a dataset that exists independently of the person who acquired it; a radiologist reading a CT weeks later sees exactly what was there. Ultrasound does not work this way. What reaches the interpreting physician is a small set of frames selected, in real time, by the person holding the transducer, from an effectively infinite set of possible images.

A structure that was never insonated does not exist in the record. A stenosis interrogated at the wrong angle produces a velocity that is wrong and looks right. A gallbladder scanned only supine may hide a stone lodged in the neck.

This is not a caveat to be acknowledged and moved past. It is why credentialing exists, why documentation standards specify what must be demonstrated rather than what must be concluded, why ergonomic injury is epidemic in this profession, and why medicolegal exposure concentrates on the person who decided what could be seen. Everything in the nineteen chapters after the first exists to reduce the distance between what is present in the patient and what appears in the report.

Each chapter opens with learning objectives and then with a short framing section that states the chapter's central problem — what makes this region difficult, which question the examination actually answers, or which technical fact governs everything that follows. These are not summaries. They are the argument the chapter is making, and they are worth reading before the detail.

The body is divided into numbered subchapters covering anatomy, protocol, and pathology in that order, because protocol determines what pathology you will be in a position to find.

Each chapter closes with three things:

Key points — decision rules rather than summaries. Each one is something that changes what you do at the machine or what you write in the report.

Registry check — questions in the style of credentialing examinations, with answers and a short rationale for each. They are written to test judgement rather than recall, and several deliberately turn on the traps described in the chapter.

Chapter notes for the editorial pass — a section addressed to the production team rather than the reader, listing verification items, cross-references, and figure requirements. It is retained in this edition because it makes explicit what has and has not been sourced.

If you are learning a region for the first time, read the opening frame, then the anatomy and protocol sections, then scan the pathology. The protocol sections are where the book differs most from a conventional text, and they repay close reading.

If you are looking something up, go to the numbered subchapter. Each is written to stand alone, with cross-references where a concept is developed elsewhere rather than repeated.

If you are preparing for an examination, the key points and registry checks across all twenty chapters constitute a condensed revision text in themselves.

Two conventions worth knowing before you start

Verification tags. Throughout the book you will find bracketed VERIFY markers attached to numerical thresholds, classification criteria, and management recommendations. They mark values that are guideline-defined, revised periodically, and often jurisdiction-specific — velocity criteria for carotid stenosis, endometrial thickness thresholds in postmenopausal bleeding, viability criteria in early pregnancy, hip classification angles.

They are deliberate. A handbook that prints a remembered threshold gives it the authority of the page, and a stale number applied in practice does harm. Where a value drives a decision — whether someone has an operation, whether a pregnancy is managed as failed — this book directs you to the current source rather than supplying a figure that may have moved.

You should treat an unresolved tag as an instruction, not an omission.

Classification systems. Six areas in this book use competing formal classification systems that differ materially in their thresholds: thyroid nodules, urinary tract dilatation, developmental hip dysplasia, carotid stenosis velocity criteria, adnexal lesion risk, and second-trimester soft markers. The text describes the framework and the reasoning without adopting a system, because a department must select one and apply it consistently. Reporting a category from one system against the thresholds of another produces recommendations that are internally incoherent.

It does not replace practice parameters. Where a professional society specifies the required content of an examination, that document governs, and this book is written to be consistent with the reasoning behind such parameters rather than to substitute for them.

It does not make you competent at a technique you have not performed. The dynamic components in particular — graded compression, the sliding sign, provoked outflow obstruction, cord motion, hip stress testing — are described as precisely as prose allows, and prose is not sufficient. They are learned at the machine, under supervision.

It is not a substitute for clinical judgement, and it is not a legal standard. It is a description of good practice, written to be useful.

Several sections of this book are shorter than their clinical weight warrants. Musculoskeletal ultrasound supports whole textbooks; it occupies two subchapters here. The female pelvis and the second and third trimesters are each compressed into a single chapter where the material would justify two. Where that has happened, the text says so, and the editorial notes identify where a future edition would divide.

Equally, the book states its limits where the modality has them. Ultrasound cannot exclude endometrial carcinoma. A normal-appearing placenta does not exclude abruption. A negative focused assessment does not exclude solid organ injury. A non-visualised appendix is not a normal appendix. These statements recur because the report that omits them is the report that causes harm, and because writing them is a skill in itself.

The measurements, protocols, and criteria in this book exist to make one person's examination comparable to another's, and to make today's study comparable to the one performed six months ago. That comparability is what allows disease to be tracked, treatment to be assessed, and a finding to be believed.

But none of it operates on its own. The machine records what the operator chose to look at, in the plane the operator chose, at the moment the operator froze the image.

The sonographer's judgement is the instrument. Everything else is apparatus.

Chapter 1: Foundations, Patient Care, and Professional Practice

Learning Objectives

On completing this chapter you should be able to:

1. Explain why operator dependence is the defining property of diagnostic ultrasound and trace its consequences through credentialing, documentation, and medicolegal exposure.
2. Situate the major technical transitions in sonography's development and explain what each one changed about clinical practice.
3. Distinguish the sonographer's scope of practice from that of the interpreting physician, and describe the credentialing architecture that governs it.
4. Conduct a pre-examination assessment that materially alters the protocol you perform.
5. Apply the Spaulding classification to transducer reprocessing and select the correct level of disinfection for any given probe and application.
6. Produce a documented examination that will survive audit, comparison, and litigation.
7. Identify the biomechanical exposures that cause work-related musculoskeletal disorders in sonographers and apply specific countermeasures at the equipment, technique, and workload level.
8. Interpret the thermal and mechanical indices, name the mode that carries the highest acoustic output, and apply ALARA to a real examination.
9. Respond appropriately to unexpected, critical, and incidental findings within scope.

The Property That Governs Everything Else

Every other imaging modality produces a dataset that exists independently of the person who acquired it. A CT scanner acquires a volume; a radiologist reads that volume weeks later and sees exactly what was there. If the technologist positioned the patient poorly, the images are still complete — reconstructable, reformattable, reviewable.

Ultrasound does not work this way. What reaches the interpreting physician is a small set of static frames and clips selected, in real time, by the person holding the transducer, from an effectively infinite set of possible images. The examination *is* the sonographer's judgment. A lesion that was never insonated does not exist in the record. A stenosis interrogated at the wrong Doppler angle produces a velocity that is wrong and looks right. A gallbladder scanned only supine may hide a stone lodged in the neck.

This is not a caveat to be acknowledged and moved past. It is the structural fact from which the entire content of this chapter follows. Credentialing exists because acquisition is a skill that must be verified. Documentation standards exist because the record must demonstrate what was and was not examined. Ergonomic injury is epidemic because the acquisition is physical labor performed under sustained static load. Medicolegal exposure concentrates on the sonographer because the sonographer made the decisions that determined what could be seen.

Hold this in mind through everything below.

1.1 Scope and Evolution of Diagnostic Medical Sonography

What ultrasound is for

Diagnostic medical sonography uses pulsed high-frequency sound to generate cross-sectional images and flow information from within the body, without ionizing radiation. In current practice it serves four distinct functions, and confusing them is a common source of protocol error.

Diagnosis. The examination answers a specific clinical question — is there a stone, is the appendix inflamed, is this mass cystic or solid. The protocol is driven by the question.

Screening. The examination is performed on an asymptomatic population to detect disease before it declares itself — abdominal aortic aneurysm screening, the fetal anatomic survey, carotid screening in defined risk groups. The protocol is standardized and complete rather than focused, because you do not know what you are looking for.

Guidance. Ultrasound provides real-time visualization for a procedure — vascular access, biopsy, drainage, regional anesthesia, amniocentesis. The imaging is subordinate to the procedure and the technical demands are different: needle conspicuity matters more than tissue characterization.

Monitoring. Serial examinations track change over time — fetal growth, transplant surveillance, aneurysm size, follicular development. Here reproducibility of technique matters more than image beauty, because the measurement must be comparable to the one taken eight weeks ago by someone else.

Where ultrasound wins and where it loses

Ultrasound's advantages are structural: no ionizing radiation, real-time acquisition, portability to the patient, dynamic assessment (compressibility, peristalsis, ligament stress, valve motion, fetal movement), direct patient interaction during acquisition, high spatial resolution in superficial structures, and cost. Nothing else lets you press on a point of maximal tenderness while watching the structure underneath it.

Its limitations are equally structural. Sound does not cross gas or bone at diagnostic frequencies, so the retroperitoneum behind bowel, the lung parenchyma, and the adult brain are largely inaccessible by conventional approach. Penetration falls as frequency rises, imposing a hard trade-off between resolution and depth that body habitus can make unwinnable. Field of view is narrow, which makes whole-region survey and communication with non-sonographers harder. And the modality is operator-dependent in both acquisition and interpretation.

Knowing when to stop and recommend cross-sectional imaging is a clinical skill, not an admission of failure. A report that reads *"technically limited by body habitus and overlying bowel gas; pancreatic body and tail not visualized; CT recommended if clinical concern persists"* is a good report. A report that describes a normal pancreas that was never adequately seen is a dangerous one.

Development of the modality

Medical ultrasound descends from industrial and military applications — flaw detection in metal, and sonar. The piezoelectric effect had been described in the 1880s, but it was the mid-twentieth century convergence of pulse-echo electronics with clinical curiosity that produced diagnostic imaging.

The earliest medical application is generally credited to the Austrian neurologist Karl Dussik, who in the early 1940s attempted to image the cerebral ventricles using through-transmission ultrasound. The technique was unsuccessful — the skull attenuated and refracted the beam far more than appreciated — but it established the premise.

The 1950s produced the modality's foundational lines of work, largely in parallel and largely independently. **John Wild and John Reid** in Minnesota demonstrated that pulse-echo ultrasound could differentiate normal from malignant tissue, and produced early two-dimensional images of breast lesions. **Douglass Howry and Joseph Holmes** in Denver built immersion-tank scanners that generated recognizable cross-sectional anatomy, at the cost of requiring the patient to sit in a water bath. **Inge Edler and Carl Hertz** in Lund adapted an industrial flaw detector to record cardiac motion, founding echocardiography. **Shigeo Satomura** in Osaka applied the Doppler principle to blood flow and cardiac wall motion, opening the entire hemodynamic branch of the field.

Ian Donald and colleagues in Glasgow made the decisive clinical translation in the late 1950s, applying contact B-mode scanning to abdominal and pelvic masses and then to obstetrics. Obstetric sonography became the modality's first mass application, and it remains the context in which most of the public encounters ultrasound.

The transitions since then are worth understanding as *changes in what clinicians could do*, not as a parts list:

Transition	What it changed
A-mode → static B-mode	From a one-dimensional trace requiring inference to a recognizable anatomic image
Static → real-time scanning	Motion became visible; examination became interactive and dramatically faster; dynamic signs (peristalsis, compressibility, cardiac motion) entered diagnosis
Continuous-wave → pulsed and duplex Doppler	Flow could be localized to a specific vessel at a specific depth, rather than summed along a line

Transition	What it changed
Analog → digital beam forming	Electronic focusing, steering, and consistent image quality; the end of mechanical scan heads
Fundamental → tissue harmonic imaging	Substantially improved image quality in technically difficult patients, particularly large body habitus
Addition of microbubble contrast	Pure intravascular tracer allowing true perfusion assessment and lesion characterization
Elastography and quantitative methods	Tissue stiffness and attenuation as measurable parameters rather than subjective impressions
Miniaturization and point-of-care ultrasound	Ultrasound moved to the bedside, the field, and non-imaging specialties — with consequences for quality and credentialing discussed in §1.2
Machine learning integration	Automated measurement, view recognition, and quality feedback; accountability questions addressed in §1.8

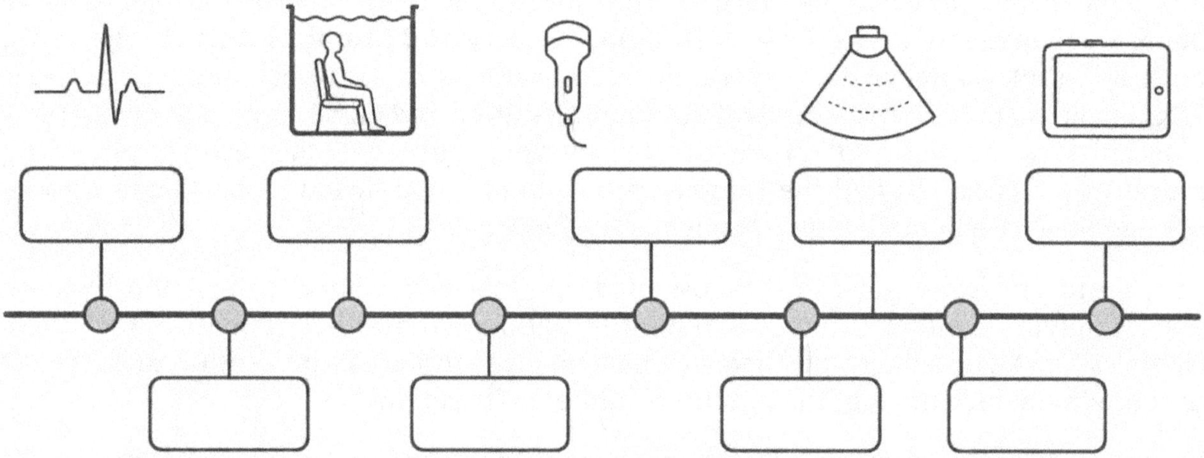

1.2 The Sonographer's Role, Scope of Practice, and Credentialing

What the sonographer actually does

The role is commonly described as "acquiring images for physician interpretation." This is accurate and badly incomplete. In practice the sonographer performs at least five distinct cognitive tasks during a single examination:

Protocol selection and modification. The order says "abdominal ultrasound." The patient says the pain is right upper quadrant, worse after eating, and that they had a normal gallbladder ultrasound two years ago. You are now performing a different examination than the one you would have performed on a patient with painless jaundice.

Real-time interpretation. You cannot decide what to image next without provisionally interpreting what you are seeing now. A sonographer who does not recognize a dilated common bile duct will not go looking for the level of obstruction. Interpretation during acquisition is not scope creep — it is a prerequisite for competent acquisition.

Search extension. When something abnormal appears, the examination expands. You find a renal mass; you now assess the renal vein and IVC, the contralateral kidney, and the liver. The protocol does not tell you to do this. Pattern knowledge does.

Technical adequacy judgment. Deciding that an image is good enough, or that it is not and no further manipulation will make it so, and documenting that.

Communication and escalation. Deciding that a finding cannot wait for routine reporting, and knowing who to tell.

The boundary

The sonographer does not render the diagnosis, does not issue the report, and does not communicate diagnostic findings to the patient. This boundary is real and it is protective — of the patient, who deserves findings delivered by the clinician who can contextualize and act on them, and of the sonographer, who has neither the clinical picture nor the professional indemnity to carry that conversation.

Most institutions permit and expect a **preliminary written observation** or worksheet communicated to the interpreting physician: objective descriptive findings and measurements, not a diagnosis. The distinction is between *"6 mm echogenic focus in the gallbladder lumen with posterior shadowing, mobile with position change"* and *"cholelithiasis."* The first is within scope everywhere. The second is a diagnosis.

Practice varies internationally and this variation is substantive, not cosmetic. In the United Kingdom, Australia, and several other systems, appropriately qualified sonographers routinely issue written reports as a defined extended role, with formal training and governance. In the United States this is generally not the model. Know which system you are in and what your institution's policy actually says in writing. Verbal custom is not scope.

The patient's question

Patients ask what you see. They ask during the exam, at its most anxious moments, and they ask because you are the only clinician in the room and you are looking at their body on a screen.

Deflecting badly causes real harm. Silence, evasion, or a sudden change in your demeanor communicates catastrophe more efficiently than words. The workable approach is honest about the structure of the process, delivered before the anxiety builds:

> "I'm going to be quiet while I concentrate on getting complete images — that's normal and it doesn't mean anything about what I'm finding. Everything gets

reviewed by the radiologist, and Dr. [name] will have the results and go over them with you. I'm not able to give you results myself, but I'll make sure they get them quickly."

Say this at the start, not when asked. Then be consistent. A sonographer who chats freely through a normal exam and goes silent when a mass appears has told the patient everything without saying anything.

Educational and credentialing architecture

Entry to the profession in the United States is generally through a programmatically accredited educational program — CAAHEP-accredited programs reviewed by the Joint Review Committee on Education in Diagnostic Medical Sonography — followed by credentialing examination. Alternative eligibility pathways exist for individuals with prior allied health credentials or clinical experience. Program accreditation matters practically: some credentialing prerequisites and many employers require it. [VERIFY: current CAAHEP/JRC-DMS program requirements and ARDMS prerequisite pathways]

The principal credentialing bodies are:

Body	Representative credentials	Domain
ARDMS	RDMS, RDCS, RVT, RMSKS	General, cardiac, vascular, musculoskeletal sonography
CCI	RCS, RVS, RCCS, RPhS	Cardiovascular and phlebology
ARRT	Sonography (S), Vascular Sonography (VS), Breast (BS)	Post-primary pathway for radiologic technologists

Credentials are typically constructed from a **physics and instrumentation examination** plus one or more **specialty examinations** — abdomen, obstetrics and gynecology, breast, pediatric, adult echocardiography, fetal echocardiography, vascular technology, musculoskeletal. Maintenance requires ongoing continuing medical education and periodic attestation. [VERIFY: current ARDMS, CCI, and ARRT examination structures, prerequisite routes, and CME requirements — these change and must be checked at time of publication]

State licensure exists in some jurisdictions and not others, and where it exists it may impose requirements beyond national credentialing. This is a genuine patchwork; verify locally rather than assuming.

Practice parameters — the documents describing what constitutes a complete examination of a given region — come principally from professional societies rather than credentialing bodies: AIUM, ACR, ACOG, SRU, SVU, ASE, and their international equivalents. Accreditation of the *practice* (as opposed to the individual) generally requires demonstrated adherence to these parameters. Chapter-specific protocols throughout this handbook are built on them, and every threshold drawn from them is flagged for verification against the current edition.

Point-of-care ultrasound and the quality question

Ultrasound performed by the treating clinician at the bedside — emergency medicine, critical care, anesthesia, obstetrics, primary care, and increasingly most specialties — is now a large fraction of all ultrasound performed. It is genuinely valuable: a focused question answered in ninety seconds at the bedside can change management before a formal study could be scheduled.

It also creates real tension. PoCUS credentialing is specialty-defined and heterogeneous, image archiving and quality assurance are inconsistently implemented, and the scope of a "focused" examination is easy to exceed unintentionally. The sonographer's professional position on this should be neither territorial nor naive. The defensible principles are that any diagnostic ultrasound should be archived and auditable; that the person performing it should be credentialed for the specific application; and that a focused examination must be reported as focused, so that a negative focused scan is not mistaken for a negative complete one.

1.3 Essentials of Patient Care and Communication

The pre-examination assessment is part of the examination

Before the transducer touches the patient, you should know the answers to a specific set of questions, because several of them change what you are about to do.

Identity and order verification. Two patient identifiers against the requisition, and the requisition against what the patient believes they are having done. Discrepancies here are common and are the cheapest error to catch.

The indication, in the patient's words. The requisition says "abdominal pain." The patient says it is left-sided, radiating to the groin, and that they have passed stones before. You are now going to interrogate the ureterovesical junctions carefully and look for a twinkling artifact, which the requisition never told you to do.

Relevant history that alters protocol. Prior surgery — an absent gallbladder saves you twenty minutes of searching and reframes any ductal dilatation you find. Prior imaging and its findings. Known malignancy. Pregnancy status where it affects the examination or its urgency. Anticoagulation before a guided procedure. Latex allergy before an endocavitary examination. Recent barium studies before an abdominal scan.

Preparation status. Fasting for gallbladder and abdominal aorta; bladder filling for transabdominal pelvic imaging. A patient who ate two hours ago has a contracted gallbladder and you need to decide, before you start, whether to proceed and caveat the report or rebook.

Mobility, positioning tolerance, and lines. Can this patient lie flat, roll into a left lateral decubitus, hold a breath, stand for a reflux study? A drain, a stoma, a wound, a recent surgical site — all change your acoustic windows and your approach.

Take this history yourself even when it appears in the chart. The three minutes it costs is repaid in the protocol you avoid getting wrong.

Positioning, exposure, and dignity

Expose only the region being scanned, and only for as long as you are scanning it. Use draping deliberately — a towel tucked at the waistband for an abdominal scan, a sheet across the chest for an upper abdominal study. Warm gel where available; cold gel makes patients tense their abdominal wall, which is both uncomfortable and technically counterproductive.

Explain each position change before you make it, and explain why. "I need you to roll onto your left side — it moves the gallbladder into a better window and shifts any stones so I can see whether they move." Patients cooperate far better with a reason than an instruction.

Chaperones. Offer a chaperone for any examination involving intimate areas — endocavitary, breast, scrotal, transabdominal pelvic in some contexts — and document the offer and the response, including declines. This is patient protection and practitioner protection simultaneously, and the documentation is not optional.

Endocavitary examinations require explicit verbal consent, an explanation of what will happen, and an unambiguous statement that the patient can stop the examination at any moment. Wherever practicable, offer the patient the option of self-inserting the transducer. Never proceed on assumed consent because the referrer ordered it.

Communicating during the examination

Three failure modes recur:

Undisclosed silence. Explained in advance (§1.2), silence is fine. Unexplained, it is terrifying.

Reflexive reassurance. "Everything looks great!" said early, before the study is complete, is a promise you cannot keep and a serious problem when the report says otherwise. Do not offer reassurance you are not authorized to give.

Reactive body language. Sharp intake of breath, a long pause on one image, calling a colleague into the room without explanation, repeatedly re-measuring one structure. Patients read all of it. If you need a second opinion mid-study, say so neutrally: "I'm going to ask a colleague to look at a couple of images with me — that's a normal part of how we work."

Populations that require adapted approach

Pediatric. Explain to both child and caregiver, at the child's level. Let a young child touch the transducer and see the gel. Keep the caregiver in view. Scan the least tolerable part last where the protocol permits. Distraction — a screen, a caregiver's phone, a toy — is a legitimate clinical tool. For neonates, thermal management and minimal handling are part of the examination, not courtesies.

Cognitively impaired or delirious patients. Short sentences, one instruction at a time, no ambiguity. Identify the person who can consent and involve them. Consider whether a modified or abbreviated protocol answering the essential question is more appropriate than a distressing complete one.

Patients with limited English proficiency. Use a professional interpreter service, in person or by phone. Family members — particularly children — are not appropriate interpreters for clinical consent or history, and using them is both a quality failure and, in many jurisdictions, a regulatory one.

Large body habitus. Adjust technique, not attitude. Lower frequency, harmonic imaging, appropriate depth and focal placement, patient positioning to bring the target closer to the transducer, and the use of the patient's own hands or an assistant to displace tissue where appropriate and consented. Ensure the table's weight rating is adequate and that transfer is safe. Comment on technical limitation in the record where it exists; do not editorialize about the patient.

Critically ill and portable examinations. You are scanning in a hostile environment — lines, monitors, ventilator, limited access, poor lighting, and a patient who cannot be repositioned. Establish before you start what the essential question is, so you can answer it if the study has to be abbreviated. Do not disconnect, move, or silence anything without the nurse's involvement.

The sonographer as observer

You spend twenty to forty uninterrupted minutes with a patient, watching them closely, in a dim quiet room. You will sometimes be the first person to notice deterioration — new confusion, worsening dyspnea, pallor, diaphoresis, a rigid abdomen, chest pain during positioning, escalating pain with transducer pressure.

Vasovagal episodes during endocavitary and prolonged supine examinations are common enough to plan for. Know where the emergency call system is in every room you work in. Know how to lower the head of the table. Know your institution's escalation pathway. This awareness is part of the job.

1.4 Infection Control and Transducer Reprocessing

The machine is a fomite

Ultrasound equipment is touched by every operator, contacts every patient, is rarely fully cleaned between cases, and lives in warm rooms. Contamination has been demonstrated on transducers, cables, keyboards, control panels, gel bottles, and the machine chassis. Cables in particular are systematically undercleaned — they contact the patient, drape across the bed, and are almost never included in a between-patient wipe.

Standard precautions apply to every patient, always. Hand hygiene before patient contact, after patient contact, after contact with the patient's surroundings, and after glove removal — gloves are not a substitute for hand hygiene, and removing gloves contaminates hands.

Gel is a documented vector. Outbreaks have been traced to contaminated multi-use gel containers, including refilled bottles and warmers. Single-use sachets are preferred for any procedure involving non-intact skin, mucous membranes, sterile fields, or immunocompromised patients. Never top up a partially used bottle. Never allow the bottle nozzle to contact the patient or the transducer face. Sterile single-use gel is required for guided invasive procedures.

Between every patient, clean the transducer face and housing, the cable to the strain relief, and the control surfaces you touched, using a product compatible with the manufacturer's instructions for use. Incompatible disinfectants degrade the acoustic lens and the housing seal, and lens damage is both an image quality failure and an infection control failure, because a cracked lens cannot be reliably disinfected.

Spaulding classification applied to transducers

Reprocessing level is determined by what the device contacts, not by what it looks like or how dirty it seems. The Spaulding framework classifies devices into three tiers, and every transducer application maps to one of them.

Noncritical — contacts intact skin only. Routine external abdominal, vascular, small parts, obstetric transabdominal, echocardiography. Requires cleaning followed by **low-level disinfection**.

Semicritical — contacts mucous membranes or non-intact skin. Endovaginal, endorectal, transesophageal, endocavitary of any kind; external transducers used on broken skin, open wounds, burns, ulcers, or rashes; intraoperative probes used in a sheathed non-sterile-tissue application. Requires cleaning followed by **high-level disinfection**. A protective sheath does *not* downgrade the requirement — sheaths fail, at rates high enough that reprocessing policy must assume failure has occurred.

Critical — contacts sterile tissue, the bloodstream, or a sterile field. Intraoperative probes on sterile tissue, biopsy and vascular access guidance within a sterile field, needle guides that penetrate tissue. Requires **sterilization**, or high-level disinfection combined with a sterile sheath and sterile gel where the device cannot be sterilized. Reusable needle guides that penetrate tissue must be sterilized between uses; single-use guides must be discarded.

The single most consequential practical point: **the application determines the level, not the probe.** A curvilinear abdominal transducer used on intact skin is noncritical. The same transducer used on a burn, an open wound, or a surgical incision is semicritical for that use and must undergo high-level disinfection afterwards.

The reprocessing workflow

The sequence is not negotiable and no step substitutes for another. Disinfectant applied to a soiled probe does not disinfect it; organic material shields organisms and inactivates the agent.

1. **Point-of-use removal.** Remove and discard the sheath and gel immediately, at the bedside, before the probe leaves the room. Wipe visible soil. Do not allow bioburden to dry, which makes subsequent cleaning substantially less effective.
2. **Cleaning.** Manual or automated cleaning with an appropriate enzymatic or approved detergent. This is the step that determines whether everything downstream works.

3. **Disinfection or sterilization.** To the level determined above, using a product and contact time validated for that device. Automated reprocessing systems reduce variability and operator chemical exposure and are preferred where available.
4. **Rinse.** With water of the quality specified for the agent used — residual disinfectant causes chemical mucosal injury, a documented and entirely preventable patient harm.
5. **Dry.** Residual moisture supports microbial growth during storage.
6. **Store.** Clean, dry, hanging where possible to protect the lens and avoid recontamination. Do not return a reprocessed probe to a drawer with unprocessed equipment.
7. **Document.** Record the device identifier, operator, method, date and time, linked to the patient episode. Traceability is what allows a contamination event to be investigated rather than guessed at.

Two overriding rules. **Manufacturer instructions for use take precedence** over general guidance for any specific device — chemical compatibility is device-specific and using an unapproved agent voids validation and may destroy the probe. And **the disinfection log is a clinical record**; treat it as one.

Additional considerations

Transducers used on patients with transmissible spongiform encephalopathy, or in outbreak conditions, may require handling beyond standard protocols; escalate to infection prevention rather than improvising.

Damaged probes must be removed from service. A crack in the lens or housing, a compromised cable strain relief, or a delaminating membrane makes reliable reprocessing impossible regardless of the protocol followed.

Personal protective equipment during reprocessing protects the operator from high-level disinfectants, which are respiratory and dermal irritants. Ventilation requirements for open-soak systems are a real occupational health issue, not a formality.

1.5 Patient Safety, Informed Consent, and Documentation

Identification and the pre-scan pause

Wrong-patient and wrong-side errors in ultrasound are less discussed than in surgery and are not rare. The controls are simple and must be performed rather than assumed:

- Two independent identifiers, verified against the requisition, spoken by the patient rather than confirmed by them. Ask "what's your date of birth" rather than "is your date of birth the fourth of June."
- Requisition matched to the modality, region, **and side**.
- For any invasive or guided procedure, a formal time-out with the proceduralist: correct patient, correct site, correct side, correct procedure, consent verified, relevant coagulation status and allergies known.

Laterality deserves particular emphasis. A mislabelled left kidney is not a clerical error — it is a finding attributed to the wrong organ, and it can generate an operation on the wrong side. Label at the moment of acquisition, not retrospectively at the end of the study when you are reconstructing from memory.

Consent

Implied consent covers routine external examinations: the patient attends, is told what will happen, and cooperates. This is sufficient for transabdominal work on intact skin.

Explicit consent is required whenever the examination is invasive, intimate, carries risk, or departs from what the patient expects. Endocavitary examinations, contrast administration, any guided invasive procedure, and any examination being recorded or observed for teaching or research all require it.

For endocavitary examination specifically, the patient must be told what the transducer is, where it goes, that a sheath and lubricant are used, roughly how long it takes, that it is usually uncomfortable rather than painful, and that they may stop it at any point. Consent obtained after the patient is already undressed and on the table is a poor consent, and a patient who feels unable to decline has not consented.

Contrast agents require explicit consent, screening for contraindications, a documented administering clinician, and immediate availability of resuscitation equipment and personnel. Reactions are uncommon but the response capability must exist before administration, not be arranged after.

Pediatric consent is given by the legal guardian; assent should still be sought from a child capable of giving it, and a child's sustained refusal warrants reassessment rather than restraint. Local law on the age and circumstances of independent minor consent varies and must be known locally.

The image as legal record

Every image you archive is a permanent medical and legal document. It will be reviewed by an interpreting physician, potentially by other clinicians for years afterwards, potentially by a court.

Minimum labeling for every stored image:

- Patient identifiers and date of examination
- Institution and, per local policy, the operator's identity or initials
- **Anatomic site and laterality**
- **Image orientation** — transverse, longitudinal, sagittal, coronal, or the named standard plane
- Transducer and, where relevant, the approach used
- Measurement calipers visible with their values, and the measurement clearly attributable to the structure measured

Machine settings — depth, frequency, gain, focal position, Doppler angle, PRF, wall filter — are recorded automatically and form part of the record. For any Doppler velocity measurement, the **angle correction cursor must be visible and correctly aligned** in the archived image, because a velocity without a demonstrable angle is an uninterpretable number.

Documenting completeness — and incompleteness

A complete examination is defined by the applicable practice parameter for that study, and the archived image set must demonstrate that each required element was assessed. "I looked at it but didn't store an image" does not exist as a defensible position; if it is not in the archive, it was not examined.

The harder discipline is documenting what you could *not* see. A study that omits a required structure without comment reads, to anyone reviewing it later, as a study in which that structure was normal. State the limitation explicitly and specifically:

> *"Pancreatic tail obscured by overlying bowel gas despite repositioning and graded compression; not evaluated."*

not

> *"Technically difficult study."*

The second sentence tells the interpreting physician nothing actionable. The first tells them exactly what is missing and lets them decide whether it matters.

Document positive negatives that the clinical question demands — for a suspected DVT study, the absence of thrombus in each interrogated segment; for an acute abdomen, the visualized appendix or the explicit statement that it was not identified. "Appendix not visualized" is a finding with a defined and non-trivial meaning; leaving it out is a serious omission.

Preliminary communication and critical findings

Institutions differ in how sonographers communicate preliminary findings, but every institution must have a defined pathway for findings that cannot wait. The sonographer's obligation is to recognize such a finding and to escalate it immediately, in person or by direct voice contact, not by leaving a note in a worksheet.

Findings that warrant immediate escalation across most practices include: ruptured or leaking abdominal aortic aneurysm; ectopic pregnancy with haemodynamic concern; testicular or ovarian torsion; large pericardial effusion with tamponade physiology; extensive proximal deep venous thrombosis; absent fetal cardiac activity where previously present; significant free intraperitoneal fluid in trauma; and acute arterial occlusion of a limb. This list is illustrative — your institution's list governs, and you should know it without looking it up. [VERIFY: institutional critical results policy and any applicable accreditation-mandated reporting timeframes]

Document the escalation itself: what was communicated, to whom by name, at what time, and by what means.

Retention, amendment, and comparison

Archived studies are retained per institutional and jurisdictional policy, typically for years and longer for pediatric and obstetric studies. Images and reports are amended by **addendum**, never by alteration — an altered record is presumptively suspect and destroys the evidentiary value of the entire study.

For serial examinations, retrieve and review the prior study *before* scanning, not after. Reproducing the prior technique — same plane, same landmark, same caliper convention — is what makes the comparison meaningful. A growth measurement taken in a different plane by a different convention is not a comparison, it is two unrelated numbers, and the difference between them will be attributed to disease.

1.6 Ergonomics and Work-Related Musculoskeletal Injury

The scale of the problem

Work-related musculoskeletal disorder is the dominant occupational hazard of this profession. Survey data across multiple countries and decades consistently report that a large majority of practising sonographers scan in pain, that a substantial fraction sustain injury severe enough to alter or end their career, and that symptoms frequently begin within the first few years of practice — including during training. [VERIFY: current SDMS Industry Standards for the Prevention of Work-Related Musculoskeletal Disorders in Sonography, and current prevalence figures from published survey literature]

Two consequences follow, and both are underappreciated. First, this is a patient safety issue as much as a workforce issue: a sonographer in pain shortens examinations, avoids the awkward angles that difficult windows require, and applies less transducer pressure than a study needs. Second, it is not a problem of individual carelessness. It is produced by equipment design, room layout, workload, and scheduling, and it is not solvable by telling individuals to sit up straight.

Mechanism

Sonographic injury is not acute trauma. It is cumulative, arising from **sustained low-level static muscular loading** — muscle held in continuous contraction without the alternating relaxation that permits perfusion and metabolite clearance. Under sustained contraction, intramuscular pressure impedes capillary flow; the smallest motor units recruited first remain active continuously and are selectively damaged.

This explains why a sonographer can be injured by an activity that looks physically undemanding, and why "it doesn't feel heavy" is not reassurance. It also explains why brief, frequent posture changes are more protective than long rest breaks: the requirement is *interruption of static load*, not total load reduction.

The specific exposures

Five biomechanical exposures account for most of the risk. They compound; a sonographer with three of them simultaneously is at substantially greater risk than the sum of the individual contributions suggests.

Shoulder abduction. The dominant single risk factor. Abduction beyond roughly 30 degrees, sustained, loads the supraspinatus and reduces subacromial perfusion. Abduction above 60 degrees for prolonged periods is a well-recognized high-risk posture. This is what produces the rotator cuff pathology, biceps tendinopathy, and subacromial impingement that characterize the profession. [VERIFY: specific abduction angle thresholds in current SDMS industry standards]

Sustained grip force. Transducers are gripped far harder than the task requires, particularly by anxious or inexperienced operators, and grip force rises with cable drag, poor probe geometry, and gel on the housing. Sustained gripping drives lateral epicondylitis, De Quervain tenosynovitis, carpal tunnel syndrome, and thumb-base pain.

Transducer pressure. Force applied through a pinched wrist and abducted shoulder, sustained for minutes at a time — most severe in large body habitus, deep vascular work, and graded compression techniques.

Reach and trunk twisting. Scanning across a bed that is too wide or too high, with the machine on one side and the patient on the other, forces trunk rotation combined with reach. This is the classic portable-examination posture and it is the worst combination available.

Sustained neck and spine posture. Static neck rotation or flexion toward a poorly placed monitor; unsupported lumbar spine; prolonged standing with weight asymmetrically loaded.

Add to these the environmental contributors: cold rooms increasing muscle tension, poor lighting driving forward head posture, foot pedals producing asymmetric standing, and cable weight loading the scanning wrist all day.

The countermeasures that actually work

Room and equipment geometry. The principle is that the patient, the machine, and the monitor should be arranged so that you can scan with the arm close to the body and the head facing forward.

- Bed height adjustable and set so your scanning forearm is roughly horizontal when the transducer is on the patient. Sitting and standing require different heights; change it between patients rather than tolerating a compromise.
- Bring the patient toward you — to the near edge of the bed — rather than reaching across. This single change eliminates a large fraction of abduction and reach exposure and costs nothing.
- Monitor directly in front of you at approximately eye level, at a comfortable viewing distance, tilted to avoid glare. Not off to one side.

- Control panel within easy reach at approximately elbow height, adjustable independently of the monitor on any machine that permits it.
- Chair with adjustable height, a supportive back, and either no arms or arms that do not prevent close approach to the bed. Foot support if your feet do not reach the floor at the required height.

Support the scanning arm. Rest the forearm or elbow on the bed, on the patient where appropriate and comfortable, or on a support cushion. An unsupported arm is the entire problem; a supported arm is a different job. Elevating the bed rail, using a rolled towel, or asking the patient to move rather than reaching are all legitimate.

Reduce grip force deliberately. Hold the transducer with the minimum force that maintains control. Support the cable — drape it over your forearm, use a cable support arm, or clip it — so that its weight is not carried by the scanning hand. Vary the grip through the examination. Wipe gel off the housing rather than gripping harder to compensate for slipperiness.

Generate pressure from the body, not the shoulder. Where sustained compression is needed, lean using body weight through a relatively neutral arm rather than pressing with an abducted, internally rotated shoulder.

Alternate hands. Genuine ambidextrous scanning capability is the most protective single skill a sonographer can develop, and it is realistically acquired only by deliberate practice during training rather than after symptoms appear.

Microbreaks and task rotation. Brief interruptions of static posture — seconds, several times within an examination — plus varied examination types across a shift. A schedule of six consecutive technically difficult vascular studies is an ergonomic exposure, and it is a scheduling decision, not a fact of nature.

Portable and bedside scanning deserves specific attention because it defeats every control above. Before starting, take the time to raise the bed, lower the rail, move furniture, reposition the machine so you are not twisting, and move the patient toward you. Thirty seconds of setup on a portable study is the highest-value ergonomic intervention available, and it is the one most often skipped because the environment feels provisional.

Report symptoms early. Persistent pain is a pathological signal, not a normal consequence of a busy week. Early modification and treatment preserve careers; the injuries that end them are typically ones that were scanned through for months.

1.7 Bioeffects, ALARA, and the Thermal and Mechanical Indices

The honest position on safety

Diagnostic ultrasound has been in widespread clinical use for decades without a confirmed causal association with harm in humans at diagnostic exposure levels. That is a strong record and it should be stated plainly to anxious patients.

It is not the same as a proof of harmlessness, and the difference matters professionally. Ultrasound deposits energy in tissue. Bioeffects are demonstrable in laboratory and animal systems at and near diagnostic output levels. Acoustic output permitted by current equipment is substantially higher than that of the machines on which much of the reassuring epidemiology was gathered, particularly in Doppler modes. Detecting a small effect on a low-frequency outcome — subtle neurodevelopmental effects from first-trimester exposure, for example — is beyond the power of the available studies.

The professional response to this is neither alarm nor complacency. It is ALARA: *as low as reasonably achievable*. Use the output you need to answer the clinical question, for the time you need, and not more. This is a positive obligation on every operator, on every examination.

Mechanisms of bioeffect

Thermal. Absorbed acoustic energy converts to heat. Tissue temperature rise depends on the intensity delivered, the absorption coefficient of the tissue, the dwell time, and the perfusion available to carry heat away. The determinants that matter at the machine are:

- **Bone absorbs far more strongly than soft tissue**, and heats disproportionately. Bone adjacent to sensitive structures — fetal cranium adjacent to developing brain, neonatal skull — is the principal thermal concern.
- **Poorly perfused tissue** cannot dissipate heat. The embryo before the establishment of substantial circulation, the eye, and any tissue in a febrile patient are more vulnerable.
- **Dwell time** is a primary determinant and the one entirely under your control. A stationary beam heats; a moving beam distributes the energy.

Mechanical (non-thermal). These arise from the pressure oscillation itself rather than heating.

- **Cavitation.** Pre-existing or acoustically nucleated gas bodies oscillate in the sound field. *Stable* cavitation produces sustained oscillation with microstreaming and shear at the bubble surface. *Inertial* cavitation is violent collapse, with locally extreme transient temperature and pressure and free radical generation. Cavitation risk rises with peak negative pressure and falls with frequency, which is exactly what the mechanical index encodes.
- **Radiation force and acoustic streaming.** Momentum transfer produces displacement and fluid motion — the basis of shear-wave elastography, and a mechanism of effect in its own right.

Gas bodies are the key variable. Tissue containing gas — lung, bowel — and tissue containing introduced microbubbles are the settings in which mechanical effects are plausible at diagnostic levels.

The output display standard

Modern equipment displays two indices in real time. Both are calculated estimates under assumed conditions, not measurements in the patient.

Mechanical index (MI) estimates the likelihood of cavitation-related effect. It is derived from the derated peak rarefactional (negative) pressure divided by the square root of the transducer centre frequency. Higher MI means higher peak negative pressure relative to frequency, and therefore greater potential for cavitation.

Thermal index (TI) estimates the potential temperature rise: broadly, the ratio of the acoustic power being used to the power estimated to produce a 1 °C rise under a defined model. A TI of 2 does not mean the tissue is 2 °C warmer. It means the conditions are such that a rise of that order is possible under the model's assumptions.

TI is displayed in one of three forms, and the machine selects based on the application preset. Using the wrong preset gives you the wrong index, which is a common and silent error:

Index	Model	When displayed
TIS — soft tissue	Homogeneous soft tissue, no bone in beam	General abdominal, small parts, early first trimester before ossification
TIB — bone at focus	Bone at or near the focal zone	Second- and third-trimester obstetric imaging, where the beam traverses soft tissue and encounters fetal bone
TIC — cranial bone	Bone at or near the transducer face	Transcranial imaging, neonatal cranial imaging

Regulatory ceilings apply to output for most applications, with substantially lower limits for ophthalmic imaging, where the poorly perfused lens and vitreous cannot dissipate heat. [VERIFY: current FDA acoustic output limits including ISPTA.3 and MI ceilings, and separate ophthalmic limits]

Output by mode — the point most often missed

Acoustic output is not uniform across modes, and the ranking is counterintuitive to anyone who assumes that a bigger picture means more energy:

B-mode distributes pulses widely across the image plane and rapidly. Any single location receives relatively little energy. Output is lowest.

M-mode concentrates pulses along a single line but with low duty cycle. Output is modest.

Colour and power Doppler interrogate a limited region of interest with multiple pulses per line. Output rises, and rises further as the colour box is made smaller — the same energy delivered to less tissue.

Spectral (pulsed-wave) Doppler holds a stationary sample volume and delivers a high pulse repetition frequency to that single small location for as long as you keep the trace running. **This is the highest-intensity mode in routine diagnostic use, and it is the one you should think about before deploying.**

The practical rule follows directly: in any sensitive application — first-trimester obstetrics above all, but also neonatal cranial and ophthalmic imaging — B-mode is the default, colour is used briefly and purposefully, and spectral Doppler is used only when the clinical question genuinely requires a velocity or waveform, for the shortest possible trace.

Embryonic cardiac activity should be documented by M-mode or by B-mode observation, **not** by spectral Doppler placed over the embryo. This is a specific, widely endorsed recommendation and it is the single most important ALARA point in the entire modality. [VERIFY: current AIUM and ISUOG statements on Doppler use in the first trimester]

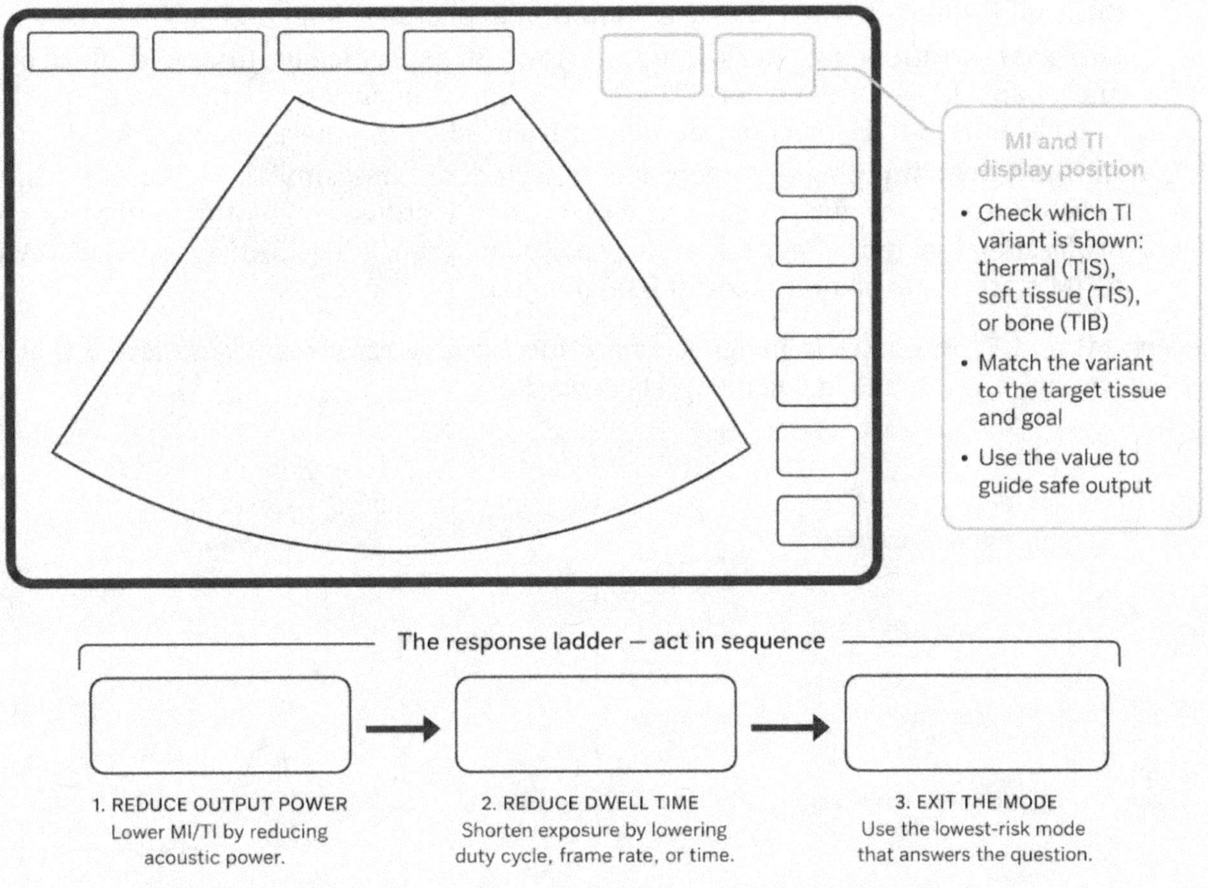

ALARA in practice

ALARA is a sequence of concrete actions, in this order:

1. **Optimize with receiver gain before transmit power.** Increasing overall gain amplifies the returning signal and costs the patient nothing. Increasing transmit

power delivers more energy into tissue. Reach for gain first; most images can be adequately brightened without touching output.

2. **Choose the correct preset.** Presets set output limits and TI variant appropriate to the application. A first-trimester obstetric study performed on a general abdominal preset is operating under the wrong constraints and displaying the wrong index.
3. **Minimize dwell.** Keep the beam moving. Do not leave the transducer on the patient, transmitting, while you speak to them, look up a value, or think. **Freeze the image or lift the probe.** Frozen frames can be measured and annotated with no further exposure — measure on a frozen image, not a live one.
4. **Use Doppler deliberately.** Colour only where flow information is needed; spectral only where a waveform or velocity is needed; short traces.
5. **Watch the indices, in obstetric and neonatal work especially.** If TI rises above the level your department's policy defines as requiring attention, reduce output or shorten exposure and be able to justify continuing. [VERIFY: institutional and society thresholds for TI-driven exposure limitation in obstetric imaging]
6. **Contrast studies** are performed at low MI specifically to avoid destroying microbubbles — a case where ALARA and image quality point the same direction. Where higher-MI destruction sequences are used deliberately, keep them brief.
7. **Non-medical imaging** — keepsake fetal videos and similar — has no clinical indication and therefore no exposure that can be justified. Regulatory authorities and professional societies have taken clear positions against it. [VERIFY: current FDA and AIUM statements on non-medical fetal imaging]

Record MI and TI in obstetric imaging where local policy requires it, and know that the settings are archived in the image metadata regardless.

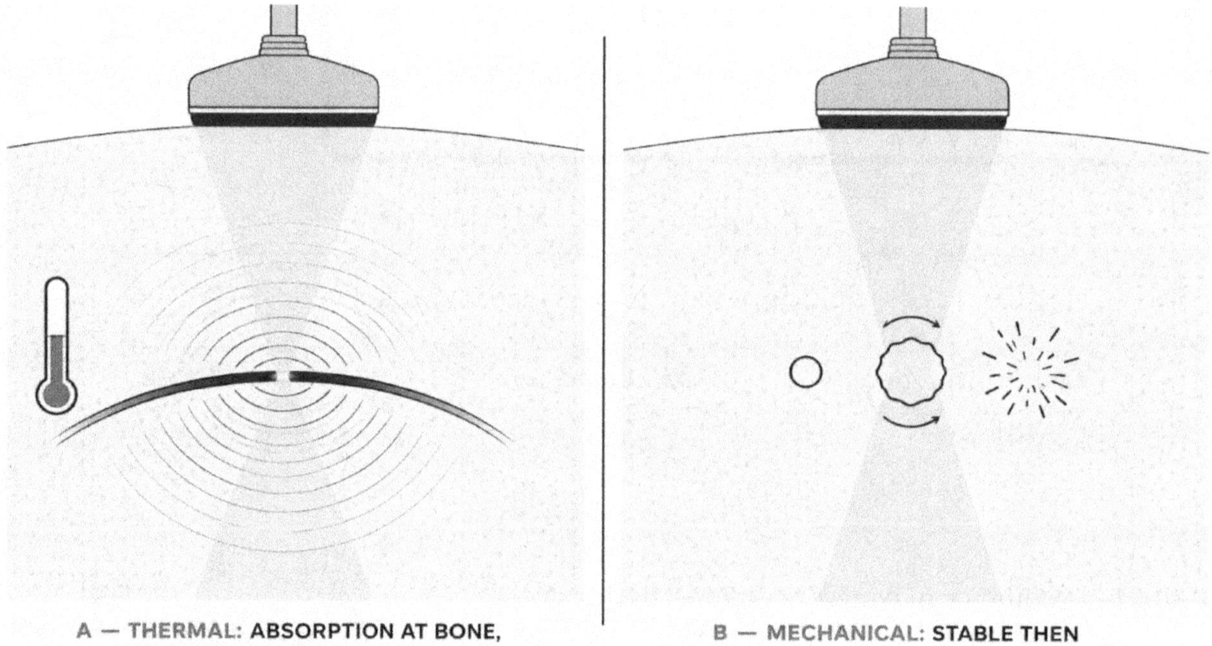

A — THERMAL: ABSORPTION AT BONE, HEAT SPREAD, TRACKED BY TI

B — MECHANICAL: STABLE THEN INERTIAL CAVITATION, TRACKED BY MI

Answering the patient

Patients ask whether ultrasound is safe, and the question deserves a real answer rather than a reflex.

> "Ultrasound doesn't use radiation — it's sound waves, and it's been used in pregnancy for decades without any evidence of harm. It does put a small amount of energy into the tissue, so we're trained to use the lowest settings that still give us a diagnostic image, and to keep the exam no longer than it needs to be. That's why I'm not going to linger anywhere I don't need to."

This is accurate, it is not falsely absolute, and it explains a behaviour the patient will otherwise interpret as haste.

1.8 Professional Ethics and Medicolegal Responsibility

The ethical frame

Professional codes of ethics for sonography — the SDMS code and its international counterparts — converge on a small set of obligations: provide competent care within your scope, protect patient privacy and dignity, act honestly, maintain and demonstrate competence, and place the patient's welfare ahead of institutional or personal convenience. [VERIFY: current SDMS Code of Ethics for the Profession of Diagnostic Medical Sonography]

The clinical ethics of obstetric imaging are substantial enough to be addressed separately in Chapter 18. What follows are obligations that apply across the whole of practice.

Confidentiality

Patient information is protected by law — HIPAA in the United States, equivalent regimes elsewhere — and by professional obligation independent of law. In sonography the recurring failure points are specific:

- **Images on personal devices.** Photographing a screen with a phone, for teaching, for a colleague's opinion, or for interest, is a breach unless performed within a sanctioned, consented, de-identified pathway. This includes images you believe are anonymous; a rare finding, a date, a device serial number, or a distinctive anatomy can identify.
- **Social media.** Posting cases — however educationally intended and however de-identified you believe them to be — has ended careers. If it originated from a patient encounter, it does not go on a personal account.
- **Conversation.** Corridors, lifts, cafeterias, shared workrooms with the door open. Volume is not privacy.
- **Screens and worksheets** left visible to the next patient entering the room. Lock the workstation; clear the desk.
- **Family members in the room.** The patient's consent to their presence is not consent to disclosure of every finding, and it is the interpreting physician who will have that conversation regardless.

Teaching and research use of images requires a defined consent process and de-identification, not an assumption of implied permission.

Disclosure of findings

Covered in scope terms in §1.2; the ethical dimension is separate. The obligation is not to withhold, but to route. The patient is entitled to their results; they are not entitled to receive them from a person who cannot contextualize them, and delivering a finding without the ability to answer "what happens now" is a harm, not a kindness.

Two situations recur and both have defensible answers.

Absent fetal cardiac activity. The patient in front of you will very often know before you speak, from the screen and from your pause. Institutional policy varies on whether the sonographer may confirm; many practices permit or require that the sonographer stop the examination, obtain the interpreting physician promptly, and remain with the patient. What is not acceptable is completing the study in silence and leaving the room. Know your institution's policy in advance, because you will not want to be improvising in that moment.

Direct questions with a clear answer. "Is it a boy or a girl?" — governed by institutional policy, which in some settings restricts disclosure; know it. "Is there a heartbeat?" in an otherwise unremarkable study — commonly permitted. "Is the mass cancer?" — never; that is a diagnosis, and it is one you frequently cannot make from images alone.

Unexpected, critical, and incidental findings

Critical findings require immediate escalation, as set out in §1.5.

Unexpected findings outside the requested study — an aortic aneurysm found during a renal scan, a large adnexal mass found during an appendix study — must be documented and communicated. The examination expands to characterize them adequately. Reporting only what was asked for, when you have seen something significant, is indefensible.

Incidental findings of uncertain significance — a small simple renal cyst, a tiny hepatic haemangioma, a subcentimetre thyroid nodule — present the opposite problem. They are documented and reported, but proportionately: over-characterizing a benign incidental finding generates anxiety, further imaging, and occasionally biopsy, with real cost and no benefit. The judgment about follow-up belongs to the interpreting physician, and the sonographer's task is accurate documentation without inflation.

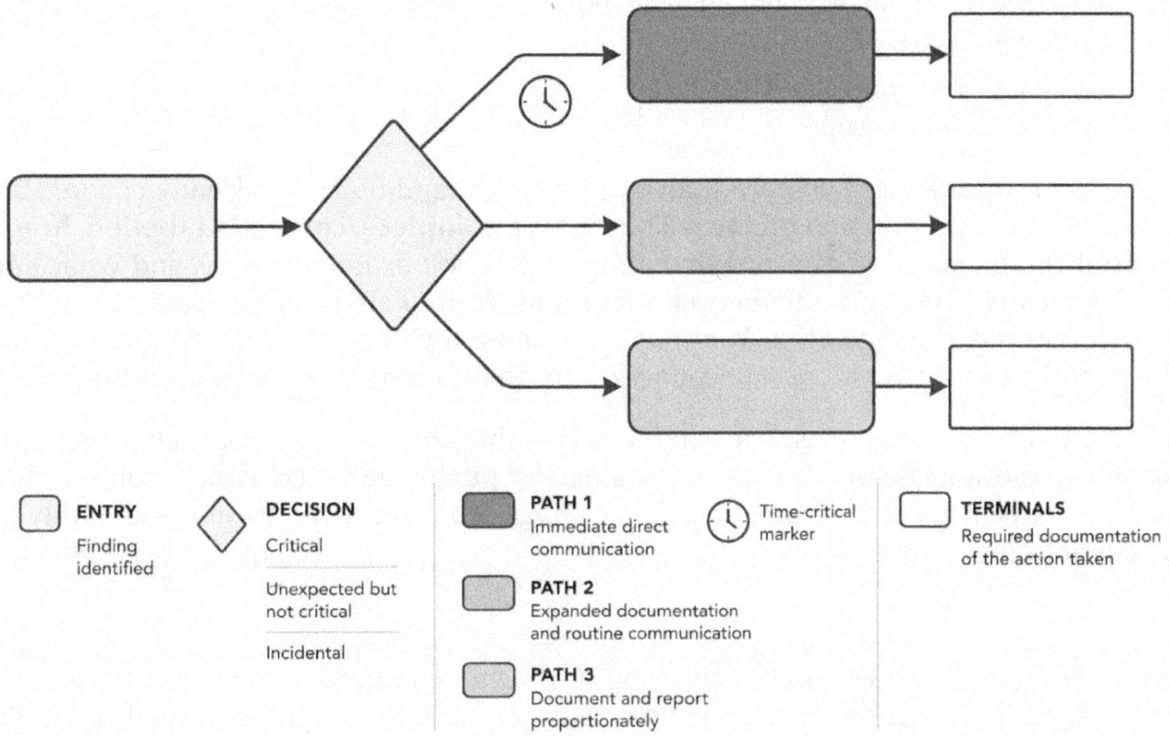

The impaired or unsafe colleague, and pressure on scope

Two situations test professional courage rather than knowledge.

A colleague whose practice is unsafe — through impairment, deteriorating competence, or persistent shortcut-taking — creates an obligation. The obligation is to raise it through the defined route, not to cover for it and not to broadcast it. Institutions that have a route and a culture of using it have fewer catastrophic events.

Pressure to exceed scope is more common and more insidious. It arrives as workload — a schedule that permits eight minutes for a study requiring twenty — or as a request to give a result to a patient because the physician is unavailable, or to omit part of a protocol to keep the list moving. The response is to document the constraint rather than absorb it silently. A study performed in insufficient time should say so. The sonographer who quietly compresses protocols to meet an impossible schedule is the person who will be named when a finding is missed.

Medicolegal exposure

Sonographers are named in malpractice actions, most commonly in obstetric and vascular practice, and the allegations cluster into a small number of patterns:

- A finding present on stored images that was not documented or communicated
- An examination documented as complete that the image set does not support

- A measurement that was performed incorrectly and relied upon — a Doppler velocity acquired at an uncorrected angle, a biometric measurement in the wrong plane
- Mislabelled laterality
- Failure to escalate a critical finding
- Practice beyond scope

Two things reduce exposure more than anything else, and both are already covered above because both are simply good practice. The first is a **complete, correctly labelled, honestly caveated image set** — the record that shows what you examined, how, and what limited you. The second is **contemporaneous documentation** of anything unusual: the limitation you encountered, the escalation you made, the person you spoke to, the time. Documents created at the time are evidence. Recollection reconstructed two years later is not.

Standard of care is judged against what a reasonably competent sonographer would have done in comparable circumstances — informed by published practice parameters, which is a further reason to know the ones governing your specialty rather than only your department's local worksheet.

Emerging accountability: automation and AI

Machine learning tools are now embedded in routine equipment — automated biometry, view recognition, ejection fraction estimation, nodule risk assignment, quality feedback. They are useful and they will become more so.

The accountability position is currently unambiguous and worth stating clearly: **an automated measurement you accept becomes your measurement.** Auto-generated biometry placed on the wrong plane, an automatically traced Doppler envelope that has captured noise, an algorithmic assessment applied to an image outside its validated population — all remain the operator's responsibility, because the operator accepted them. Verify automated output at the same standard you would apply to a trainee's, and reject it as readily.

Key Points

1. Ultrasound is operator-dependent in acquisition as well as interpretation; a structure that was not insonated does not exist in the record, and every professional obligation in this chapter follows from that fact.
2. Take the history yourself before you scan. It changes the protocol often enough to justify the three minutes every time.
3. Explain your silence at the beginning of the examination, then be consistent — inconsistent demeanour communicates findings you are not permitted to disclose.
4. Reprocessing level is set by the application, not the probe. A transducer used on non-intact skin is semicritical for that use and requires high-level disinfection, sheath or no sheath.
5. Cleaning precedes disinfection and cannot be replaced by it; disinfectant applied to a soiled probe does not disinfect it.

6. Document what you could not see, specifically. An unremarked omission reads as a normal finding to everyone who reviews the study afterwards.
7. Label laterality and orientation at the moment of acquisition, never retrospectively.
8. Bring the patient to you and support your scanning arm. Sustained shoulder abduction is the dominant biomechanical risk in the profession, and room geometry determines it before you touch the transducer.
9. Reach for receiver gain before transmit power, and freeze the image before you measure — neither costs the patient any exposure.
10. Spectral Doppler carries the highest acoustic output of any routine mode. In the first trimester, document cardiac activity with M-mode or B-mode, not spectral Doppler over the embryo.
11. A finding you accept from an automated tool is your finding. Verify automated measurements to the same standard you would apply to your own.
12. Contemporaneous documentation of limitations, escalations, and communications is the single strongest medicolegal protection available to you.

Registry Check

1. A curvilinear transducer is used to image a fluctuant collection beneath an open surgical wound. Which reprocessing level is required after the examination?

A. Low-level disinfection, as the probe is an external transducer **B.** Low-level disinfection, provided a sheath was used **C.** High-level disinfection **D.** Sterilization

> **Answer: C.** Contact with non-intact skin places this use in the semicritical category regardless of the probe type or the use of a sheath. Sheaths are assumed to fail and do not downgrade the reprocessing requirement.

2. Which mode delivers the highest acoustic intensity to a given location in tissue?

A. B-mode **B.** M-mode **C.** Colour Doppler **D.** Spectral pulsed-wave Doppler

> **Answer: D.** Spectral Doppler holds a stationary sample volume and delivers a high pulse repetition frequency to one small location for the duration of the trace. B-mode distributes pulses across the whole image plane and delivers the least energy to any single point.

3. During a second-trimester obstetric examination, which thermal index should the machine display?

A. TIS **B.** TIB **C.** TIC **D.** MI

> **Answer: B.** TIB models bone at or near the focal zone, which is the situation once fetal ossification has occurred. TIS applies where no bone is in the beam, TIC where bone is at the transducer face as in transcranial and neonatal cranial imaging, and MI is not a thermal index at all.

4. A patient undergoing an abdominal ultrasound asks whether the mass you are imaging is cancer. The most appropriate response is to:

A. Explain that the appearances favour a benign process **B.** State that you are not able to give results, and confirm who will provide them and when **C.** Continue the examination without responding **D.** Tell the patient the radiologist will explain everything, and change the subject

> **Answer: B.** Rendering a diagnosis exceeds scope, and A does so. C is non-responsive and will be read as bad news. D is closer but evasive. The defensible response names the boundary, names who will provide the result, and does not leave the patient to interpret silence.

5. The biomechanical exposure most strongly associated with shoulder injury in sonographers is:

A. Sustained transducer grip force **B.** Sustained shoulder abduction **C.** Prolonged standing **D.** Repetitive foot pedal use

> **Answer: B.** Sustained abduction, particularly beyond approximately 30 degrees and markedly beyond 60, loads the supraspinatus and reduces subacromial perfusion. Grip force is a major contributor to distal upper limb pathology rather than shoulder injury.

6. The pancreatic tail could not be visualized during an abdominal examination despite repositioning. The correct documentation is to:

A. Omit reference to the pancreatic tail **B.** Record that the study was technically difficult **C.** Record specifically that the pancreatic tail was obscured by bowel gas and not evaluated **D.** Record the pancreatic tail as normal, since no abnormality was seen

> **Answer: C.** An unremarked omission is read by subsequent reviewers as a normal finding, and D states this explicitly and dangerously. B is too vague to act on. The interpreting physician needs to know precisely what is missing to decide whether further imaging is warranted.

7. Which of the following most appropriately requires explicit rather than implied consent?

A. Transabdominal renal ultrasound **B.** Transvaginal pelvic ultrasound **C.** Carotid duplex examination **D.** Transabdominal obstetric ultrasound in the third trimester

> **Answer: B.** Endocavitary examination is invasive and intimate, and requires explicit verbal consent including an explanation of the procedure and a clear statement that the patient may stop at any point. The remaining options are external examinations on intact skin, covered by implied consent.

8. An automated software tool places biometric calipers on a stored image. The measurement appears in the report and is later shown to have been acquired in an incorrect plane. Responsibility for the measurement rests with:

A. The equipment manufacturer **B.** The software vendor **C.** The sonographer who accepted the measurement **D.** No individual, as the measurement was automated

> **Answer: C.** An automated output accepted into the record becomes the operator's measurement. Automated tools require verification at the same standard applied to any other assistance, and acceptance transfers responsibility to the person who accepted it.

Chapter Notes for the Editorial Pass

Verification queue. Every [VERIFY: ...] tag in this chapter must be resolved against a current primary source before layout. They cluster in §1.2 (credentialing structures and prerequisites), §1.4 (reprocessing guidance), §1.6 (prevalence figures and abduction thresholds), and §1.7 (regulatory output limits and first-trimester Doppler statements). None of these should be published as written; all are placeholders indicating where a real, dated, cited source is required.

Society documents to cite directly. SDMS Scope of Practice and Clinical Standards; SDMS Code of Ethics; SDMS Industry Standards for the Prevention of Work-Related Musculoskeletal Disorders in Sonography; AIUM guidelines for cleaning and preparing external and internal ultrasound transducers; AIUM Official Statements on prudent use, non-medical use, and safety in obstetric imaging; FDA guidance on diagnostic ultrasound acoustic output; CDC guideline for disinfection and sterilization in healthcare facilities.

Figure count: 8 (all Lane A). No Lane B sonographic images are required in this chapter, which is expected — Chapter 1 contains no diagnostic imaging content. Lane B demand begins in Chapter 2 with artifact demonstration.

Word count: approximately 10,400 excluding image prompt blocks, learning objectives, registry questions, and these notes.

Chapter 2: Physics, Instrumentation, Technique, and Artifacts

Learning Objectives

On completing this chapter you should be able to:

1. Predict how a given tissue interface will behave acoustically from its impedance mismatch and geometry, and explain why that prediction governs image appearance.
2. Distinguish axial, lateral, elevational, contrast, and temporal resolution, and name the parameter that controls each.
3. Select transducer frequency, footprint, and array geometry from the clinical task rather than from habit.
4. Manipulate gain, TGC, depth, focus, and dynamic range deliberately, and explain what each does and does not do to the underlying data.
5. State the mechanism, benefit, and cost of harmonic imaging and spatial compounding, including the circumstances in which compounding is harmful.
6. Apply the Doppler equation to explain angle dependence, and optimize a spectral trace to produce a velocity that means something.
7. Describe the five assumptions the scanner makes about sound propagation, and derive every major artifact from the violation of one of them.
8. Identify each principal artifact, state whether it is diagnostically useful, and perform the specific maneuver that resolves it.
9. Explain the difference between strain and shear-wave elastography and name the confounders that invalidate a stiffness measurement.

The Organizing Idea

Everything in this chapter reduces to a single premise. The scanner does not know what is inside the patient. It makes **five assumptions** about how sound behaved, converts returning echoes into an image on that basis, and displays the result with complete confidence whether or not the assumptions held.

The assumptions are:

1. Sound travels in a **straight line** along the beam axis, out and back.
2. Sound travels at a **constant 1,540 m/s**.
3. Echoes originate **only from structures on the beam axis**.
4. Echo depth is proportional to **round-trip time**, and each pulse produces one round trip.
5. Attenuation is **uniform** across the field.

Sections 2.1 through 2.6 explain how the machine builds an image when the assumptions hold. Sections 2.7 through 2.9 are, in their entirety, an inventory of what appears on screen when they do not. There is no separate body of knowledge called "artifacts" — there is only physics, observed at the moment it stops matching the model.

Learn the artifacts this way and you will never have to memorize a list. Given a finding, you ask which assumption is being violated, and the answer tells you both what you are looking at and what maneuver will resolve it.

2.1 Acoustic Principles and Tissue Interaction

The pulse and the range equation

Diagnostic ultrasound is a pulse-echo technique. The transducer emits a brief pulse, then listens for far longer than it transmitted — the listening interval is roughly 99% of each cycle. Nothing is imaged while the pulse is being emitted.

The machine calculates depth from the round-trip time using assumption 2:

depth = (c × t) / 2, with c taken as 1,540 m/s

The division by two accounts for the out-and-back path. Every pixel's vertical position on your screen is this calculation, and nothing else. When the actual propagation speed differs from 1,540 m/s — through fat, which is slower, or through some pathological tissue — the structure is placed at the wrong depth. That is speed-error artifact, and it is assumption 2 failing.

A useful consequence: **13 microseconds of round-trip time corresponds to 1 cm of depth**. Deeper imaging therefore requires waiting longer between pulses, which caps how many pulses per second you can send, which caps frame rate. Depth, pulse repetition frequency, and temporal resolution are locked together by the speed of sound, and no amount of processing escapes it.

Impedance and what happens at an interface

Acoustic impedance (Z) is the product of tissue density and propagation speed. It is not a property you can palpate or infer clinically — it is the acoustic property that determines what happens when a pulse meets a boundary.

At an interface, the proportion of energy reflected depends on the **difference** in impedance between the two media:

- **Small mismatch** — most soft tissue-to-soft tissue boundaries. A small fraction of energy reflects; the great majority transmits onward. This is the regime in which imaging is possible at all. Liver against kidney, muscle against fat: visible boundaries, plenty of sound continuing deeper.
- **Large mismatch** — soft tissue against bone or calcium, and soft tissue against gas. A very large fraction reflects at the surface. Almost nothing continues beyond. This is why you cannot image through bowel gas or the ribs, and why a stone is a bright line with nothing behind it.

Gas is the more extreme case, because the impedance mismatch is so severe that essentially all energy reflects, chaotically, at the surface. Bone reflects strongly *and* absorbs strongly, producing shadowing with a somewhat different character.

Two other behaviors matter clinically:

Specular versus diffuse reflection. A large, smooth interface relative to the wavelength — diaphragm, bladder wall, vessel wall, fascial plane — reflects like a mirror, sending energy back along the angle of incidence. These interfaces are brilliantly bright when insonated perpendicularly and **disappear entirely when insonated obliquely**. This is why a tendon vanishes when you rock the probe a few degrees, and why the near and far walls of a vessel are bright while the side walls are not. When a structure you know exists suddenly is not there, the first thing to change is your angle of incidence, not your gain.

Scattering. Interfaces small relative to the wavelength — the internal architecture of parenchymal organs, red blood cells — scatter energy in all directions. Only a small fraction returns, but it returns from *any* insonation angle. Scattering is what gives liver, spleen, and renal cortex their characteristic uniform internal texture, and it is what makes parenchymal echogenicity comparable between patients and over time. It is also angle-independent, which is why parenchyma looks the same as you rock the probe while the specular boundaries flash in and out.

Speckle is the interference pattern produced by scattered echoes arriving in and out of phase. It looks like tissue texture and is often described as such, but it is not a map of histology — it is an interference pattern, and it changes if you move the probe slightly. This distinction matters when you evaluate speckle-reduction and compounding methods in §2.4.

Attenuation

Sound loses intensity with depth through absorption (conversion to heat — the dominant mechanism, and the origin of the thermal bioeffects in Chapter 1), reflection, and scattering.

The clinically indispensable relationship is that **attenuation increases with both frequency and depth**. In soft tissue, a working figure is approximately 0.5 dB per centimetre per megahertz of path length. A 10 MHz pulse travelling 4 cm is attenuated far more severely than a 3 MHz pulse travelling the same distance.

This single relationship generates the central trade-off of the entire modality:

> **Higher frequency gives better resolution and worse penetration. Lower frequency gives better penetration and worse resolution.**

Every transducer selection decision is a position taken on this trade-off. There is no setting that escapes it and no processing that undoes it.

Attenuation is also tissue-dependent and non-uniform, which is assumption 5. Fluid attenuates far less than solid tissue; that non-uniformity produces posterior acoustic enhancement (§2.7). Calcium and gas attenuate severely; that produces shadowing.

"Resolution" without a qualifier is not a useful word. Five distinct resolutions matter, and confusing them leads to reaching for the wrong control.

Axial resolution — the ability to separate two structures lying one behind the other along the beam. Determined by **spatial pulse length**: the shorter the pulse, the finer the axial detail. Shorter pulses come from higher frequency and from heavy damping of the crystal. Axial resolution is the best of the resolutions, is constant with depth, and improves directly with frequency.

Lateral resolution — the ability to separate two structures lying side by side, perpendicular to the beam. Determined by **beam width**. Beam width varies with depth, being narrowest at the focus. Lateral resolution is therefore depth-dependent and is always worse than axial resolution. This is why you should place your focal zone at the level of the structure of interest — a control discussed in §2.3 and constantly neglected in practice.

Elevational resolution — the ability to resolve in the third dimension, perpendicular to the imaging plane. Determined by **slice thickness**, which is fixed by the physical height of the array and its lens. This is the resolution operators forget exists, and it produces the section-thickness artifact of §2.7 — the pseudo-sludge in a gallbladder or the false debris in a simple cyst. Matrix and 1.5D arrays with electronic focusing in elevation improve it.

Contrast resolution — the ability to distinguish tissues of similar echogenicity. Governed by dynamic range, processing, harmonic imaging, and compounding.

Temporal resolution — the ability to resolve events in time, determined by frame rate. Improved by reducing depth, narrowing the sector, reducing line density, and using a single focal zone. It matters most in echocardiography and any moving-target application, and it trades directly against spatial resolution.

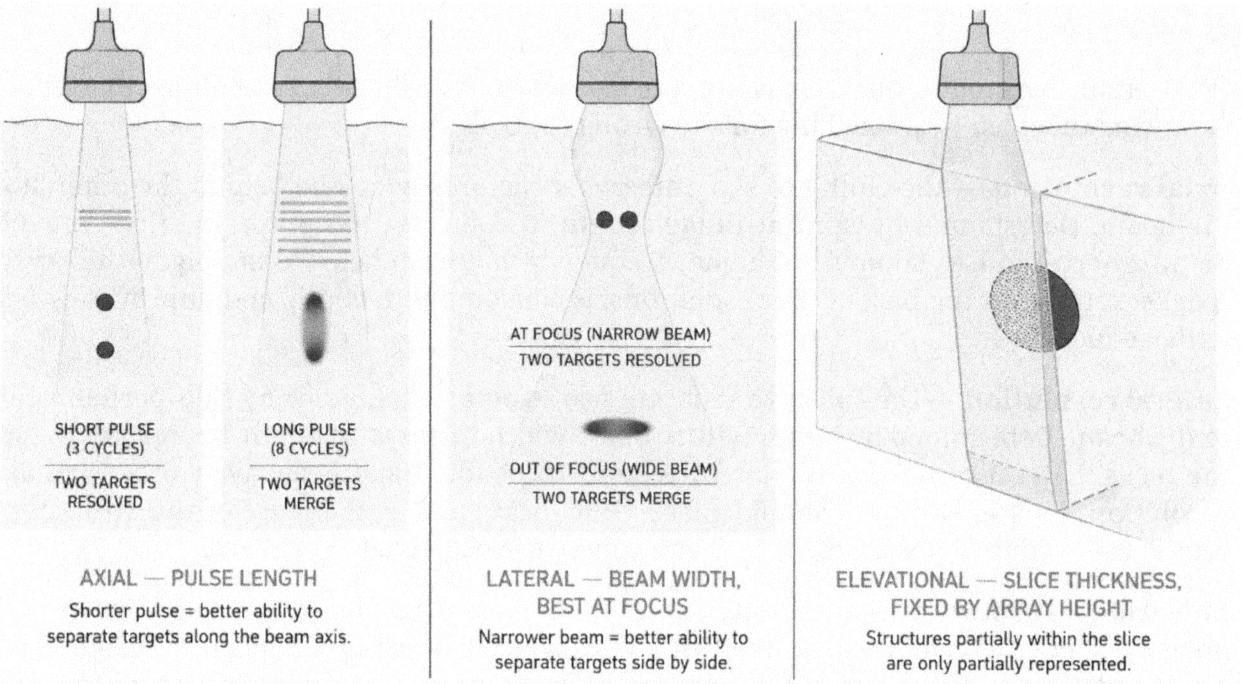

2.2 Transducer Design, Frequency, and Selection

Construction

A transducer converts electrical energy to acoustic energy and back, using the piezoelectric effect. The elements — historically lead zirconate titanate, increasingly single-crystal and composite materials with superior efficiency and bandwidth — deform when voltage is applied and generate voltage when deformed.

Four components determine performance:

The active element array. Element count, size, and pitch determine beam-forming capability and lateral resolution.

The matching layer sits between element and patient. Element impedance is vastly higher than skin's; without an intermediate layer, most energy would reflect at the transducer face and never enter the patient. Coupling gel serves the same purpose at the final boundary — eliminating the air gap, which would otherwise reflect essentially everything. **Gel is not a lubricant.** It is an impedance-matching medium, and this is why an inadequately gelled probe produces a poor image rather than merely an uncomfortable one.

The damping (backing) layer absorbs rearward energy and shortens the ringdown of the element after excitation. Shorter pulse means better axial resolution and wider bandwidth, at some cost in sensitivity. Damping is why modern broadband probes can operate across a frequency range rather than at a single frequency.

The acoustic lens and housing shape the beam in elevation and provide the patient-contact surface. The lens is the part that cracks, and a cracked lens cannot be reliably disinfected — the infection control point from Chapter 1 §1.4 is a physics consequence.

Array geometries and their clinical logic

Array	Footprint / beam	Chosen for
Linear	Flat, rectangular field	Superficial work: vascular, small parts, breast, MSK, thyroid, scrotum, needle guidance. High frequency, excellent near-field resolution, no field divergence
Curvilinear	Convex, diverging sector	Abdomen, obstetrics, general. Wide far field from a modest footprint; near-field resolution inferior to linear
Phased (sector)	Small footprint, wide diverging sector	Cardiac and intercostal work. Fits between ribs and through the small acoustic windows of the chest; poor near field
Endocavitary	Compact, high-frequency, wide sector	Transvaginal, transrectal. Proximity to target permits high frequency; excellent resolution of pelvic structures
Matrix / 2D	Electronically steered in both planes	Volume acquisition, biplane, improved elevational focusing

Intracavitary and specialist probes — transesophageal, intravascular, laparoscopic, hockey-stick linear for small-part and MSK work — extend the same principles to constrained access.

Selecting frequency

The choice follows directly from §2.1's trade-off, and the correct approach is to **start at the highest frequency that penetrates to your target and step down only as far as necessary**. Operators habitually work at too low a frequency, having selected once for the most difficult patient and never revisited.

Typical starting points:

Application	Working range
Superficial vascular, thyroid, MSK, small parts	High frequency linear
Breast	High frequency linear, adjusted for depth
General adult abdomen	Mid-range curvilinear
Large body habitus abdomen	Lower frequency curvilinear
Adult echocardiography	Low frequency phased

Application	Working range
Neonatal and pediatric abdomen	Substantially higher than adult equivalents
Endocavitary pelvic	High frequency endocavitary

The pediatric point is worth emphasizing because it is routinely missed: a child scanned with adult settings is being under-resolved for no reason. Small patients permit high frequencies, and the resolution gain is dramatic.

Broadband transducers operate across a range and permit frequency shift within a single probe — often labelled as resolution, general, and penetration settings. Use them. Shifting to the penetration setting mid-examination for a deep structure and back up for a superficial one is faster than changing probes and is chronically underused.

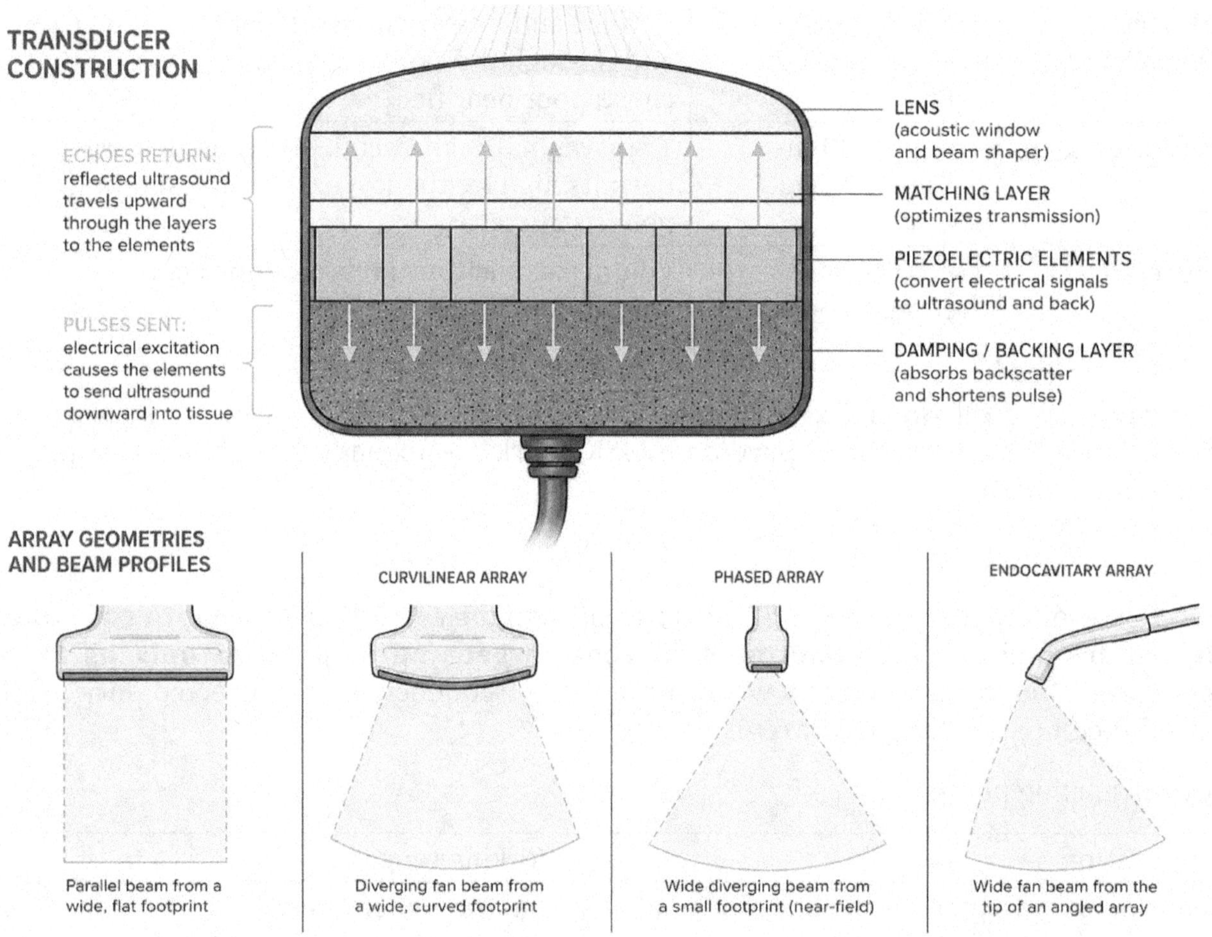

2.3 System Controls: Gain, TGC, Depth, Focus, Dynamic Range

Controls divide into two categories, and knowing which is which changes how you use them.

Transmit controls alter the pulse sent into the patient — output power, frequency, focal position, line density, sector width. They change the data acquired. Output power also changes patient exposure (Chapter 1 §1.7).

Receive controls alter the processing of echoes already returned — overall gain, TGC, dynamic range, gray map, post-processing. They change the display of existing data and cost the patient nothing.

The consequence, stated in Chapter 1 and worth repeating because it is the most common ALARA failure: **exhaust receive controls before increasing transmit power.**

Overall gain

Uniform amplification of all returning echoes. Set it so that fluid-filled structures are genuinely anechoic and parenchyma has a mid-gray texture with visible internal detail.

Both failure modes cause diagnostic error. **Excessive gain** fills cysts and vessels with false internal echoes, obscures low-level shadowing, and can manufacture sludge, debris, or thrombus that does not exist. **Insufficient gain** loses low-level echoes — subtle parenchymal change, low-level internal content in a complex cyst, faint plaque — and can make a solid mass look cystic.

If you are unsure whether internal echoes in a cyst are real, reduce gain until surrounding parenchyma darkens. Real internal echoes persist relative to their surroundings; noise disappears with everything else.

Time gain compensation

Attenuation means deep echoes return weaker than identical shallow echoes. TGC applies depth-dependent amplification to correct for this, so that identical tissue looks identical at all depths.

Set TGC to produce **uniform parenchymal brightness from near field to far field.** The classic errors are a visible bright or dark horizontal band where an individual slider is misaligned, and a globally over-compensated far field that makes deep structures brighter than shallow ones.

TGC is a correction for a physical process, so its correct setting changes with the patient and the depth. Slider positions carried over from the previous patient are a specific, common, and entirely avoidable source of error. Many systems offer automatic optimization; it is a good starting point and a poor final answer, particularly where a large fluid collection or a shadowing structure makes the depth-brightness relationship non-uniform.

Depth and sector width

Set depth so the structure of interest occupies most of the field, with a modest margin beyond. Excess depth wastes image area on tissue you are not assessing and — because of the range equation — lowers frame rate for no benefit.

Narrowing the sector on a curvilinear or phased array raises frame rate and line density simultaneously. It is close to free improvement when you are working on a localized structure, and it is underused.

Focus

The focal zone is where the beam is narrowest and lateral resolution is best. **Place it at, or just deep to, the structure of interest.** A focal marker left at the bottom of the screen while you assess a superficial structure is discarding lateral resolution for nothing, and it is the single most common control error in routine practice.

Multiple focal zones improve lateral resolution across a greater depth range at direct cost to frame rate, because each zone requires a separate transmit for every line. Use multiple zones for static assessment, a single zone for anything moving.

Some contemporary systems retrospectively focus across the whole field and remove this trade-off. Know whether yours does, because if it does not, the focal marker matters and if it does, it does not.

Dynamic range

Dynamic range determines how many shades of gray span the range from weakest to strongest displayed echo.

- **Wide** dynamic range gives many gray levels: a softer, smoother image with more subtle tissue differentiation. Suited to parenchymal assessment — liver texture, subtle focal lesions.
- **Narrow** dynamic range gives fewer gray levels: a higher-contrast, more black-and-white image. Suited to tasks where boundary conspicuity matters more than internal detail — needle visualization, stone identification, vascular lumen assessment.

Neither is correct in general; each is correct for a task. Adjusting dynamic range mid-examination as the task changes is a mark of a skilled operator.

The optimization sequence

A workable default order, which takes about fifteen seconds:

1. Correct preset and probe.
2. Frequency as high as penetrates.
3. Depth set to the target.
4. Focus at the target.
5. TGC for uniform brightness top to bottom.
6. Overall gain for anechoic fluid and mid-gray parenchyma.
7. Dynamic range for the task.
8. Sector width narrowed if the target is localized.
9. Harmonics on or off per §2.4.
10. Output power only if all of the above are exhausted.

id: fig-2-4
lane: A
prompt: >-

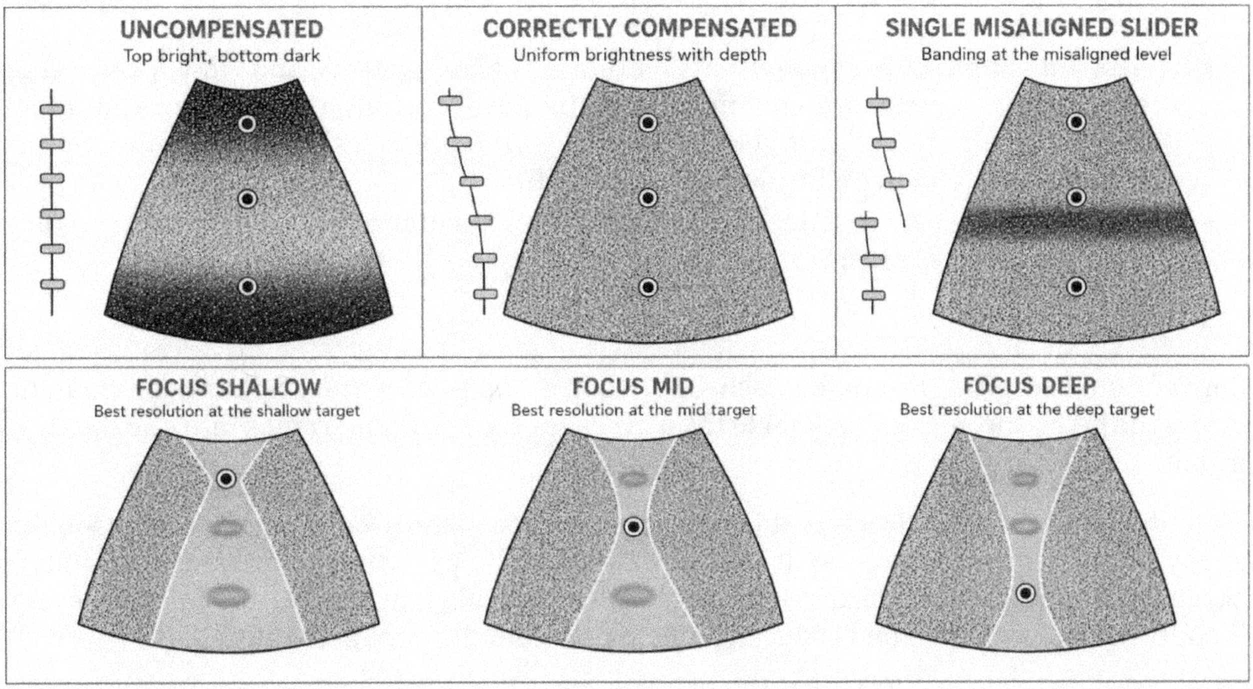

2.4 Harmonic, Spatial Compound, and Advanced Imaging Modes

Tissue harmonic imaging

Sound propagation through tissue is not perfectly linear. The compressional phase of the wave travels marginally faster than the rarefactional phase, and the waveform progressively distorts with depth. That distortion generates energy at multiples of the transmitted frequency — principally the second harmonic.

Harmonic imaging transmits at the fundamental frequency and **receives selectively at the second harmonic**, discarding the fundamental. The clinical benefit comes from the properties of the harmonic signal:

- Harmonics are generated *within tissue*, building with depth, rather than at the transducer face. Near-field reverberation and haze — which are fundamental-frequency phenomena — are largely excluded.
- The harmonic beam is narrower than the fundamental, improving lateral resolution.
- Side lobe and grating lobe energy is too weak to generate significant harmonics, so off-axis clutter is suppressed.
- Weak scatterers generate proportionally less harmonic signal, increasing contrast between fluid and tissue.

The practical result is markedly cleaner fluid spaces and better images in technically difficult patients — the improvement is greatest exactly where you need it most, in large body habitus.

The costs are real and must be understood:

- **Reduced penetration**, since harmonic signal is weaker and generated at higher frequency.
- **Altered apparent echogenicity.** Contrast is enhanced and low-level echoes suppressed. A structure containing genuine low-level internal content can appear anechoic on harmonics. If you are deciding whether a lesion is a simple cyst or a complex one, **check on fundamental as well.**
- Possible frame rate cost depending on the implementation (pulse inversion methods require multiple transmits per line).

Spatial compounding

Conventional imaging insonates each line from a single direction. Spatial compounding steers the beam through several angles and averages the resulting frames into one displayed frame.

Benefits: **speckle reduction** (speckle is an interference pattern and changes with insonation angle, so averaging suppresses it while real structure persists), improved continuity of curved and specular boundaries — a vessel wall or capsule that would drop out at one angle is captured at another — and reduced angle-dependent dropout generally.

The costs are more consequential than most operators realize:

- **Reduced temporal resolution.** Several acquisitions per displayed frame. Poor for anything moving.
- **Blurring of moving structures** for the same reason.
- **Suppression of shadowing and enhancement.** This is the one that causes diagnostic error. Insonating from multiple angles fills in the shadow behind a stone and washes out enhancement behind a cyst. **A stone may lose its shadow, and a cyst may lose its enhancement, under compounding.**

The rule that follows: **turn compounding off when the shadow is the diagnosis.** Assessing for cholelithiasis, renal calculi, or any calcification, or using enhancement to confirm a cyst, switch to conventional imaging before you conclude. A great many "non-shadowing" stones are shadowing stones under compounding.

Frequency compounding averages across sub-bands of the received bandwidth and reduces speckle without the temporal cost, at some expense in resolution.

Adaptive speckle-reduction processing applies edge-preserving filtering to suppress speckle while retaining boundaries. It is a display process; it does not add information, and aggressive settings smooth away subtle texture — precisely the texture you may be assessing in diffuse parenchymal disease.

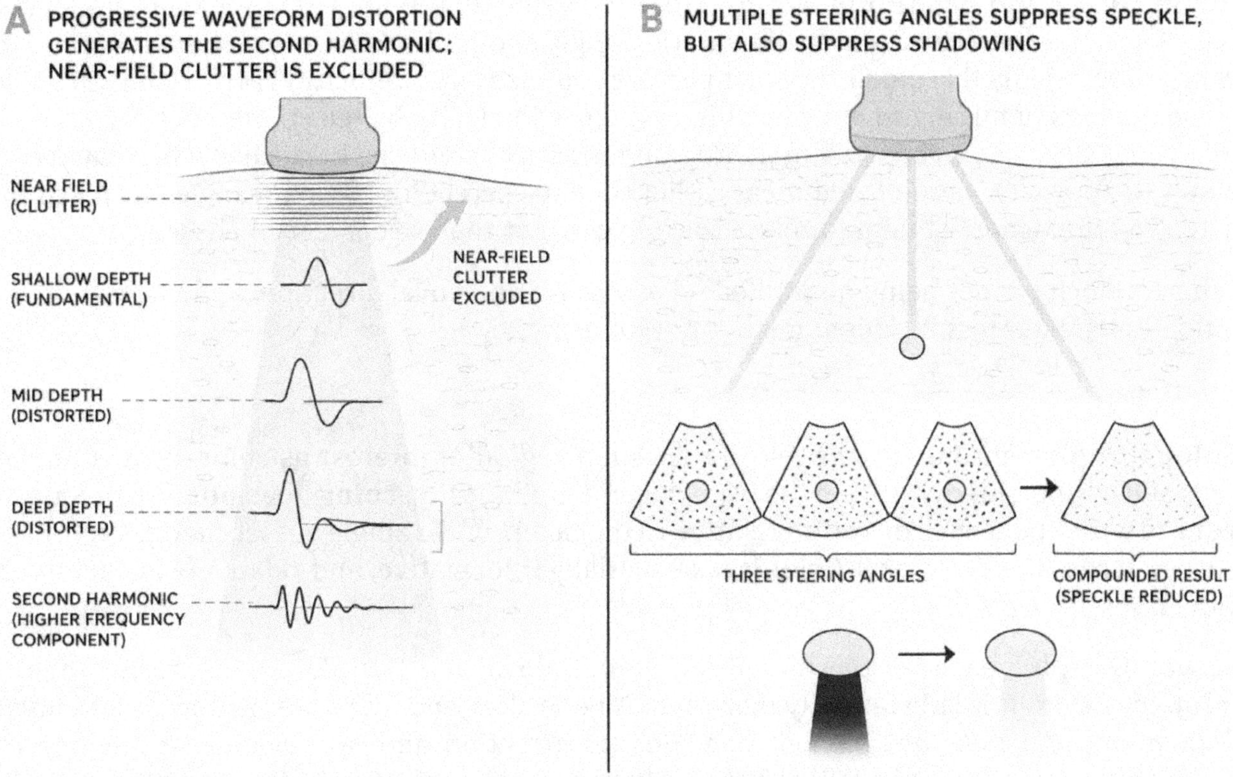

2.5 Doppler Principles: Color, Power, and Spectral

The Doppler equation and what it obliges you to do

A sound wave reflected from a moving target returns at a shifted frequency. The magnitude of the shift is:

$$f\_d = (2 \cdot f_0 \cdot v \cdot \cos\theta) / c$$

where f_0 is the transmitted frequency, v the target velocity, θ the angle between beam and flow direction, and c the propagation speed.

Three consequences govern all Doppler practice.

Angle dependence is absolute. Because the shift scales with cos θ, and cos 90° = 0, **flow perpendicular to the beam produces no Doppler shift at all.** A patent vessel insonated at 90° shows no color and no spectral trace. This is not equipment failure and it is not occlusion. It is the single most important fact in Doppler imaging, and mistaking it for absent flow is a serious and recurrent error.

The correction is geometric, not electronic. To get flow, change the angle: heel-toe the probe, use the sector steering control on a linear array, approach from a different window, or ask the patient to change position. Increasing gain or color sensitivity will not create a shift that physics has set to zero.

Angle correction has limits. For quantitative velocity, the angle cursor must be aligned parallel to the vessel axis and the insonation angle should be **60° or less.** Beyond 60°, cos θ changes so rapidly that small alignment errors produce large velocity errors — at high angles a few degrees of misalignment can shift a measured velocity by tens of percent, which is the difference between a reported moderate and a critical stenosis. In cardiac work, where the aim is to approach parallel alignment rather than to correct for a known angle, the discipline is to seek the window that minimizes the angle rather than to correct a bad one.

Where velocity is not being quantified — assessing presence, direction, and pattern of flow only — angle matters for detection but not for accuracy.

The Doppler modes

Color Doppler encodes mean velocity within a region of interest as color, conventionally red toward and blue away from the transducer. Emphatically: **color does not encode artery versus vein.** It encodes direction relative to the beam, and a single vessel changes color as it curves across the beam axis. Color is fast, spatially informative, and relatively insensitive to slow flow.

Power Doppler encodes the integrated amplitude of the Doppler signal rather than its frequency shift. It is substantially more sensitive to slow and low-volume flow, is less angle-dependent, and does not alias. It provides no direction and no velocity, and it is more susceptible to motion artifact. Use it for perfusion questions — testicular or ovarian viability, low-flow parenchymal perfusion, small vessel detection — and where you need to demonstrate that any flow exists at all.

Spectral pulsed-wave Doppler samples a specific location defined by the sample volume and displays the full velocity spectrum against time. It gives quantitative velocity and waveform morphology, at the price of a Nyquist limit (below) and the highest acoustic output of any routine mode.

Continuous-wave Doppler transmits and receives continuously on separate elements. It cannot localize depth — it records everything along the line — but it has **no aliasing limit** and can therefore measure very high velocities. Essential in echocardiography for high-velocity jets.

Optimizing a spectral trace

A spectral trace is a measurement instrument, and a badly optimized one produces confidently wrong numbers.

Scale (PRF). Set so the waveform fills roughly two-thirds to three-quarters of the vertical display. Too low and the trace aliases; too high and low velocities are compressed into an uninterpretable band near baseline.

Baseline. Shift to allocate display space to the direction of interest, which also buys headroom against aliasing.

Sample volume size. Small enough to sample the intended vessel without including adjacent flow; large enough to capture the range of velocities present. Typically positioned mid-lumen for peak velocity, but note that a very small sample volume in a large vessel can miss the true peak.

Angle correction cursor aligned to the vessel axis, angle at or below 60°, and **visible in the archived image** (Chapter 1 §1.5).

Doppler gain raised until faint background speckle just appears, then reduced slightly. Excessive gain broadens the spectrum artificially and inflates measured peak velocity by capturing noise.

Wall filter set to exclude low-frequency wall motion without eliminating genuine low-velocity flow. A high wall filter can erase diastolic flow entirely — creating an apparent absent-diastolic-flow pattern that is a machine setting, not a physiological finding. This matters intensely in umbilical artery Doppler, where absent or reversed end-diastolic flow is a management-changing finding.

Reading a waveform

The morphology carries most of the diagnostic information, independent of the absolute numbers:

- **Low-resistance** waveforms show continuous forward flow throughout diastole, characteristic of beds requiring constant perfusion — internal carotid, renal, hepatic, splenic, and the uterine artery in pregnancy.
- **High-resistance** waveforms show sharp systolic peaks with little, absent, or reversed diastolic flow — the external carotid and resting peripheral limb arteries.
- **Triphasic** peripheral arterial waveforms indicate healthy compliant vessels with high peripheral resistance; loss of the reverse component and progression to monophasic, damped, delayed forms indicates proximal disease.
- **Venous waveforms** show respiratory phasicity, cardiac pulsatility near the heart, and response to augmentation and Valsalva. Loss of phasicity implies proximal obstruction — the point developed at length in Chapter 16.

Standard measurements — peak systolic velocity, end-diastolic velocity, resistive index, pulsatility index, systolic/diastolic ratio, acceleration time — are defined and applied in the relevant clinical chapters, with their thresholds verified against the governing society criteria.

2.6 Scanning Technique, Terminology, and Image Labeling Convention

Transducer movements

Five movements, with distinct names because they do distinct things:

Sliding — translating the probe across the skin, keeping orientation constant. Moves the imaging plane to a new location.

Rocking (heel-toe) — tilting within the plane of the image, along the probe's long axis. Steers the field of view forward or back within the same plane, and changes angle of incidence on specular structures. This is the movement that recovers a tendon or vessel wall that has dropped out.

Angling (sweeping) — tilting perpendicular to the image plane. Moves the imaging plane through the tissue like turning pages, and is how you survey a volume.

Rotating — turning the probe about its own axis. Converts transverse to longitudinal and finds oblique planes such as the long axis of a vessel or the renal hilum.

Compression — applying pressure. A diagnostic maneuver in its own right: displacing bowel gas, testing venous compressibility, assessing focal tenderness, evaluating lesion mobility and compressibility, and reducing depth to the target.

Competent scanning is continuous, purposeful combination of these. The commonest technical fault in trainees is scanning statically — holding the probe still and adjusting controls when the correct response is a small rocking or rotating movement.

Planes and orientation

Sagittal / longitudinal — divides left from right; the long axis of the body or of an organ. **Transverse / axial** — divides superior from inferior; perpendicular to the long axis. **Coronal** — divides anterior from posterior; often the best window for the kidney and spleen via a flank approach. **Oblique** — any plane between, named by the structure it is aligned to (subcostal oblique, intercostal oblique).

Note that "longitudinal" for an organ means aligned to *that organ's* long axis, which is frequently oblique to the body's. A longitudinal renal image is not a sagittal body image.

The orientation convention

Every transducer carries a physical orientation marker corresponding to an indicator on one side of the screen image. The convention, followed with near-universal consistency in general sonography:

- **Sagittal / longitudinal:** marker toward the patient's head. Cephalad appears on the left of the screen.
- **Transverse:** marker toward the patient's right. The patient's right appears on the left of the screen, as with CT.
- **Screen top** is always superficial; depth increases downward.

Echocardiography uses different conventions, and endocavitary imaging requires its own careful orientation discipline. Both are addressed in their chapters.

Before you begin any examination on an unfamiliar machine, **verify the marker-to-screen relationship** by touching a finger to one edge of the probe face and observing which side of the image moves. This takes two seconds and prevents laterality errors of the kind discussed in Chapter 1 §1.5.

Echogenicity is described *relative to a named reference*, never in absolute terms:

- **Anechoic** — no internal echoes; simple fluid
- **Hypoechoic** — darker than the reference tissue
- **Isoechoic** — same as the reference
- **Hyperechoic / echogenic** — brighter than the reference
- **Complex** — mixed cystic and solid components
- **Heterogeneous / homogeneous** — variable or uniform internal texture

Always name the comparator: *"hypoechoic relative to adjacent renal cortex"*, *"echogenic relative to liver"*. Standard hierarchies — renal sinus brighter than liver, liver brighter than or equal to renal cortex, renal cortex brighter than medulla — are the basis of most parenchymal assessments, and a comparison without a stated reference is not interpretable by anyone reading the report later.

Describe lesions systematically: location, size in three dimensions, shape, margin, internal echogenicity and texture, posterior acoustic features, vascularity, and relationship to adjacent structures. This ordering appears throughout the clinical chapters.

PROBE MARKER ORIENTATION AND THE RESULTING SCREEN CONVENTION

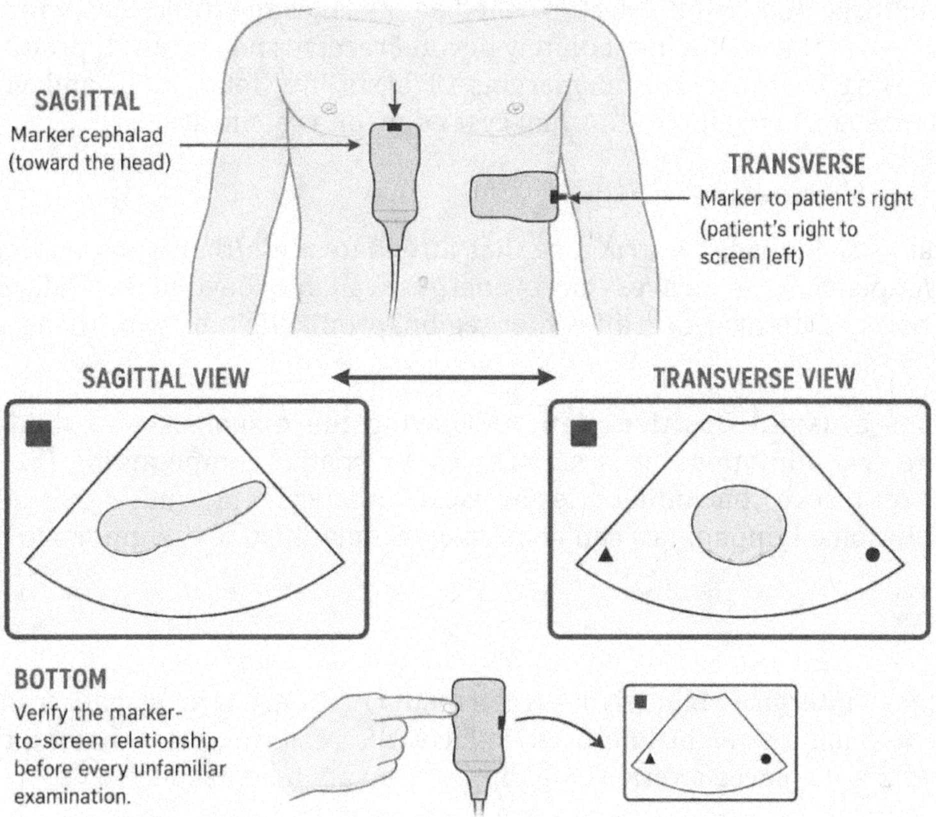

2.7 Propagation and Attenuation Artifacts

These arise from violations of assumptions 1, 2, and 5 — sound does not travel in a straight line, does not travel at 1,540 m/s, and is not attenuated uniformly.

Acoustic shadowing

Severe attenuation or reflection at a structure leaves insufficient energy to image beyond it, producing a hypoechoic or anechoic band deep to the structure. Assumption 5 fails.

The **distinction between clean and dirty shadowing** is a genuine diagnostic tool and is frequently taught poorly:

Clean shadowing — sharply marginated, uniformly anechoic, arising from calcium, stone, or bone. Energy is reflected and absorbed at a smooth interface with little scatter, so the region behind is genuinely empty of signal.

Dirty shadowing — ill-defined, containing internal echoes and reverberation, arising from gas. The chaotic multiple reflections at the gas interface fill the shadow with low-level noise.

The discrimination matters constantly: gallstone versus duodenal gas at the gallbladder neck; renal calculus versus bowel; abscess containing gas versus calcified mass.

Edge (refractive) shadowing is a different mechanism entirely — assumption 1 rather than 5. At the curved edge of a round structure, the beam strikes the interface at a critical angle and refracts away, so the region immediately beyond receives no energy. It produces narrow shadows extending from the lateral margins of cysts, the fetal skull, and vessel walls. Recognizing it prevents mistaking a normal cyst edge for a calcification.

Posterior acoustic enhancement

The reciprocal of shadowing. A structure that attenuates less than surrounding tissue — most often simple fluid — leaves more energy available beyond it. TGC, set for the surrounding tissue, then over-amplifies that region, producing a brighter band deep to the structure.

Enhancement is a **useful positive sign**, supporting the diagnosis of a fluid-containing structure. Note two limitations: it is suppressed by spatial compounding (§2.4), so turn compounding off before concluding a lesion lacks enhancement; and highly cellular solid masses, notably some lymphomas, can show enhancement, so it is supportive rather than diagnostic.

Refraction

Sound crossing an interface obliquely between media of different propagation speed bends. The machine, assuming straight-line travel, places the resulting echoes along the original axis. Structures are displaced laterally, and duplication artifacts result.

The classic case is refraction at the rectus abdominis muscles, which can produce a **double image of a single structure** — a duplicated gestational sac or aorta in a transverse epigastric view. Recognizing this prevents a diagnosis of twins or of a dissection flap where neither exists. Changing the scanning window or angle resolves it, and a duplicate that disappears when the approach changes was never there.

Speed-error (propagation speed) artifact

Fat propagates sound more slowly than 1,540 m/s; some tissues faster. Slower travel means longer round-trip time, and the machine places the structure deeper than it is. Across a fat-containing region, an interface can appear stepped or discontinuous where it is in fact straight — described in breast imaging beyond a lipoma, and at fatty planes generally.

Section thickness (partial volume)

The elevational limitation of §2.1. The imaging plane has thickness, and echoes from within that thickness are all displayed as if arising from a plane of zero width. A small anechoic structure narrower than the slice thickness therefore has adjacent tissue echoes superimposed on it.

This is the mechanism of **pseudo-sludge** in the gallbladder and false internal echoes within small cysts and the bladder. The resolving maneuver is to rescan in an orthogonal plane or from a different window; true internal content persists, section-thickness artifact does not.

Side lobes and grating lobes

Assumption 3 fails: energy exists outside the main beam. **Side lobes** are inherent to any aperture; **grating lobes** are additional and arise from the regular spacing of array elements. Echoes returned from these off-axis lobes are displayed as though they came from the main beam, appearing as faint curved bands or false echoes in structures that should be anechoic — the classic false debris in the bladder or gallbladder lying in a curved arc.

Harmonic imaging substantially suppresses lobe artifacts, because off-axis energy is too weak to generate harmonics. This is the fastest practical test: if the internal echoes disappear on harmonics, they were lobe artifact.

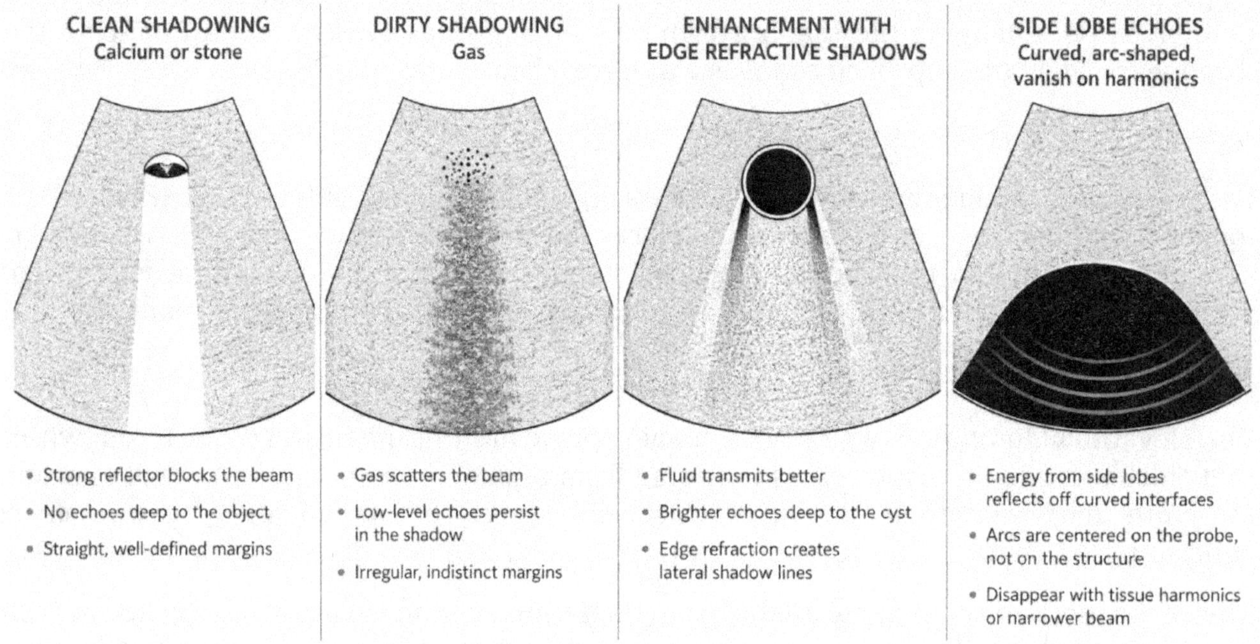

2.8 Reflection Artifacts: Reverberation, Comet Tail, Ring-Down, Mirror Image

All arise from violation of assumption 4 — the pulse makes more than one round trip before returning, so the machine, timing a longer path, places the echo deeper than its source.

Reverberation

The pulse bounces repeatedly between two strong parallel reflectors — commonly the transducer face and a superficial strong interface, or two closely spaced tissue interfaces. Each successive round trip takes proportionally longer and is placed proportionally deeper.

The appearance is a series of **equally spaced parallel bright lines** at progressively decreasing intensity, extending into the far field. The equal spacing is the diagnostic feature; the interval equals the separation of the two reflectors.

Near-field reverberation ("near-field clutter") degrades the most superficial centimetre of the image and is a common cause of false echoes in superficial structures. Countermeasures: harmonic imaging (highly effective, since the artifact is a fundamental-frequency phenomenon), adequate standoff or gel, changing angle to break the parallel geometry, and adjusting near-field gain.

Comet tail

A form of reverberation between two very closely spaced reflectors. Because the separation is tiny, the individual reverberations are so closely spaced that they merge into a **discrete tapering trail** of decreasing width and intensity, extending a short distance and terminating.

Sources include cholesterol crystals in the gallbladder wall — the finding underlying adenomyomatosis — surgical clips, metallic foreign bodies, and IUDs.

Ring-down

Frequently conflated with comet tail, and mechanistically different. Ring-down arises from a **trapped fluid or gas configuration** — classically a small collection of gas bubbles with fluid trapped between them — which is set into continuous resonant oscillation by the incident pulse and emits a sustained signal back to the transducer.

Because emission is sustained rather than a sequence of discrete echoes, the appearance is a **continuous, uninterrupted, non-tapering band** extending deep into the far field, uniform in width.

The practical discrimination:

	Comet tail	Ring-down
Mechanism	Reverberation between closely spaced reflectors	Resonance of trapped fluid/gas
Appearance	Discrete bands, tapering, terminates	Continuous solid band, non-tapering, extends far
Typical source	Cholesterol crystals, clips, metal	Gas collections, bowel, abscess gas

Distinguishing them is clinically consequential: comet-tail artifact within a thickened gallbladder wall supports adenomyomatosis, a benign entity, while ring-down from gas in the wall raises emphysematous cholecystitis, a surgical emergency.

Mirror image

A strong, large, curved specular reflector — the diaphragm above all — acts as an acoustic mirror. The pulse travels to a structure, reflects to the diaphragm, reflects again, returns to the structure, and only then returns to the transducer. Timing the longer path, the machine places a duplicate of the structure **deep to the reflector, at a distance equal to the true structure's distance in front of it.**

The classic appearance is apparent liver tissue and hepatic lesions "above" the diaphragm, in the thorax. Recognizing it prevents a diagnosis of a pulmonary or subpulmonic lesion. The mirrored copy is always deeper than the reflector, at equal perpendicular distance, and generally somewhat less echogenic.

Mirror artifact also occurs in Doppler, producing a symmetrical spectral trace above and below the baseline where flow is unidirectional — usually from excessive Doppler gain or a near-perpendicular angle. Reducing gain and improving angle resolves it.

Resolving maneuvers for all mirror artifact: change the angle of incidence on the reflector, or use a different acoustic window. A structure that changes position or disappears with a different approach was never there.

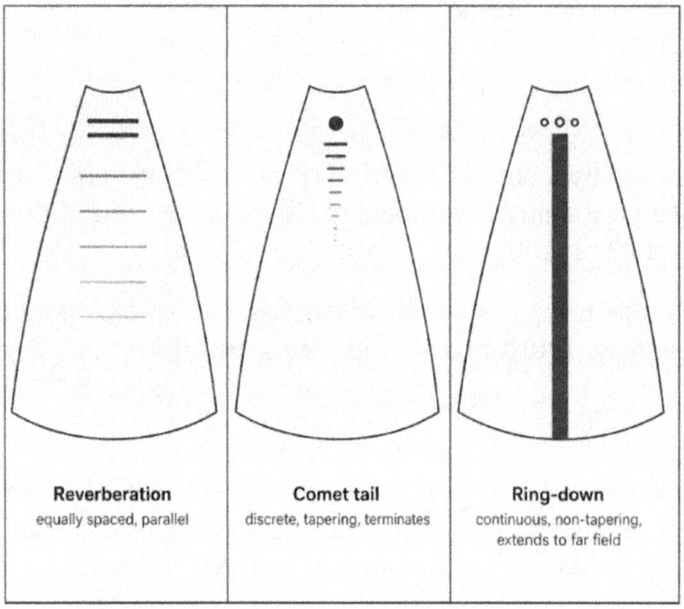

Mirror image artifact

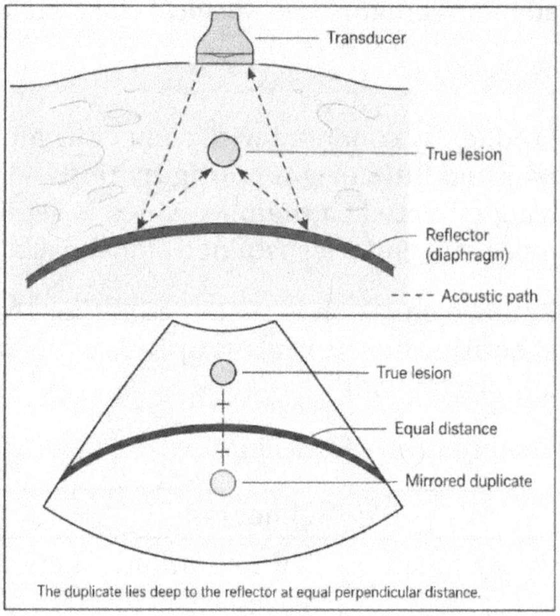

2.9 Doppler Artifacts: Aliasing, Twinkling, Blooming, Flash

Aliasing

Pulsed Doppler samples flow intermittently, and any sampled system can only unambiguously represent frequencies below half its sampling rate. The **Nyquist limit** is therefore **PRF / 2**. A Doppler shift exceeding it is misrepresented — displayed as flow in the opposite direction.

On **spectral** display, the peaks of the waveform are cut off and reappear ("wrap around") below the baseline. On **color** display, the center of a high-velocity jet shows the opposite color, producing a mosaic or a color reversal in mid-vessel that does not correspond to any anatomic boundary.

Aliasing must be distinguished from genuine flow reversal. In aliasing, the color transition passes through the *lightest* shades of both colors — because the represented velocity has wrapped through the maximum — whereas true flow reversal at a boundary passes through **black**, the zero-velocity color, since flow must decelerate through zero to reverse. This is a reliable discriminator and worth internalizing.

Aliasing is not always a nuisance. Persistent focal aliasing is a useful flag for a high-velocity jet, and is used deliberately to locate stenoses and to find small vessels.

The correction ladder, in order of preference:

1. **Increase the scale (PRF).** The direct fix, limited by depth — deep structures cannot support high PRF because of the round-trip time.

2. **Shift the baseline** toward the direction of flow, allocating more of the display range to it. Costs nothing.
3. **Increase the insonation angle** toward 90°, reducing the shift. Use with caution: it degrades velocity accuracy and invalidates quantitative measurement above 60°.
4. **Select a lower transmit frequency**, which reduces the shift for the same velocity.
5. **Switch to continuous-wave Doppler**, which has no Nyquist limit. The definitive solution where high velocities must be quantified, at the cost of range resolution.

Twinkling

A rapidly alternating mosaic of color, often with an associated disorganized spectral signal, appearing **behind a strongly reflective granular or crystalline surface** — most characteristically a calculus. The mechanism relates to intrinsic machine noise and phase jitter in the returning signal from a rough interface, not to genuine motion.

Twinkling is a **valuable positive finding**, not a nuisance. It identifies stones that are small, poorly shadowing, or in a location where shadowing is ambiguous, and it is used routinely in renal and ureteric assessment. Its sensitivity depends strongly on machine settings — it is favored by higher color write priority and appropriate PRF, and can be lost or created by changing them. Know your machine's behavior before relying on presence or absence.

Blooming (color bleed)

Color signal extending beyond the true vessel lumen into surrounding tissue. Caused by excessive color gain, excessive color write priority, or high signal intensity following contrast administration. It obscures the true lumen boundary and can conceal wall thrombus or plaque.

Correction: reduce color gain until color just fills the lumen without spilling, and check the lumen boundary on B-mode.

Flash artifact

A sudden burst of color filling a large region, produced by motion of the tissue or transducer rather than blood flow — respiration, cardiac transmission, bowel peristalsis, patient movement, or operator hand movement.

Correction: raise the wall filter, reduce color gain, hold the probe still, and scan during suspended respiration. Power Doppler, being more motion-sensitive, is more susceptible.

Other Doppler artifacts

Spectral broadening — a filled-in spectral window, indicating a wide range of velocities within the sample volume. Genuinely present in turbulent post-stenotic flow, and *artifactually* produced by an oversized sample volume, excessive Doppler gain, or a sample volume placed near the vessel wall. Distinguishing real from artifactual broadening requires checking those settings before calling turbulence.

Doppler mirror image — symmetrical spectral display above and below the baseline with unidirectional flow, from excessive gain or near-perpendicular angle.

Directional ambiguity at 90° insonation, where the trace appears symmetrically bidirectional because the shift is at the boundary between the two directions.

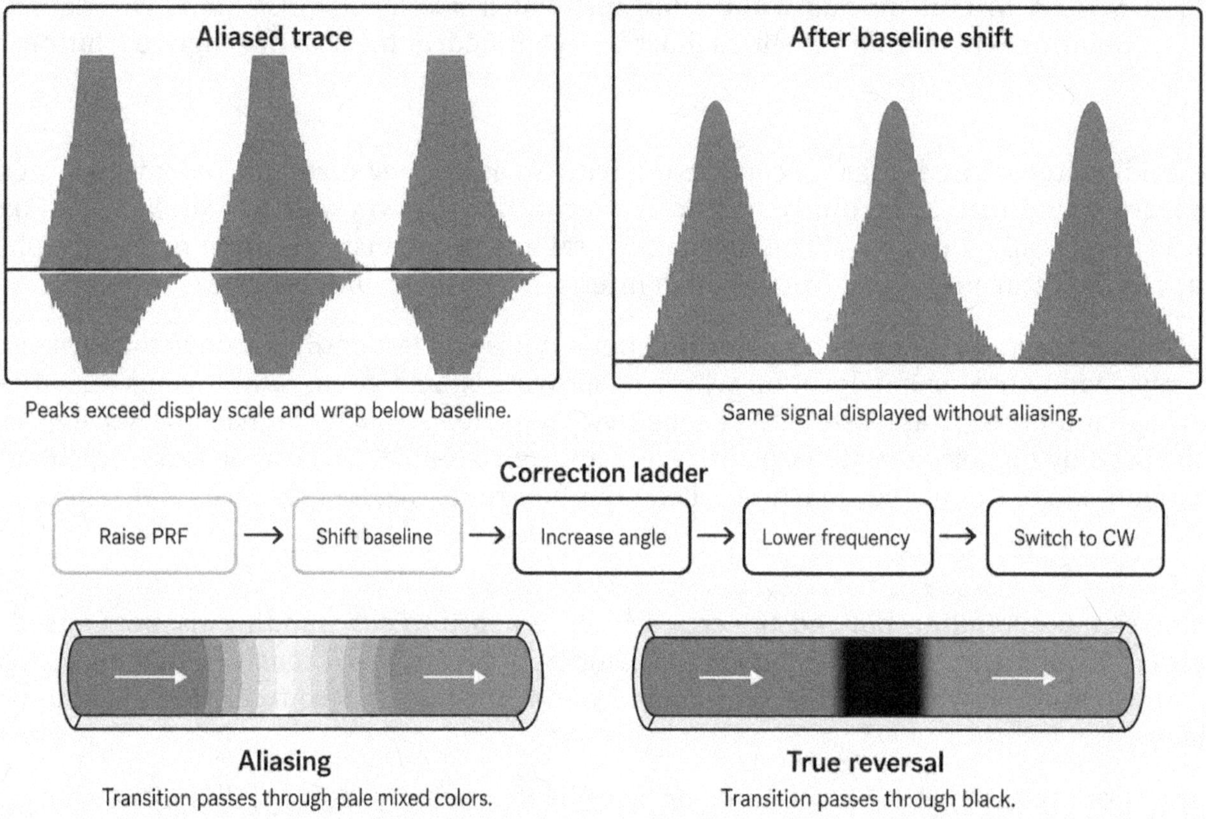

Aliasing, its correction ladder, and the discriminator from true flow reversal.

2.10 Elastography and Quantitative Ultrasound

Why stiffness

Palpation has been a diagnostic method for as long as medicine has existed, and it works because pathology changes tissue mechanical properties — fibrosis, desmoplastic tumor stroma, and inflammation all alter stiffness, often before they alter B-mode appearance. Elastography measures what the examining hand has always been reaching for, quantitatively and at depth.

Strain elastography

Method. Tissue is compressed — by light rhythmic transducer pressure, or by intrinsic physiological motion such as cardiac pulsation — and the system tracks tissue displacement, computing relative strain. Stiff tissue deforms less than soft tissue under the same stress.

Output. A color-coded map overlaid on B-mode showing relative stiffness. Because the applied stress is unknown, the output is **qualitative or semi-quantitative**: it tells you a lesion is stiffer than surrounding tissue, not how stiff it is in absolute units. A **strain ratio** comparing lesion to a reference region provides semi-quantitative comparison.

Limitations. Highly operator-dependent — the result varies with the compression applied. Not comparable between operators, machines, or time points in any rigorous way. Depth-limited, since applied stress attenuates.

Shear-wave elastography

Method. A focused acoustic radiation force "push" pulse displaces tissue at a target location, generating transverse shear waves propagating perpendicular to the beam. The system measures shear wave propagation **speed**, which is directly related to tissue stiffness.

Output. Quantitative, in metres per second or, converted through Young's modulus, in kilopascals. Displayed as a numeric value with a quality or reliability metric, and optionally as a two-dimensional stiffness map.

Advantages. Operator-independent applied stress, quantitative, reproducible, and therefore usable for longitudinal monitoring and for comparison against published thresholds.

Applications. Liver fibrosis staging — the dominant clinical use, now embedded in hepatology pathways as an alternative to biopsy in many contexts; thyroid and breast nodule characterization as an adjunct to B-mode features; and a growing range of applications in kidney, spleen, prostate, and musculoskeletal tissue.

The confounders — and why they matter more than the number

A stiffness value obtained under invalid conditions is not a less accurate number; it is a meaningless one, and it will be acted upon as though it were valid. For liver stiffness specifically, the following invalidate or distort measurement:

- **Non-fasting state.** Postprandial hepatic blood flow raises measured stiffness. Fasting is required. [VERIFY: current recommended fasting interval before liver stiffness measurement]
- **Hepatic inflammation.** Elevated transaminases raise stiffness independent of fibrosis, and can push a non-fibrotic liver into a range suggesting advanced disease.
- **Hepatic congestion.** Right heart failure raises stiffness substantially. A stiff liver in decompensated cardiac failure is a congested liver, not necessarily a fibrotic one.
- **Cholestasis** and extrahepatic biliary obstruction raise stiffness.
- **Ascites.** Shear waves do not propagate through fluid. Measurement through ascites fails or produces invalid results.
- **Obesity and deep measurement depth** degrade reliability.
- **Measurement location.** Too close to the capsule, across a large vessel, or through a rib shadow produces invalid values. Measurements are taken at a specified depth

below the capsule in a homogeneous region free of large vessels, typically through an intercostal approach with the patient in a defined position and breath-hold state.

- **Vendor differences.** Thresholds are not interchangeable between manufacturers or between shear-wave and transient elastography systems.

Thresholds for fibrosis staging vary by etiology, by technique, and by vendor, and must be taken from the current guideline applicable to the specific system and disease being assessed. [VERIFY: current society guidance on liver stiffness thresholds by etiology and platform — do not publish generic kPa cut-offs]

Report stiffness with the technique, the platform, the number of acquisitions, the reliability metric, and the conditions under which it was obtained. A bare number is not a result.

Attenuation-based quantification

A newer family of tools estimates the **ultrasound attenuation coefficient**, which correlates with hepatic fat content, offering a quantitative alternative to the subjective B-mode grading of steatosis discussed in Chapter 4. Vendor implementations differ in name and in output units, and thresholds are platform-specific. Treat them as promising and platform-bound rather than as interchangeable measurements. [VERIFY: current evidence and thresholds for ultrasound attenuation-based hepatic steatosis quantification]

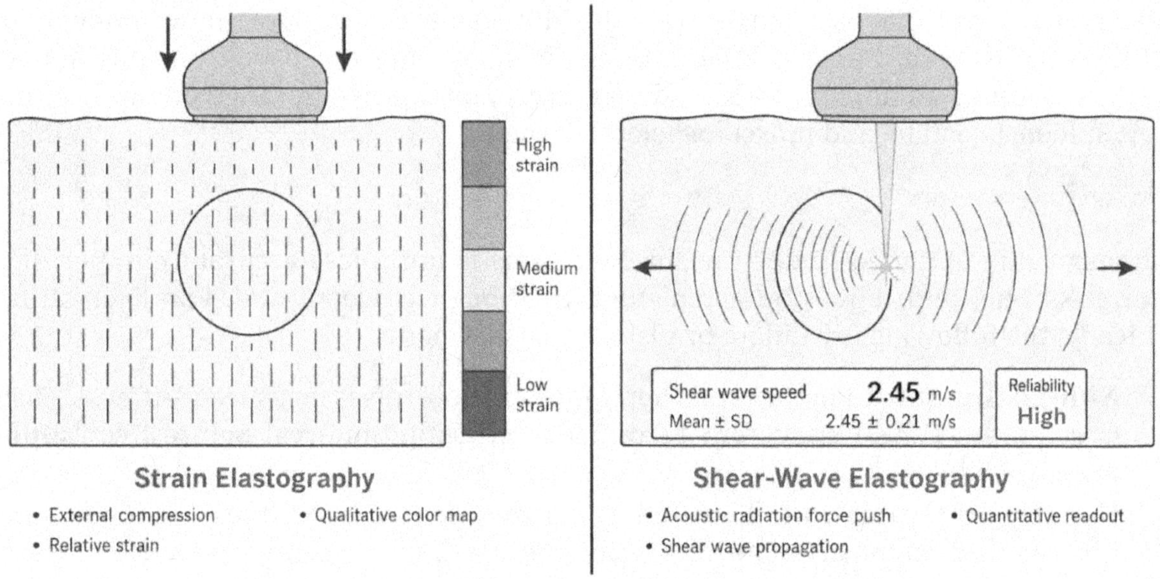

Elastography Techniques

Strain elastography measures relative deformation; shear-wave elastography measures propagation speed.

Key Points

1. Every artifact is a violated assumption. Ask which of the five failed, and you have both the diagnosis and the resolving maneuver.
2. Higher frequency buys resolution and costs penetration. This trade-off is not escapable by any control or processing algorithm.

3. Specular reflectors are angle-dependent and vanish when insonated obliquely; scatterers are not. When a known structure disappears, change your angle before you change your gain.
4. Axial resolution is set by pulse length and is constant with depth; lateral resolution is set by beam width and is best at the focus. Move the focal marker to the structure you are assessing.
5. Elevational slice thickness is the resolution operators forget, and it is the mechanism of pseudo-sludge and false cyst contents. Rescan orthogonally.
6. Exhaust receive controls before touching transmit power — gain costs the patient nothing, output does not.
7. Harmonic imaging suppresses near-field clutter and side lobes, but also suppresses genuine low-level echoes. Check a possibly complex cyst on fundamental too.
8. Spatial compounding suppresses shadowing and enhancement. Turn it off before concluding that a stone does not shadow or a lesion does not enhance.
9. Flow perpendicular to the beam produces no Doppler shift. Absent color at 90° is geometry, not occlusion.
10. Keep the insonation angle at or below 60° for any velocity you intend to report, and archive the image with the angle cursor visible.
11. Aliasing transitions through the palest shades of both colors; true flow reversal transitions through black.
12. Comet tail is discrete and tapering; ring-down is continuous and non-tapering. Gallbladder wall: the first suggests adenomyomatosis, the second suggests gas.
13. Twinkling is a positive finding for calculus, not a nuisance — but its presence depends on machine settings.
14. A shear-wave stiffness value obtained non-fasting, through ascites, in a congested or inflamed liver, or at the wrong depth is not an approximate result. It is an invalid one.

Registry Check

1. A 6 mm echogenic focus in the gallbladder shows no posterior shadowing. Before concluding that it does not shadow, the operator should first:

A. Increase overall gain **B.** Disable spatial compounding **C.** Switch to power Doppler **D.** Increase the dynamic range

> **Answer: B.** Spatial compounding insonates from multiple angles and fills in acoustic shadows, frequently abolishing the shadow behind a genuine stone. Increasing gain would further obscure a subtle shadow, and widening dynamic range reduces contrast.

2. A patent internal carotid artery demonstrates no color filling on a transverse image. The most likely explanation is:

A. Complete occlusion **B.** Insufficient color gain **C.** Insonation at approximately 90° to flow **D.** Wall filter set too low

Answer: C. The Doppler shift is proportional to cos θ, and cos 90° equals zero, so flow perpendicular to the beam produces no detectable shift regardless of gain. A transverse image insonates a longitudinally running vessel at close to 90°. The correction is geometric — heel-toe, steer, or image longitudinally.

3. Equally spaced parallel bright lines extending into the far field from a superficial interface represent:

A. Comet tail artifact **B.** Ring-down artifact **C.** Reverberation artifact **D.** Side lobe artifact

Answer: C. Equal spacing is the signature of reverberation, the interval corresponding to the separation of the two reflectors. Comet tail tapers and terminates; ring-down is continuous and non-segmented; side lobe echoes appear as curved arcs.

4. A structure appearing above the diaphragm, identical to a lesion below it and at equal perpendicular distance, is explained by violation of which assumption?

A. Sound travels at 1,540 m/s **B.** Each pulse produces a single round trip **C.** Attenuation is uniform **D.** Echoes arise only from the beam axis

Answer: B. Mirror artifact results from a multiple-bounce path off a strong curved specular reflector. The longer transit time places the duplicate deeper than the reflector at a distance equal to the true structure's distance in front of it.

5. Aliasing on a spectral Doppler trace is best addressed first by:

A. Increasing Doppler gain **B.** Increasing the pulse repetition frequency **C.** Reducing the sample volume size **D.** Increasing the insonation angle beyond 60°

Answer: B. Aliasing occurs when the Doppler shift exceeds the Nyquist limit of PRF/2, so raising the PRF is the direct correction. Baseline shift is the next step. Increasing the angle beyond 60° does reduce the shift but degrades velocity accuracy unacceptably, and gain and sample volume do not affect the Nyquist limit.

6. Low-level echoes within the dependent portion of the gallbladder that disappear when the patient is rescanned in an orthogonal plane most likely represent:

A. Biliary sludge **B.** Section thickness artifact **C.** Ring-down artifact **D.** Hemobilia

Answer: B. Elevational slice thickness superimposes echoes from adjacent tissue onto a narrow anechoic structure, producing pseudo-sludge. Genuine sludge persists across planes, layers dependently, and moves with position change.

7. A liver stiffness value of markedly elevated magnitude is obtained in a patient with decompensated right heart failure and normal transaminases. The most appropriate interpretation is:

A. Advanced fibrosis is confirmed **B.** The measurement is unreliable because inflammation is absent **C.** Hepatic congestion raises stiffness independent of fibrosis, and the value cannot be interpreted as a fibrosis stage **D.** The value should be converted from kPa to m/s before interpretation

> **Answer: C.** Congestion is a well-recognized confounder that elevates liver stiffness independent of fibrosis. Other confounders include the non-fasting state, inflammation, cholestasis, and ascites. Unit conversion does not address the validity problem.

8. Tissue harmonic imaging improves image quality principally because:

A. Harmonic frequencies penetrate more deeply than the fundamental **B.** Harmonics are generated within tissue, so near-field clutter and off-axis lobe artifact are excluded **C.** It increases frame rate **D.** It widens the dynamic range of the display

> **Answer: B.** Harmonic energy builds progressively within tissue rather than originating at the transducer face, and weak off-axis energy generates negligible harmonic signal. Penetration is reduced rather than improved, and frame rate may fall with multi-pulse implementations.

Chapter Notes for the Editorial Pass

Verification queue. [VERIFY] tags cluster in §2.10 — fasting interval before liver stiffness measurement, fibrosis thresholds by etiology and platform, and attenuation-based steatosis quantification. Do not publish generic kPa cut-offs; these are etiology- and vendor-specific and a generic figure printed in a handbook will be applied wrongly. The attenuation coefficient figure of approximately 0.5 dB/cm/MHz in §2.1 is a conventional working value and should be presented as such rather than as a precise constant.

Figure count: 14 Lane A, 2 Lane B (`fig-2-9` compounding paired images; `fig-2-13` twinkling). The two Lane B slots are the chapter's acquisition dependency and both require paired acquisitions on the same machine — these are difficult to source from open archives and are strong candidates for the author's own de-identified captures.

Cross-reference targets to fix at layout: §2.1 resolution → Chapter 3 vascular technique; §2.4 compounding → Chapter 5 cholelithiasis; §2.5 waveform morphology → Chapter 16; §2.7 dirty shadowing → Chapter 5 emphysematous cholecystitis; §2.9 twinkling → Chapter 7 nephrolithiasis; §2.10 elastography → Chapter 4 diffuse liver disease.

Word count: approximately 10,300 excluding image prompt blocks, learning objectives, registry questions, and these notes.

Chapter 3 Sectional Anatomy and the Vascular System

Learning Objectives

On completing this chapter you should be able to:

1. Assign any abdominal organ to its peritoneal or retroperitoneal compartment and predict where fluid arising from it will collect.
2. Name the dependent recesses of the peritoneal cavity and state which is most dependent in a given patient position.
3. Correlate a sonographic image with the corresponding CT or MR section, and explain where the orientation conventions of the three modalities agree and where they do not.
4. Select the acoustic window and patient position that will open a given structure, and explain the anatomic reason each one works.
5. Identify the aorta and its major branches by their sonographic landmarks, and use the vascular landmarks to locate non-vascular structures.
6. Trace the inferior vena cava and its tributaries, and recognize the normal anatomic relationships that generate compression syndromes.
7. Distinguish portal from hepatic veins by wall character and drainage direction, and describe normal portal hemodynamics.
8. Recognize the normal Doppler waveform signature of each major abdominal vascular bed and explain what determines it.
9. Measure an abdominal aortic aneurysm correctly and distinguish mural thrombus from dissection and from a periaortic process.

Why the Vessels Come First

Sonographic navigation of the abdomen is vascular navigation. The organs are variable in position, size, and appearance; they move with respiration and posture; and several of them look alike. The great vessels are constant. They run in predictable planes, they are anechoic and therefore instantly recognizable, and they carry named branches that arise at fixed levels.

Everything you will do in Chapters 4 through 9 depends on this. You do not find the pancreas by looking for the pancreas — you find the splenic vein and the superior mesenteric artery, and the pancreas is the tissue between and around them. You do not find the adrenal by searching the upper pole; you find the IVC and the crus and look in the space between. You do not identify a mass as retroperitoneal by its appearance, but by whether it displaces the aorta and IVC anteriorly or is displaced by them.

This chapter therefore treats sectional anatomy and vascular anatomy as one subject, because in practice they are.

3.1 Anatomic and Physiologic Relationships of the Abdominopelvic Cavity

The two compartments

The peritoneum is a continuous serous membrane. Its parietal layer lines the abdominal wall; its visceral layer invests the organs. The potential space between them is the peritoneal cavity, normally containing only a trace of lubricating fluid.

Organs are classified by their relationship to this membrane, and the classification is not academic — it determines where a disease process spreads, where fluid collects, and how you will approach the structure.

Intraperitoneal — invested by peritoneum and suspended by a mesentery or ligament: liver, gallbladder, spleen, stomach, first part of the duodenum, jejunum, ileum, appendix, transverse colon, sigmoid colon, and the tail of the pancreas within the splenorenal ligament.

Retroperitoneal — lying behind the peritoneum, covered on the anterior surface only: kidneys, ureters, adrenal glands, aorta, inferior vena cava, the pancreas apart from its tail, the second through fourth parts of the duodenum, the ascending and descending colon, and the upper rectum.

The retroperitoneal position of the pancreas is the reason it is technically difficult and the reason pancreatitis produces the fluid distributions it does. The retroperitoneal position of the aorta and IVC is the reason a mass that lifts them forward is retroperitoneal and one they compress from in front is not.

The retroperitoneal spaces

The retroperitoneum is divided by the renal fascia into three compartments, and knowing them lets you localize a collection by its shape and boundaries rather than by guesswork.

Anterior pararenal space — between the posterior parietal peritoneum and the anterior renal fascia. Contains the pancreas, the retroperitoneal duodenum, and the ascending and descending colon. This is where pancreatitis collections begin, and it communicates across the midline, which is why pancreatic fluid tracks bilaterally.

Perirenal space — enclosed by the anterior and posterior layers of the renal fascia (Gerota's fascia). Contains the kidney, adrenal, and perinephric fat. It is cone-shaped and relatively confined, which is why a perinephric collection has a characteristic conforming shape.

Posterior pararenal space — between the posterior renal fascia and the transversalis fascia. Contains only fat and vessels. It communicates with the properitoneal fat of the flank, and blood here tracks laterally.

The peritoneal recesses — where fluid goes

Free intraperitoneal fluid obeys gravity and the anatomy of the recesses. The clinically important collections, and their significance:

Morison's pouch (hepatorenal recess) — between the right lobe of the liver and the right kidney. **The most dependent portion of the upper abdomen in the supine patient**, and consequently the highest-yield single view in trauma assessment. Fluid from anywhere in the upper abdomen collects here first.

Subphrenic spaces — right and left, beneath the diaphragm above the liver and spleen. The right subphrenic space communicates with Morison's pouch.

Lesser sac (omental bursa) — behind the stomach and in front of the pancreas, communicating with the greater sac only through the narrow epiploic foramen. Because that communication is restricted, fluid here is usually locally generated — pancreatitis, gastric or duodenal perforation — rather than tracked in from elsewhere. A collection confined to the lesser sac is a meaningful localizing finding.

Paracolic gutters — lateral to the ascending and descending colon, providing the vertical channel along which fluid travels between the upper abdomen and the pelvis. The right gutter is the deeper and more continuous of the two.

Pelvic recesses — the rectouterine pouch (pouch of Douglas) in women, the rectovesical pouch in men. **The most dependent portion of the entire peritoneal cavity in the upright or semi-upright patient**, and the site where small volumes of free fluid accumulate first.

The practical rule: **fluid in the upper abdomen collects in Morison's pouch; fluid overall collects in the pelvis.** Both are searched in any assessment for free fluid, and the pelvis requires an adequately filled bladder or a transvaginal approach to be assessed properly.

Physiologic relationships that matter at the machine

Respiration. The diaphragm descends on inspiration, displacing the liver, spleen, and kidneys caudally by several centimetres. This is exploited constantly: deep inspiration brings the liver below the costal margin and the right kidney into view; it also pushes the pancreas away from a subcostal approach, which is why some pancreatic imaging is better in suspended expiration. Learn to direct respiration deliberately rather than reflexively asking for a deep breath.

Gastric and bowel content. Gas rises. In the supine patient, gas accumulates in the antrum and transverse colon, directly over the pancreas — hence the value of fasting, of graded compression, of the left lateral decubitus position, and of a water-filled stomach as an acoustic window.

Vascular pulsation and transmitted motion are used diagnostically: a structure that pulsates with the aorta may be adherent to it, and transmitted pulsation distinguishes a mass abutting the aorta from one arising within its wall.

Bladder filling provides a pelvic acoustic window and displaces bowel superiorly, at the cost of distorting pelvic anatomy when overfilled.

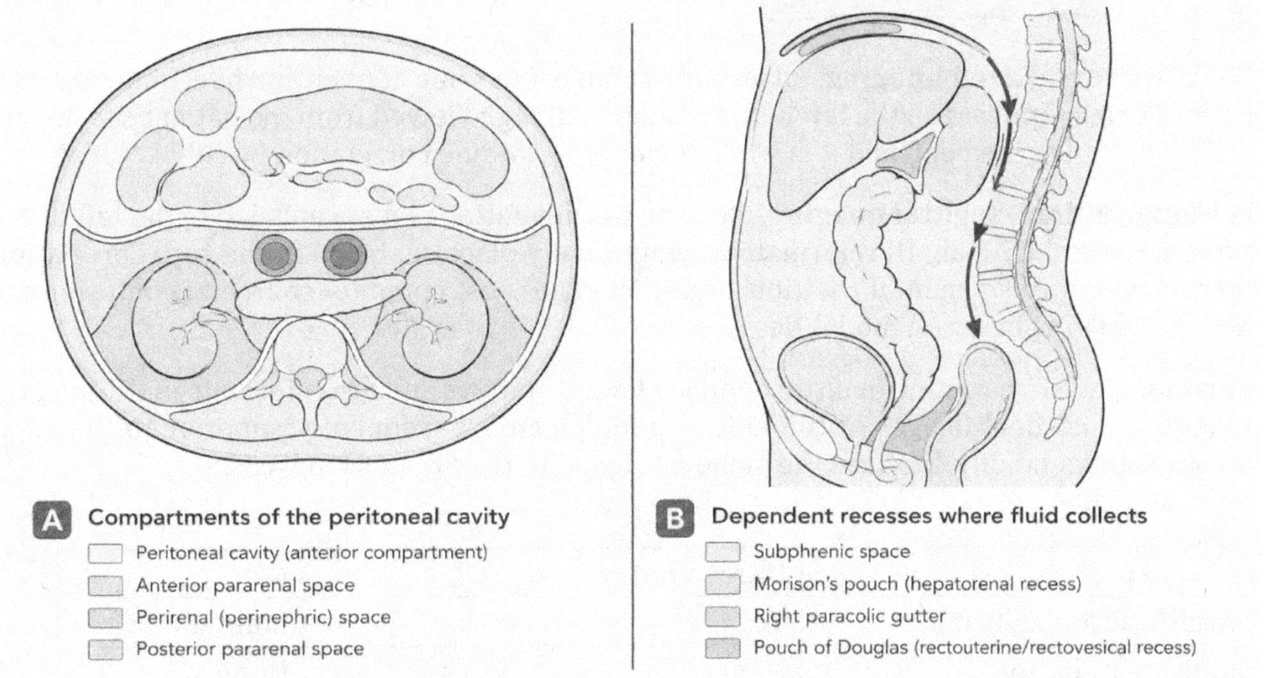

3.2 Comparative Sectional Anatomy: Ultrasound, CT, and MRI

Why the correlation is a working skill

You will constantly be asked to find something a CT reported, to explain why your images do not show what a CT showed, or to target a biopsy to a lesion described in cross-sectional terms. Reading CT and MR sections fluently is therefore part of the job, not an adjacent specialty.

The differences that matter to you are these.

Field of view. CT and MR display the entire cross-section at a fixed anatomic level. Ultrasound displays a narrow sector in an operator-chosen, frequently oblique plane. A CT axial section at the level of the renal hila shows the aorta, IVC, both kidneys, pancreas, and duodenum simultaneously. No single ultrasound image does. This is why correlating requires you to reconstruct the CT's whole-section view from several ultrasound images, and why your labeling convention (§2.6) has to be exact.

Plane discipline. CT sections are true axial, orthogonal to the scanner axis. Your "transverse" is frequently an oblique angled subcostally, and your "longitudinal" of an organ is aligned to that organ rather than to the body. A pancreas imaged in the standard oblique transverse is not in a plane CT ever produces.

Contrast mechanism. Ultrasound displays acoustic impedance and scattering; CT displays X-ray attenuation; MR displays proton density and relaxation behavior. Structures that are conspicuous in one may be invisible in another. Calcium is conspicuous on both CT and ultrasound. Bowel gas ruins ultrasound and is unremarkable on CT. Fluid-fluid levels, septations, and low-level internal echoes are often better shown by ultrasound than by CT.

The orientation convention — where the modalities agree

For **transverse/axial imaging**, ultrasound follows the same convention as CT and MR: the patient's right appears on the **left** of the image, as though viewed from the patient's feet. This is the point of agreement, and it is what makes side-by-side correlation possible.

For **longitudinal/sagittal imaging**, ultrasound convention places cephalad to the **left** of the screen. Sagittal CT and MR reformats conventionally place cephalad at the **top**. Correlation therefore requires a mental rotation, and this is the most common source of confusion for trainees moving between modalities.

Coronal views are routine in ultrasound via flank windows and are reformats in CT and MR. Ultrasound coronal images of the kidney and spleen are frequently superior to the axial views of any modality, because the plane is aligned to the organ's long axis.

Choosing between them

	Ultrasound	CT	MR
Real-time and dynamic	Yes	No	Limited
Ionizing radiation	None	Yes	None
Gas and bone	Blocked	Unaffected	Unaffected
Body habitus	Degrades markedly	Minor effect	Moderate effect
Soft tissue contrast	Moderate	Moderate	Highest
Vascular flow without contrast	Yes (Doppler)	No	Yes
Portability	Yes	No	No
Operator dependence	High	Low	Low

Ultrasound's decisive advantages are the ones no reformat can replicate: real-time observation, dynamic maneuvers, direct correlation of imaging with point tenderness, and flow assessment without contrast. Its decisive weaknesses are gas, bone, depth, and operator dependence.

The report language that follows from this is covered in Chapter 1 §1.5: state the limitation specifically, so the next modality is chosen for a reason.

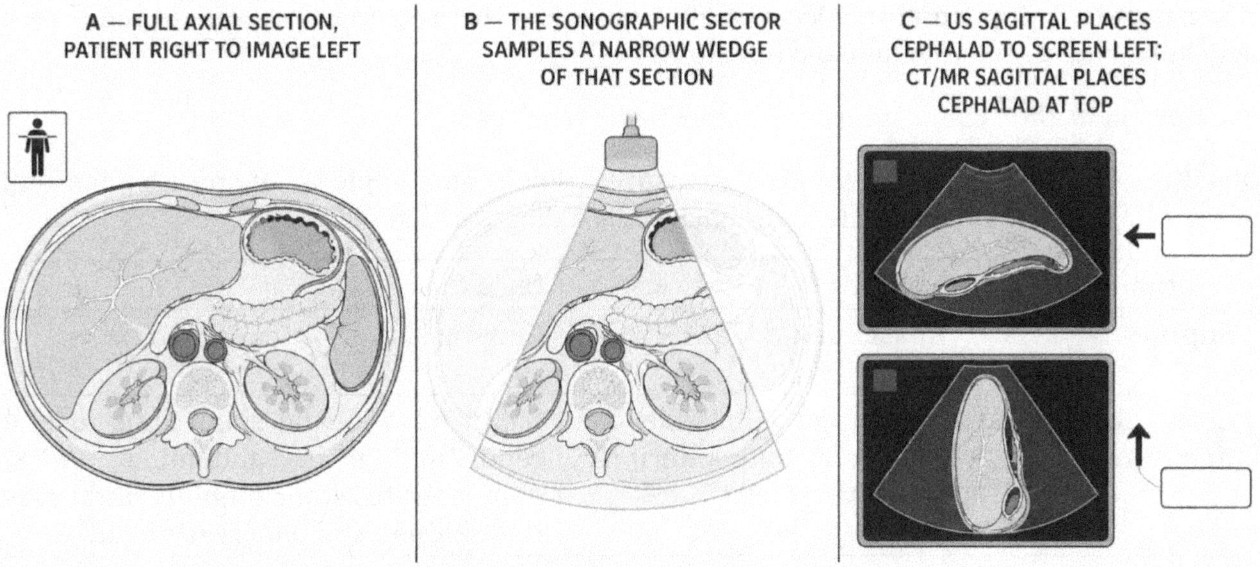

3.3 Body Planes, Acoustic Windows, and Patient Positioning

The windows

An acoustic window is a path to the target that avoids gas and bone. Learning the windows is learning the abdomen's accessible geometry.

Subxiphoid / epigastric. Through the left lobe of the liver, which acts as an acoustic window to the structures behind it — aorta, celiac axis, SMA, pancreas, portal confluence. The single most productive window in the abdomen, and dependent on the left lobe being interposed. Where the left lobe is small, this window is poor and the pancreas becomes very difficult.

Right subcostal. Angled cephalad beneath the costal margin during deep inspiration. Opens the liver dome, hepatic veins and their confluence with the IVC, and the gallbladder.

Right and left intercostal. Through the intercostal spaces, using the liver or spleen as a window. Essential for the liver dome and for the spleen, which sits high and posterior behind ribs. The transducer must be aligned along the intercostal space to avoid rib shadowing — a small rotation is often the difference between a useless image and a good one. Phased or small-footprint probes fit these spaces best.

Right and left flank (coronal). Through the liver or spleen to the kidney. The best window for renal length and for the spleen. The left flank is harder because the spleen is a smaller window than the liver and the stomach and splenic flexure interfere.

Suprapubic. Through a filled bladder to the pelvic organs, displacing bowel superiorly.

Transvaginal / transrectal. Direct high-frequency proximity, bypassing the abdominal wall and bowel entirely.

Translumbar / posterior. Occasionally used for the retroperitoneum and for renal transplant assessment in unusual positions.

Positions and what each one achieves

Position changes are not comfort measures. Each one exploits a specific anatomic consequence, and knowing which to reach for is a diagnostic skill:

Position	Effect	Used for
Supine	Baseline; gas rises anteriorly	General survey
Left lateral decubitus	Liver and gallbladder fall medially and anteriorly; gas moves left	Gallbladder — the single most useful repositioning in abdominal work; demonstrates stone mobility; improves right kidney and pancreatic head
Right lateral decubitus	Spleen falls medially; gas moves right	Spleen, left kidney, pancreatic tail
Erect / semi-erect	Organs descend; fluid moves to the pelvis; gallbladder stones settle to the fundus	Confirming stone mobility, demonstrating small volumes of pelvic fluid, hernia assessment
Prone	Direct posterior renal access	Renal biopsy guidance, difficult renal windows, some pediatric spine imaging
Reverse Trendelenburg / standing	Increases venous filling in the legs	Venous reflux studies (Chapter 16)
Trendelenburg	Distends upper-body veins	Central venous access, jugular assessment
Left lateral tilt in pregnancy	Relieves aortocaval compression	Any supine obstetric examination of significant duration

The last is a safety point rather than a technical one: prolonged supine positioning in advanced pregnancy allows the gravid uterus to compress the IVC and reduce venous return. Tilt the patient or wedge the right hip.

Optimizing the window

Beyond position, four maneuvers open windows:

Respiratory control. Deep inspiration for the liver, kidneys, and diaphragm; suspended expiration for some pancreatic and epigastric work; quiet breathing for uncooperative patients and for structures degraded by motion.

Graded compression. Steady, progressively increasing pressure displaces bowel gas and reduces the distance to the target. It is the foundation of appendiceal and bowel imaging (Chapter 6), and it is applied gradually — abrupt pressure causes guarding, which defeats it.

Filling the stomach with water creates an acoustic window to the pancreas and the gastric wall. Underused, and highly effective where the standard epigastric window fails.

Probe rotation into the intercostal plane — as above, and worth restating because rib shadowing is so often accepted as unavoidable when a few degrees of rotation would resolve it.

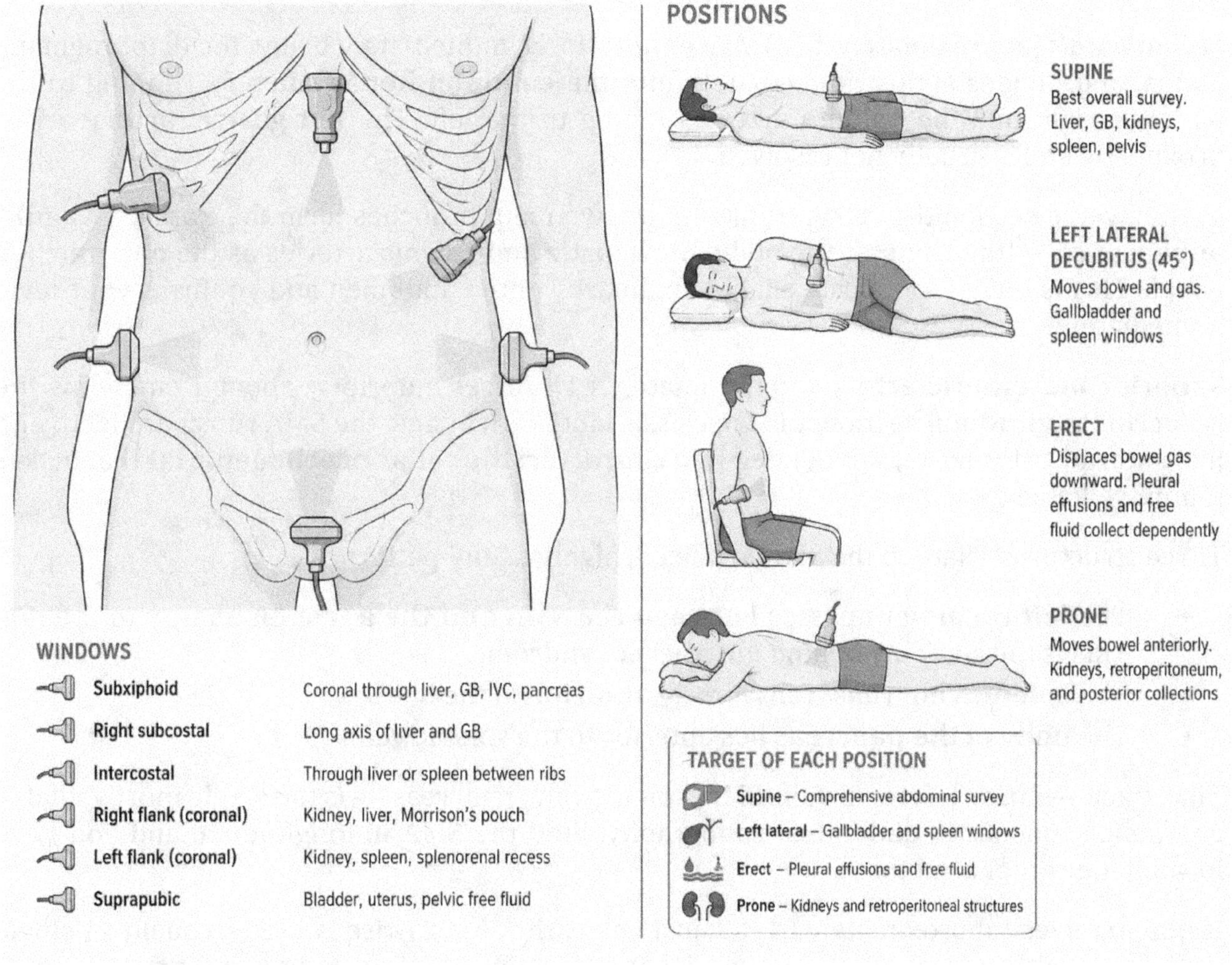

3.4 The Aorta and Its Major Branches

Course and normal appearance

The abdominal aorta enters through the diaphragmatic hiatus at approximately the level of T12 and descends slightly left of midline, anterior to the vertebral bodies, **tapering progressively** as it gives off branches. It bifurcates into the common iliac arteries at approximately L4 — roughly the level of the umbilicus, and a useful surface landmark.

Sonographically it is an anechoic tubular structure with **thick, bright, pulsatile walls**, lying to the left of the IVC and anterior to the vertebral bodies, whose bright anterior surfaces and posterior shadowing form a reliable posterior landmark. In longitudinal section it appears straight-walled and tapering; in transverse it is round and does not compress with probe pressure.

Normal diameter is under 3 cm, decreasing distally. Measure **outer wall to outer wall**, perpendicular to the vessel's long axis — the technique detail is developed in §3.8 because getting it wrong is the commonest error in aortic imaging.

The branches, in the order you meet them

Celiac trunk (approximately T12). Arises anteriorly, immediately below the diaphragmatic hiatus, and divides almost immediately into the **common hepatic artery** running to the patient's right and the **splenic artery** running to the left. The **left gastric artery** arises proximally and is usually not resolved.

In transverse section the celiac trunk and its two main branches form the classic **"seagull" appearance** — the trunk as the body, the hepatic and splenic arteries as the outstretched wings. This is one of the most reliable landmarks in the abdomen and confirms your level immediately.

Superior mesenteric artery (approximately L1). Arises anteriorly about 1 cm below the celiac. In **longitudinal** section it is the classic landmark image: the SMA runs parallel to and just anterior to the aorta, surrounded by a **characteristic collar of echogenic fat** that makes it unmistakable.

Three structures relate to the SMA in a fixed, highly useful pattern:

- The **left renal vein** passes **between the SMA and the aorta** on its way to the IVC. This is the anatomy behind nutcracker syndrome.
- The **splenic vein** runs transversely **anterior** to the SMA.
- The **body of the pancreas** lies anterior to the splenic vein.

That stack — aorta, left renal vein, SMA, splenic vein, pancreas — is the single most valuable anatomic sequence in abdominal sonography. Find the SMA in longitudinal and you have located four other structures.

Renal arteries (approximately L1–L2, just below the SMA). Arise laterally, usually as single vessels but with accessory arteries in a substantial minority. **The right renal artery passes posterior to the IVC**, a relationship visible in transverse section and important in transplant and stenosis assessment. Origin stenosis assessment requires interrogation at the origin, mid-vessel, and hilum.

Gonadal arteries arise anterolaterally below the renals and are not routinely resolved.

Inferior mesenteric artery (approximately L3). Arises anteriorly, small, and requires deliberate searching a few centimetres above the bifurcation, slightly to the left.

Lumbar arteries arise posteriorly and are not routinely imaged.

Bifurcation (approximately L4) into the common iliac arteries, which divide into internal and external iliacs at the pelvic brim.

Using the aorta as a navigation tool

Because the branch levels are fixed, the aorta is a ruler. Working from the diaphragm downward in longitudinal section, the first anterior branch is the celiac, the second is the SMA, and the vessel between them at the aortic anterior wall in transverse is the point from which the pancreas, portal confluence, and left renal vein can all be located.

Reverse the logic for pathology: a mass that **displaces the aorta anteriorly** arises behind it; a mass that **encases** it without displacing it suggests infiltrative retroperitoneal disease such as lymphoma or fibrosis; a mass that indents it from the front is anterior retroperitoneal or intraperitoneal.

Technical approach

Fasting improves the study substantially. Scan in the **epigastrium through the left lobe of the liver**, with graded compression to displace overlying gas. Use a curvilinear probe at the highest frequency that reaches, and expect to need the lower end of the range in larger patients.

Image the aorta in **both planes throughout its length**, from the diaphragm to the bifurcation and into the proximal common iliacs. Transverse for diameter, longitudinal for contour and to confirm you are measuring perpendicular. Where bowel gas defeats the epigastric approach, a **left lateral decubitus with a left coronal approach** through the flank frequently succeeds and is the standard rescue technique.

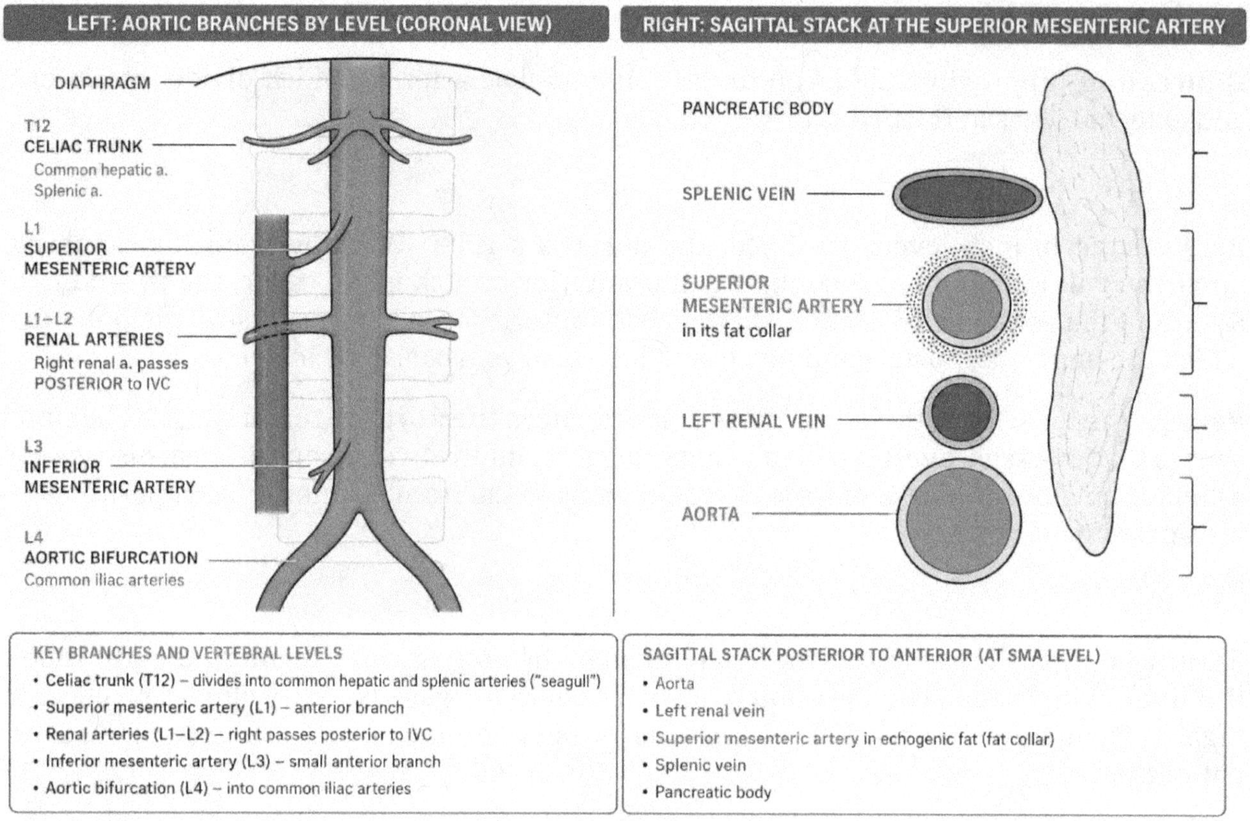

3.5 The Inferior Vena Cava and Tributaries

Course and normal appearance

The IVC is formed by the confluence of the common iliac veins at approximately L5 and ascends **to the right of the aorta**, anterior to the vertebral bodies, passing through the diaphragm at approximately T8 to enter the right atrium.

Sonographically it differs from the aorta in ways that make confusion avoidable:

	Aorta	IVC
Position	Left of midline	Right of midline
Walls	Thick, bright, distinctly echogenic	Thin, less conspicuous
Shape in transverse	Round	Oval, flattened anteroposteriorly
Compressibility	Non-compressible	Compresses readily with probe pressure
Calibre change	Tapers distally, fixed calibre otherwise	Varies with respiration and cardiac cycle
Course cephalad	Passes posterior to diaphragm	Curves anteriorly into the right atrium

	Aorta	IVC
Doppler	Pulsatile arterial	Phasic, variably pulsatile

The **anterior curve of the IVC as it approaches the diaphragm** is a definitive distinguishing feature in longitudinal section: the aorta continues straight posteriorly, the IVC hooks forward to the heart.

Tributaries

Common iliac veins — join at L5.

Renal veins. The **left renal vein is the long one**, crossing the midline **anterior to the aorta and posterior to the SMA** to reach the IVC. This anatomic sandwich is the basis of **nutcracker syndrome**, in which the left renal vein is compressed in that angle, producing left flank pain, haematuria, and in men a left varicocele. The **right renal vein is short** and enters directly.

Gonadal veins. Asymmetric drainage with real clinical consequence: the **right gonadal vein drains directly into the IVC**, while the **left gonadal vein drains into the left renal vein**. The longer, higher-pressure left pathway is why varicoceles are predominantly left-sided, and why a **new right-sided varicocele** raises concern for a retroperitoneal mass obstructing the right gonadal vein.

Hepatic veins. Right, middle, and left, converging on the IVC just below the diaphragm. The **caudate lobe drains separately by short direct veins into the IVC**, which is why the caudate hypertrophies and remains perfused in Budd-Chiari syndrome (Chapter 4).

Lumbar and phrenic veins are not routinely imaged but form important collateral pathways in IVC obstruction.

Assessment and the volume question

IVC calibre and its respiratory variation are widely used as a non-invasive surrogate for right atrial pressure and volume status, particularly in critical care and echocardiography.

The physiology: in spontaneous breathing, inspiration lowers intrathoracic pressure, increases venous return, and **collapses** the IVC. A small, highly collapsible IVC suggests low right atrial pressure; a dilated IVC with minimal respiratory variation suggests elevated right atrial pressure.

Measure in the **longitudinal plane, a defined short distance caudal to the hepatic vein confluence**, perpendicular to the vessel axis, recording maximum and minimum diameters across the respiratory cycle.

Interpret with real caution. The relationship is a correlation with wide scatter, not a measurement of pressure. It is confounded by mechanical ventilation — where the respiratory changes are **reversed**, since positive pressure inspiration increases intrathoracic pressure — by raised intra-abdominal pressure, by tricuspid disease, by pulmonary hypertension, and by athletic physiology in which a dilated IVC may be normal.

Report it as a finding with its conditions stated, not as a volume status. [VERIFY: current society thresholds for IVC diameter and collapsibility in right atrial pressure estimation]

IVC pathology in outline

Thrombus — bland thrombus from a propagating lower limb DVT, or extension from the iliac veins. Non-enhancing, no internal flow.

Tumour thrombus — direct intravascular extension of tumour, most characteristically **renal cell carcinoma extending via the renal vein into the IVC**, and hepatocellular carcinoma via the hepatic veins. The distinction from bland thrombus is important surgically and is made by demonstrating **internal arterial flow within the thrombus** on colour and spectral Doppler — bland thrombus has none. Assessing the cephalad extent, and whether it reaches the right atrium, changes the operation.

Extrinsic compression by retroperitoneal mass or lymphadenopathy.

Congenital variants — duplication, left-sided IVC, azygos continuation with interrupted IVC. Uncommon, but recognizing them prevents a normal variant being called a mass or a thrombosis.

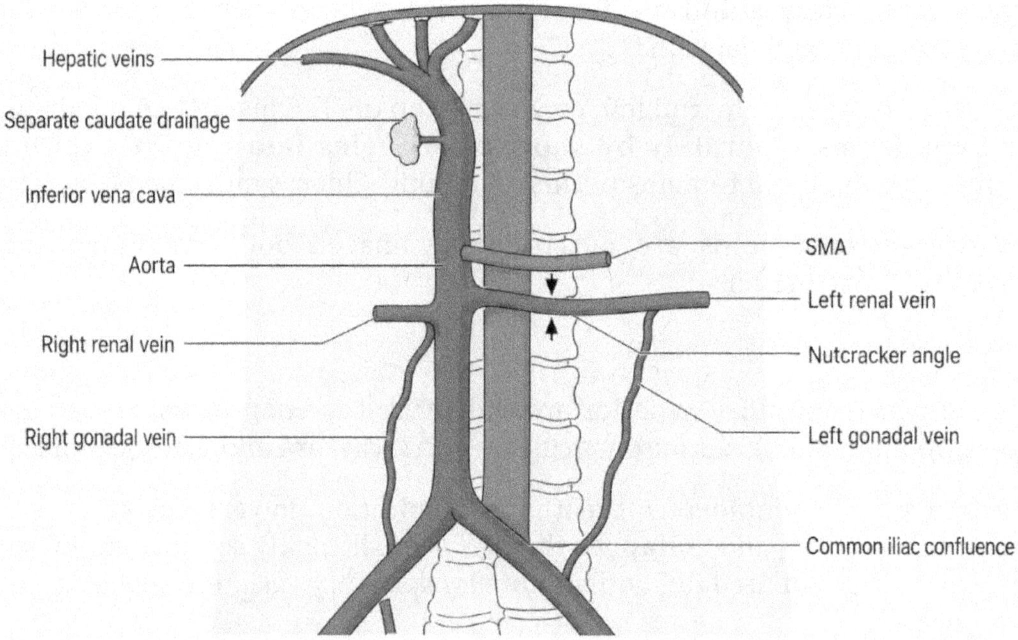

Inferior vena cava and key tributaries.

3.6 The Portal Venous System

Formation and course

The portal venous system carries nutrient-rich, partly deoxygenated blood from the gut, spleen, and pancreas to the liver. It is a **portal system** in the strict sense — a venous network beginning and ending in capillaries — and this is why its obstruction produces the distinctive collateral phenomena of portal hypertension rather than simple congestion.

The **main portal vein** is formed **posterior to the neck of the pancreas** by the confluence of the **superior mesenteric vein** and the **splenic vein**. The **inferior mesenteric vein** usually drains into the splenic vein.

The portal vein ascends to the right in the hepatoduodenal ligament and divides at the porta hepatis into **right and left portal branches**, whose distribution defines the hepatic segments (Chapter 4).

The portal triad and the identification rule

Within the liver, the portal vein branches travel with a hepatic artery branch and a bile duct, wrapped in a fibrous sheath continuous with the hepatic capsule. This sheath is the reason for the single most useful identification rule in hepatic imaging:

> **Portal veins have bright echogenic walls. Hepatic veins do not.**

Add the flow direction and the discrimination is complete:

	Portal veins	Hepatic veins
Walls	Bright, echogenic (fibrous sheath)	Imperceptible
Flow direction	Toward the liver periphery (hepatopetal)	Toward the IVC and diaphragm
Course	Accompanied by artery and duct	Run alone, between segments
Waveform	Gently undulating, continuous, above baseline	Multiphasic with flow reversal
Calibre with respiration	Increases on inspiration	Varies with cardiac cycle

Confusing the two systems is a common trainee error and it makes segmental localization impossible, because hepatic veins run **between** segments while portal branches run **within** them.

Normal portal haemodynamics

Normal flow is **hepatopetal** — toward the liver — and continuous, with gentle undulation from transmitted cardiac and respiratory variation but without the phasic reversal seen in hepatic veins.

Velocity is modest and varies physiologically, rising after meals and falling in the upright position; portal vein diameter increases on deep inspiration and in the supine position. Because of this variability, portal measurements should be taken under stated conditions — fasting, supine, quiet respiration — and compared like with like. [VERIFY: current reference ranges for main portal vein diameter and velocity, and the conditions under which they are defined]

The collateral pathways

When portal pressure rises, flow seeks routes back to the systemic circulation through portosystemic anastomoses — sites where portal and systemic venous territories meet. These are the pathways to search when portal hypertension is suspected, and finding one is often easier than measuring pressure:

Left gastric (coronary) vein — dilating and reversing to supply **oesophageal and gastric varices**. The most clinically dangerous collateral, since these are the varices that bleed.

Paraumbilical vein — recanalizing within the falciform ligament, running from the left portal vein toward the umbilicus. Produces the clinical *caput medusae*. A recanalized paraumbilical vein is a highly specific sign of portal hypertension.

Splenorenal and gastrorenal shunts — between splenic and left renal veins, often large and tortuous in the splenic hilum.

Haemorrhoidal plexus — between superior rectal (portal) and middle/inferior rectal (systemic) veins.

Retroperitoneal and omental collaterals, and recanalized veins around a previous surgical site.

In advanced disease, portal flow becomes **biphasic** and then **hepatofugal** — away from the liver. Documenting flow direction in the main portal vein is therefore a core part of any liver study, and it is a finding that changes management. The full portal hypertension complex, with its splenic, ascitic, and hepatic vein components, is developed in Chapter 4 §4.5.

Portal vein thrombosis appears as echogenic material within the lumen with absent or partial flow. Chronic occlusion is followed by **cavernous transformation** — replacement of the vein by a tangle of periportal collateral channels, which on colour Doppler produces a characteristic mass of small serpiginous vessels at the porta.

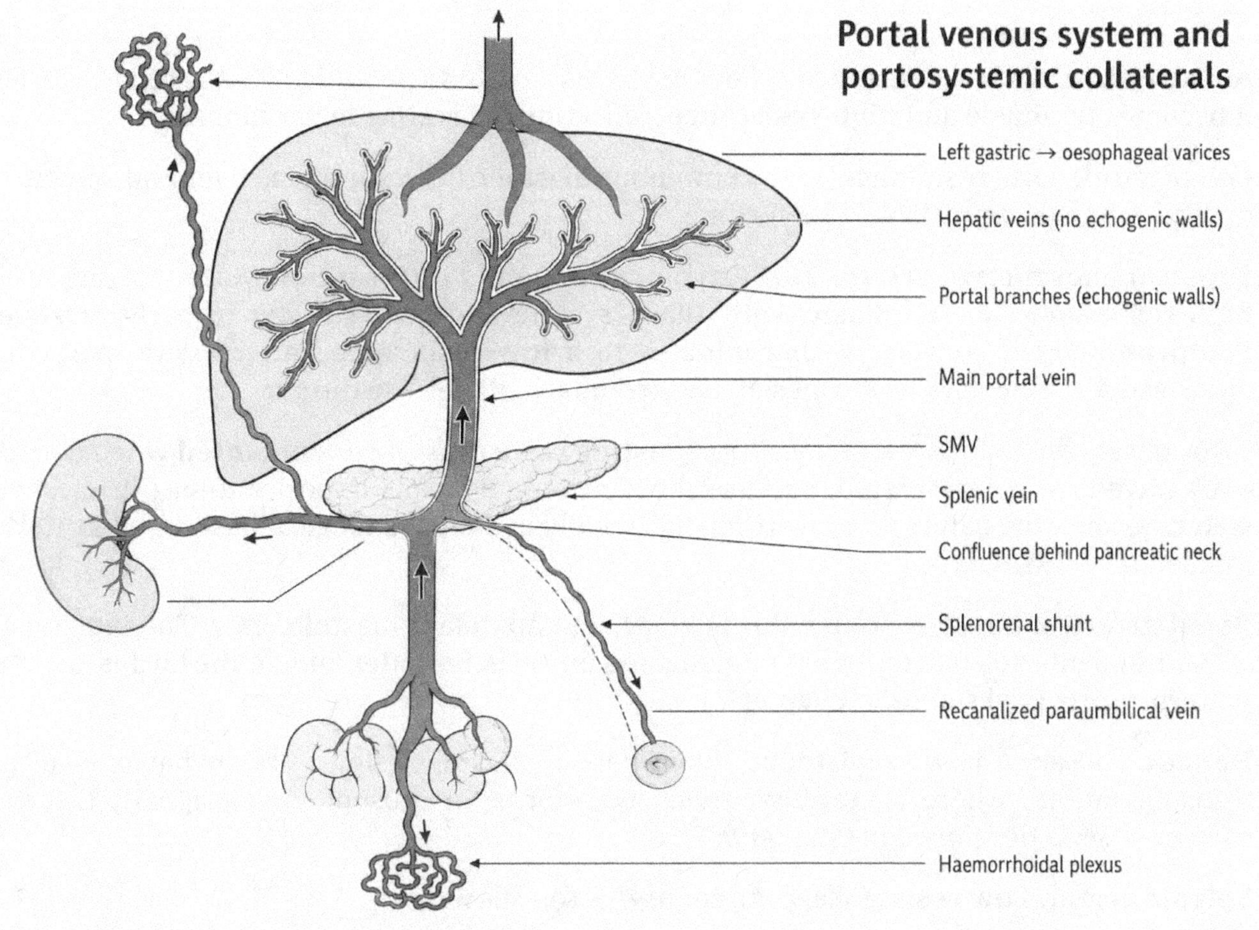

3.7 Normal Doppler Waveform Signatures by Vascular Bed

What determines a waveform

Arterial waveform shape is governed almost entirely by the **resistance of the vascular bed downstream**, modified by proximal disease and by cardiac output. Once you understand that single relationship, you can predict the normal waveform of any vessel from the organ it supplies, and you can interpret an abnormal one without memorizing a catalogue.

Low-resistance beds require continuous perfusion throughout the cardiac cycle — brain, kidney, liver, spleen, placenta, and any organ with high constant metabolic demand. Their waveforms show a rapid systolic upstroke and **continuous forward flow throughout diastole**, never returning to baseline.

High-resistance beds do not require continuous perfusion — resting skeletal muscle, and the fasting bowel. Their waveforms show a sharp systolic peak, **little or no diastolic flow**, and often a brief early diastolic **reverse component** produced by elastic recoil against a closed distal bed.

The essential insight is that resistance can change physiologically. The SMA is the clearest example and is worth internalizing as the model case.

Aorta. Proximally low-resistance, reflecting the visceral branches; distal to the renal arteries it becomes **triphasic and high-resistance**, reflecting the resting lower limbs.

Celiac trunk. Low resistance, with continuous diastolic flow, supplying liver and spleen. It does not change appreciably with feeding.

Superior mesenteric artery. The waveform depends on prandial state. Fasting, it is **high-resistance and triphasic**, with sharp systole and reverse flow in early diastole. **Postprandially** it converts within minutes to a **low-resistance** pattern with markedly increased diastolic flow, as the mesenteric bed dilates to perfuse the gut.

Two consequences follow directly. First, a **fasting state must be documented** whenever an SMA waveform is interpreted, because the same trace means opposite things in the two states. Second, the failure to convert postprandially is the physiological basis of mesenteric ischaemia assessment.

Renal arteries. Low resistance throughout, with abundant diastolic flow. The intrarenal arcuate and interlobar arteries are interrogated for resistive index and for the tardus-parvus pattern of proximal stenosis (Chapter 7).

Hepatic artery. Low resistance, continuous diastolic flow. Its behaviour after transplantation, where a tardus-parvus waveform or absent flow signals arterial compromise, is developed in Chapter 9.

Splenic artery. Low resistance, continuous diastolic flow.

Internal carotid. Low resistance — the model low-resistance vessel, contrasted with the **external carotid**, which is high-resistance with sharp peaks and minimal diastolic flow, and which can be confirmed by temporal tapping (Chapter 16).

Peripheral limb arteries at rest. Triphasic: sharp systolic peak, early diastolic reverse flow, late diastolic forward flow. Loss of the reverse component, then progression to monophasic, damped, and delayed waveforms, indicates progressively more severe proximal disease. After exercise, the peripheral bed dilates and the waveform normally becomes low-resistance — the same physiology as the SMA.

Hepatic veins. Multiphasic with flow reversal, reflecting right atrial pressure changes transmitted directly through the IVC. The normal trace has an antegrade systolic wave, an antegrade diastolic wave, and a retrograde component with atrial contraction. **Loss of phasicity — flattening toward a monophasic trace — occurs in cirrhosis** as the surrounding parenchyma stiffens and damps transmission. Increased pulsatility with prominent reversal suggests right heart failure or tricuspid regurgitation.

Portal vein. Gently undulating, continuous, hepatopetal, remaining above the baseline throughout. Increased pulsatility suggests right heart failure or tricuspid regurgitation; flattening, reversal, or biphasic flow suggests portal hypertension.

IVC. Phasic with respiration, with cardiac pulsatility increasing toward the right atrium.

Peripheral veins. Spontaneous, phasic with respiration, compressible, and augmentable. Loss of phasicity implies proximal obstruction — the central finding of Chapter 16.

Reading a waveform you do not recognize

Given an unfamiliar trace, work through four questions in order:

1. **Arterial or venous?** Pulsatile and cardiac-synchronous, or phasic and respiratory?
2. **If arterial, high or low resistance?** Look at diastole: continuous forward flow, or absent/reversed?
3. **Does that match the bed you are in?** A high-resistance renal artery is abnormal. A high-resistance fasting SMA is normal.
4. **If it does not match, is the abnormality proximal or distal?** Tardus-parvus — slow upstroke, blunted peak — indicates **proximal** stenosis. Elevated resistive index with a normal upstroke indicates **distal** parenchymal disease.

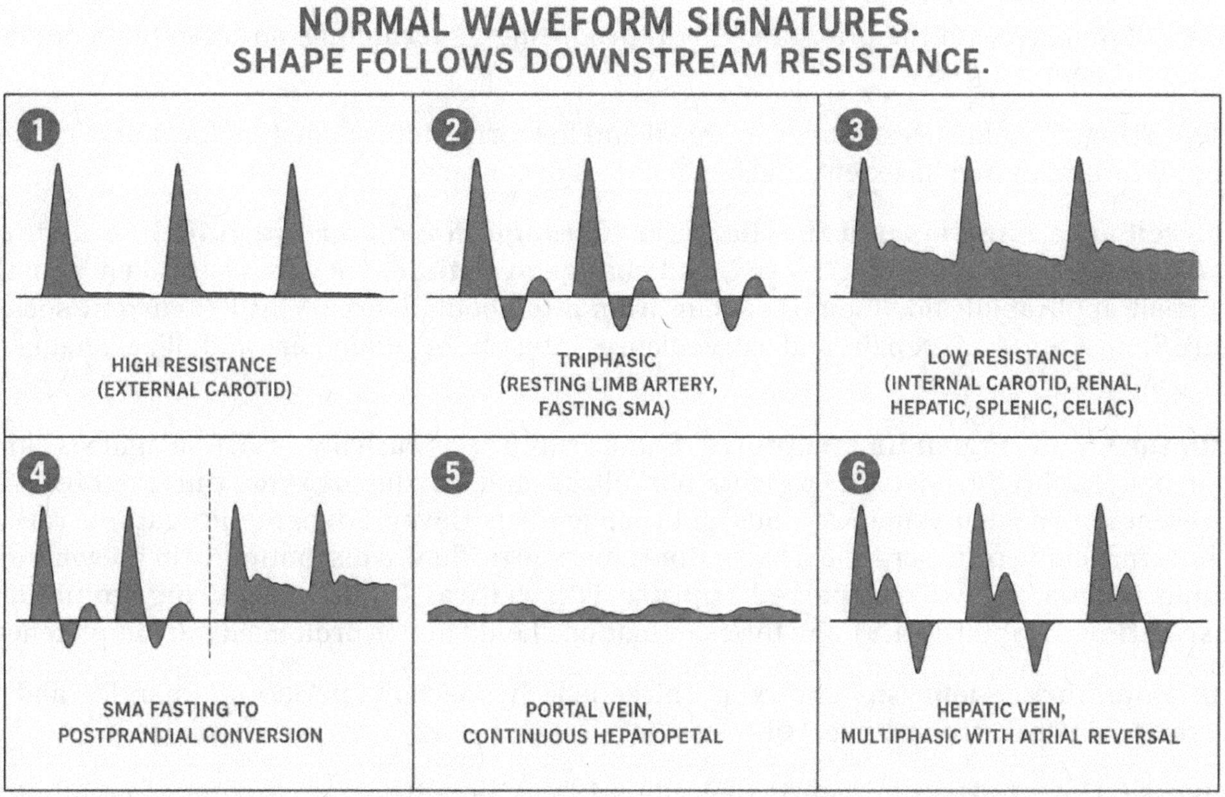

3.8 Abdominal Vascular Pathology: Aneurysm, Dissection, Thrombosis

Abdominal aortic aneurysm

Definition. Focal dilatation of the aorta, conventionally at or above **3.0 cm**, or a focal increase of 50% over the adjacent normal calibre. Below this, a mildly enlarged aorta is described as ectatic.

Measurement technique — the section that matters most. Aneurysm measurement drives surveillance intervals and repair decisions, so measurement error has direct clinical consequences. The technique:

- Measure **outer wall to outer wall**, including any mural thrombus. Measuring the residual lumen underestimates the aneurysm, sometimes grossly, because thrombus can occupy a large proportion of the sac.
- Measure the **maximum anteroposterior diameter on a true transverse image**, with the plane **perpendicular to the aortic long axis**. A tortuous aorta imaged in the body's transverse plane is cut obliquely, and an oblique cut through a cylinder is an ellipse — which overestimates diameter. Angle the probe to cut the vessel squarely.
- Confirm on the **longitudinal** image that you measured at the true maximum and that your plane was perpendicular.
- Document the **level** of the maximum, the **relationship to the renal arteries** (infrarenal, juxtarenal, suprarenal), the **craniocaudal extent**, and the **iliac arteries**, which are frequently involved.
- Compare with the prior study by reproducing its technique, not merely its number (Chapter 1 §1.5).

Reporting. Most aneurysms are infrarenal and fusiform. Note shape (fusiform or saccular), mural thrombus and its extent, and any features of concern.

Surveillance intervals and the diameter threshold for repair are guideline-defined, vary between societies and by sex, and change over time. They must be taken from the current applicable guideline rather than from a textbook figure. [VERIFY: current society thresholds for AAA repair and surveillance interval by diameter, and iliac aneurysm thresholds]

Rupture and impending rupture. Frank rupture is usually a CT diagnosis in a haemodynamically unstable patient, but ultrasound at the bedside can establish the presence of an aneurysm in seconds and change the pathway. Sonographic features raising concern include retroperitoneal haematoma, periaortic fluid, a discontinuity in the wall, and rapid interval growth. **Suspected rupture is a critical finding requiring immediate escalation** (Chapter 1 §1.5), and the examination should not be prolonged for completeness.

Inflammatory aneurysm shows a thickened, hypoechoic periaortic mantle, and is associated with retroperitoneal fibrosis.

Mycotic (infected) aneurysm is typically saccular, eccentric, rapidly growing, and often accompanied by periaortic inflammatory change.

Mural thrombus versus dissection

These are distinguished by what lies between the layers, and the discrimination is straightforward once framed correctly:

Mural thrombus is echogenic material **adherent to the wall**, reducing the lumen concentrically or eccentrically, with **no flow within it** on colour or spectral Doppler and **no**

mobile membrane. Common in aneurysms and the reason outer-wall measurement is mandatory.

Dissection is a **mobile intimal flap** separating a true and a false lumen, with **flow in both lumina** — typically differing in velocity, direction, and timing. The flap moves with the cardiac cycle in real time, which is the most reliable sign and is visible only on cine, not on a still frame. Colour Doppler shows the two lumina filling differently, sometimes with flow reversal in the false lumen.

The commonest error is calling a **reverberation or side-lobe artifact** within a large aorta a dissection flap. Apply the tests from Chapter 2: does it move independently of the wall, is there genuine flow on both sides, and does it persist when the angle and window change? An artifactual flap disappears with a change of approach; a real one does not.

Abdominal dissection is most often extension of a thoracic dissection, so assess **whether branch vessels arise from the true or false lumen** — renal and mesenteric compromise determines management — and document the proximal and distal extent visible.

Other vascular pathology of the abdomen

Aortic occlusion and stenosis — Leriche syndrome with distal aortic occlusion; atherosclerotic stenosis with velocity elevation and post-stenotic turbulence.

Median arcuate ligament syndrome — extrinsic compression of the celiac origin by the diaphragmatic crus, producing elevated velocity that **worsens in expiration and improves in inspiration**. The respiratory variation is the diagnostic manoeuvre, and a celiac velocity measured in one respiratory phase only is uninterpretable for this diagnosis.

Nutcracker syndrome — left renal vein compression between the SMA and aorta, as described in §3.5.

Renal artery stenosis — assessed by direct origin velocity and by the intrarenal tardus-parvus pattern (Chapter 7).

Portal vein thrombosis and cavernous transformation — §3.6 and Chapter 4.

Pseudoaneurysm — a contained wall rupture, typically post-procedural, showing the characteristic **yin-yang** swirling colour pattern within the sac and a **to-and-fro** spectral waveform in the connecting neck. The neck waveform is the diagnostic finding and should be documented specifically; the femoral case is developed in Chapter 16.

Arteriovenous fistula — high-velocity low-resistance arterial inflow with arterialized venous outflow and perivascular tissue vibration producing a visible colour mosaic.

Retroperitoneal lymphadenopathy — encasing rather than displacing the vessels, sometimes lifting the aorta forward off the spine, a sign described as the "floating aorta."

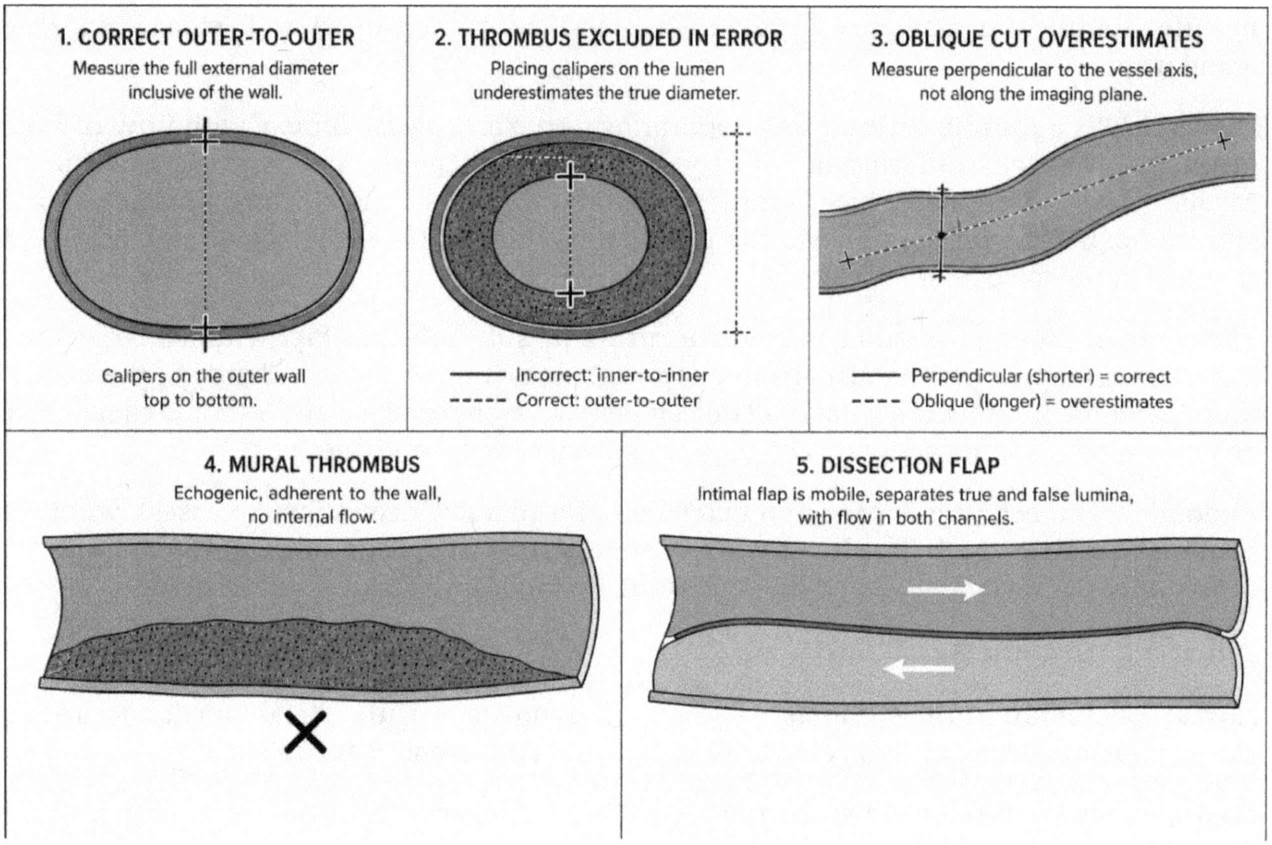

Key Points

1. Navigate by vessels, not by organs. The great vessels are constant; the organs are not.
2. A mass that displaces the aorta and IVC anteriorly arises behind them. A mass that encases without displacing suggests infiltrative retroperitoneal disease.
3. Morison's pouch is the most dependent upper abdominal space in the supine patient; the pelvis is the most dependent space overall. Search both.
4. Fluid confined to the lesser sac is locally generated, because the sac communicates with the rest of the peritoneum only through a narrow foramen.
5. Transverse ultrasound shares the CT convention — patient's right to image left. Sagittal does not: ultrasound places cephalad to screen left, CT and MR place it at the top.
6. Left lateral decubitus is the highest-yield repositioning in abdominal sonography, and it is underused.
7. The sagittal stack at the SMA — aorta, left renal vein, SMA in its fat collar, splenic vein, pancreatic body — locates five structures from one image.
8. The right renal artery passes posterior to the IVC; the left renal vein passes between the aorta and the SMA; the left gonadal vein drains to the left renal vein rather than the IVC. Each asymmetry has a clinical consequence.
9. Portal veins have echogenic walls and flow toward the periphery; hepatic veins have imperceptible walls and flow toward the IVC. Portal branches run within segments, hepatic veins between them.

10. Arterial waveform shape follows downstream resistance. The SMA is high-resistance fasting and low-resistance postprandially — document the prandial state or the trace cannot be interpreted.
11. Tardus-parvus indicates proximal stenosis; an elevated resistive index with a normal upstroke indicates distal parenchymal disease.
12. Measure an aneurysm outer wall to outer wall, perpendicular to the vessel axis. Measuring the lumen understates it and an oblique cut overstates it.
13. Mural thrombus is adherent with no internal flow; a dissection flap is mobile with flow in both lumina. A "flap" that vanishes when you change window was an artifact.
14. Suspected aneurysm rupture is a critical finding. Establish the aneurysm, escalate immediately, and do not prolong the examination for completeness.

Registry Check

1. A large mass in the upper abdomen displaces the aorta and inferior vena cava anteriorly, away from the vertebral bodies. This indicates the mass is:

A. Intraperitoneal **B.** Retroperitoneal, arising posterior to the great vessels **C.** Within the lesser sac **D.** Arising from the pancreatic head

> **Answer: B.** Anterior displacement of the great vessels off the spine indicates origin posterior to them. An intraperitoneal or anterior retroperitoneal mass would indent or displace the vessels posteriorly, and lymphomatous disease characteristically encases the vessels and may lift the aorta forward — the "floating aorta" sign.

2. In a longitudinal epigastric image, a vessel is identified running parallel and immediately anterior to the aorta, surrounded by a conspicuous collar of echogenic fat. The structure passing between this vessel and the aorta is the:

A. Splenic vein **B.** Left renal vein **C.** Common bile duct **D.** Right renal artery

> **Answer: B.** The vessel described is the superior mesenteric artery, and the left renal vein crosses the midline between the SMA and the aorta on its way to the IVC — the anatomy underlying nutcracker syndrome. The splenic vein runs anterior to the SMA, not behind it.

3. A new right-sided varicocele in an adult male should prompt evaluation for:

A. Left renal vein compression **B.** A retroperitoneal mass obstructing the right gonadal vein **C.** Portal hypertension **D.** Testicular torsion

> **Answer: B.** The right gonadal vein drains directly into the IVC by a short route, so right-sided varicoceles are uncommon and a new one raises concern for obstruction by a retroperitoneal process. Left-sided varicoceles are common because the left gonadal vein drains into the left renal vein by a longer, higher-pressure route.

4. Within the liver, a tubular anechoic structure with bright echogenic walls carrying flow toward the periphery is a:

A. Hepatic vein **B.** Portal vein branch **C.** Bile duct **D.** Hepatic artery branch

> **Answer: B.** The fibrous sheath of the portal triad produces the echogenic walls, and normal portal flow is hepatopetal — toward the liver periphery. Hepatic veins lack perceptible walls, run between segments, and drain toward the IVC.

5. A superior mesenteric artery waveform shows a sharp systolic peak with early diastolic flow reversal and minimal forward diastolic flow. The most appropriate interpretation is:

A. Mesenteric ischaemia **B.** Normal, if the patient is fasting **C.** Normal, if the patient has recently eaten **D.** Median arcuate ligament syndrome

> **Answer: B.** The fasting SMA supplies a high-resistance bed and normally shows a triphasic waveform. Postprandially it converts to a low-resistance pattern with abundant diastolic flow. The prandial state must therefore be documented, because the same trace is normal fasting and abnormal after a meal.

6. An abdominal aortic aneurysm contains extensive concentric mural thrombus. Measuring only the residual patent lumen will:

A. Overestimate the aneurysm diameter **B.** Underestimate the aneurysm diameter **C.** Have no effect on the measurement **D.** Be the preferred technique for surveillance

> **Answer: B.** Aneurysm diameter is measured outer wall to outer wall and includes mural thrombus. Excluding the thrombus can understate the true diameter substantially, potentially delaying surveillance escalation or repair.

7. Loss of normal phasicity in the hepatic vein waveform, producing a flattened monophasic trace, is characteristically associated with:

A. Right heart failure **B.** Tricuspid regurgitation **C.** Cirrhosis **D.** Portal vein thrombosis

> **Answer: C.** Hepatic vein phasicity depends on transmission of right atrial pressure changes through compliant surrounding parenchyma. Cirrhotic stiffening damps this transmission and flattens the waveform. Right heart failure and tricuspid regurgitation produce the opposite — increased pulsatility with exaggerated reversal.

8. Elevated peak systolic velocity at the celiac artery origin that worsens during expiration and improves during inspiration suggests:

A. Atherosclerotic celiac stenosis **B.** Median arcuate ligament syndrome **C.** Aliasing artifact **D.** Hepatic artery aneurysm

> **Answer: B.** Compression of the celiac origin by the diaphragmatic crus varies with diaphragmatic position, worsening in expiration. The respiratory variation

distinguishes it from fixed atherosclerotic stenosis, and a velocity recorded in a single respiratory phase cannot make the distinction.

Chapter Notes for the Editorial Pass

Verification queue. `[VERIFY]` tags cover IVC diameter and collapsibility thresholds for right atrial pressure estimation (§3.5), portal vein diameter and velocity reference ranges with their defining conditions (§3.6), and AAA repair and surveillance thresholds including sex-specific and iliac criteria (§3.8). The AAA thresholds are the most consequential in the chapter — they are guideline-defined, differ between societies, and have changed within recent editions. Do not publish a generic figure.

Vertebral levels given for aortic branch origins (§3.4) are conventional approximations with normal individual variation and should be presented as such rather than as fixed values.

Figure count: 8 Lane A, 2 Lane B (`fig-3-5` celiac seagull with paired longitudinal; `fig-3-10` AAA with mural thrombus and calipers). Both Lane B slots are standard acquisitions likely available from the author's own archive and are lower-risk than the paired-settings acquisitions required in Chapter 2.

Cross-reference targets to fix at layout: §3.1 recesses → Chapter 8 FAST; §3.4 SMA stack → Chapter 6 pancreas; §3.5 tumour thrombus → Chapter 7 renal neoplasms; §3.6 collaterals → Chapter 4 portal hypertension; §3.7 tardus-parvus → Chapter 7 and Chapter 9; §3.8 pseudoaneurysm → Chapter 16.

Word count: approximately 10,200 excluding image prompt blocks, learning objectives, registry questions, and these notes.

Chapter 4: The Liver

Learning Objectives

On completing this chapter you should be able to:

1. Assign a hepatic lesion to a Couinaud segment in real time using the hepatic veins and portal bifurcation as landmarks.
2. Perform a complete hepatic protocol, naming the acoustic window and respiratory maneuver appropriate to each region.
3. Interpret hepatic laboratory patterns as hepatocellular, cholestatic, or synthetic-failure, and use that pattern to direct the examination.
4. Recognize the sonographic features of steatosis, chronic hepatitis, and cirrhosis, and state the limits of B-mode assessment for each.
5. Identify the components of the portal hypertension complex and document flow direction in the main portal vein.
6. Characterize the principal benign and malignant focal lesions, including their contrast enhancement behavior.
7. State the single discriminator between hepatocellular carcinoma and metastasis on contrast-enhanced ultrasound.
8. Recognize hepatic infection patterns and their epidemiologic associations.
9. Distinguish bland from tumor thrombus, and recognize Budd-Chiari syndrome.
10. Distinguish focal fatty change from a true lesion using geometry, margins, and vessel behavior.

The Two Orders

Almost every hepatic ultrasound arrives from one of two clinical situations, and they require different examinations.

Abnormal liver function tests. The question is diffuse disease: is there steatosis, is there evidence of cirrhosis, is there biliary obstruction, is the portal system patent. The examination is a systematic survey with attention to echotexture, surface contour, vascular flow, and the biliary tree.

A lesion found on another modality. The question is characterization: is this the same lesion, is it solid or cystic, what are its vascular characteristics, and does it need contrast. The examination is targeted, and its most important output is often a decision about whether ultrasound can answer the question at all.

Recognizing which examination you are performing, before you start, determines your protocol and your report.

4.1 Normal Anatomy, Couinaud Segments, and Vascular Landmarks

Gross anatomy and surface landmarks

The liver occupies the right upper quadrant, extending across the midline. Its diaphragmatic surface is smooth and convex; its visceral surface carries impressions from the adjacent organs and the porta hepatis.

The classical division into right and left lobes by the falciform ligament is a **surface** anatomy that does not correspond to the functional anatomy and should not be used for lesion localization. The functional division is by vascular territory, described below.

Two ligamentous landmarks are sonographically useful:

- **Ligamentum teres** — the obliterated umbilical vein, running in the free edge of the falciform ligament. Seen in transverse section as a round echogenic focus in the left lobe, frequently mistaken for a lesion or for a stone. It is a normal structure and the commonest hepatic pseudolesion.
- **Ligamentum venosum** — the obliterated ductus venosus, appearing as an echogenic line separating the caudate lobe from the left lobe. It is the landmark that defines the caudate.

Normal variants worth recognizing so they are not reported as pathology include **Riedel's lobe** — an inferior tongue-like extension of the right lobe, more common in women, extending below the costal margin and easily mistaken for hepatomegaly — and diaphragmatic slips, which produce hypoechoic bands along the liver surface.

Hepatic size is conventionally assessed by craniocaudal span in the midclavicular line, but the measurement is unreliable in isolation: it is affected by body habitus, respiration, plane obliquity, and lobar variation. Contour, echotexture, and lobar proportion carry more information than a single number. [VERIFY: current reference ranges for hepatic craniocaudal span and their measurement conditions]

Normal echotexture

Normal hepatic parenchyma is **homogeneous, fine, and mid-gray**, with echogenicity **equal to or slightly greater than the adjacent right renal cortex** and roughly comparable to the spleen. Vessels traverse it as anechoic channels, and the portal branches carry bright walls (Chapter 3 §3.6).

Because these comparisons are relative, always acquire an image containing **both liver and right kidney in the same frame at the same depth and gain**. A statement that the liver is echogenic, made without the kidney visible for comparison, cannot be verified by anyone reading the study afterwards, and this single image is the foundation of the steatosis assessment in §4.4.

The functional anatomy divides the liver into eight segments, each with its own portal inflow, arterial supply, biliary drainage, and hepatic venous outflow. This makes each segment independently resectable, which is why surgeons work in these terms and why your localization must too.

Construction, in the two planes that matter:

The **three hepatic veins** run in the vertical planes between sectors, dividing the liver into four vertical sectors:

- **Right hepatic vein** separates the right posterior sector (segments VI, VII) from the right anterior sector (segments V, VIII).
- **Middle hepatic vein** runs in the principal plane (Cantlie's line) separating the functional right and left lobes — the true lobar division, running from the gallbladder fossa to the IVC, not along the falciform ligament.
- **Left hepatic vein** separates the left lateral sector (segments II, III) from segment IV.

The **portal bifurcation plane** — horizontal, at the level of the right and left portal branches — divides each sector into a superior and an inferior segment.

The resulting map:

Segment	Location
I	Caudate lobe, between IVC and ligamentum venosum
II	Left lateral, superior
III	Left lateral, inferior
IVa / IVb	Left medial, superior / inferior
V	Right anterior, inferior
VI	Right posterior, inferior
VII	Right posterior, superior
VIII	Right anterior, superior

The practical method at the machine. Do not attempt to recall the map abstractly. Work in two steps:

1. Find the **hepatic vein confluence** in a transverse subcostal view angled cephalad. The three veins fan toward the IVC and divide the superior liver into its sectors — this single image assigns segments II, IVa, VIII, and VII.
2. Drop caudally to the **portal bifurcation**. Below this level, the same sectoral divisions now correspond to segments III, IVb, V, and VI.

Above the portal bifurcation, the segment numbers are the "superior" set; below it, the "inferior" set. That is the whole system.

The caudate lobe and why it is special

Segment I sits between the IVC posteriorly and the ligamentum venosum anteriorly. It has two distinguishing features:

- **Dual portal inflow** from both right and left portal branches.
- **Separate venous drainage** by short veins passing directly into the IVC, bypassing the three main hepatic veins.

This separate drainage is why the caudate is spared, and characteristically **hypertrophies**, in Budd-Chiari syndrome (§4.9), and why caudate size relative to the right lobe is used as a morphological marker of cirrhosis (§4.4).

Vascular supply

The liver has a **dual blood supply**: roughly three-quarters of inflow from the **portal vein**, and one-quarter from the **hepatic artery**, which supplies a disproportionate share of oxygen and — critically for lesion characterization — is the sole supply of most tumors and the dominant supply of the biliary tree.

The **hepatic artery** arises from the celiac trunk via the common hepatic artery, ascends in the hepatoduodenal ligament, and divides at the porta. Variant anatomy is common: a **replaced right hepatic artery from the SMA**, or a **replaced left hepatic artery from the left gastric**, occur frequently enough that their recognition matters in transplant and surgical planning (Chapter 9).

Portal and hepatic vein discrimination is covered in Chapter 3 §3.6 and is assumed here: portal branches have echogenic walls, run within segments, and flow hepatopetally; hepatic veins have imperceptible walls, run between segments, and flow toward the IVC.

COUINAUD SEGMENTS, BUILT FROM THE THREE HEPATIC VEINS AND THE PORTAL BIFURCATION PLANE

Segments I–VIII; right, middle, and left hepatic veins; principal plane; portal bifurcation; caudate with separate IVC drainage

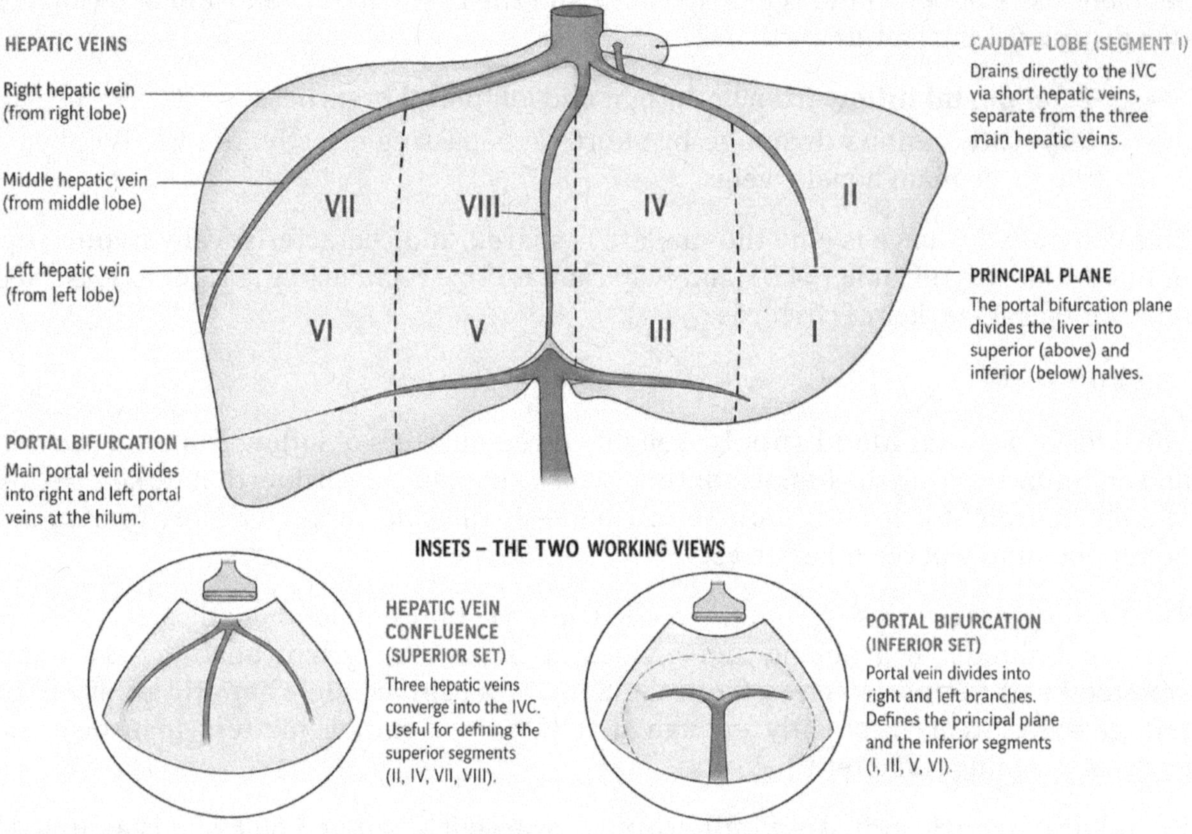

4.2 Scanning Protocol and Technical Considerations

Preparation and setup

Fasting for a documented interval improves the study by reducing bowel gas and, where the gallbladder is being assessed concurrently, by ensuring it is distended. [VERIFY: institutional fasting interval for hepatobiliary ultrasound]

Transducer. Curvilinear at the highest frequency that penetrates. A **high-frequency linear probe** should be available and used deliberately for two purposes: assessing the **surface contour** for nodularity in suspected cirrhosis, and evaluating **subcapsular lesions** lost in the near field of the curvilinear probe. Both are commonly omitted and both change conclusions.

Settings. Harmonic imaging on as default. **Turn spatial compounding off** when assessing for shadowing or when characterizing a possibly cystic lesion by its enhancement (Chapter 2 §2.4). Focal zone at the depth of interest. Depth adjusted between the near-field and dome assessments rather than left at one setting.

The sweep

The liver is surveyed in overlapping sweeps through complementary windows, not from a single approach:

Subcostal transverse, angled cephalad, in deep inspiration. Sweeps from the dome down. This is the view that yields the hepatic vein confluence and the superior segments.

Subcostal longitudinal. Sweeps from the left lateral segment across to the right lateral margin, covering the left lobe, the IVC and caudate, the porta, and the right lobe.

Intercostal, probe rotated to align with the rib space. Essential for the dome and the posterior right lobe, which subcostal approaches cannot reach in most patients. Segments VII and VIII are the most commonly under-imaged regions of the liver and this is the window that covers them.

Right coronal/flank. Provides the liver-kidney comparison image and the posterior right lobe.

Respiratory maneuvers. Deep inspiration lowers the liver below the costal margin. In patients who cannot cooperate, scan in quiet respiration and use more intercostal windows.

Required documentation

A complete hepatic examination should demonstrate, at minimum: the left lobe in two planes; the right lobe in two planes including the dome; the hepatic vein confluence; the portal vein at the porta with **spectral Doppler documenting flow direction**; the main portal vein diameter; the liver-and-right-kidney comparison image; the hepatic surface contour; and any focal lesion in two planes with measurements and Doppler.

Document flow direction in the main portal vein on **every** liver study, not only when portal hypertension is suspected. It takes fifteen seconds and it is the finding most likely to change management.

Where a region cannot be seen — most often the dome behind ribs, or the posterior right lobe in a large patient — **say so specifically** (Chapter 1 §1.5). "Dome not fully evaluated due to rib shadowing" is a real and useful statement; a silent omission is read as a normal dome.

4.3 Hepatic Function and Correlative Laboratory Values

You are not interpreting the laboratory data, but recognizing the pattern tells you what to look for and frequently changes your protocol. Three patterns matter.

The hepatocellular pattern

Predominant elevation of the **transaminases (ALT, AST)**, reflecting hepatocyte injury and leakage.

Directs attention to parenchymal disease: steatosis, viral or autoimmune hepatitis, drug injury, alcohol-related disease, ischemic injury. Very high values suggest acute injury — viral, toxic, or ischemic. Modest chronic elevation suggests steatohepatitis or chronic viral hepatitis.

What it changes: examine echotexture, echogenicity relative to the kidney, surface contour, and vascular patency carefully. Note that transaminase elevation independently raises measured liver stiffness (Chapter 2 §2.10), so an elastography value in this setting must be reported with that caveat.

The cholestatic pattern

Predominant elevation of **alkaline phosphatase and gamma-glutamyl transferase**, with or without **bilirubin**, reflecting biliary obstruction or cholestasis.

What it changes: the examination becomes a biliary study. Interrogate the intrahepatic ducts for dilatation, follow the common duct through its full course, measure it, identify the level of obstruction, and assess the pancreatic head. A cholestatic picture with a normal-caliber duct is itself a useful finding, pointing toward intrahepatic cholestasis or early or intermittent obstruction. This work is developed in Chapter 5.

Note that **GGT rises with alcohol and with enzyme-inducing drugs** independent of obstruction, and that an isolated alkaline phosphatase elevation may be of bone rather than hepatic origin.

The synthetic-failure pattern

Prolonged prothrombin time / raised INR, low albumin, and rising bilirubin indicate loss of synthetic function — a marker of severity, not of etiology.

What it changes: it raises the prior probability of cirrhosis and portal hypertension substantially, so the examination should include a deliberate search for the collateral pathways, splenic size, ascites, and portal flow direction (§4.5). It also matters procedurally: **coagulopathy is a relative contraindication to biopsy**, and any guided procedure requires the coagulation status to be known before the time-out (Chapter 1 §1.5).

Other correlations

Serum tumor markers — a rising alpha-fetoprotein in a cirrhotic patient raises concern for hepatocellular carcinoma and should heighten the care of the focal search. **Iron studies and ferritin** relate to hemochromatosis, which ultrasound cannot assess directly. **Viral serology** identifies the population under surveillance.

The general point: read the request and the available laboratory data before scanning, and let them direct the examination. A patient with a cholestatic picture needs a different scan from one with transaminitis, even though both requests may say "liver ultrasound."

4.4 Diffuse Disease: Steatosis, Hepatitis, Fibrosis, Cirrhosis

Hepatic steatosis

Findings, in the order they become apparent:

1. **Increased parenchymal echogenicity** relative to the right renal cortex — the primary sign, assessed on the paired liver-kidney image.
2. **Increased posterior attenuation**, with the deep liver appearing progressively darker and the diaphragm poorly defined or invisible.
3. **Loss of definition of the portal vein walls**, whose normal brightness is progressively obscured as the surrounding parenchyma brightens toward it.
4. **Blurring of the intrahepatic vascular architecture** generally.
5. **Hepatomegaly**, in more advanced cases.

Grading into mild, moderate, and severe is conventional and is **subjective and poorly reproducible between operators**. Report it as an impression, not a measurement.

Limitations you must state honestly. B-mode is relatively insensitive to low-grade steatosis and may be normal until a substantial fraction of hepatocytes are involved. It cannot distinguish fat from fibrosis, both of which raise echogenicity. It cannot grade reliably. And it cannot exclude steatohepatitis or fibrosis in a bright liver.

Attenuation-based quantification (Chapter 2 §2.10) offers a quantitative alternative, is platform-specific in its thresholds, and is the direction of travel for this assessment. [VERIFY: current evidence and platform-specific thresholds for ultrasound attenuation quantification of hepatic steatosis]

Acute hepatitis

Frequently **sonographically normal** — an important negative to be comfortable reporting, because a normal-appearing liver does not exclude significant acute hepatitis.

When abnormal, findings include a **decrease** in parenchymal echogenicity with consequent accentuation of the bright portal triads — the **"starry sky"** appearance — hepatomegaly, **gallbladder wall thickening** with a collapsed lumen (a reactive finding, not cholecystitis, and a common source of misdiagnosis), and periportal lymphadenopathy.

Starry sky is not specific to hepatitis and can occur in other conditions and in normal livers with certain settings. Treat it as supportive, not diagnostic.

Chronic hepatitis and fibrosis

Progressive **coarsening of the echotexture**, loss of the normal fine homogeneity, and **reduced brightness of the portal vein walls**. These are insensitive and non-specific, and B-mode cannot stage fibrosis.

Elastography is the tool for fibrosis assessment, and its confounders — non-fasting state, inflammation, congestion, cholestasis, ascites, obesity, measurement depth, vendor variation — are set out fully in Chapter 2 §2.10 and must accompany any reported value.

Cirrhosis

The morphological endpoint, and it is diagnosed on a **combination** of findings rather than any single one:

Surface nodularity. The most specific sign. Best demonstrated with a **high-frequency linear transducer** along the anterior liver surface, and especially conspicuous where ascites provides contrast. A curvilinear probe at abdominal settings frequently misses it entirely — this is the single most common reason cirrhosis is under-called.

Coarse, heterogeneous echotexture with regenerative nodules.

Lobar redistribution. Atrophy of the right lobe and segment IV, with **hypertrophy of the caudate lobe and the left lateral segment**. The **caudate-to-right-lobe ratio** measured on transverse section is a conventional quantitative expression of this. [VERIFY: current caudate-to-right-lobe ratio threshold and measurement technique]

Widening of the fissures and the porta hepatis, and enlargement of the gallbladder fossa, as the surrounding parenchyma atrophies.

Hepatic vein waveform flattening — loss of the normal multiphasic pattern toward a monophasic trace, as the stiffened parenchyma damps transmission of right atrial pressure (Chapter 3 §3.7).

Signs of portal hypertension (§4.5), which frequently accompany but are not required for the diagnosis.

The surveillance obligation. Cirrhosis is a premalignant state, and patients enter **periodic surveillance for hepatocellular carcinoma**. This changes how you scan them: a cirrhotic liver is nodular throughout, which makes a small HCC genuinely difficult to detect, and it demands a slower, more systematic focal search with attention to the dome and posterior segments. Any new or enlarging nodule in a cirrhotic liver is significant until proven otherwise. [VERIFY: current surveillance interval and modality recommendations for HCC in cirrhosis]

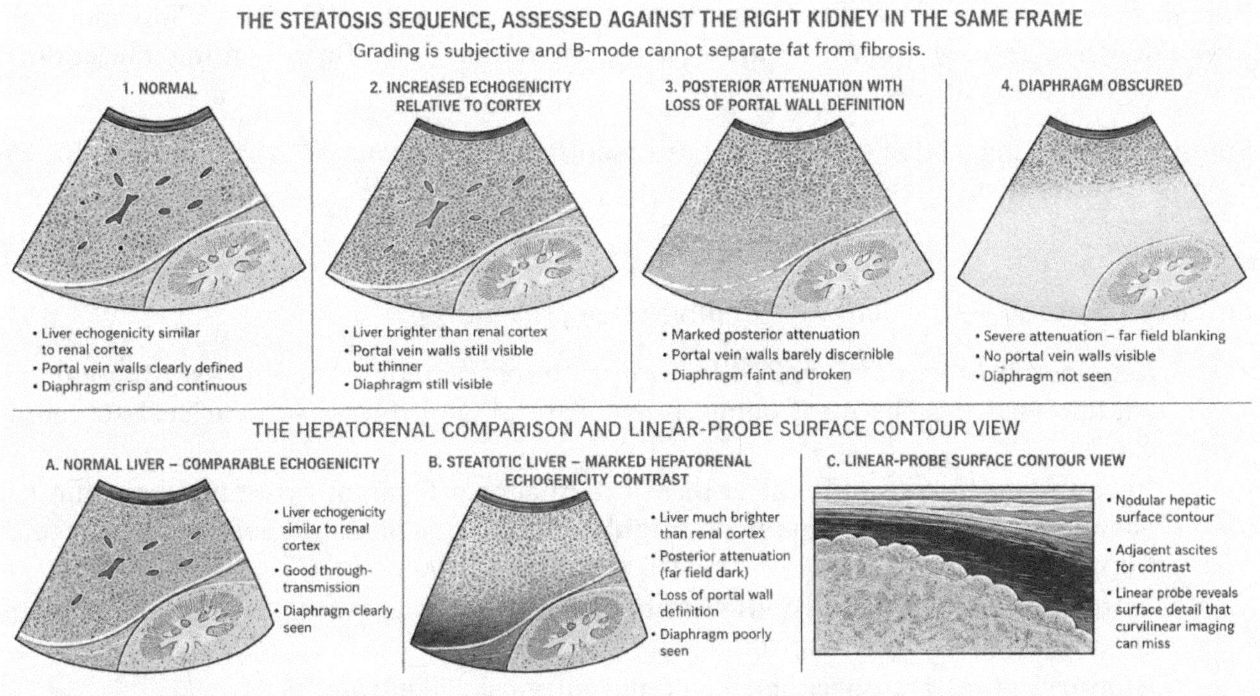

4.5 Portal Hypertension and Collateral Pathways

The mechanism

Portal hypertension is raised pressure in the portal system, most often from increased intrahepatic resistance in cirrhosis. Because the portal system begins and ends in capillary beds, elevated pressure cannot decompress by simple congestion — it must find **portosystemic anastomoses**, and it is these collaterals that produce both the diagnostic signs and the principal complication.

Causes are conventionally classified by the site of resistance: **prehepatic** (portal or splenic vein thrombosis), **intrahepatic** (cirrhosis, schistosomiasis, congenital fibrosis), and **posthepatic** (Budd-Chiari, right heart failure, constrictive pericarditis). The classification matters because it directs where you look — a patient with portal hypertension and a normal-appearing liver requires careful interrogation of the portal vein and the hepatic veins.

The sonographic complex

No single finding establishes the diagnosis. The following constitute the complex, and the more that are present the more confident the assessment:

Portal vein caliber. Dilatation of the main portal vein, with **loss of the normal respiratory variation** in the caliber of the splenic vein and SMV — normally these enlarge on inspiration. Loss of that variation is an early and useful sign. [VERIFY: current threshold values for main portal vein diameter and for the respiratory caliber change]

Portal velocity and flow direction. Velocity falls as resistance rises. Flow becomes **biphasic**, then frankly **hepatofugal** — away from the liver. Documenting direction is mandatory on every study.

Splenomegaly. Congestive enlargement, frequently the most conspicuous finding. [VERIFY: current threshold for splenic length]

Ascites.

Collateral vessels — the definitive finding when present:

- **Left gastric (coronary) vein** dilatation with reversed flow, feeding **esophageal and gastric varices**. The most dangerous collateral, and the reason variceal screening exists.
- **Recanalized paraumbilical vein** in the falciform ligament, running from the left portal vein toward the umbilicus. **Highly specific** for portal hypertension. On color Doppler it is unmistakable — a vessel where none should be.
- **Splenorenal and gastrorenal shunts** — large tortuous vessels in the splenic hilum connecting to the left renal vein.
- **Hemorrhoidal**, retroperitoneal, and postsurgical collaterals.

Hepatic vein waveform flattening, as in §4.4.

Gallbladder wall thickening from venous congestion and hypoalbuminemia — again, not cholecystitis, and a recurrent misinterpretation.

Search technique

Collaterals are found by deliberate search, not incidentally. Use **color Doppler with a low velocity scale and appropriately low wall filter**, since collateral flow is slow. Interrogate: the falciform ligament and the region between the left portal vein and the anterior abdominal wall; the region posterior to the left lobe and around the gastroesophageal junction; the splenic hilum; and the region around the pancreas.

A collateral is confirmed by demonstrating **flow** within it, not by its appearance alone.

TIPS and shunt surveillance

A transjugular intrahepatic portosystemic shunt creates an artificial channel between portal and hepatic venous systems. Surveillance assesses shunt patency by direct interrogation of velocities within the stent at defined positions, along with the direction of flow in the intrahepatic portal branches — which should reverse toward the shunt — and the main portal vein velocity. Deviations from the baseline study performed after insertion are more informative than absolute values, which reinforces the comparison discipline of Chapter 1 §1.5. [VERIFY: current velocity criteria for TIPS stenosis, which are stent-type and institution dependent]

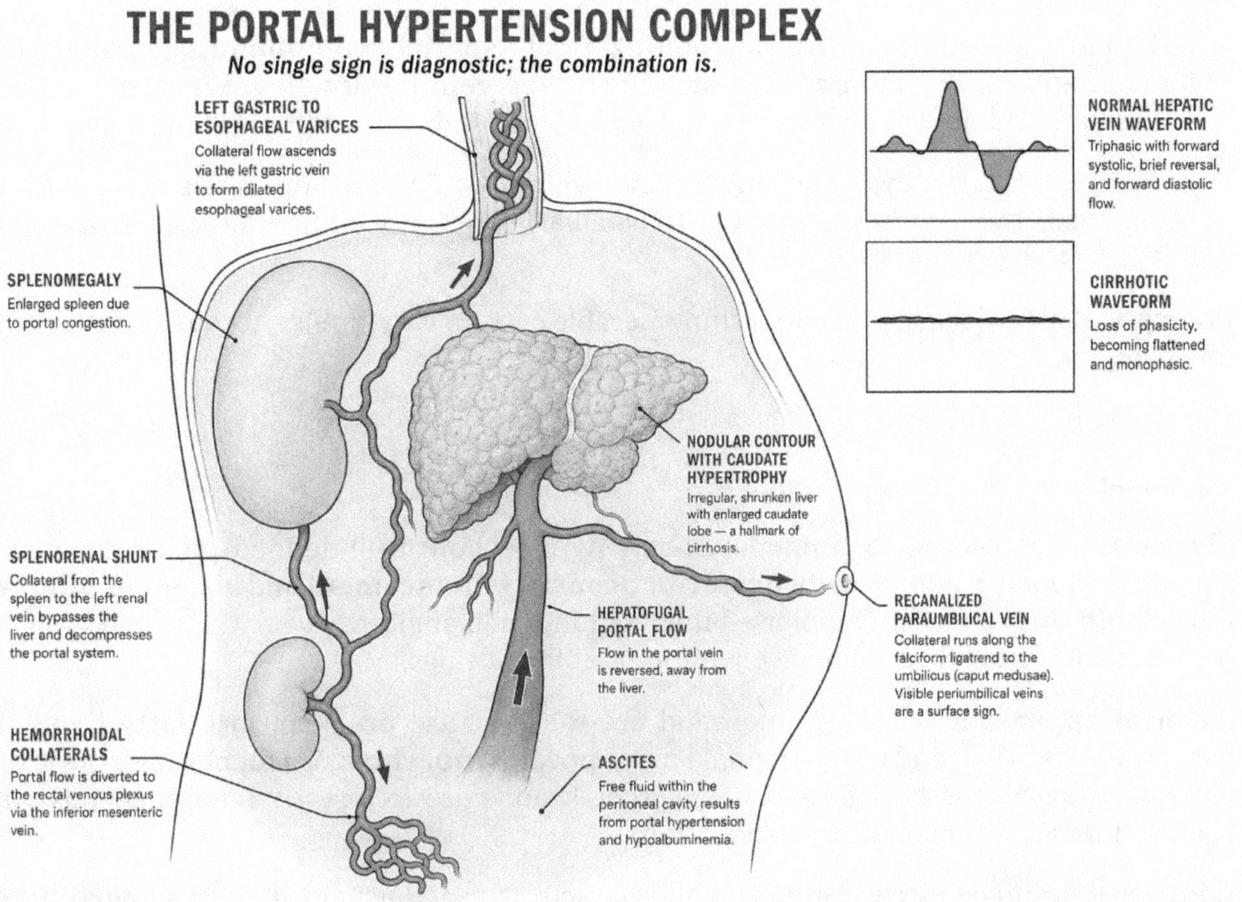

4.6 Benign Focal Lesions

The characterization framework

Every focal lesion is described in the same order, and the sequence should become automatic: **location by segment, size in three dimensions, shape, margin, internal echogenicity relative to adjacent parenchyma, internal texture, posterior acoustic features, vascularity on color and spectral Doppler, and relationship to vessels and capsule.**

Then two questions determine the next step: **does the background liver put the patient at risk of HCC**, and **can ultrasound characterize this lesion or does it need contrast or MRI?** A lesion in a cirrhotic liver is approached with entirely different suspicion from the same lesion in a normal one.

Simple hepatic cyst

Findings. Anechoic, thin imperceptible wall, sharply marginated, **posterior acoustic enhancement**, edge refractive shadows, no internal flow.

The three criteria that define a simple cyst — anechoic, thin-walled, enhancing — must all be present. Remember from Chapter 2 that **spatial compounding suppresses enhancement** and **harmonic imaging suppresses genuine low-level internal echoes**: check a questionable cyst on fundamental with compounding off before calling it simple.

Features that make a cyst **not** simple, and which require further assessment: thick or irregular wall, mural nodule, septations (particularly thick or vascular ones), internal debris that layers, and any internal flow.

Polycystic liver disease presents as innumerable cysts of varying size, frequently with renal involvement.

Hemangioma

The commonest benign hepatic tumor.

Classic appearance. Small, **homogeneously hyperechoic**, well-defined, often lobulated or slightly scalloped in outline, with **posterior acoustic enhancement** and **absent or minimal detectable flow** on color Doppler — flow within a hemangioma is very slow and typically below the detection threshold of conventional color settings.

Atypical appearances are common and are the practical problem. In a **fatty liver**, the background is bright and a hemangioma may appear **hypoechoic or isoechoic** — the lesion has not changed, the background has. Larger lesions are frequently heterogeneous with central fibrosis, thrombosis, or calcification.

Contrast-enhanced ultrasound is highly characteristic and usually definitive: **peripheral, nodular, discontinuous enhancement** in the arterial phase, progressing by **centripetal fill-in** toward the center over the portal venous and late phases, with **no washout**. The globular peripheral pattern is the signature.

Focal nodular hyperplasia

A hyperplastic response to a vascular anomaly rather than a true neoplasm. More common in women; **not associated with malignant transformation and not prone to hemorrhage** — which is the entire reason distinguishing it from adenoma matters.

Findings. Frequently **isoechoic or nearly so**, which makes it easy to miss on B-mode; detected by mass effect on vessels or by a subtle contour change. A **central scar** may be visible as a hypoechoic or hyperechoic linear or stellate area, though it is inconsistently seen.

Color Doppler may show the characteristic **central feeding artery with a spoke-wheel radiating pattern**, which is highly suggestive when present.

CEUS is characteristic: **marked arterial hyperenhancement filling centrifugally from the center outward** — often in a spoke-wheel pattern — with **sustained enhancement and no washout** in the portal venous and late phases.

Hepatocellular adenoma

A true benign neoplasm, associated with **estrogen exposure (oral contraceptives), androgen use, and glycogen storage disease.** It matters clinically because of **hemorrhage risk** and a recognized potential for **malignant transformation**, so it is managed very differently from FNH.

Findings. Variable and non-specific: often heterogeneous, may be hyperechoic where fat-containing, may contain anechoic areas of hemorrhage. There is no reliable B-mode discriminator from FNH.

CEUS shows arterial hyperenhancement filling **centripetally** — from the periphery inward, the opposite of FNH — with sustained or mildly reduced enhancement and typically **no marked washout**. The distinction from FNH on CEUS is real but can be difficult, and **contrast-enhanced MRI with a hepatobiliary agent is frequently the definitive study.** Recognizing that ultrasound may not resolve this question, and saying so, is the correct professional response.

Other benign entities

Biliary hamartomas (von Meyenburg complexes) — multiple tiny lesions, often with comet-tail artifact, a benign incidental finding.

Focal fatty change — dealt with fully in §4.10, because it is a pseudolesion rather than a lesion.

Regenerative nodules in cirrhosis — the background against which HCC must be detected, and the reason that detection is difficult.

Hepatic lipoma, angiomyolipoma, and post-traumatic or post-procedural collections complete the benign differential.

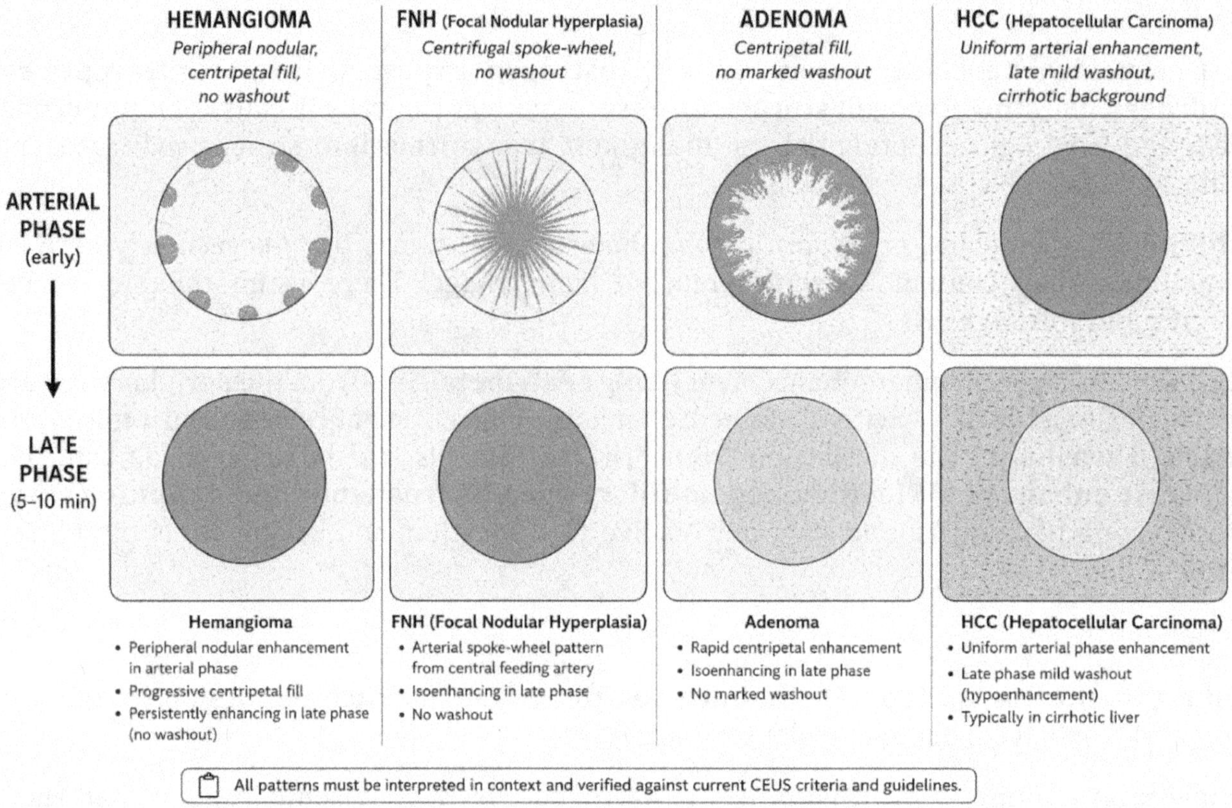

4.7 Malignant Focal Lesions

Hepatocellular carcinoma

Context is the first diagnostic fact. HCC arises overwhelmingly in a background of chronic liver disease — cirrhosis of any etiology, and chronic hepatitis B even without cirrhosis. A solid lesion in a cirrhotic liver is HCC until proven otherwise; the same lesion in a normal liver has a very different differential.

B-mode findings. Highly variable, which is the difficulty. Small lesions are often hypoechoic; larger ones become heterogeneous with a **mosaic** internal architecture. A thin hypoechoic **capsule or halo** may be present. Fatty change within the tumor can make it hyperechoic. In a nodular cirrhotic liver, a small HCC may be nearly indistinguishable from a regenerative nodule — which is why surveillance requires deliberate, slow, complete coverage rather than a survey.

Vascular invasion is a defining behavior and must be sought specifically. HCC characteristically invades the **portal vein**, and less commonly the hepatic veins and IVC. The finding that distinguishes tumor thrombus from bland thrombus is **arterial flow within the thrombus** on color and spectral Doppler; tumor thrombus also tends to **expand** the vein. This distinction changes staging and operability and is developed in §4.9.

CEUS. Arterial-phase hyperenhancement followed by **washout that is late and mild** — beginning after the early portal venous phase and remaining relatively subtle. **This washout**

timing is the single most valuable discriminator in hepatic contrast imaging, and it separates HCC from metastasis (below). [VERIFY: current CEUS washout timing criteria distinguishing HCC from non-hepatocellular malignancy]

Metastases

The commonest malignant hepatic lesions overall, and typically **multiple**.

Appearances vary with the primary, and the associations are useful:

Appearance	Typical primaries
Hyperechoic	Colorectal, neuroendocrine, renal
Hypoechoic	Breast, lung, lymphoma, pancreatic
Target / bull's-eye (hypoechoic halo around an echogenic center)	Any; a highly suspicious pattern in any liver
Calcified	Mucinous colorectal, some neuroendocrine, ovarian
Cystic / necrotic	Ovarian, sarcoma, neuroendocrine, treated metastases
Diffuse infiltrative	Breast, lung, melanoma — the most difficult pattern, producing only heterogeneity without a discrete mass

The hypoechoic halo is the most important single sign: a peripheral rim of low echogenicity around a lesion suggests malignancy and should raise the level of concern regardless of the lesion's internal appearance.

CEUS. Arterial enhancement is variable — often rim-like — but the diagnostic feature is **early and marked washout**, typically well within the portal venous phase, producing a conspicuous dark lesion against an enhancing liver. The late phase is the most sensitive for detecting additional lesions, which is a genuine clinical advantage of CEUS in staging.

The HCC-versus-metastasis discriminator, stated plainly: both enhance in the arterial phase; **HCC washes out late and mildly, metastasis washes out early and markedly.** Combined with the background liver and the clinical context, this is the core of hepatic contrast interpretation.

Cholangiocarcinoma

Intrahepatic (mass-forming) — an irregular infiltrative mass, often with **capsular retraction** and **peripheral biliary dilatation** distal to the lesion. Enhancement is typically **peripheral rim arterial enhancement with progressive central filling**, and washout behavior differs from HCC.

Hilar (Klatskin) — at the confluence of the right and left hepatic ducts, frequently small and difficult to see directly, presenting as **intrahepatic biliary dilatation with a non-united right and left system** and a normal-caliber distal common duct. The pattern of ductal dilatation localizes the lesion even when the mass is invisible.

Biliary malignancy is developed further in Chapter 5.

Other malignancies

Lymphoma — hypoechoic, sometimes strikingly so, and occasionally nearly anechoic enough to be mistaken for a cyst; may show posterior enhancement despite being solid, a pitfall noted in Chapter 2 §2.7.

Angiosarcoma and other primary sarcomas — rare, heterogeneous, vascular.

Hepatoblastoma — the principal pediatric primary, covered in Chapter 12.

Reporting a focal lesion

The report should carry: segment, size, morphology, vascularity, background liver, comparison with any prior imaging, and a clear statement of whether ultrasound has characterized the lesion. Where it has not — which is often — say so and recommend the modality that will. A confident-sounding descriptive report on an uncharacterized lesion in a cirrhotic liver is a worse outcome than an honest statement of limitation.

4.8 Infectious and Inflammatory Processes

Pyogenic abscess

Origin. Biliary (ascending cholangitis, the commonest route), portal (from intra-abdominal sepsis such as appendicitis or diverticulitis), arterial, direct extension, or traumatic.

Findings. Highly variable and **evolving**, which is the diagnostic trap. Early lesions may appear as an ill-defined region of altered echogenicity resembling a solid mass. As liquefaction proceeds they become complex fluid collections with irregular thick walls, internal debris, septations, and fluid-fluid levels.

Gas within an abscess is highly suggestive and produces **dirty shadowing or ring-down artifact** (Chapter 2 §2.8) — the discrimination from clean shadowing matters here.

Doppler shows no internal flow within the liquefied cavity, with peripheral hyperemia.

Abscess is a strong indication for **image-guided aspiration or drainage** (Chapter 9), and the ultrasound frequently drives that decision directly.

Amebic abscess

Entamoeba histolytica, with a travel or residence history in an endemic area. Characteristically a **solitary, round or oval, hypoechoic lesion with low-level homogeneous internal echoes, located peripherally in the right lobe near the capsule**, with a relatively thin wall and minimal surrounding inflammation compared with a pyogenic abscess.

Serology is the diagnostic test. Management is usually medical, so the distinction from a pyogenic abscess — which usually requires drainage — is clinically consequential, and the epidemiologic history is often the deciding factor.

Hydatid disease

Echinococcus granulosus, with exposure to dogs and livestock in endemic regions. The sonographic appearances are staged, and the staging directs management:

- **Simple unilocular cyst** with a fine wall, indistinguishable from a simple cyst without epidemiologic context.
- **Cyst with detached endocyst membrane** floating within the fluid — the **"water lily" sign**, effectively pathognomonic.
- **Multivesicular cyst with daughter cysts** in a honeycomb or rosette arrangement — the classic and most recognizable form.
- **Heterogeneous, degenerating cyst** with a solid appearance.
- **Calcified, inactive cyst** with dense wall calcification and shadowing.

"Hydatid sand" — mobile echogenic debris within the cyst that shifts with position change — is a supportive sign.

Aspiration carries a risk of anaphylaxis and of dissemination and is not undertaken casually; the sonographic recognition matters precisely because it changes the procedural decision. A formal staging classification exists and should be used. [VERIFY: current WHO-IWGE classification of cystic echinococcosis and its management implications]

Fungal infection

Hepatosplenic candidiasis occurs in profoundly immunocompromised patients, particularly during neutrophil recovery in hematologic malignancy. The classic descriptions are the **"wheel within a wheel"** appearance and the **bull's-eye lesion**, evolving to uniformly hypoechoic lesions and eventually to echogenic calcified scars.

The clinical context — persistent fever in a neutropenic patient despite antibacterial therapy — is often what prompts the study, and the lesions may only become apparent as the neutrophil count recovers.

Schistosomiasis

Endemic in large parts of Africa, the Middle East, South America, and Asia, and a major global cause of **non-cirrhotic portal hypertension**.

The characteristic finding is **marked periportal fibrosis** — thickened, brightly echogenic bands surrounding the portal branches, described as a mosaic or "turtle-back" pattern. Crucially, the **liver parenchyma between the fibrotic bands is relatively preserved**, and the presentation is portal hypertension with **relatively preserved synthetic function** — a pattern that should prompt consideration of schistosomiasis where the epidemiology fits, rather than an assumption of cirrhosis.

Granulomatous and other inflammatory disease

Tuberculosis and sarcoidosis produce small hypoechoic lesions or, in healed disease, calcified granulomas with clean shadowing. **Hepatic involvement in inflammatory bowel disease**, **primary sclerosing cholangitis**, and **autoimmune hepatitis** are recognized in their biliary and parenchymal patterns, with PSC developed in Chapter 5.

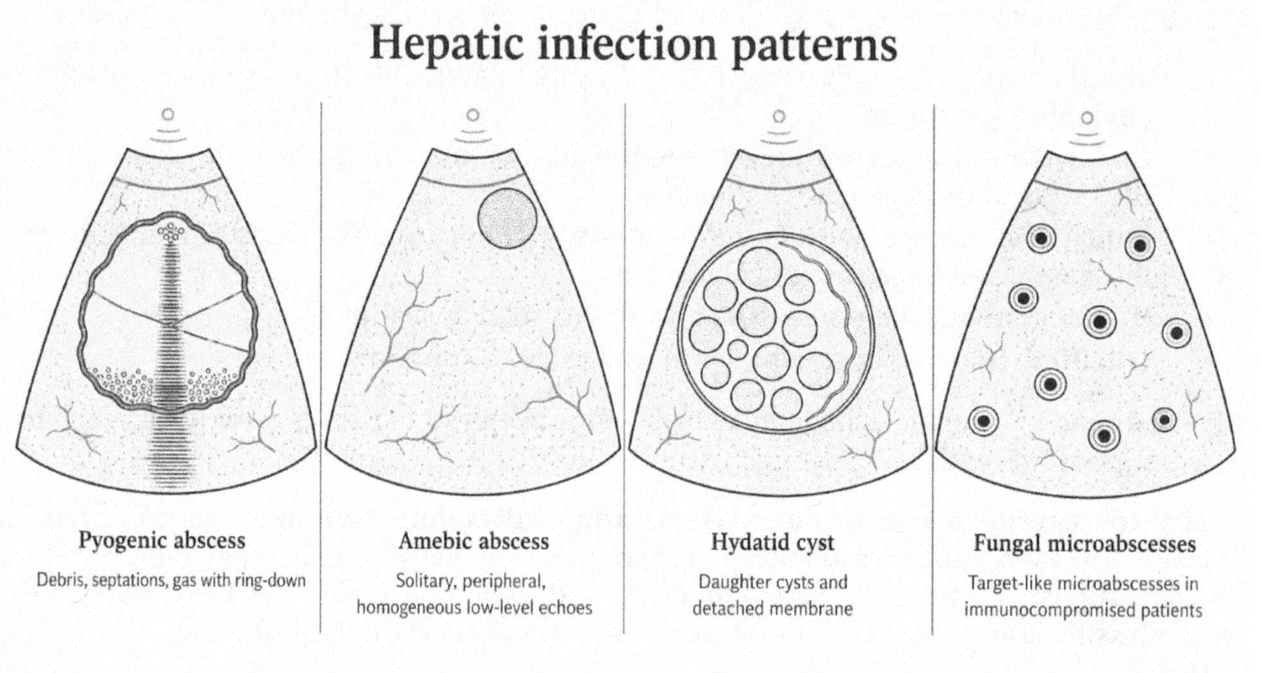

4.9 Vascular Disorders: Portal Vein Thrombosis and Budd-Chiari Syndrome

Portal vein thrombosis

Causes divide usefully into three groups: **cirrhosis and portal hypertension** (the commonest), **local inflammatory or infective processes** (pancreatitis, cholangitis, appendicitis, diverticulitis — pylephlebitis), and **prothrombotic states and malignancy**.

Findings. Echogenic material within the portal lumen with **absent or partial flow** on color and spectral Doppler. Acute thrombus may be nearly anechoic and therefore **easily missed on B-mode alone** — this is a case where color Doppler is not optional. The vein may be expanded. Where the thrombus is occlusive, no flow is detected; where partial, flow is seen around a filling defect.

The critical distinction — bland versus tumor thrombus:

	Bland thrombus	Tumor thrombus
Internal flow	**None**	**Arterial flow within the thrombus**

	Bland thrombus	Tumor thrombus
Vein caliber	Normal or mildly expanded	Characteristically **expanded**
Context	Any of the causes above	Adjacent HCC, or HCC elsewhere in the liver
Contrast behavior	No enhancement	Enhances in the arterial phase

Demonstrating **arterial signal within the thrombus** establishes tumor thrombus. This is a staging determination that affects operability and transplant candidacy, and it must be sought deliberately with a low-velocity color setting and spectral confirmation.

Cavernous transformation is the chronic sequel of occlusion: the thrombosed vein is replaced by a tangle of periportal collateral channels. On color Doppler this appears as a **mass of small serpiginous vessels at the porta** where a single portal vein should be — an appearance that is unmistakable once seen and easily misread as a mass on B-mode alone.

Budd-Chiari syndrome

Hepatic venous outflow obstruction, at the level of the hepatic veins, the IVC, or both. Causes include prothrombotic states, malignancy, membranous webs, and extrinsic compression.

Findings:

- **Absent, reversed, or turbulent flow in the hepatic veins**, with loss of the normal multiphasic waveform.
- Hepatic veins that are **narrowed, non-visualized, or filled with echogenic thrombus**.
- **Intrahepatic collateral "spider-web" vessels** — a highly characteristic tangle of small collaterals connecting obstructed hepatic veins.
- **Caudate lobe hypertrophy**, because its separate direct venous drainage into the IVC is preserved — the anatomic point from §4.1 becoming a diagnostic sign.
- **Ascites**, often prominent and early.
- Altered hepatic echotexture, with the caudate relatively spared.
- In IVC involvement, thrombus or narrowing of the IVC with reversed or absent flow.

The combination of ascites, altered hepatic veins, and a hypertrophied caudate should prompt explicit interrogation of hepatic venous flow, which is otherwise easily overlooked.

Other hepatic vascular conditions

Portal venous gas. Echogenic foci moving within the portal flow, and characteristically distributed **peripherally**, extending to within a short distance of the capsule, because portal flow carries them outward. This distinguishes it from **pneumobilia**, which is **central** and moves toward the porta. The distinction is critical: **portal venous gas in an adult suggests bowel ischemia or necrosis and is a critical finding requiring immediate escalation**

(Chapter 1 §1.5), whereas pneumobilia is often an expected post-procedural or post-sphincterotomy finding.

Hepatic artery pseudoaneurysm — post-traumatic, post-procedural, or infective, showing the yin-yang swirling color pattern and a to-and-fro neck waveform (Chapter 3 §3.8).

Arterioportal shunting — from trauma, biopsy, cirrhosis, or tumor, producing arterialized portal flow.

Sinusoidal obstruction syndrome (veno-occlusive disease) — following stem cell transplantation or certain chemotherapies, with hepatomegaly, ascites, gallbladder wall thickening, and reduced or reversed portal flow.

Hereditary hemorrhagic telangiectasia — with characteristic hepatic vascular malformations and shunting.

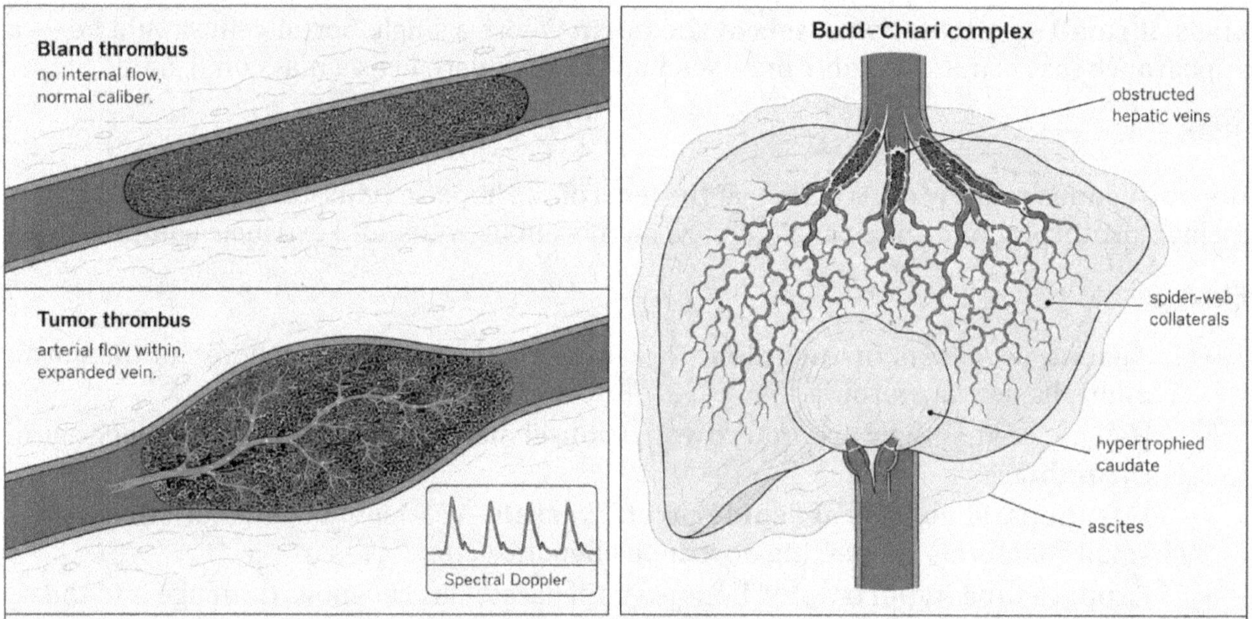

Bland versus tumor thrombus, and the Budd–Chiari complex.

4.10 Pitfalls, Pseudolesions, and Focal Fatty Change

Focal fatty sparing and focal fatty infiltration

The commonest pseudolesions in abdominal sonography, and the source of a large volume of unnecessary follow-up imaging.

Focal fatty sparing — an island of normal parenchyma within a diffusely steatotic liver, appearing **hypoechoic** against the bright background.

Focal fatty infiltration — a region of focal fat within an otherwise normal liver, appearing **hyperechoic**.

Both occur in **characteristic locations**, which is the first and best discriminator. These are regions with anomalous venous supply — perfused partly by systemic rather than portal blood — and the pattern is consistent:

- **Adjacent to the gallbladder fossa**
- **Anterior to the porta hepatis, in segment IV**
- **Adjacent to the falciform ligament and ligamentum teres**
- **Subcapsular regions**

The discriminating features, applied together:

	Focal fatty change	True lesion
Location	Characteristic sites above	Anywhere
Shape	**Geometric** — wedge, band, or sheet with straight, angular margins	Rounded, convex
Margins	Conform to no anatomic or vascular boundary; may be sharply linear	Defined by the lesion's own edge
Mass effect	**None** — vessels run undisturbed straight through the region	Displaces or deforms vessels
Contour	Does not bulge the capsule	May bulge the capsule
Doppler	Normal vessels traversing	May show its own vascularity

The single most reliable sign is the absence of mass effect. A vessel that passes straight through a region of altered echogenicity without deviation is passing through altered parenchyma, not through a mass. Look for it deliberately.

Where doubt persists, **CEUS resolves it** — focal fatty change enhances identically to surrounding liver in all phases.

Other pseudolesions and technical pitfalls

Ligamentum teres. In transverse section, a round echogenic focus in the left lobe, sometimes with posterior shadowing, routinely mistaken for a calcified lesion or a stone. Resolved by scanning longitudinally, where it is clearly a linear structure running to the umbilicus.

Segment IV pseudolesion. The area anterior to the porta, subject to focal fatty change as above, and a recurrent source of false-positive reports.

Riedel's lobe. An inferior extension of the right lobe, easily called hepatomegaly. Recognize it by its continuity with the right lobe and normal echotexture.

Diaphragmatic slips. Hypoechoic bands indenting the hepatic surface, mistaken for subcapsular lesions or fluid.

Hypertrophied caudate in cirrhosis, mistaken for a mass at the porta.

The dome. Segments VII and VIII are the most under-imaged regions of the liver. Rib shadowing and near-field position conspire against them, and a lesion here is the classic miss. **Use intercostal windows with the probe rotated into the rib space**, and use deep inspiration.

Near-field subcapsular lesions. Lost in the curvilinear probe's poor near field. **Switch to a high-frequency linear probe** for the anterior surface. This is the same maneuver that demonstrates surface nodularity in §4.4, and it is omitted far more often than it should be.

Mirror image above the diaphragm. Hepatic tissue and lesions duplicated into the thorax (Chapter 2 §2.8). Recognized by the equal-distance geometry and resolved by changing the window.

Side-lobe and section-thickness echoes within cysts and the gallbladder, producing false internal content (Chapter 2 §2.7). Rescan orthogonally and check on harmonics.

Compounding-suppressed enhancement making a simple cyst appear solid or a stone appear non-shadowing (Chapter 2 §2.4). Turn compounding off before concluding.

Key Points

1. Determine which examination you are performing — diffuse disease survey or lesion characterization — before you start, because they require different protocols and different reports.
2. Localize by segment using two views: the hepatic vein confluence gives the superior set, the portal bifurcation gives the inferior set.
3. The functional lobar division runs in the principal plane along the middle hepatic vein, not along the falciform ligament.
4. Acquire a liver-and-right-kidney image in the same frame at matched depth and gain on every study. Without it, a statement about echogenicity cannot be verified.
5. Use the high-frequency linear probe for the anterior surface. It is how you detect cirrhotic nodularity and how you find subcapsular lesions, and it is routinely omitted.
6. Document portal flow direction on every liver study. It takes fifteen seconds and is the finding most likely to change management.
7. B-mode cannot grade steatosis reliably, cannot separate fat from fibrosis, and cannot exclude significant fibrosis in a bright liver. Say so.
8. Gallbladder wall thickening in hepatitis, cirrhosis, and hypoalbuminemia is reactive, not cholecystitis.
9. A hemangioma in a fatty liver may be hypoechoic. The lesion has not changed; the background has.
10. FNH does not hemorrhage or transform; adenoma does both. Ultrasound often cannot separate them, and saying so is the correct report.
11. HCC washes out late and mildly; metastasis washes out early and markedly. This is the core discriminator of hepatic contrast imaging.
12. A hypoechoic halo around a lesion is a malignancy sign and should raise concern regardless of internal appearance.

13. Arterial flow within a portal vein thrombus establishes tumor thrombus, which changes staging and operability. Look for it deliberately.
14. Portal venous gas is peripheral and suggests bowel ischemia — a critical finding. Pneumobilia is central and often benign.
15. Focal fatty change is geometric, sits in characteristic locations, and exerts no mass effect. A vessel running straight through a region of altered echogenicity is running through parenchyma, not a mass.
16. Segments VII and VIII are the most commonly under-imaged regions of the liver. Use rotated intercostal windows and deep inspiration.

Registry Check

1. A hepatic lesion lies superior to the portal bifurcation plane and between the right and middle hepatic veins. It occupies segment:

A. V **B.** VI **C.** VII **D.** VIII

> **Answer: D.** The right and middle hepatic veins bound the right anterior sector, which contains segments V and VIII. Above the portal bifurcation the segment is VIII; below it, V. Segments VI and VII lie in the right posterior sector, lateral to the right hepatic vein.

2. A 2 cm hyperechoic, well-defined, lobulated lesion with posterior acoustic enhancement and no detectable color Doppler flow is found incidentally in a normal liver. On CEUS it shows peripheral nodular discontinuous arterial enhancement with centripetal fill-in and no washout. This is:

A. Hepatocellular carcinoma **B.** Hemangioma **C.** Focal nodular hyperplasia **D.** Metastasis

> **Answer: B.** Peripheral nodular discontinuous enhancement progressing centripetally without washout is the characteristic and essentially diagnostic contrast pattern of hemangioma. FNH fills centrifugally in a spoke-wheel pattern; HCC and metastasis both wash out, at different times and to different degrees.

3. The single most useful feature distinguishing hepatocellular carcinoma from metastasis on contrast-enhanced ultrasound is:

A. Arterial phase enhancement **B.** Lesion size **C.** Timing and degree of washout **D.** Presence of posterior acoustic enhancement

> **Answer: C.** Both enhance in the arterial phase, so that feature does not discriminate. HCC washes out late and mildly; metastasis washes out early and markedly. Combined with the background liver and clinical context, this is the core of hepatic contrast interpretation.

4. Echogenic foci are seen moving within hepatic vessels and extending peripherally to within a short distance of the liver capsule. This finding indicates:

A. Pneumobilia, likely post-sphincterotomy **B.** Portal venous gas, requiring urgent escalation **C.** Hepatic artery calcification **D.** Comet-tail artifact from biliary hamartomas

> **Answer: B.** Portal flow carries gas outward, so portal venous gas is distributed peripherally. Pneumobilia is central and moves toward the porta because bile flows inward. Portal venous gas in an adult suggests bowel ischemia or necrosis and is a critical finding.

5. A hypoechoic region with straight angular margins is seen adjacent to the gallbladder fossa in a diffusely echogenic liver. A portal branch traverses the region without deviation and the hepatic capsule above it is undistorted. The most likely diagnosis is:

A. Metastasis **B.** Hepatocellular carcinoma **C.** Focal fatty sparing **D.** Abscess

> **Answer: C.** Geometric margins, a characteristic location, and — decisively — the absence of mass effect on the traversing vessel and the capsule identify focal fatty sparing. A true lesion displaces vessels and may bulge the contour.

6. Which finding most strongly supports a diagnosis of cirrhosis?

A. Increased parenchymal echogenicity **B.** Hepatomegaly **C.** Nodular surface contour on high-frequency linear imaging **D.** Gallbladder wall thickening

> **Answer: C.** Surface nodularity is the most specific sonographic sign of cirrhosis and is best demonstrated with a high-frequency linear probe along the anterior surface. Increased echogenicity indicates fat or fibrosis non-specifically; gallbladder wall thickening is a reactive finding with many causes.

7. Echogenic material expands the main portal vein, and color Doppler demonstrates pulsatile arterial signal within it. This indicates:

A. Bland thrombus **B.** Tumor thrombus **C.** Cavernous transformation **D.** Slow flow artifact

> **Answer: B.** Bland thrombus contains no flow. Arterial signal within the thrombus, particularly with expansion of the vein, establishes tumor thrombus — most often from hepatocellular carcinoma — and is a staging determination affecting operability and transplant candidacy.

8. A patient presents with ascites and hepatomegaly. Hepatic veins are narrowed with absent flow, a tangle of fine intrahepatic collaterals is seen, and the caudate lobe is enlarged. The diagnosis is:

A. Cirrhosis with portal hypertension **B.** Budd-Chiari syndrome **C.** Portal vein thrombosis **D.** Right heart failure

> **Answer: B.** Hepatic venous outflow obstruction with spider-web collaterals and caudate hypertrophy defines Budd-Chiari syndrome. The caudate enlarges because its short veins drain directly into the IVC, bypassing the obstructed main hepatic veins. Right heart failure produces dilated hepatic veins with increased pulsatility, not obstruction.

Chapter Notes for the Editorial Pass

Verification queue. The tags in this chapter carry more clinical weight than in any preceding chapter, and none should be published as written. In priority order: **CEUS washout timing criteria** (§4.6, §4.7) — the chapter's central discriminator, and the criteria are formally defined and periodically revised; **HCC surveillance interval and modality** (§4.4); **caudate-to-right-lobe ratio threshold and technique** (§4.4); **portal vein diameter and splenic length thresholds** (§4.5); **TIPS velocity criteria**, which are stent-type and institution dependent (§4.5); **WHO-IWGE echinococcosis classification** (§4.8); hepatic span reference ranges (§4.1); and attenuation-quantification thresholds for steatosis (§4.4, carried from Chapter 2).

Terminology note for the editorial pass. This chapter deliberately does not use a formal lesion-reporting classification system for HCC, since those systems are jurisdiction- and modality-specific and are revised on their own cycle. If the book is to reference one, it should be introduced once with its version and date, and applied consistently — a decision to make before Chapter 9 rather than after.

Figure count: 6 Lane A, 3 Lane B. Lane B demand is rising as predicted: the hepatorenal comparison set (`fig-4-3`), the pseudolesion-versus-lesion pair (`fig-4-9`), and — not yet specified — a CEUS phase sequence, which should be added if a source can be secured. CEUS clips are difficult to license and the author's own archive is the realistic route.

Cross-reference targets to fix at layout: §4.1 caudate drainage → §4.9 Budd-Chiari; §4.3 cholestatic pattern → Chapter 5; §4.4 elastography confounders → Chapter 2 §2.10; §4.5 collaterals → Chapter 3 §3.6; §4.7 biliary malignancy → Chapter 5; §4.9 transplant vascular assessment → Chapter 9; §4.10 artifact pitfalls → Chapter 2 §2.7–2.8.

Word count: approximately 10,400 excluding image prompt blocks, learning objectives, registry questions, and these notes.

Chapter 5: The Gallbladder and Biliary System

Learning Objectives

On completing this chapter you should be able to:

1. Identify the gallbladder and biliary tree using the main lobar fissure and portal triad landmarks, and recognize the normal variants that mimic disease.
2. Perform a hepatobiliary protocol that demonstrates stone mobility, elicits a sonographic Murphy sign, and measures the wall and duct correctly.
3. Apply the three criteria for cholelithiasis and distinguish stones from polyps, sludge, and adjacent duodenal gas.
4. Assemble the sonographic diagnosis of acute cholecystitis from its component findings and state which carries the most weight.
5. Recognize gangrenous, emphysematous, and perforated cholecystitis, and identify which constitute critical findings.
6. Work through a differential for gallbladder wall thickening that begins with the commonest cause rather than the most serious.
7. Distinguish adenomyomatosis, cholesterol polyp, and carcinoma, and state the artifact that identifies the first.
8. Determine the level of biliary obstruction from the pattern of ductal dilatation and gallbladder distension.
9. Describe the technical approaches that improve visualization of the distal common bile duct, and state the modality's limits.
10. Recognize normal postoperative appearances and the complications of cholecystectomy.

The Highest-Volume Study in the Abdomen

Right upper quadrant pain is one of the commonest reasons an ultrasound is ordered anywhere in the world, and the gallbladder is the structure this modality assesses better than any other. CT is inferior for stones. MRI is superior for the ducts but slower, costlier, and not available at the bedside. For the gallbladder itself, **ultrasound is the reference standard**, and the diagnosis usually rests entirely on your images.

That places unusual weight on technique. Almost every diagnostic failure in this chapter is a technical failure: a stone missed because the patient was not repositioned, a wall called thick in a patient who had eaten, a Murphy sign not elicited, a distal duct not pursued past bowel gas. The pathology in this chapter is not subtle. The scanning is.

5.1 Normal Anatomy and Physiology

The gallbladder

A pear-shaped reservoir on the inferior surface of the liver, lying in the gallbladder fossa at the interface between the right and left functional lobes. It is described in four parts:

- **Fundus** — the rounded blind end, projecting beyond the inferior hepatic margin
- **Body** — the main reservoir
- **Neck** — narrowing toward the cystic duct
- **Infundibulum (Hartmann's pouch)** — a dilatation at the junction of neck and cystic duct, where stones characteristically impact

The **cystic duct** contains the **spiral valves of Heister**, a mucosal fold arrangement that keeps the duct patent but which is rarely resolved sonographically and makes the cystic duct itself difficult to follow.

The main lobar fissure is the key landmark. This echogenic line runs from the right portal vein to the gallbladder neck, and it is the most reliable way to locate a contracted, stone-filled, or otherwise inconspicuous gallbladder. When you cannot find the gallbladder, find the right portal vein and follow the fissure.

Normal measurements. The wall is thin and measures under 3 mm **when the gallbladder is adequately distended** — a qualification that carries most of the diagnostic weight in §5.6. Length is conventionally under 10 cm and transverse diameter under 4–5 cm. [VERIFY: current reference values for gallbladder wall thickness, length, and transverse diameter, and the distension conditions under which they apply]

Normal variants

These are common and each is regularly misreported:

Phrygian cap — a fold of the fundus back on itself, producing an apparent septation at the fundus. Entirely normal.

Junctional folds — kinks at the body-neck junction, which can appear as a septation or trap a stone.

Septations and duplication — true septate or duplicated gallbladders, uncommon but reported.

Agenesis and ectopic position — including intrahepatic and left-sided gallbladders. Before diagnosing agenesis, exclude a contracted stone-filled gallbladder, which is far more common and can be nearly invisible except for its wall-echo-shadow signature (§5.3).

A fold produces an apparent discontinuity that **changes with position and plane**; a true septation does not. Rescan in a second plane before reporting either.

The biliary tree

Bile drains from the intrahepatic ducts, which run **within the portal triads alongside the portal vein branches**, to the **right and left hepatic ducts**, which unite at the porta to form the **common hepatic duct**. The **cystic duct** joins to form the **common bile duct**, which descends in the hepatoduodenal ligament, passes **through the head of the pancreas**, and enters the duodenum at the **ampulla of Vater**, usually after joining the pancreatic duct, under the control of the **sphincter of Oddi**.

Sonographic landmarks:

The portal triad at the porta hepatis in transverse section gives the classic **"Mickey Mouse"** configuration: the portal vein forms the face, and the **common bile duct (anterolateral, to the patient's right)** and **hepatic artery (medial)** form the two ears. Distinguishing duct from artery is done with **color Doppler**, which should be applied routinely rather than reserved for doubt — the two are of similar caliber and the error is easy.

In longitudinal section, the CBD runs anterior to the portal vein. The **right hepatic artery** commonly crosses **between** the CBD and the portal vein, and is a recurrent source of confusion.

Normal duct caliber. The common duct is conventionally measured at or near the porta, and the normal upper limit is small — around 6 mm in most adults, with two caveats that matter constantly: the duct **enlarges after cholecystectomy**, and duct caliber is widely held to **increase modestly with age**, though the extent of the age effect is debated. [VERIFY: current normal upper limits for common bile duct diameter, the post-cholecystectomy allowance, and the evidence for age-related increase]

Intrahepatic ducts are normally not visible or barely so. When they become apparent alongside portal branches, the result is the **"parallel channel"** or **"double-barrel"** appearance, and on a broader survey the impression of **"too many tubes"** in the liver — both signs of dilatation, and both confirmed by demonstrating absence of flow with color Doppler.

Physiology

The liver secretes bile continuously. Between meals, the sphincter of Oddi is closed and bile is diverted into the gallbladder, which **concentrates it substantially** by absorbing water and electrolytes.

Fat and protein entering the duodenum trigger release of **cholecystokinin**, which causes the gallbladder to contract and the sphincter to relax.

Two practical consequences follow, and both are central to this chapter:

1. **A recently fed patient has a contracted gallbladder with an apparently thick wall.** This is the commonest single cause of "gallbladder wall thickening" reported anywhere, and it is not disease.
2. **A contracted gallbladder cannot be assessed for stones or wall thickness.** If the patient has eaten, the correct response is to state the limitation and rebook, not to report findings from an uninterpretable organ.

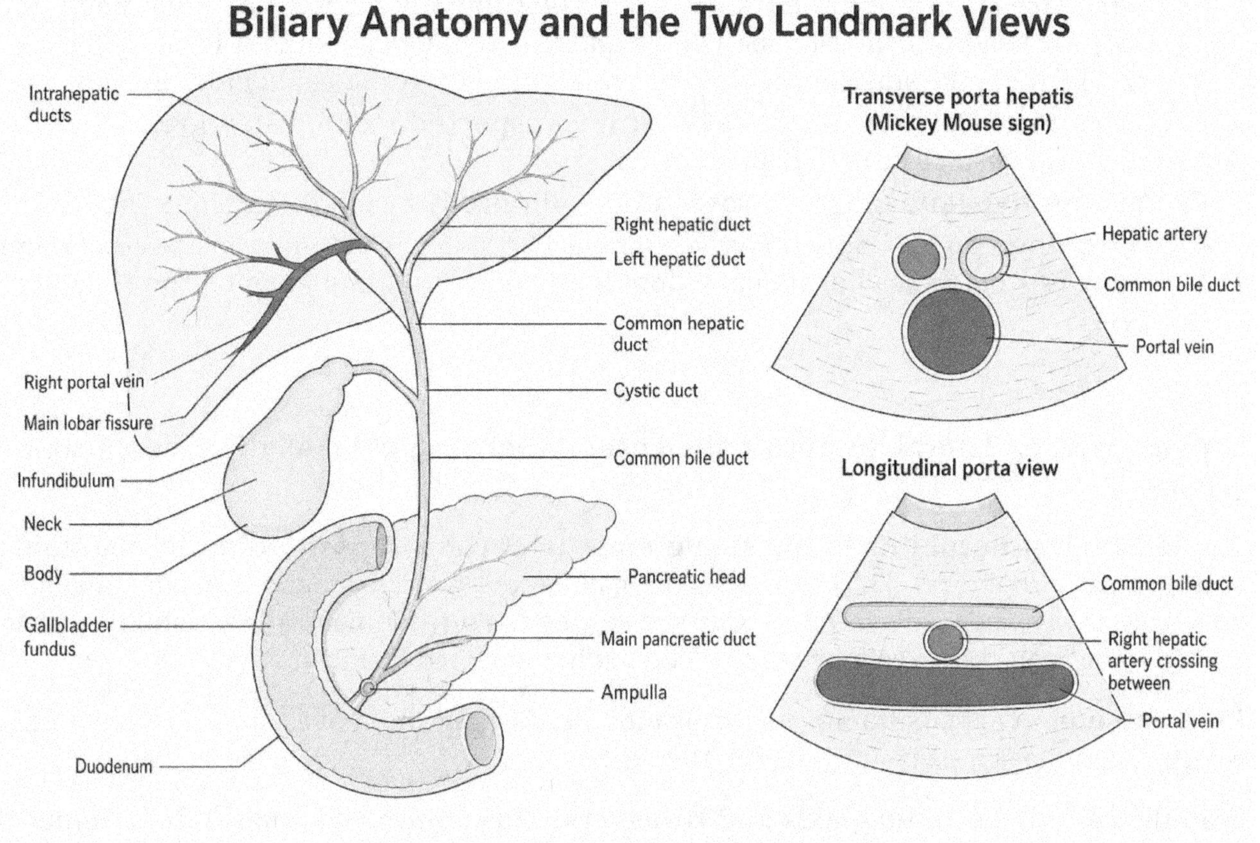

Left: biliary anatomy. Right: the two classic sonographic landmark views.

5.2 Scanning Protocol and Patient Preparation

Preparation

Fasting is not optional for this study. The patient should have taken nothing by mouth for a defined interval so that the gallbladder is distended and its wall assessable. [VERIFY: institutional fasting interval for hepatobiliary ultrasound]

Where the patient has eaten, you have two defensible options: perform the study and **report explicitly that the gallbladder was contracted and could not be assessed for calculi or wall thickness**, or rebook. What is not defensible is reporting a thick wall or a stone-free gallbladder from a contracted organ.

Transducers and settings

Curvilinear for the survey. **High-frequency linear** for the anterior wall, for small polyps, and for wall detail — the same discipline as the hepatic surface in Chapter 4, and equally often skipped.

Settings that matter here more than anywhere:

- **Turn spatial compounding OFF when assessing for stones.** Compounding fills in acoustic shadows and can abolish the shadow behind a genuine calculus (Chapter 2 §2.4). This is the single most consequential setting error in gallbladder imaging.
- **Place the focal zone at the level of the suspected stone.** Lateral resolution and shadow conspicuity both depend on it.
- **Narrow dynamic range** improves stone conspicuity by increasing contrast.
- **Harmonics on** to suppress near-field reverberation and side-lobe echoes that mimic sludge — but check questionable low-level content on fundamental too (Chapter 2 §2.4).

The examination

Supine, then left lateral decubitus, then erect where possible. All three, as a matter of routine.

The **left lateral decubitus is the single most important repositioning in abdominal sonography** (Chapter 3 §3.3). It brings the gallbladder anteriorly and medially, displaces bowel gas away, and — decisively — **causes stones to roll**, demonstrating mobility. A stone that has not been shown to move has not been distinguished from a polyp.

Erect or semi-erect positioning confirms mobility further and moves stones to the fundus, which can unmask a stone impacted in the neck.

Scan the gallbladder in **long axis and transverse throughout its length**, from fundus to neck, using **subcostal in deep inspiration** and **intercostal** windows. The **neck and infundibulum must be seen specifically** — an impacted stone here is the classic miss, because it does not move, sits in the least accessible part of the organ, and is often obscured by adjacent duodenal gas.

Three measurements and one sign

Wall thickness. Measure the **anterior wall**, perpendicular to it, on a distended gallbladder. Measuring the posterior wall is unreliable because posterior acoustic enhancement alters its apparent thickness.

Gallbladder dimensions, where distension or contraction is relevant.

Common bile duct diameter. Measured at or near the porta, perpendicular to the duct axis, **inner wall to inner wall**. Confirm with color Doppler that you are measuring the duct and not the hepatic artery.

The sonographic Murphy sign. Elicited by locating the gallbladder, then applying graded pressure **directly over it** while watching the patient's response, and comparing with pressure applied elsewhere in the right upper quadrant. It is positive when maximal tenderness is reproducibly localized to the gallbladder itself.

This is an active maneuver requiring you to elicit and interpret it, and it is the finding that most often converts a set of ambiguous images into a diagnosis. It is also the finding most often not performed. Its value falls in patients who have received analgesia, in the obtunded, and — importantly — in gangrenous cholecystitis, where mural necrosis may abolish it (§5.5).

Documentation

At minimum: gallbladder long axis and transverse; the neck and infundibulum specifically; any calculus with its shadow, plus an image in a second position demonstrating mobility; anterior wall thickness measurement; pericholecystic region; the CBD at the porta with measurement and color Doppler confirmation; the intrahepatic ducts; the visualized portion of the distal CBD; and the pancreatic head where seen.

State what was not seen — most often the distal duct — rather than omitting it silently.

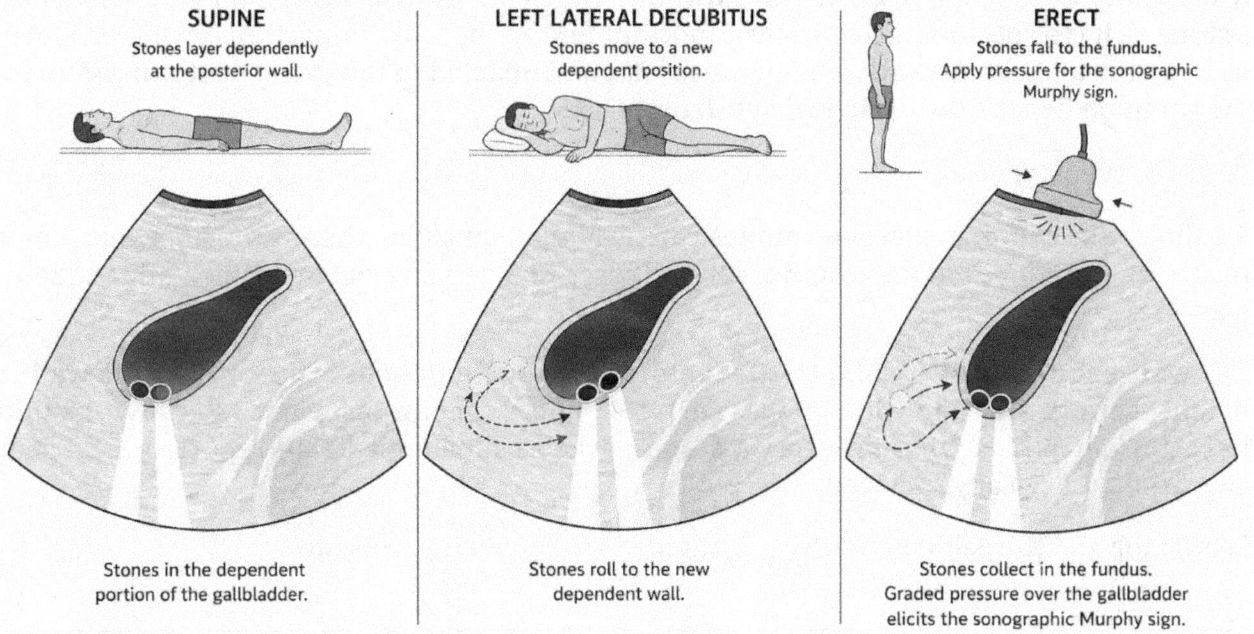

5.3 Cholelithiasis and Its Mimics

The three criteria

A gallstone satisfies three criteria, and all three should be sought:

1. **Echogenic focus** within the lumen
2. **Posterior acoustic shadowing**
3. **Mobility** with change in patient position

Meeting all three is diagnostic. Failing any one requires explanation.

When the shadow is absent

Small stones frequently fail to shadow convincingly, and the response is technical rather than interpretive. Before concluding that a focus does not shadow:

- **Turn spatial compounding off.** This alone recovers the shadow in a substantial proportion of cases.
- **Move the focal zone to the level of the stone.** A stone in the far field of a beam focused elsewhere sits in a wide beam that fills the shadow laterally.
- **Increase the frequency** if penetration allows — shadowing improves.
- **Narrow the dynamic range** to increase contrast.
- **Reposition** so the stone lies within the beam rather than at the edge of the sector.

Only after all of these should a focus be described as non-shadowing.

When mobility is absent

A stone impacted at the **neck or infundibulum** does not move. This is not evidence against a stone — it is a specific and clinically important finding, because impaction is what produces obstruction and cholecystitis, and because a stone impacted in the cystic duct can compress the common hepatic duct (**Mirizzi syndrome**, §5.5).

The wall-echo-shadow complex

A gallbladder contracted around stones can be almost invisible: there is no anechoic lumen to attract attention, and the whole organ collapses to a curved echogenic line with a shadow behind it.

The **wall-echo-shadow (WES) triad** identifies it: a thin **hypoechoic outer line** (the wall), a **bright echogenic line** (the stone surface), and a **clean acoustic shadow** behind. Recognizing WES is what prevents a stone-packed gallbladder being reported as absent, agenetic, or surgically removed.

Search for it at the gallbladder fossa, located via the main lobar fissure.

The mimics

Mimic	Distinguishing features
Polyp	Non-mobile, attached to the wall, **no shadow**, may show internal flow with a vascular stalk, usually small
Sludge	Mobile but **slowly**, layers dependently with a **fluid-fluid level**, **no shadow**, conforms to the lumen shape, may swirl with movement
Tumefactive sludge	A rounded sludge ball mimicking a mass — non-shadowing, **no internal flow**, and changes shape and position over minutes and with repositioning
Adjacent duodenal gas	Produces **dirty** shadowing rather than clean, lies **outside** the wall, and **changes appearance over seconds** as gas moves. Watch it in real time
Gallbladder wall calcification (porcelain)	Wall-based rather than intraluminal, may show a broad shadow following the wall contour

Mimic	Distinguishing features
Folds and septations	Change with plane and position
Side-lobe and section-thickness artifact	Curved arcs or low-level echoes with no shadow; resolve on harmonics or in an orthogonal plane (Chapter 2 §2.7)

The gas discrimination deserves emphasis. The clean-versus-dirty shadow distinction from Chapter 2 §2.7 is used here more than anywhere else in the body: a stone at the gallbladder neck and duodenal gas behind it look similar on a still image and completely different in real time and on shadow character.

Related entities

Cholesterolosis ("strawberry gallbladder") — cholesterol deposition in the mucosa, usually invisible sonographically or producing tiny non-shadowing mural echogenic foci.

Milk of calcium bile — a suspension of calcium salts that layers dependently and can be strikingly echogenic with shadowing, mimicking a stone-filled gallbladder but shifting as a fluid level.

Porcelain gallbladder — mural calcification, historically associated with carcinoma, though the strength of that association is now regarded as lower than once taught. [VERIFY: current understanding of the porcelain gallbladder–carcinoma association and management recommendations]

5.4 Acute and Chronic Cholecystitis

Acute calculous cholecystitis

The pathophysiology is obstruction: a stone impacts in the neck or cystic duct, the gallbladder cannot empty, pressure rises, the wall becomes inflamed and then ischemic. The sonographic findings follow that sequence, and none of them is diagnostic alone.

The findings, in descending order of usefulness:

1. Positive sonographic Murphy sign. Maximal, reproducible tenderness localized to the gallbladder under direct transducer pressure. Combined with the presence of stones, this is the highest-yield combination available and is the reason the maneuver must actually be performed. Its value is reduced by analgesia, altered consciousness, and mural necrosis (§5.5).

2. Cholelithiasis, particularly a stone impacted at the neck or in the cystic duct. The great majority of acute cholecystitis is calculous.

3. Gallbladder wall thickening beyond 3 mm on the anterior wall of a **distended** gallbladder. Non-specific in isolation — the whole of §5.6 exists because of this.

4. Pericholecystic fluid — a rim of fluid outside the wall, in the absence of generalized ascites.

5. Gallbladder distension, with a rounded rather than pear-shaped contour under tension.

6. Mural hyperemia on color Doppler, reflecting inflammation. Useful when present; its absence does not exclude the diagnosis and, in a thick-walled tender gallbladder, **absent** flow should raise concern for gangrene.

7. Striated or layered wall, which may indicate edema — or, when marked and irregular, gangrene.

The diagnosis is a composite. Report the components you found, and be explicit about the constellation rather than issuing a bare label. "Cholelithiasis with a stone impacted at the neck, anterior wall thickness 5 mm, pericholecystic fluid, and a strongly positive sonographic Murphy sign" is a far more useful report than "acute cholecystitis," because it lets the surgeon weigh the evidence.

Acalculous cholecystitis

Cholecystitis without stones, occurring in **critically ill patients** — major trauma, burns, sepsis, prolonged fasting and total parenteral nutrition, mechanical ventilation, and the postoperative state.

It is **substantially more difficult to diagnose**, for compounding reasons: the reassuring anchor of stones is absent; the sonographic Murphy sign is usually unobtainable in a sedated or ventilated patient; and the same population has many alternative causes of wall thickening (§5.6) — hypoalbuminemia, fluid overload, heart failure, and prolonged fasting itself, which produces a distended, sludge-filled gallbladder as a normal consequence.

Rely on the combination of marked wall thickening, distension, pericholecystic fluid, sludge, and mural changes, interpreted against the clinical picture, and communicate the degree of diagnostic uncertainty honestly. Mortality in this group is high and the threshold for escalation should be low.

Chronic cholecystitis

Repeated episodes of inflammation produce a **contracted, thick-walled, stone-containing gallbladder**, often with the WES appearance. The wall may be uniformly thickened and fibrotic, and the organ fails to distend even after fasting.

The distinction from acute cholecystitis rests on the absence of tenderness, distension, and pericholecystic fluid — a small firm gallbladder rather than a tense inflamed one.

Xanthogranulomatous cholecystitis is an uncommon chronic form with intramural hypoechoic nodules, marked wall thickening, and a propensity to mimic carcinoma both sonographically and at surgery.

5.5 Complicated Cholecystitis: Gangrenous, Emphysematous, Perforated

These are surgical emergencies and their recognition changes management immediately. All three warrant prompt communication rather than routine reporting (Chapter 1 §1.5).

Gangrenous cholecystitis

Mural ischemia and necrosis following sustained raised intraluminal pressure. It carries substantially higher morbidity than uncomplicated cholecystitis and often requires urgent surgery.

Findings:

- **Intraluminal membranes** — sloughed mucosa appearing as fine linear echoes floating within the lumen, **not attached to the wall along their length** and **not casting shadows**. This is the most specific sign and is the one to look for deliberately.
- **Marked, irregular, asymmetric wall thickening** with loss of the normal layered appearance.
- **Striated wall** with alternating hypoechoic and echogenic bands.
- **Focal wall defects or irregularity** of the mucosal contour.
- **Absent mural flow** on color Doppler in the necrotic segment — an important reversal of expectation, since inflammation ordinarily increases flow.
- **Pericholecystic fluid**, often prominent.
- **A negative or absent sonographic Murphy sign** in a patient who looks unwell. Mural nerve destruction can abolish tenderness, so a **falling** tenderness in a deteriorating patient is a warning sign rather than reassurance.

That last point is the trap: the sign that supported the diagnosis of uncomplicated cholecystitis can disappear precisely as the disease worsens.

Emphysematous cholecystitis

Gas-forming infection of the gallbladder wall and lumen. It is associated with **diabetes mellitus**, is more common in men, and carries a high risk of perforation and a high mortality. It is a **critical finding**.

Findings:

- **Gas within the gallbladder wall or lumen**, producing **dirty shadowing** and **ring-down artifact** (Chapter 2 §2.8). The clean-versus-dirty shadow discrimination and the comet-tail-versus-ring-down discrimination both do real work here.
- Echogenic foci **within the wall itself**, following its contour — the appearance sometimes described as a **"champagne" or "effervescent" gallbladder** when bubbles rise through the lumen.
- **Non-dependent** echogenic foci that **move to the highest point** with repositioning — gas rises, stones fall. This is the maneuver that distinguishes intraluminal gas from stones, and it is definitive.
- Often relatively **little pain** relative to the severity, which contributes to delayed diagnosis.

The differential is a stone-filled gallbladder or porcelain gallbladder, and it is resolved by shadow character and by the direction the foci move on repositioning.

Perforation

The consequence of untreated gangrene, and it may be contained, free, or into an adjacent viscus.

Findings:

- **A focal wall defect** — a discontinuity in the wall, sometimes called the **"hole sign"**. It is the direct sign and it requires deliberate careful inspection of the whole wall to find.
- **Pericholecystic collection or abscess** adjacent to the defect, often complex with debris.
- **Free intraperitoneal fluid**.
- Collapse of a previously distended gallbladder.

Cholecystoenteric fistula may follow, allowing gas to enter the biliary tree (**pneumobilia**, §5.10) and, occasionally, a stone to enter the bowel and obstruct it — **gallstone ileus**, classically with the triad of pneumobilia, small bowel obstruction, and an ectopic calculus.

Other complications

Empyema — the gallbladder filled with pus: distended, thick-walled, with echogenic non-shadowing debris filling the lumen and marked tenderness.

Mirizzi syndrome — a stone impacted in the cystic duct or gallbladder neck compressing the adjacent common hepatic duct, producing **obstructive jaundice with intrahepatic dilatation and a normal-caliber distal common bile duct**. The pattern is distinctive and is easily attributed to a distal lesion if the cystic duct region is not inspected. It matters surgically because it changes the operation and carries a higher risk of bile duct injury.

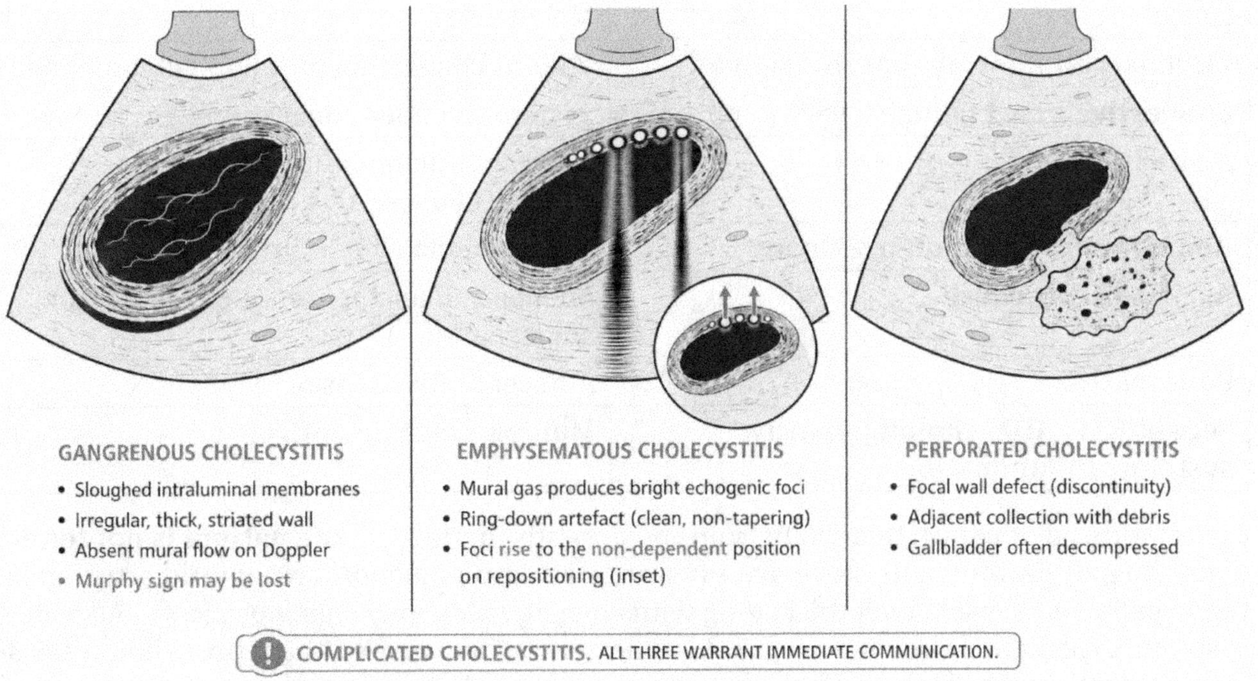

5.6 Gallbladder Wall Thickening: A Differential Approach

The reasoning error to avoid

Gallbladder wall thickening is the finding most likely to be over-interpreted in abdominal sonography. It is a **non-specific response** to a long list of local and systemic conditions, and its most common cause is not disease of the gallbladder at all.

The correct reasoning order is therefore:

1. **Is the gallbladder distended?** If contracted — because the patient ate — the wall is thick as a normal consequence and **the finding is uninterpretable**. This is the commonest explanation and it should be excluded first, every time.
2. **Is the thickening focal or diffuse?**
3. **If diffuse, is there a systemic cause?**
4. **If diffuse with no systemic cause, is there evidence of gallbladder inflammation?**
5. **If focal, is it adenomyomatosis, polyp, or carcinoma?**

Diffuse thickening with a systemic cause

In each of the following, the gallbladder wall is thick because of a process elsewhere, and the gallbladder is a bystander:

Cause	Mechanism
Recent food intake	Physiologic contraction — the commonest cause overall
Hypoalbuminemia	Reduced oncotic pressure, mural edema

Cause	Mechanism
Cirrhosis and portal hypertension	Venous congestion plus hypoalbuminemia
Congestive heart failure	Systemic venous congestion
Acute hepatitis	Adjacent inflammation and reactive edema (Chapter 4 §4.4)
Renal failure and fluid overload	Mural edema
Ascites of any cause	Edema, and an apparent thickening from adjacent fluid
Pancreatitis	Adjacent inflammation
Sepsis, HIV/AIDS cholangiopathy, systemic inflammation	Multiple mechanisms

Two features distinguish this group from cholecystitis in practice: **the patient is not tender over the gallbladder**, and **there are no stones and no pericholecystic fluid** attributable to the gallbladder itself. Wall thickening with a negative Murphy sign, no calculi, and a clear systemic explanation should be reported as a reactive finding, and the report should say so explicitly rather than leaving a bare measurement for a clinician to over-read.

Diffuse thickening from gallbladder disease

Acute cholecystitis (§5.4) — with stones, tenderness, distension, and pericholecystic fluid.

Chronic cholecystitis — contracted, fibrotic, stone-containing, non-tender.

Gangrenous cholecystitis (§5.5) — irregular, striated, with membranes and absent mural flow.

Adenomyomatosis, diffuse form (§5.7) — with intramural comet-tail artifact.

Carcinoma, infiltrative form (§5.7) — irregular, asymmetric, with loss of wall layering and often mass formation.

Focal thickening

Focal thickening carries a different differential and a higher threshold for concern:

- **Adenomyomatosis**, most often fundal, identified by comet-tail artifact
- **Polyp**, identified by its intraluminal projection and absent shadow
- **Carcinoma**, identified by irregularity, size, asymmetry, vascularity, and hepatic invasion
- **Xanthogranulomatous cholecystitis**, which mimics carcinoma
- **Adjacent inflammation** from hepatic or pancreatic disease

Reporting

State the measurement, the distension state, the presence or absence of stones, tenderness, pericholecystic fluid, and any systemic explanation available to you. A measurement reported without those qualifiers invites an incorrect conclusion, and providing them costs one sentence.

5.7 Adenomyomatosis, Polyps, and Carcinoma

Adenomyomatosis

A benign hyperplastic condition in which the mucosa invaginates into a thickened muscular layer, forming **Rokitansky-Aschoff sinuses**. Cholesterol crystals precipitate within these sinuses and produce the diagnostic artifact.

The identifying finding is comet-tail artifact arising from within the gallbladder wall. From Chapter 2 §2.8: comet tail is **discrete, tapering, and terminates**, arising from reverberation between closely spaced reflectors — here, cholesterol crystals. This is the finding that establishes the diagnosis, and it is why the comet-tail-versus-ring-down distinction earns its place in the physics chapter.

The contrast matters clinically. Comet tail in a thickened gallbladder wall indicates adenomyomatosis, a benign condition. **Ring-down** from the same wall indicates **gas** — emphysematous cholecystitis, a surgical emergency. The two look superficially alike and mean opposite things.

Forms:

- **Focal (fundal)** — the commonest, a rounded fundal thickening with comet tails, easily mistaken for a mass
- **Segmental (annular)** — a circumferential band producing an **hourglass** gallbladder
- **Diffuse** — generalized wall thickening with scattered comet tails

Small anechoic intramural spaces representing the sinuses themselves may be visible, sometimes with tiny echogenic foci within them.

Adenomyomatosis is benign. A historically debated association with carcinoma, particularly in the segmental form, is not firmly established. [VERIFY: current evidence and management recommendations regarding adenomyomatosis and gallbladder carcinoma risk]

Polyps

Cholesterol polyps account for the majority of gallbladder polyps. They are small, often multiple, attached to the wall, and represent mucosal cholesterol deposits rather than neoplasia.

Distinguishing a polyp from a stone, restated because it is the daily task: a polyp is **immobile with position change, casts no shadow**, is **attached to the wall**, and **may demonstrate internal vascular flow** in a stalk. A stone is mobile, shadows, and has no flow. Where a stone is impacted and therefore immobile, the shadow and the absence of flow settle it.

Adenomatous polyps are true neoplasms with malignant potential, and cannot be reliably distinguished from cholesterol polyps by ultrasound alone.

Features that raise concern and drive management: **larger size, solitary rather than multiple, sessile rather than pedunculated, demonstrable growth on follow-up, internal vascularity**, associated **wall thickening**, older patient age, and coexisting primary sclerosing cholangitis.

Size thresholds determine whether a polyp is followed, followed more closely, or removed, and these thresholds are guideline-defined and have been revised. They must be taken from the current applicable guideline. [VERIFY: current size thresholds and surveillance intervals for gallbladder polyps, including risk-stratified criteria]

Report polyps with size, number, location, morphology, stalk, and vascularity — the parameters the guideline will be applied to.

Gallbladder carcinoma

Uncommon, aggressive, and frequently advanced at diagnosis because early disease is silent and mimics benign conditions.

Risk associations include **gallstones** (present in the large majority), chronic inflammation, large polyps, primary sclerosing cholangitis, and anomalous pancreaticobiliary junction.

Three sonographic patterns, in roughly ascending order of stage:

1. **Focal or diffuse irregular wall thickening**, asymmetric, with loss of the normal wall layering. This is the pattern that overlaps most with benign disease and is the hardest to call.
2. **An intraluminal polypoid mass**, typically larger than a benign polyp, with internal vascularity, and immobile.
3. **A mass replacing the gallbladder fossa**, often engulfing stones and **invading the adjacent liver** with an indistinct interface — the most recognizable and the most advanced.

Assess and report: hepatic invasion and its extent, biliary obstruction, portal or hepatic vein involvement, regional lymphadenopathy, and hepatic metastases. These determine resectability.

The diagnostic trap is that xanthogranulomatous cholecystitis, chronic cholecystitis, and complicated inflammation can all produce irregular thickening indistinguishable from early carcinoma. Ultrasound frequently cannot resolve this, and the correct report says so and recommends cross-sectional imaging.

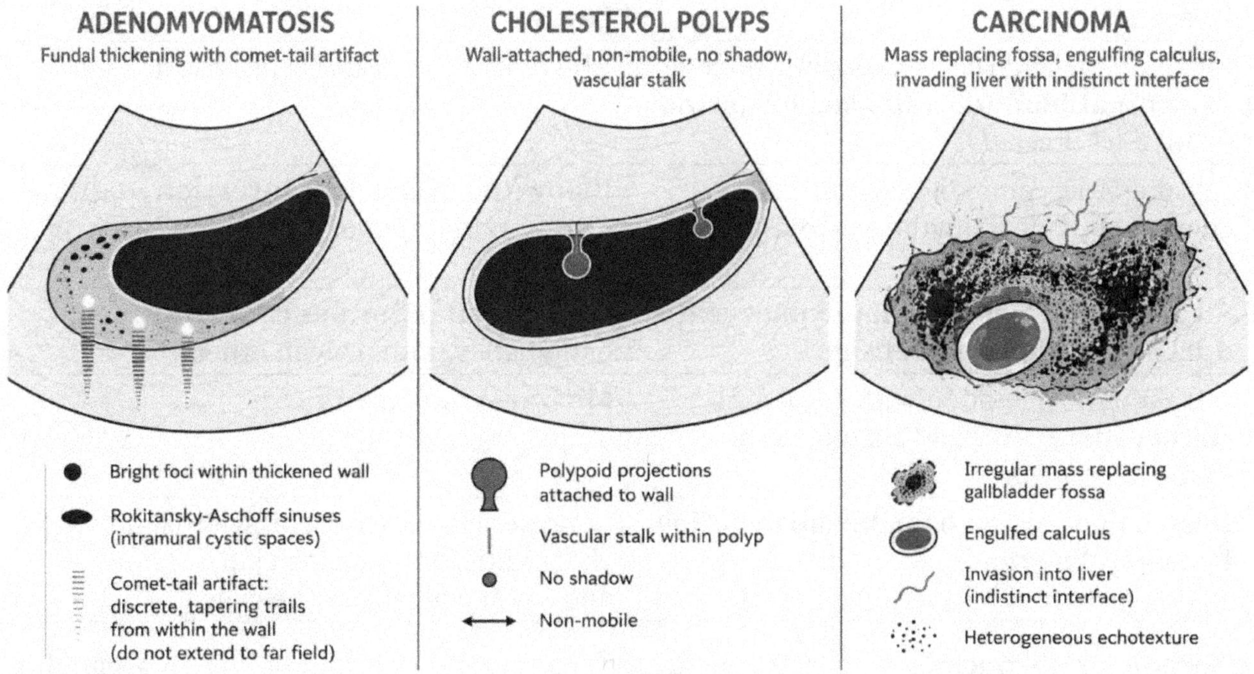

5.8 Biliary Obstruction and Ductal Dilatation

Recognizing dilatation

Intrahepatic ducts become visible as anechoic tubular structures **running alongside the portal branches**, producing the **parallel channel** or **double-barrel** appearance, and on survey the impression of **too many tubes**. Dilated ducts branch irregularly, converge toward the porta, may show **acoustic enhancement** posteriorly, and — decisively — **contain no flow on color Doppler**.

Always apply color Doppler before calling a tubular structure a dilated duct. Hepatic arteries in a cirrhotic or hyperdynamic liver can be conspicuous enough to mimic ducts, and the distinction takes one button press.

Extrahepatic duct dilatation is assessed by measuring the common duct at the porta, inner wall to inner wall, perpendicular to its axis. The thresholds and their caveats are in §5.1 and must be verified.

Determining the level — the core skill

The **pattern** of what is dilated and what is not localizes the obstruction, often precisely, even when the causative lesion is invisible. Work through it systematically:

Pattern	Level of obstruction
Intrahepatic ducts dilated, **right and left systems not communicating**, extrahepatic duct normal	**Hilar** — at or above the confluence (Klatskin tumor, hilar stricture)

Pattern	Level of obstruction
Intrahepatic and common hepatic duct dilated, **gallbladder collapsed or normal**, distal duct normal	**Above the cystic duct insertion**
Intrahepatic, common hepatic, and common bile duct dilated, **gallbladder distended**	**Below the cystic duct insertion** — distal CBD or periampullary
All of the above **plus a dilated pancreatic duct** — the **"double duct sign"**	**Periampullary or pancreatic head** — malignancy until proven otherwise
Intrahepatic dilatation with a **normal-caliber distal CBD** and a stone at the cystic duct/neck	**Mirizzi syndrome** (§5.5)
Dilated ducts with **no visible obstructing lesion and no mass**	Consider stone, stricture, sclerosing cholangitis, or an unseen small tumor — and say the level, not the cause

Courvoisier's principle — a palpable, distended, non-tender gallbladder in a jaundiced patient suggests malignant distal obstruction rather than stone disease, on the reasoning that a chronically stone-diseased gallbladder is fibrotic and cannot distend. It is a useful heuristic with recognized exceptions, not a rule.

The double duct sign deserves particular weight. Simultaneous dilatation of the common bile duct and the pancreatic duct localizes the obstruction to the periampullary region and carries a high probability of malignancy. It should be sought specifically whenever the CBD is dilated, and it should be communicated clearly.

Causes of obstruction

Intraluminal — choledocholithiasis (much the commonest), sludge, blood clot, parasites.

Mural — cholangiocarcinoma, benign stricture (postoperative, post-inflammatory), primary sclerosing cholangitis, AIDS cholangiopathy, choledochal cyst.

Extrinsic — pancreatic head carcinoma, pancreatitis, periportal lymphadenopathy, Mirizzi syndrome, ampullary tumor, duodenal tumor.

Dilatation without jaundice, and jaundice without dilatation

Both occur and both must be interpreted with care.

Dilated ducts with normal bilirubin may reflect a post-cholecystectomy state, prior obstruction now relieved, intermittent obstruction from a ball-valve stone, or early obstruction before biochemical change.

Jaundice with normal-caliber ducts may reflect hepatocellular disease, intrahepatic cholestasis, very early obstruction, or obstruction in a stiff non-compliant biliary system as in **primary sclerosing cholangitis** — where ducts are strictured and may not dilate despite significant obstruction. This is an important exception and prevents a false reassurance.

5.9 Choledocholithiasis, Cholangitis, and Cholangiocarcinoma

Choledocholithiasis

The technical problem. The distal common bile duct passes behind the duodenum, and duodenal gas obscures it in a large proportion of patients. This is where the study most often fails, and the failure is under-acknowledged.

Technique to improve visualization, applied in sequence:

1. **Left lateral decubitus and erect positions**, moving gas away from the duct.
2. **Right lateral decubitus** or a **right lateral intercostal approach**, using the liver as a window and approaching the duct from the patient's right.
3. **Graded compression** over the duodenum to displace gas.
4. **Water ingestion** to fill the duodenum with fluid rather than gas, converting an obstacle into an acoustic window.
5. **Frequency and focus optimization**, and **compounding off** to preserve the stone's shadow.

Findings. An echogenic focus within the duct, usually with shadowing, and duct dilatation proximal to it. Small stones may not shadow, and a stone at the ampulla may be surrounded by little bile and therefore poorly contrasted.

State the limits honestly. Ultrasound has meaningful but imperfect sensitivity for common duct stones, and a negative study does not exclude them — particularly with a dilated duct, deranged cholestatic laboratory values, or a poorly visualized distal segment. The correct report describes the visualized extent, the caliber, and the limitation, and the onward pathway is **MRCP or endoscopic ultrasound**. Reporting "no common duct stone" when the distal duct was never seen is a serious and common error.

Acute cholangitis

Bacterial infection of an obstructed biliary system. It is a **medical emergency** with a high mortality if decompression is delayed.

Clinically it presents with **Charcot's triad** — fever, jaundice, right upper quadrant pain — progressing in severe disease to include hypotension and altered mental status.

Sonographic findings are often unimpressive relative to the severity, which is itself a hazard: biliary dilatation, duct wall thickening, echogenic material or pus within the ducts, an identifiable obstructing stone or stricture, and in advanced disease hepatic abscesses.

The examination's role is to establish obstruction and identify its level and cause, so that decompression — usually endoscopic — can proceed. **Suspected cholangitis is a critical finding requiring immediate communication** (Chapter 1 §1.5), and the study should not be prolonged for completeness once the essential question is answered.

Recurrent pyogenic cholangitis (oriental cholangiohepatitis), endemic in parts of East and Southeast Asia, produces intrahepatic pigment stones, duct strictures with disproportionate dilatation of the extrahepatic relative to the peripheral intrahepatic ducts, and segmental atrophy.

Primary sclerosing cholangitis

Chronic fibrosing inflammation producing multifocal strictures and intervening dilatation. Strongly associated with **inflammatory bowel disease**, particularly ulcerative colitis.

Findings include irregular duct wall thickening, a beaded pattern of alternating strictures and dilated segments, and — importantly — **ducts that may not dilate despite obstruction** because they are fibrotic and non-compliant. MRCP is the imaging reference standard.

PSC carries a substantially increased risk of **cholangiocarcinoma** and of gallbladder polyps and carcinoma, which raises the significance of any new mass or dominant stricture in these patients.

Cholangiocarcinoma

Classified by location, and the location determines both appearance and management:

Intrahepatic (peripheral, mass-forming) — an irregular hepatic mass, often with **capsular retraction** and **peripheral biliary dilatation** distal to it. Covered also in Chapter 4 §4.7.

Hilar (Klatskin) — at the confluence of the right and left hepatic ducts. Frequently **small and difficult or impossible to see directly**, diagnosed by the pattern: **intrahepatic dilatation with non-communicating right and left systems and a normal distal duct**. The pattern is the diagnosis. Extent of involvement of the right and left ducts determines resectability and is described by a formal classification. [VERIFY: current classification system for hilar cholangiocarcinoma extent and its surgical implications]

Distal — in the extrahepatic duct, producing dilatation above and often a visible intraductal or periductal mass, with a distended gallbladder.

Periductal infiltrating growth produces duct wall thickening and stricture rather than a mass, and is the hardest to detect.

Assess and report: the level and extent of ductal involvement, vascular encasement (portal vein and hepatic artery), lobar atrophy, nodal disease, and hepatic metastases.

Other biliary conditions

Choledochal cysts — congenital cystic dilatation of the biliary tree, classified by a formal system, presenting in childhood or adulthood, carrying a malignancy risk. Developed in Chapter 12. [VERIFY: current choledochal cyst classification]

Biliary parasites — *Ascaris lumbricoides* appearing as a long tubular structure within the duct, sometimes with visible movement, and *Clonorchis sinensis* producing duct wall thickening and peripheral dilatation. Both are important in endemic regions and are easily unrecognized elsewhere.

AIDS cholangiopathy — papillary stenosis with duct wall thickening and dilatation in advanced immunosuppression.

5.10 The Postcholecystectomy and Postoperative Biliary Tract

Normal postoperative appearances

Absent gallbladder. The gallbladder fossa contains fat and occasionally a small amount of fluid or fibrous tissue. Before reporting an absent gallbladder as surgical, **confirm the history** — a contracted stone-filled gallbladder with a WES complex (§5.3) can be mistaken for an empty fossa, and agenesis exists.

Surgical clips appear as small bright echogenic foci in the fossa and along the cystic duct stump, frequently with **shadowing or comet-tail artifact**. They are expected and should not be reported as calculi.

Mild common duct dilatation is common after cholecystectomy and is generally accepted as physiologic, on the reasoning that the duct assumes some reservoir function. The permissible caliber is larger than in an intact patient, and interpreting a post-cholecystectomy duct against the standard threshold generates false positives. [VERIFY: current accepted upper limit for common bile duct diameter after cholecystectomy]

Small perihepatic or subhepatic fluid collections are expected in the early postoperative period and generally resolve.

Pneumobilia — gas within the biliary tree — is expected after sphincterotomy, biliary stenting, or a surgical biliary-enteric anastomosis. It appears as echogenic foci with reverberation or ring-down artifact, distributed **centrally** and moving **toward the porta**, in contrast to the **peripheral** distribution of portal venous gas (Chapter 4 §4.9). The distinction is critical and is made on distribution and direction of movement.

Complications

Retained or recurrent stone. A stone left in the duct at surgery, or formed subsequently. Presents with pain, cholestasis, or cholangitis. The distal duct problem of §5.9 applies fully.

Bile leak and biloma. A collection of bile, typically in the gallbladder fossa or subhepatic space, appearing as an anechoic or minimally complex collection without a defined wall early on. Distinguishing a biloma from a seroma, hematoma, or abscess on ultrasound alone is often impossible; the clinical picture and aspiration decide. Suspected bile leak in a symptomatic patient warrants prompt communication.

Bile duct injury and stricture. The most serious complication of cholecystectomy. Presents early with leak or late with obstruction. Sonographically: biliary dilatation to the level of the stricture, with the level determined by the §5.8 method. Requires cholangiographic assessment.

Dropped gallstones. Stones spilled into the peritoneal cavity during laparoscopic cholecystectomy, which may remain inert or produce an abscess, sometimes years later, in unexpected locations including subhepatic, subphrenic, and abdominal wall sites. An echogenic shadowing focus within a collection remote from the biliary tree, in a patient with a cholecystectomy history, should raise this possibility.

Cystic duct remnant — a residual stump, occasionally containing a stone and producing recurrent symptoms.

Abscess and hematoma in the fossa or subhepatic space.

Other postoperative biliary states

Biliary stents appear as echogenic tubular structures within the duct, frequently with reverberation. Assess for **patency** — indicated by duct decompression relative to prior imaging — and for **occlusion or migration**, indicated by recurrent dilatation above the stent or by the stent lying outside the expected course.

Biliary-enteric anastomosis (hepaticojejunostomy, choledochojejunostomy, and the reconstruction after pancreaticoduodenectomy) produces expected **pneumobilia** and mild ductal dilatation. The diagnostic question in these patients is usually **anastomotic stricture**, indicated by increasing dilatation on serial studies — which again makes the comparison discipline of Chapter 1 §1.5 the operative skill.

Transplant biliary complications are covered in Chapter 9.

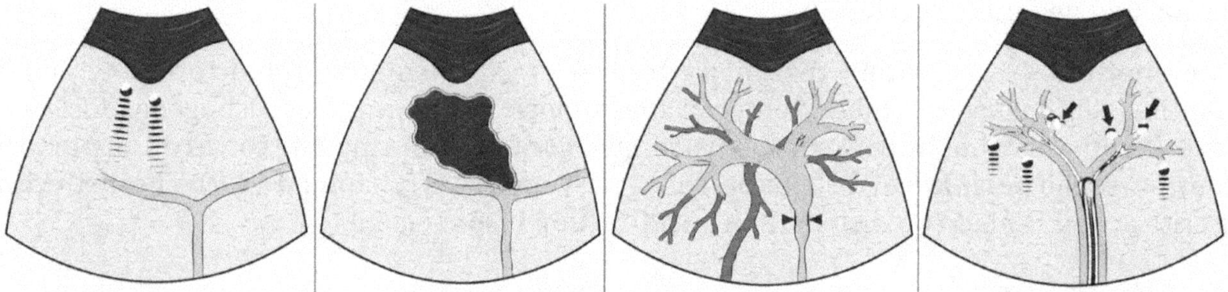

1. SURGICAL CLIPS WITH COMET-TAIL ARTIFACT, NORMAL DUCT

- Two echogenic foci in the gallbladder fossa.
- Short comet-tail (ring-down) artifact beneath each clip.
- Common bile duct normal in caliber.

2. BILOMA IN THE GALLBLADDER FOSSA

- Irregular anechoic collection in the gallbladder fossa.
- Extends beneath the liver edge.
- Common bile duct remains narrow.

3. BILE DUCT STRICTURE WITH DILATATION TO THE LEVEL OF INJURY

- Intrahepatic ducts and common duct are markedly dilated.
- Short narrowing at the level of injury (stricture).
- Duct distal to stricture is normal caliber.

4. BILIARY STENT WITH PNEUMOBILIA – CENTRAL DISTRIBUTION

- Linear stent within the common bile duct.
- Echogenic foci with comet-tail in intrahepatic ducts.
- Arrows indicate gas moving toward the porta hepatis.
- Central pattern distinguishes pneumobilia from portal venous gas.

Key Points

1. Fasting is not optional. A contracted gallbladder cannot be assessed for stones or wall thickness, and reporting findings from one is an error rather than a limitation.

2. Turn spatial compounding off when looking for stones. It is the single most consequential setting error in gallbladder imaging.
3. The left lateral decubitus position is mandatory. A stone that has not been shown to move has not been distinguished from a polyp.
4. Examine the neck and infundibulum specifically. An impacted stone there is the classic miss, and impaction is what causes the disease.
5. Elicit the sonographic Murphy sign actively. It is the finding that most often converts ambiguous images into a diagnosis, and it is the one most often not performed.
6. Recognize the wall-echo-shadow complex, or a stone-packed gallbladder will be reported as absent.
7. Duodenal gas produces dirty shadowing, lies outside the wall, and changes within seconds. Watch it in real time before calling it a stone.
8. Acute cholecystitis is a composite diagnosis. Report the components, not just the label.
9. In gangrenous cholecystitis the Murphy sign may be lost and mural flow may be absent. Falling tenderness in a deteriorating patient is a warning, not reassurance.
10. Comet tail from the gallbladder wall means adenomyomatosis, a benign condition. Ring-down from the wall means gas, and a surgical emergency.
11. Before working up wall thickening, ask whether the gallbladder is distended. The commonest cause of a thick wall is a recent meal.
12. Wall thickening with no stones, no tenderness, and a systemic explanation is a reactive finding — say so in the report rather than leaving a bare measurement.
13. The pattern of ductal dilatation localizes the obstruction even when the lesion is invisible. Non-communicating right and left systems mean hilar; a distended gallbladder means below the cystic duct; a dilated pancreatic duct too means periampullary.
14. The double duct sign carries a high probability of malignancy and should be sought whenever the CBD is dilated.
15. A negative ultrasound does not exclude a common duct stone, particularly when the distal duct was not seen. Report the visualized extent and the limitation, and let MRCP or EUS answer the question.
16. Pneumobilia is central and moves toward the porta; portal venous gas is peripheral. One is often expected, the other is a critical finding.

Registry Check

1. An echogenic focus is seen in the gallbladder lumen without posterior shadowing. Before concluding it is a polyp, the operator should first:

A. Increase the overall gain **B.** Disable spatial compounding and place the focal zone at the level of the focus **C.** Apply power Doppler **D.** Measure the wall thickness

> **Answer: B.** Compounding fills in acoustic shadows and a focus lying outside the focal zone sits in a wide beam that fills the shadow laterally. Both must be corrected

before a focus is described as non-shadowing. Increasing gain would further obscure a subtle shadow.

2. A gallbladder is contracted with a wall measuring 4 mm in a patient who ate two hours before the examination. The correct interpretation is:

A. Acute cholecystitis **B.** Chronic cholecystitis **C.** Adenomyomatosis **D.** The wall is uninterpretable in a contracted gallbladder, and the finding should be reported as such

Answer: D. Physiologic contraction after a meal produces apparent wall thickening and is the commonest cause of this finding. The gallbladder must be distended for wall thickness to be assessable, and the correct response is to state the limitation and repeat after adequate fasting.

3. Echogenic foci are seen within the gallbladder wall producing continuous, non-tapering bands extending to the far field. The most likely diagnosis is:

A. Adenomyomatosis **B.** Cholesterolosis **C.** Emphysematous cholecystitis **D.** Porcelain gallbladder

Answer: C. Continuous non-tapering ring-down artifact indicates gas. Adenomyomatosis produces comet-tail artifact — discrete, tapering, and terminating — from cholesterol crystals in Rokitansky-Aschoff sinuses. The distinction separates a benign condition from a surgical emergency with high mortality.

4. Fine linear echoes are seen floating freely within the lumen of a thick-walled gallbladder, unattached to the wall and casting no shadow, with absent mural flow on color Doppler. This suggests:

A. Sludge **B.** Gangrenous cholecystitis with sloughed mucosal membranes **C.** Septations **D.** Side-lobe artifact

Answer: B. Intraluminal membranes representing sloughed mucosa are the most specific sign of gangrenous cholecystitis, and absent mural flow supports mural necrosis. Sludge layers dependently and does not form linear membranes; septations are attached to the wall.

5. Ultrasound shows dilated intrahepatic ducts in which the right and left systems do not communicate, with a normal-caliber common bile duct and a collapsed gallbladder. The obstruction is:

A. At the ampulla **B.** In the distal common bile duct **C.** At the hilar confluence **D.** In the cystic duct

Answer: C. Non-communicating right and left intrahepatic systems with a normal extrahepatic duct localizes the obstruction to the confluence — the pattern of hilar cholangiocarcinoma, which is frequently invisible directly. The pattern is the diagnosis.

6. Simultaneous dilatation of the common bile duct and the pancreatic duct indicates:

A. Chronic pancreatitis **B.** Obstruction at the periampullary region, with a high probability of malignancy **C.** Post-cholecystectomy change **D.** Primary sclerosing cholangitis

> **Answer: B.** The double duct sign localizes obstruction to the point where both ducts converge and carries a high probability of malignancy — pancreatic head or ampullary carcinoma. It should be sought specifically whenever the common duct is dilated.

7. A jaundiced patient has intrahepatic biliary dilatation, a normal-caliber distal common bile duct, and a stone impacted at the gallbladder neck. This describes:

A. Choledocholithiasis **B.** Mirizzi syndrome **C.** Gallstone ileus **D.** Acalculous cholecystitis

> **Answer: B.** A stone impacted in the cystic duct or gallbladder neck compressing the adjacent common hepatic duct produces obstruction above with a normal duct below. It changes the surgical approach and carries a higher risk of bile duct injury, so recognizing the pattern matters.

8. Echogenic foci with reverberation artifact are seen within the biliary tree, distributed centrally and moving toward the porta hepatis, in a patient who underwent endoscopic sphincterotomy. This represents:

A. Portal venous gas, requiring urgent escalation **B.** Pneumobilia, an expected finding **C.** Intrahepatic calculi **D.** Hepatic artery calcification

> **Answer: B.** Bile flows toward the porta, so biliary gas is distributed centrally and moves inward — the reverse of portal venous gas, which is carried peripherally to within a short distance of the capsule. Pneumobilia after sphincterotomy, stenting, or biliary-enteric anastomosis is expected

Chapter Notes for the Editorial Pass

Verification queue. In priority order: **gallbladder polyp size thresholds and surveillance intervals** (§5.7) — these are guideline-defined, risk-stratified, and have been revised, and a stale figure printed here would drive real management decisions; **common bile duct upper limits**, including the post-cholecystectomy allowance and the disputed age effect (§5.1, §5.10); **gallbladder wall, length, and diameter reference values with their distension conditions** (§5.1); **fasting interval** (§5.2); **hilar cholangiocarcinoma classification** (§5.9); **choledochal cyst classification** (§5.9); the **porcelain gallbladder–carcinoma association**, where the historical teaching has been substantially revised downward (§5.3); and the **adenomyomatosis–carcinoma question** (§5.7), which should be presented as unsettled rather than resolved in either direction.

Cross-modality note. This chapter repeatedly recommends MRCP and EUS as the onward pathway for the distal duct. If the book is to include a standing modality-selection appendix, the biliary tree is the strongest candidate section for it, and Appendix B in the current back matter plan could absorb it.

Figure count: 7 Lane A, 3 Lane B. The comet-tail versus ring-down pair (`fig-5-8`) is the highest-value Lane B acquisition in the chapter and directly supports the Chapter 2 §2.8 physics — securing both halves from the same machine would strengthen both chapters.

Cross-reference targets to fix at layout: §5.1 physiology → §5.6 wall thickening; §5.2 compounding → Chapter 2 §2.4; §5.3 dirty shadowing → Chapter 2 §2.7; §5.5 ring-down → Chapter 2 §2.8; §5.6 hepatitis and cirrhosis → Chapter 4 §4.4–4.5; §5.9 intrahepatic cholangiocarcinoma → Chapter 4 §4.7; §5.9 choledochal cyst → Chapter 12; §5.10 pneumobilia versus portal venous gas → Chapter 4 §4.9; §5.10 transplant biliary complications → Chapter 9.

Word count: approximately 10,300 excluding image prompt blocks, learning objectives, registry questions, and these notes.

Chapter 6: The Pancreas, Spleen, and Gastrointestinal Tract

Learning Objectives

On completing this chapter you should be able to:

1. Locate the pancreas using its vascular landmarks and apply the technical maneuvers that open the epigastric window.
2. State the actual role of ultrasound in acute pancreatitis, and classify the fluid collections that follow it.
3. Recognize the features of chronic pancreatitis and its principal vascular complication.
4. Distinguish the major solid and cystic pancreatic neoplasms, and state where ultrasound cannot characterize a cystic lesion.
5. Identify the spleen and its normal variants, and avoid the errors those variants generate.
6. Assess splenic size, recognize infarction by its geometry, and describe the sonographic findings of splenic trauma.
7. Characterize splenic focal lesions in their clinical context.
8. Name the five layers of the gut signature and use loss of stratification as a discriminator.
9. Perform graded compression for appendicitis, apply the diagnostic criteria, and report non-visualization correctly.
10. Recognize small bowel obstruction, intussusception, and the inflammatory bowel patterns.

Three Organs, One Window Problem

These three structures are grouped not because they share physiology but because they share a technical adversary: **bowel gas**. The pancreas sits behind the stomach and transverse colon. The spleen sits behind ribs with the splenic flexure in front of it. The gut is itself the gas.

Consequently, this chapter is more about maneuver than any other in the book. Graded compression, patient repositioning, respiratory control, water ingestion, and window selection are not refinements here — they are the difference between a diagnostic study and a non-diagnostic one. A sonographer who accepts the first obscured view will fail these organs consistently.

6.1 Pancreatic Anatomy and Acoustic Windows

Position and parts

The pancreas is **retroperitoneal**, lying in the **anterior pararenal space** (Chapter 3 §3.1), oriented obliquely with the head inferior and to the patient's right and the tail superior and to the left. This obliquity is why the standard pancreatic view is an **oblique transverse** plane rather than a true transverse one.

Head — nestled in the C-loop of the duodenum, to the right of the midline. **Uncinate process** — the hook-like extension of the head passing **posterior and inferior to the superior mesenteric vein**. **Neck** — the narrow segment anterior to the portal confluence. **Body** — crossing the midline anterior to the aorta and SMA. **Tail** — extending toward the splenic hilum, and the only part that is **intraperitoneal**, lying within the splenorenal ligament.

The vascular landmarks

You do not find the pancreas by looking for the pancreas. You find its vessels, and the pancreas is the tissue in the defined relationships around them.

The splenic vein is the single most useful landmark. It runs transversely along the **posterior surface of the body and tail**, and in the standard oblique transverse view it appears as a long anechoic channel with the pancreas draped anteriorly over it. Find the splenic vein and you have found the pancreas.

The portal confluence — where the splenic vein and superior mesenteric vein meet to form the portal vein — lies **directly behind the neck**. It is the pivot of the whole anatomy.

The SMA lies **posterior to the body**, surrounded by its distinctive echogenic fat collar (Chapter 3 §3.4).

Other constant relationships:

Structure	Relationship to pancreas
Aorta	Posterior to the body
IVC	Posterior to the head
Left renal vein	Between the SMA and aorta, posterior to the body
Common bile duct	Runs through the **posterolateral head**
Gastroduodenal artery	At the **anterolateral head**
Stomach and transverse colon	Anterior — the source of all technical difficulty

The CBD and GDA together bracket the head and are a useful pair: seeing both in cross-section confirms you are at the pancreatic head.

Echotexture, duct, and variants

Normal parenchyma is **homogeneous and iso- to hyperechoic relative to the adjacent liver**. Echogenicity **increases with age** as fatty replacement occurs, so a bright pancreas in an older patient is usually normal and should not be reported as pathological.

The **main pancreatic duct (of Wirsung)** may be visible as a fine anechoic line or a pair of echogenic parallel lines within the body, and is normally small. Measure inner-to-inner in the body, perpendicular to its axis. [VERIFY: current upper limit of normal for main pancreatic duct diameter and its measurement site]

Variants worth recognizing: **pancreas divisum** (failure of ductal fusion, a predisposing factor for pancreatitis, and generally an MRCP diagnosis), **annular pancreas** (encircling the duodenum, presenting with obstruction usually in infancy), and ectopic pancreatic tissue.

Opening the window

The pancreas is the most technically demanding solid organ in the abdomen, and the following are applied in sequence rather than as alternatives:

1. **Fasting**, to reduce gastric and colonic gas and content.
2. **Epigastric approach through the left lobe of the liver**, which acts as the acoustic window. Where the left lobe is small, this window is poor and the study will be difficult — a limitation worth stating in the report.
3. **Graded compression**, applied slowly to displace overlying gas.
4. **Suspended respiration**, trying both deep inspiration and expiration — they move the gland differently and one will usually be better.
5. **Sitting or erect position**, which lowers the gland and moves gas superiorly.
6. **Water ingestion** — 300–500 mL taken slowly, filling the stomach to create a fluid acoustic window directly over the gland. This is the most effective single rescue maneuver and is markedly underused. Scan in the erect or right lateral decubitus position after drinking so the fluid sits over the head and body.
7. **For the tail specifically**, a **left coronal intercostal approach through the spleen or left kidney**, since the tail is frequently invisible from the front.

The tail is the most commonly non-visualized part of the pancreas, and a study in which it was not seen must say so. "Pancreatic tail obscured by bowel gas and not evaluated" is a real statement with consequences; silence is read as normality (Chapter 1 §1.5).

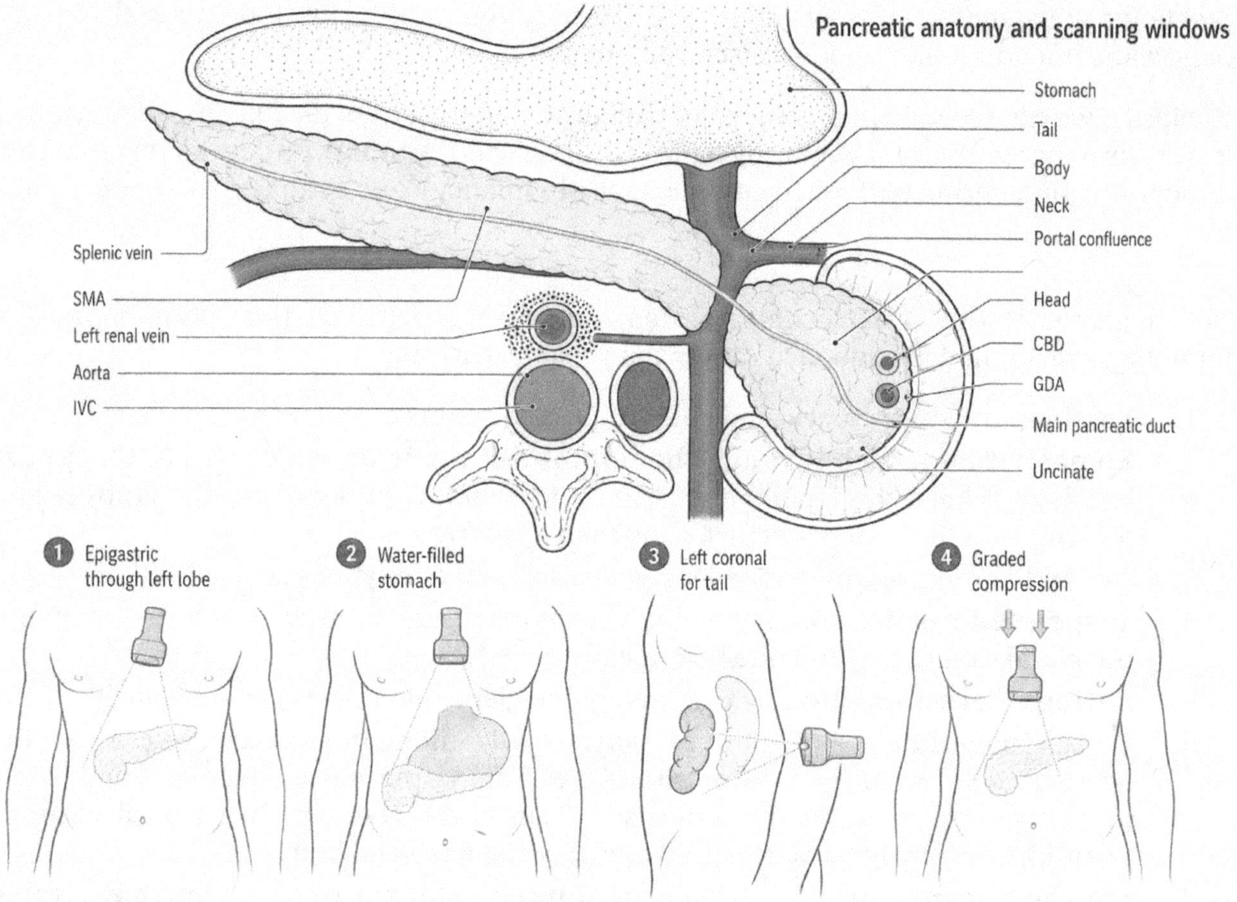

6.2 Acute Pancreatitis and Its Complications

What ultrasound is actually for

Acute pancreatitis is a clinical and biochemical diagnosis, established by characteristic pain with elevated serum lipase or amylase. Ultrasound does not make the diagnosis and frequently does not support it — the gland is normal in a substantial proportion of cases, and in many others it is simply not visible because of the ileus that accompanies the illness.

The examination has a different and well-defined purpose:

1. **Identify gallstones as the etiology.** This is the primary indication. Biliary pancreatitis changes management — it leads to cholecystectomy, and to consideration of ERCP where there is concurrent obstruction. Examining the gallbladder and biliary tree is therefore the highest-priority component of the study.
2. **Assess the biliary tree** for duct dilatation and choledocholithiasis (Chapter 5 §5.8–5.9).
3. **Detect and follow fluid collections**, particularly for drainage planning.
4. **Detect vascular complications**.

Say this in the report where relevant: a study that documents gallstones and a dilated duct has succeeded, even if the pancreas itself was never adequately seen.

Severity assessment and necrosis detection are CT territory, and the report should direct there rather than implying that a normal-looking pancreas on ultrasound means mild disease.

Findings when the gland is visible

- **Diffuse or focal enlargement** with **decreased echogenicity** from edema
- **Indistinct, poorly defined margins** as peripancreatic fat becomes inflamed
- **Peripancreatic fluid**
- **Ileus** with gas-filled loops obscuring the gland — itself an indirect sign
- **Focal pancreatitis** may produce a hypoechoic mass-like area that is genuinely difficult to distinguish from carcinoma, and this ambiguity should be stated rather than resolved by assertion

Fluid collections — classification matters for drainage

Collections following acute pancreatitis are classified by **two variables: the presence of necrosis, and time**. The distinction determines whether and how a collection can be drained, and using the terms loosely causes real problems.

	Under ~4 weeks	**Over ~4 weeks (encapsulated)**
No necrosis (interstitial edematous pancreatitis)	Acute peripancreatic fluid collection — anechoic, no defined wall, conforms to fascial planes	**Pseudocyst** — well-defined wall, anechoic contents, no solid debris
With necrosis (necrotizing pancreatitis)	Acute necrotic collection — heterogeneous, contains solid material	**Walled-off necrosis** — defined wall, contains **non-liquefied solid debris**

The sonographic discriminator is internal content. A collection that appears simple and anechoic is a pseudocyst; one containing echogenic non-dependent solid debris is walled-off necrosis. This matters because **percutaneous catheter drainage of a collection full of solid necrotic material fails** — the catheter blocks — and the correct approach is endoscopic or surgical necrosectomy. Reporting "pseudocyst" for a collection containing debris misdirects the procedure.

Look specifically for internal echogenic material, and describe it. [VERIFY: current revised Atlanta classification definitions, terminology, and time thresholds for pancreatic fluid collections]

Vascular and other complications

Splenic artery pseudoaneurysm — the most feared vascular complication, arising when enzymatic digestion erodes the arterial wall. On color Doppler, a cystic-appearing structure adjacent to the pancreas that demonstrates **internal swirling yin-yang flow**, with a **to-and-fro** waveform in the neck (Chapter 3 §3.8). **A "pseudocyst" must be interrogated with color Doppler before it is called a pseudocyst** — this takes seconds and prevents the puncture of an aneurysm.

Splenic vein thrombosis — common in pancreatic inflammation, and it produces **left-sided (sinistral) portal hypertension** with gastric varices and splenomegaly while the portal vein and liver remain normal. Interrogate the splenic vein in every pancreatitis study.

Portal and mesenteric venous thrombosis.

Biliary obstruction from head edema or a stone.

Infected collection or abscess — suggested by gas within a collection producing dirty shadowing or ring-down (Chapter 2 §2.8), though the diagnosis is usually clinical plus aspiration.

Ascites and pleural effusion, the latter typically left-sided.

Hemorrhage into a collection, appearing as heterogeneous echogenic material, sometimes with a fluid-fluid level.

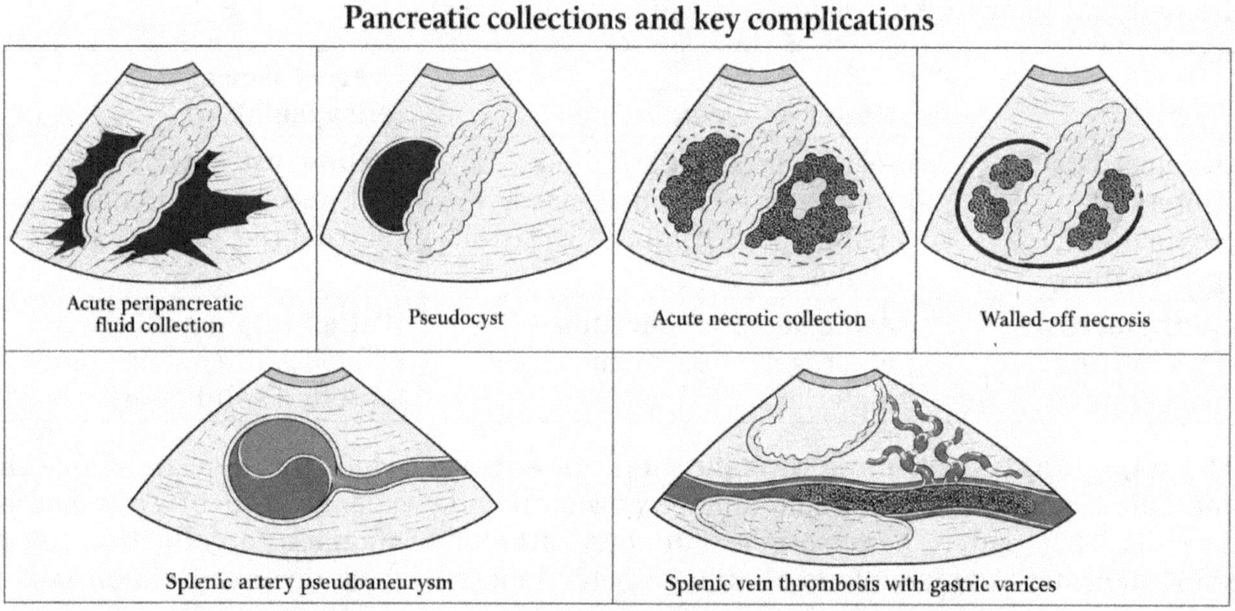

Different pancreatic collections are distinguished by wall formation and internal debris. Before drainage, exclude pseudoaneurysm and splenic vein thrombosis.

6.3 Chronic Pancreatitis

Findings

Chronic pancreatitis is progressive irreversible fibrosis with loss of exocrine and eventually endocrine function. The sonographic features, in descending order of specificity:

Parenchymal calcifications — echogenic foci, often with **shadowing** when large enough. The most specific sign. As always, disable spatial compounding before concluding that a focus does not shadow (Chapter 2 §2.4).

Intraductal calculi — echogenic shadowing foci within a dilated duct.

Main pancreatic duct dilatation, characteristically **irregular and beaded** rather than smoothly tapered — the irregularity distinguishes it from the smooth uniform dilatation of a distal obstructing tumor.

Gland atrophy with reduced anteroposterior dimensions.

Heterogeneous, coarsened echotexture with increased echogenicity.

Pseudocysts, which may persist from prior acute episodes.

Contour irregularity.

The gland may also be **focally enlarged**, producing a mass-like appearance that is genuinely difficult to distinguish from carcinoma — an important limitation given that chronic pancreatitis is itself a risk factor for pancreatic malignancy.

The vascular complication to seek

Splenic vein thrombosis occurs in chronic as well as acute pancreatitis, and produces the same **left-sided portal hypertension**: gastric and short gastric varices, splenomegaly, and collateral flow, with a normal liver and a normal portal vein. This is a genuinely reversible cause of variceal bleeding — splenectomy is curative — so identifying it matters.

Interrogate the splenic vein along its course in every chronic pancreatitis study, and if it cannot be followed, say so.

Other complications

Biliary stricture from fibrosis in the head, producing obstructive jaundice with a smoothly tapered distal duct — and creating the differential with carcinoma again.

Duodenal obstruction.

Increased risk of pancreatic ductal adenocarcinoma, which raises the significance of any new focal lesion or new duct dilatation in a known chronic pancreatitis patient.

Autoimmune pancreatitis

Worth distinguishing because it is treatable with steroids and is frequently mistaken for carcinoma, sometimes leading to unnecessary resection.

Type 1 is the pancreatic manifestation of IgG4-related disease. Sonographically, the classic form is a **diffusely enlarged, uniformly hypoechoic gland with a smooth "sausage-like" contour** and loss of the normal lobulation, sometimes with a hypoechoic **capsule-like rim**.

The main duct is characteristically **narrowed rather than dilated** — the opposite of what obstruction from a tumor produces, and a useful discriminator.

A focal form exists and is far harder, mimicking a mass. Serology, other organ involvement, and response to treatment resolve it; ultrasound raises the possibility.

6.4 Pancreatic Solid and Cystic Neoplasms

Ductal adenocarcinoma

The dominant pancreatic malignancy, with a poor prognosis largely because it presents late.

Findings. A **hypoechoic, ill-defined mass**, most commonly in the **head**. Head lesions present earlier because they obstruct — producing painless jaundice — while body and tail lesions present late and larger.

The secondary signs are often more conspicuous than the mass, and should be sought actively:

- **Double duct sign** — simultaneous dilatation of the common bile duct and main pancreatic duct (Chapter 5 §5.8). In a patient with painless jaundice this is a high-probability finding for periampullary malignancy.
- **Abrupt duct cut-off** with upstream dilatation
- **Distended gallbladder** (Courvoisier)
- **Upstream gland atrophy**
- **Vascular involvement** — encasement or occlusion of the SMA, celiac axis, SMV, splenic vein, or portal vein
- **Liver metastases and regional lymphadenopathy**
- **Ascites**, suggesting peritoneal disease

Report for resectability. The determinants are the relationship to the arterial and venous structures, the presence of metastases, and nodal disease. Describe **the degree of vessel contact** and whether the vessel appears narrowed or occluded. Definitive staging is by contrast-enhanced CT, and EUS provides both superior local assessment and tissue sampling.

Neuroendocrine tumors

Typically **well-defined, rounded, and hypervascular** on Doppler — a marked contrast to the hypovascular, ill-defined adenocarcinoma. They may be **functioning** (insulinoma, gastrinoma, and others, presenting with hormonal syndromes and often very small) or non-functioning (presenting late and large).

Small functioning tumors are frequently below transabdominal ultrasound's detection threshold; EUS and dedicated cross-sectional or nuclear imaging are the tools.

Cystic lesions — the practical differential

Pancreatic cystic lesions are found with increasing frequency as incidental findings, and their differential is the area where ultrasound most often cannot give a final answer.

Lesion	Typical features
Pseudocyst	History of pancreatitis; unilocular; no septations, no mural nodules, no wall enhancement; may contain debris
Serous cystadenoma	**Microcystic**, honeycomb of many tiny cysts, sometimes with a **central scar with calcification**; may appear almost solid because the cysts are below resolution; older women; essentially benign
Mucinous cystic neoplasm	**Macrocystic**, few large locules, **thick wall**, septations, **peripheral eggshell calcification**; **body and tail**; middle-aged women; **malignant potential**
IPMN, branch duct	Cystic lesion **communicating with the pancreatic duct**; often multifocal; malignant potential varying with features
IPMN, main duct	**Diffuse main duct dilatation** without an obstructing mass, sometimes with a patulous ampulla; higher malignant risk
Solid pseudopapillary neoplasm	Mixed solid and cystic, often large with hemorrhage; young women; low-grade malignant

Features that raise concern across the cystic lesions include an **enhancing mural nodule, thick or enhancing septations, main duct involvement or dilatation, larger size,** associated lymphadenopathy, and demonstrable growth on follow-up.

Size and feature thresholds drive surveillance and resection decisions, are guideline-defined, differ between guidelines, and have been revised. They must be taken from the current applicable guideline. [VERIFY: current management guideline thresholds for pancreatic cystic lesions, including worrisome features and high-risk stigmata]

State the limitation. Transabdominal ultrasound frequently cannot distinguish these lesions from one another, cannot reliably demonstrate ductal communication, and cannot exclude a small mural nodule. Describe what you see — size, location, locularity, wall and septal thickness, calcification, solid components, duct caliber, duct communication if demonstrable — and direct to **MRI/MRCP or EUS**, which can also sample cyst fluid.

6.5 Splenic Anatomy and Normal Variants

Position and appearance

The spleen is **intraperitoneal**, lying in the left upper quadrant, posterolateral, beneath the diaphragm and behind the **ninth to eleventh ribs**. It has a convex diaphragmatic surface and a concave visceral surface with the **hilum**, through which the splenic artery and vein pass. It is related to the stomach, the splenic flexure of the colon, the left kidney, and the pancreatic tail.

Echotexture is homogeneous and fine, **slightly more echogenic than the adjacent left kidney** and roughly comparable to or slightly greater than the liver. As with the liver-kidney pair, acquire an image containing **spleen and left kidney together** at matched settings so the comparison can be verified.

Size is assessed by **maximum length in the coronal plane** through the hilum, and this is the measurement that must be reproduced on serial studies. [VERIFY: current upper limit of normal for splenic length, and any accepted volumetric alternative]

The window

The spleen is behind ribs, so the approach is a **left lateral intercostal coronal** window with the transducer **rotated to align with the rib space** (Chapter 3 §3.3). The **right lateral decubitus** position brings the spleen medially and anteriorly.

Respiration requires experiment. Deep inspiration brings the spleen down but also brings aerated lung into the window; suspended expiration sometimes gives a better view for that reason. Try both rather than assuming.

The splenic flexure lies anterior and is a common source of obscuring gas.

Normal variants

Accessory spleen (splenule) — a common variant, usually a small rounded structure **near the hilum**. It is identified by having **exactly the same echotexture as the spleen** and **its own vascular pedicle** demonstrable on color Doppler. It is regularly reported as a lymph node, a pancreatic tail mass, or an adrenal lesion; the echotexture match and the vascular pedicle prevent the error.

Its clinical relevance: after splenectomy for a hematologic indication, a hypertrophied accessory spleen can cause **disease recurrence**, so its identification is specifically requested in that context.

Splenules and polysplenia — multiple splenic tissue masses, the latter part of a heterotaxy syndrome with associated cardiac and situs anomalies (Chapters 12 and 15).

Wandering spleen — an abnormally mobile spleen on a long mesentery, at risk of **torsion**, and found in an unexpected location. If the left upper quadrant is empty, look elsewhere before concluding asplenia.

Splenosis — autotransplanted splenic tissue after traumatic rupture or splenectomy, appearing as multiple peritoneal nodules with splenic echotexture, and easily mistaken for peritoneal metastases.

Splenic clefts and lobulation — normal contour indentations, mistaken for lacerations in the trauma setting. A cleft has smooth echogenic margins; a laceration is irregular and accompanied by hemoperitoneum.

6.6 Splenomegaly, Infarction, and Trauma

Splenomegaly

Enlargement is common, non-specific, and its causes group usefully by mechanism:

Mechanism	Causes
Congestive	Portal hypertension (much the commonest), splenic vein thrombosis, right heart failure, Budd-Chiari
Infiltrative / hematologic	Lymphoma, leukemia, myeloproliferative disease, myelofibrosis
Infective	Infectious mononucleosis, malaria, tuberculosis, endocarditis, visceral leishmaniasis, HIV
Hemolytic	Sickle cell disease (early; late the spleen autoinfarcts and shrinks), thalassemia, spherocytosis
Storage / infiltrative	Gaucher, Niemann-Pick, amyloidosis, sarcoidosis
Inflammatory	Systemic lupus, rheumatoid disease (Felty syndrome)

Assess alongside the spleen: the liver echotexture and contour, portal vein caliber and flow direction, the splenic vein, collateral vessels, and ascites. Splenomegaly with a nodular liver and hepatofugal portal flow is a portal hypertension picture (Chapter 4 §4.5); splenomegaly with a normal liver and a thrombosed splenic vein is left-sided portal hypertension from pancreatic disease (§6.2–6.3); splenomegaly with a normal liver and normal veins directs attention to hematologic and infective causes.

Gamna-Gandy bodies — small punctate echogenic foci from organized microhemorrhages, seen in longstanding portal hypertension, and a useful supporting sign.

A practical caution: an enlarged spleen in acute infectious mononucleosis is at increased risk of rupture, and the examination should be performed gently. This is one of the few settings where transducer pressure itself carries a risk.

Infarction

The geometry is diagnostic. A splenic infarct is characteristically a **peripheral wedge-shaped lesion with its base at the capsule and its apex directed toward the hilum**, following the territory of an end artery.

- **Acute** — hypoechoic, sometimes barely perceptible, with absent internal flow on color Doppler.
- **Evolving** — becomes more heterogeneous.
- **Chronic** — becomes **echogenic and contracts**, producing a **capsular retraction** and a permanent contour notch.

Causes include cardiac and aortic emboli, endocarditis, atrial fibrillation, sickle cell disease, splenic vein or artery thrombosis, torsion of a wandering spleen, pancreatitis, and hematologic malignancy.

Contrast-enhanced ultrasound is particularly good here, showing a sharply demarcated non-enhancing wedge in all phases, and it resolves the frequent B-mode ambiguity of a subtle acute infarct.

Trauma

The spleen is the most commonly injured solid abdominal organ in blunt trauma.

Findings:

Subcapsular hematoma — a crescentic collection conforming to and **flattening or indenting the splenic contour**, lying between the capsule and the parenchyma. Its echogenicity changes with age: acute blood may be echogenic and become progressively more hypoechoic and then complex.

Parenchymal laceration — an irregular hypoechoic or heterogeneous linear defect. Acute lacerations can be nearly isoechoic and therefore **easily missed on B-mode**.

Intraparenchymal hematoma — a focal heterogeneous region.

Perisplenic and free intraperitoneal fluid — often the most conspicuous finding, and frequently the only one. In the FAST examination (Chapter 8), the left upper quadrant view seeks precisely this.

Active bleeding — demonstrable on CEUS as extravasation of contrast.

The honest position on ultrasound in splenic trauma:

- **FAST is a screening test for free fluid**, not an organ-injury assessment. A negative FAST does not exclude splenic injury, and this must be understood rather than assumed.
- **Contrast-enhanced CT is the reference standard** for grading solid organ injury in the stable patient.
- **CEUS has a growing evidence-supported role** in selected settings — hemodynamically stable patients, follow-up of known conservatively managed injury, and pediatric trauma where radiation avoidance is a priority — and performs substantially better than B-mode for parenchymal injury. [VERIFY: current society guidance on CEUS in blunt abdominal trauma, including pediatric recommendations]
- **Delayed rupture** of a contained subcapsular hematoma is a recognized event, which is why conservatively managed injuries are followed.

Free fluid in the trauma setting is a critical finding and warrants immediate communication (Chapter 1 §1.5); the examination should not be prolonged once it is established.

6.7 Splenic Focal Lesions

Splenic lesions are less common than hepatic ones and their differential is narrower, which makes clinical context unusually decisive.

Cystic lesions

True (epithelial/congenital) cyst — anechoic, thin-walled, with posterior enhancement; may have thin septations or wall calcification.

Post-traumatic pseudocyst — the commoner cystic lesion, following prior injury; wall may be thick or calcified, contents may be complex.

Echinococcal cyst — as in the liver (Chapter 4 §4.8), with daughter cysts, detached membranes, or calcification; consider in endemic exposure.

Lymphangioma — multiloculated, thin-septated, often subcapsular.

Solid benign lesions

Hemangioma — the commonest benign splenic neoplasm. Typically a well-defined **hyperechoic** lesion, analogous to its hepatic counterpart, though appearances vary.

Hamartoma — well-defined, often iso- or hyperechoic, hypervascular.

Granulomas — small, echogenic, often **calcified with clean shadowing**, from prior tuberculosis, histoplasmosis, or sarcoidosis. Usually multiple and incidental.

Malignant lesions

Lymphoma is by a wide margin the commonest splenic malignancy, and it presents in three patterns:

1. **Diffuse infiltration** with splenomegaly and no discrete lesion — the commonest, and the one that looks like nothing but a big spleen
2. **Multiple hypoechoic nodules**
3. **A solitary mass**

Splenic hypoechoic nodules in a patient with known or suspected lymphoma should be reported clearly, as they affect staging.

Metastases are uncommon relative to hepatic metastases; melanoma, breast, lung, and ovarian primaries are the usual sources. Appearances are variable and may be target-like.

Angiosarcoma — rare, aggressive, heterogeneous and vascular, with a risk of rupture.

Infection

Pyogenic abscess — complex collection with debris, irregular wall, possible gas with dirty shadowing or ring-down.

Fungal microabscesses — as in the liver, in the profoundly immunocompromised, with the "wheel within a wheel" and bull's-eye appearances (Chapter 4 §4.8). The liver and spleen are typically involved together, so examine both.

Tuberculosis — multiple small hypoechoic lesions, later calcifying.

Approach to a splenic lesion

Ask three questions: **is the spleen enlarged**, **are the lesions single or multiple**, and **what is the clinical context** — immunosuppression, known malignancy, prior trauma, endemic exposure, or an incidental finding in a well patient. Those three answers narrow the differential more effectively than the sonographic appearance alone, which is frequently non-specific.

CEUS is useful for distinguishing an infarct from a lesion and for characterizing focal lesions, and biopsy of the spleen is undertaken cautiously given the bleeding risk.

id: fig-6-5
lane: A
prompt: >-

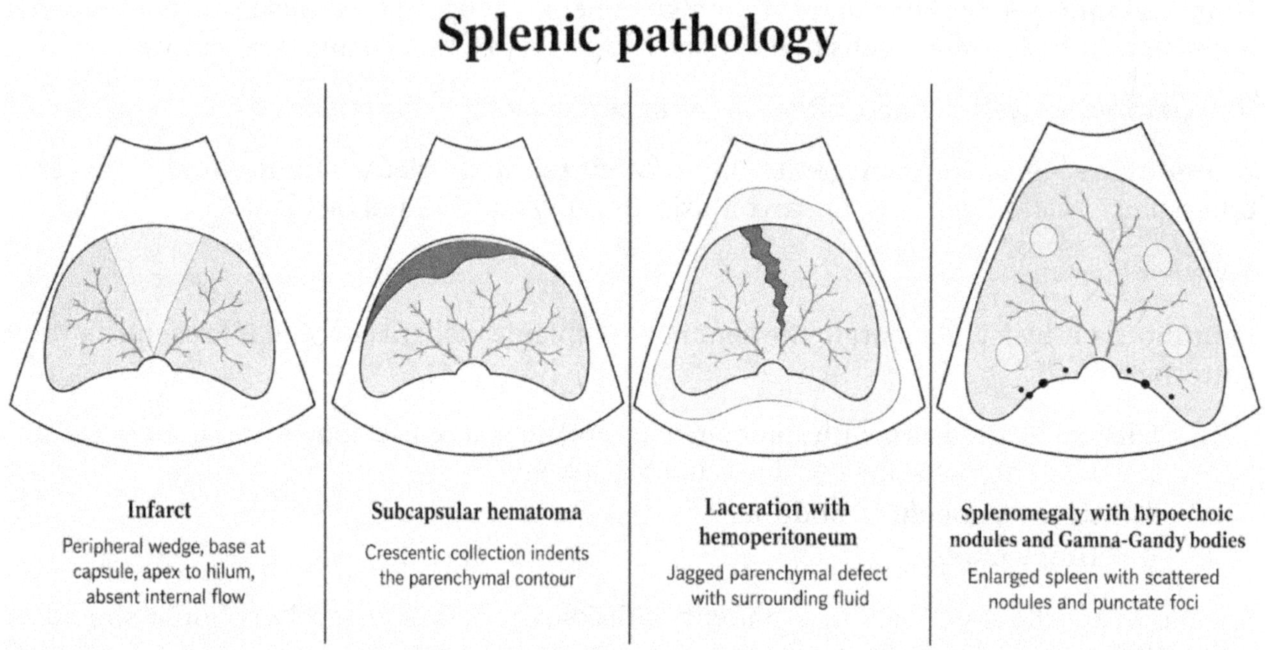

6.8 Gastrointestinal Wall Signature and Scanning Technique

The gut signature

Normal bowel wall shows a characteristic **five-layer** alternating pattern, resolvable with a high-frequency linear transducer. From the lumen outward:

Layer	Appearance	Corresponds to
1	Echogenic	Lumen–mucosa interface
2	Hypoechoic	Deep mucosa / muscularis mucosae
3	Echogenic	Submucosa
4	Hypoechoic	Muscularis propria
5	Echogenic	Serosa / adventitia

This pattern — the **gut signature** — is the reference against which all bowel pathology is judged, and the single most useful question in bowel imaging is whether it is **preserved or lost**.

> **Stratification preserved** → inflammatory processes (Crohn disease, infectious enteritis, diverticulitis) **Stratification lost** → malignancy, transmural necrosis, ischemia, severe transmural inflammation

Normal wall thickness is a few millimetres and depends on distension — a collapsed loop has an apparently thicker wall. [VERIFY: current normal thresholds for small bowel and colonic wall thickness, distended and non-distended]

Recognizing bowel and identifying which bowel

Bowel is identified by **behavior** as much as appearance, which is why real-time observation matters:

- **Peristalsis** — present in small bowel, sluggish in colon, **absent** in inflamed, obstructed-late, or ischemic bowel
- **Compressibility** — normal bowel compresses and displaces; inflamed and infiltrated bowel does not
- **Content** — fluid, gas, or particulate matter, moving in real time
- **Valvulae conniventes** — closely spaced circular folds crossing the full lumen of the jejunum, producing the **"keyboard sign"** when the bowel is fluid-filled and dilated
- **Haustra** — the sacculations of the colon, more widely spaced and not crossing the full lumen
- **Position and calibre** — colon peripheral and larger, small bowel central

Signs of abnormal bowel

Target sign — thickened bowel in cross-section, with a hypoechoic thickened wall surrounding an echogenic lumen.

Pseudokidney sign — the same thickened bowel in longitudinal section, resembling a kidney with an echogenic central lumen and a hypoechoic surrounding wall. Non-specific but reliable for "abnormal bowel here."

Echogenic surrounding fat — inflamed mesenteric or pericolic fat becomes **hyperechoic and non-compressible**, and it is often the most conspicuous finding of a localized inflammatory process. In diverticulitis and epiploic appendagitis it is the primary sign.

Mural hyperemia on color Doppler, indicating active inflammation. Set a low velocity scale.

Free fluid, abscess, and fistula as complications.

Technique

Graded compression is the core technique. Apply slow, steadily increasing pressure with the transducer to displace gas and bowel contents, bring the target closer, and test compressibility. Applied abruptly it causes guarding and fails; applied gradually over several seconds it works.

Transducer choice. Begin with a **curvilinear** probe for orientation and depth, then switch to a **high-frequency linear** probe for wall detail — the gut signature is not resolvable at abdominal frequencies. In children and thin adults the linear probe may be used throughout.

Scan systematically where the question is diffuse, and **scan the point of maximal tenderness first** where it is focal. Asking the patient to indicate the worst point with one finger, and starting there, is one of the highest-yield maneuvers in abdominal sonography — it exploits the modality's unique ability to correlate imaging with symptoms directly.

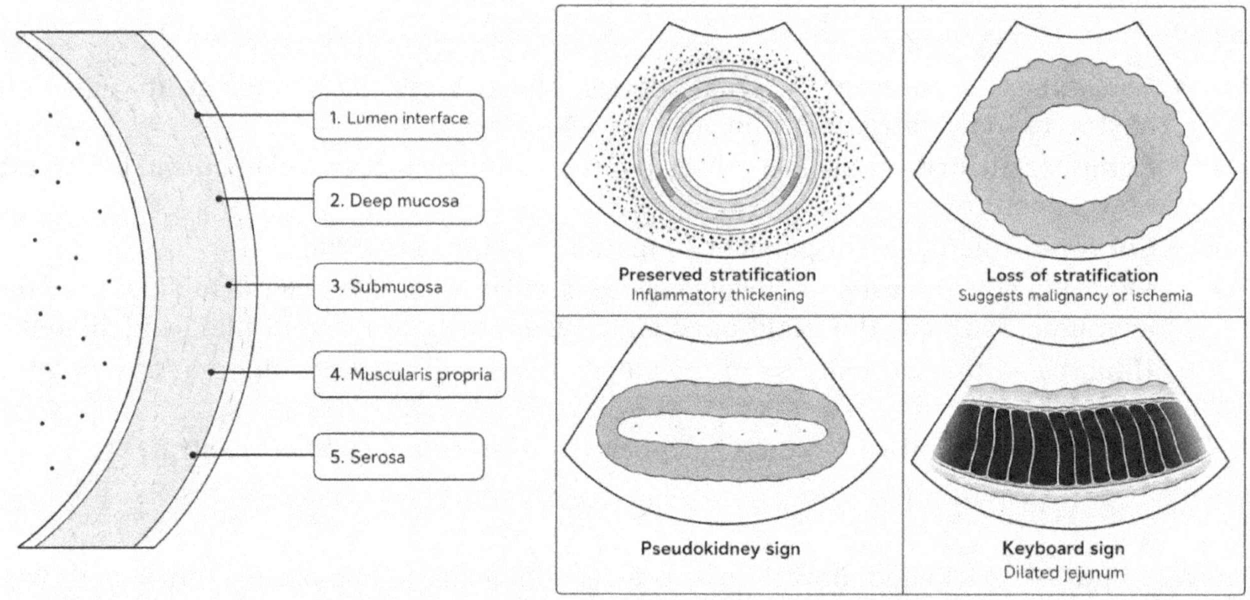

The gut signature: is stratification preserved or lost?

6.9 Appendicitis and Diverticulitis

Appendicitis — technique

Ultrasound is the first-line modality in children, young adults, and pregnancy, where radiation avoidance matters most, and it is highly operator-dependent. The technique is specific and worth performing exactly.

1. **Ask the patient to point to the worst spot with one finger**, and begin there.
2. **Curvilinear probe first** for orientation; identify the **iliac vessels**, **psoas muscle**, and **cecum** as anatomic anchors.
3. **Switch to a high-frequency linear probe** for the appendix itself.
4. **Apply graded compression** slowly, over several seconds, to displace gas and bring the appendix into the near field.
5. **Follow the cecum to its blind end** and identify the appendiceal origin at the base, then follow the appendix along its full length **to its blind tip** — a normal proximal appendix with an inflamed tip is a classic miss.
6. **Search retrocecally** — angling from the flank with the patient in left lateral decubitus — and into the pelvis, since appendiceal position varies widely.

Diagnostic criteria

The appendix is identified as a **blind-ending, non-peristaltic tubular structure arising from the cecal base**, with the gut signature in its wall and a target appearance in cross-section.

Criteria for appendicitis:

- **Outer diameter above the accepted threshold** measured in cross-section, outer wall to outer wall, under compression [VERIFY: current diameter threshold and measurement convention for appendiceal diameter, including any distinction between borderline and diagnostic values]
- **Non-compressibility** — the defining functional sign
- **Wall thickening**, with the gut signature usually preserved early
- **Appendicolith** — an echogenic focus with clean shadowing, a strong supporting finding
- **Periappendiceal fat** that is echogenic, thickened, and non-compressible
- **Mural hyperemia** on color Doppler
- **Free fluid** in the right lower quadrant
- **Focal tenderness maximal over the visualized appendix** — the sonographic equivalent of the Murphy sign, and equally valuable

Perforation is suggested by loss of wall continuity, a periappendiceal collection or phlegmon, loculated fluid, marked surrounding fat inflammation, and — paradoxically — **decreasing tenderness and loss of the previously non-compressible structure** as the appendix decompresses.

Reporting non-visualization

A non-visualized appendix does not exclude appendicitis. This is the most important reporting point in the section. The correct report states that the appendix was not identified, describes what secondary signs were present or absent — free fluid, inflamed fat, tenderness, lymphadenopathy — and states the limiting factors, such as body habitus or bowel gas.

"No appendicitis" written from a study in which the appendix was never seen is indefensible, and it is common.

The mimics

Because the study frequently identifies an alternative diagnosis, they should be actively considered:

- **Mesenteric adenitis** — clustered enlarged mesenteric nodes with a normal appendix, common in children
- **Terminal ileitis** — infectious or Crohn-related wall thickening of the terminal ileum
- **Ovarian pathology** — torsion, ruptured cyst, tubo-ovarian abscess. **In any female patient with right lower quadrant pain, the pelvis must be assessed** (Chapter 17)
- **Epiploic appendagitis** — an ovoid, non-compressible, **hyperechoic** fatty mass abutting the colon, with a hypoechoic rim, **no bowel wall thickening**, and exquisite focal tenderness. Self-limiting, and recognizing it avoids surgery
- **Omental infarction** — a larger echogenic non-compressible fatty mass, often right-sided
- **Meckel diverticulitis, cecal diverticulitis, typhlitis** in the neutropenic patient
- **Renal colic** (Chapter 7)

Diverticulitis

Typically **left lower quadrant**, involving the sigmoid, though right-sided and cecal diverticulitis occur and are more common in some populations.

Findings:

- **Focal hypoechoic or echogenic outpouching** from the colonic wall, representing the inflamed diverticulum, sometimes containing a shadowing fecolith
- **Surrounding echogenic, thickened, non-compressible pericolic fat** — often the most conspicuous sign and the one that localizes the process
- **Segmental hypoechoic colonic wall thickening**, usually with preserved stratification
- **Focal tenderness** over the abnormality
- **Mural and pericolic hyperemia**
- **Complications**: abscess (a walled collection), free gas, fistula, and obstruction

The same **point-of-tenderness graded compression** technique applies, with a linear probe.

CT remains the reference standard for staging diverticulitis and detecting complications, particularly free perforation, and the report should direct there when the clinical picture is severe or complications are suspected.

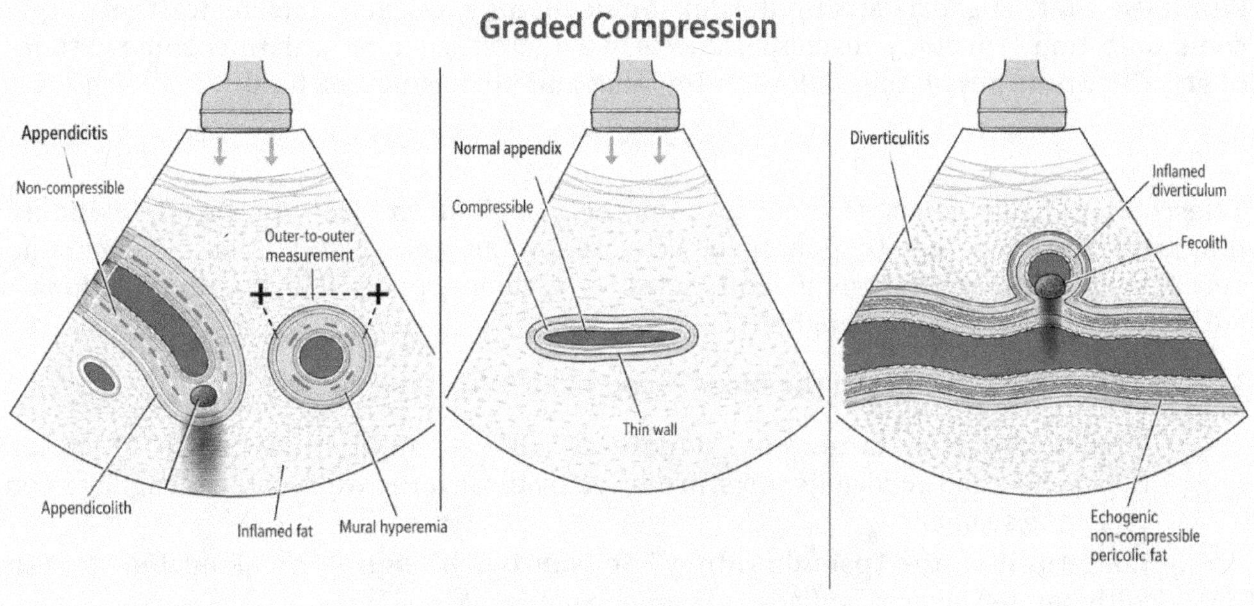

Non-compressibility is the defining functional sign.

6.10 Obstruction, Intussusception, and Inflammatory Bowel Disease

Small bowel obstruction

Ultrasound performs better in obstruction than is generally assumed, and is genuinely useful at the bedside and in patients in whom CT is being avoided.

Findings:

- **Dilated fluid-filled small bowel loops** proximal to the obstruction [VERIFY: current calibre threshold defining small bowel dilatation on ultrasound]
- **Valvulae conniventes** clearly visible against fluid, producing the **keyboard sign**
- **Altered peristalsis** — initially **increased**, with vigorous **to-and-fro** movement of contents as bowel works against the obstruction; later **absent** as the bowel decompensates
- **Collapsed bowel distal** to the obstruction — the finding that distinguishes obstruction from ileus
- **A transition point** between dilated and collapsed segments, which may localize the cause

- **Free interloop fluid**, which increases with severity and is associated with a worse outcome

Obstruction versus ileus rests principally on **peristalsis and the distal segment**: obstruction shows hyperperistalsis early and collapsed distal bowel; ileus shows generalized dilatation with absent peristalsis throughout and no transition point.

Findings that suggest strangulation or ischemia — and which warrant urgent communication — include absent peristalsis in a dilated segment, wall thickening with **loss of stratification**, absent mural flow on Doppler, and increasing free fluid.

Intussusception

Telescoping of one bowel segment into another. In children it is typically **ileocolic and idiopathic**, and is a pediatric emergency covered in Chapter 12; in adults it is uncommon and usually has a **pathological lead point** — a tumor, polyp, Meckel diverticulum, or adhesion — which must be sought.

The appearances are among the most recognizable in sonography:

- **Transverse: the "target" or "doughnut" sign** — multiple concentric alternating hypoechoic and echogenic rings, produced by the layered walls of the invaginated and receiving segments.
- **Longitudinal: the "pseudokidney" or "sandwich" sign** — an elongated structure with parallel layered walls.
- **Trapped mesenteric fat** drawn in between the layers, appearing as a crescent of echogenic material, frequently containing **entrapped lymph nodes** — a specific and useful finding.
- **Absent flow** within the entrapped mesentery on color Doppler suggests ischemia and is an adverse sign.
- **Free fluid** and trapped fluid within the intussusceptum.

Identify a **lead point** where possible, and assess for obstruction proximally.

Crohn disease

Distribution. Any part of the gastrointestinal tract, characteristically the **terminal ileum**, with **skip lesions** — discontinuous involvement.

Findings:

- **Transmural wall thickening**, usually with **stratification preserved** in active inflammatory disease and **lost** in severe transmural disease or fibrosis
- **Marked mural hyperemia** on color Doppler in active disease, which correlates with disease activity and is a genuinely useful monitoring tool
- **"Creeping fat"** — hypertrophied, echogenic, non-compressible mesenteric fat wrapping around the involved segment, a characteristic finding
- **Mesenteric lymphadenopathy**

- **Strictures** with proximal dilatation
- **Fistulae** — hypoechoic tracts extending from bowel to bowel, skin, bladder, or vagina
- **Abscess** — walled collections, often adjacent to a fistula
- **Reduced or absent peristalsis** in the involved segment

Ultrasound has an established role in monitoring Crohn disease — assessing disease activity, extent, and complications without radiation, repeatedly, in a young population with a lifelong illness. This is one of the strongest arguments for bowel ultrasound as a subspecialty skill.

Ulcerative colitis

Distribution. Continuous, beginning at the rectum and extending proximally, confined to the colon.

Findings. Wall thickening that is **more mucosal and less transmural** than in Crohn disease, generally with **preserved stratification**, loss of haustration in chronic disease, and hyperemia. The rectum is poorly assessed transabdominally, which limits the study.

Other bowel conditions

Ischemic bowel — wall thickening with **loss of stratification**, **absent mural flow**, absent peristalsis, and in advanced disease **pneumatosis intestinalis** (echogenic foci within the wall) and **portal venous gas** (Chapter 4 §4.9). This combination is a critical finding.

Pseudomembranous colitis — marked, often striking colonic wall thickening with an irregular "accordion" luminal appearance.

Infectious enterocolitis — segmental wall thickening with preserved stratification, hyperemia, reactive nodes; a common alternative diagnosis in suspected appendicitis.

Colonic carcinoma — a short, asymmetric segment of wall thickening with **loss of stratification** and an abrupt "shouldered" transition to normal bowel; may present as a pseudokidney mass or as the lead point of an intussusception.

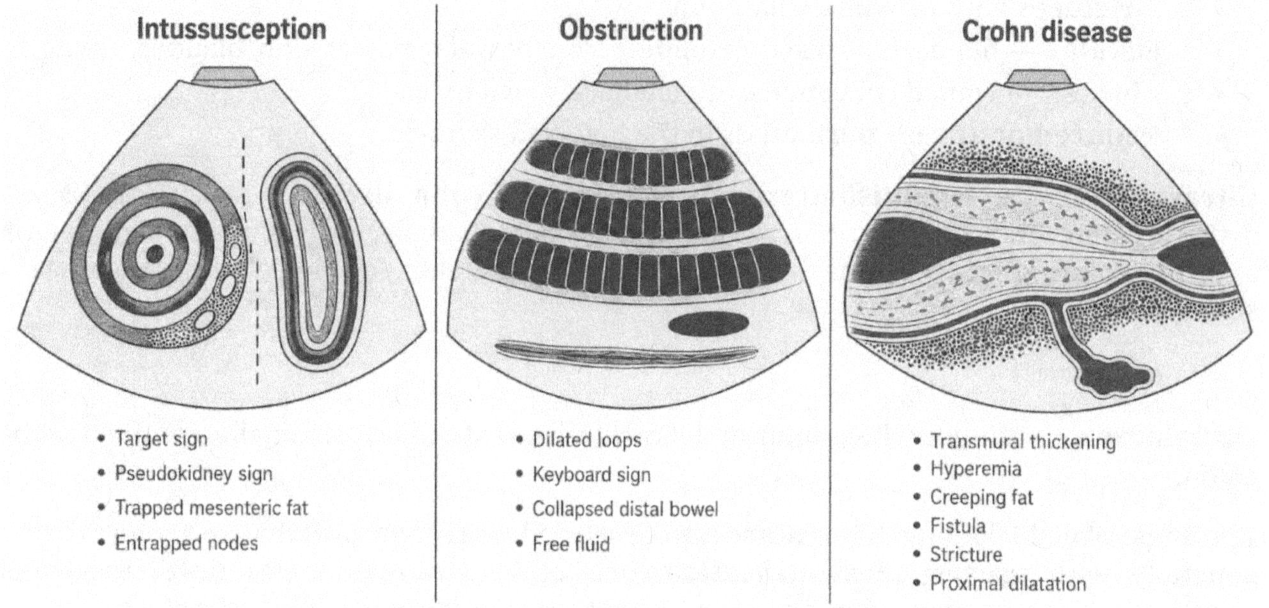

Intussusception, obstruction, and Crohn disease.

Key Points

1. Find the splenic vein and you have found the pancreas. The portal confluence sits behind the neck and anchors the whole anatomy.
2. Water ingestion is the most effective rescue maneuver for the pancreas and is markedly underused.
3. The pancreatic tail is the most commonly non-visualized part of the gland. Say so when it was not seen.
4. Ultrasound's role in acute pancreatitis is to find the gallstones, not to diagnose the pancreatitis. A study that documents biliary etiology has succeeded.
5. A collection containing solid debris is walled-off necrosis, not a pseudocyst. The distinction determines whether percutaneous drainage will work.
6. Interrogate every apparent pseudocyst with color Doppler before calling it one — a splenic artery pseudoaneurysm looks identical on B-mode.
7. Splenic vein thrombosis produces left-sided portal hypertension with gastric varices and a normal liver, and it is surgically curable. Check the splenic vein in every pancreatitis study.
8. Autoimmune pancreatitis narrows the duct; tumor obstruction dilates it. That inversion is a useful discriminator in a diffusely enlarged gland.
9. Transabdominal ultrasound frequently cannot characterize a pancreatic cystic lesion. Describe the features the guideline needs and direct to MRI/MRCP or EUS.
10. An accessory spleen has the same echotexture as the spleen and its own vascular pedicle. That is how it is distinguished from a node, a mass, or a pancreatic tail lesion.
11. A splenic infarct is a peripheral wedge with its base at the capsule. The geometry is the diagnosis.

12. A negative FAST does not exclude splenic injury. FAST screens for free fluid; CT grades organ injury.
13. The gut signature has five layers, and the most useful question in bowel imaging is whether stratification is preserved or lost. Preserved suggests inflammation; lost suggests malignancy or ischemia.
14. Ask the patient to point to the worst spot with one finger and start there. It exploits the modality's unique ability to correlate imaging with symptoms.
15. Non-compressibility is the defining sign of appendicitis, and a non-visualized appendix does not exclude it. Report what you saw, what you did not, and why.
16. Echogenic non-compressible fat is often the most conspicuous sign of a localized inflammatory process, and in diverticulitis and epiploic appendagitis it is the primary finding.
17. Collapsed distal bowel with a transition point distinguishes obstruction from ileus.
18. In any female patient with right lower quadrant pain, assess the pelvis.

Registry Check

1. In the standard oblique transverse pancreatic view, the vessel running along the posterior surface of the body and tail is the:

A. Superior mesenteric artery **B.** Splenic vein **C.** Left renal vein **D.** Portal vein

> **Answer: B.** The splenic vein runs transversely along the posterior body and tail and is the single most reliable landmark for locating the pancreas. The SMA lies posterior in cross-section with its fat collar, the left renal vein passes between SMA and aorta, and the portal vein is formed behind the neck.

2. A well-defined collection with a thick wall is seen adjacent to the pancreas six weeks after severe acute pancreatitis. It contains multiple non-dependent irregular echogenic solid masses. This represents:

A. Pseudocyst **B.** Acute peripancreatic fluid collection **C.** Walled-off necrosis **D.** Pancreatic abscess

> **Answer: C.** An encapsulated collection containing non-liquefied solid debris after necrotizing pancreatitis is walled-off necrosis. The distinction from a pseudocyst matters because percutaneous catheter drainage fails when the collection contains solid material, and endoscopic or surgical necrosectomy is required.

3. A rounded anechoic structure adjacent to the pancreatic tail demonstrates swirling internal color flow with a to-and-fro spectral waveform in its neck. This is:

A. A pseudocyst **B.** A splenic artery pseudoaneurysm **C.** A dilated splenic vein **D.** A mucinous cystic neoplasm

> **Answer: B.** Swirling yin-yang internal flow with a to-and-fro neck waveform is diagnostic of a pseudoaneurysm. Every apparent peripancreatic pseudocyst should

be interrogated with color Doppler before it is described as one, since the two are indistinguishable on B-mode and puncture of an aneurysm is catastrophic.

4. Gastric varices and splenomegaly are found in a patient with a normal liver, normal portal vein, and a thrombosed splenic vein. This is:

A. Cirrhosis with portal hypertension **B.** Budd-Chiari syndrome **C.** Left-sided (sinistral) portal hypertension **D.** Portal vein thrombosis

Answer: C. Splenic vein thrombosis, most often from pancreatic inflammation or malignancy, produces isolated left-sided portal hypertension with gastric and short gastric varices while the liver and portal vein remain normal. It is important because splenectomy is curative.

5. A wedge-shaped hypoechoic region is seen in the spleen with its base at the capsule and its apex directed toward the hilum, containing no flow on color Doppler. This represents:

A. Laceration **B.** Infarct **C.** Lymphomatous deposit **D.** Subcapsular hematoma

Answer: B. The peripheral wedge with base at the capsule and apex toward the hilum follows the territory of an end artery and is the characteristic geometry of splenic infarction. A subcapsular hematoma is crescentic and indents the parenchymal contour rather than being wedge-shaped within it.

6. A segment of bowel shows marked wall thickening with complete loss of the normal five-layer stratification, absent peristalsis, and absent mural flow. This pattern suggests:

A. Active Crohn disease **B.** Infectious enteritis **C.** Ischemia or malignancy **D.** Ulcerative colitis

Answer: C. Loss of stratification indicates transmural destruction of the wall architecture, seen in ischemia and malignancy. Inflammatory conditions including Crohn disease and infectious enteritis typically preserve stratification, at least in active inflammatory phases, and show increased rather than absent mural flow.

7. A tubular structure in the right lower quadrant is blind-ending, measures above the diagnostic threshold, does not compress under graded pressure, and is surrounded by echogenic non-compressible fat. The single most specific functional sign in this description is:

A. The blind ending **B.** The measured diameter **C.** Non-compressibility **D.** The echogenic surrounding fat

Answer: C. Non-compressibility is the defining functional sign of appendicitis and is what graded compression exists to test. Diameter alone has borderline values and is affected by measurement technique; the blind ending identifies the structure as appendix but says nothing about inflammation.

8. Dilated fluid-filled small bowel loops with visible valvulae conniventes are seen alongside collapsed distal bowel and a demonstrable transition point. This indicates:

A. Paralytic ileus **B.** Mechanical small bowel obstruction **C.** Infectious enteritis **D.** Pseudomembranous colitis

> **Answer: B.** The combination of proximal dilatation, collapsed distal bowel, and a transition point defines mechanical obstruction. Ileus produces generalized dilatation with absent peristalsis throughout and no transition point or collapsed distal segment.

Chapter Notes for the Editorial Pass

Verification queue. In priority order: **pancreatic cystic lesion management thresholds** (§6.4) — guideline-defined, differing between guidelines, revised, and directly driving surveillance and resection decisions; **appendiceal diameter threshold and measurement convention** (§6.9), including the handling of borderline values, which is contested and clinically consequential; the **revised classification of pancreatic fluid collections** with its terminology and time thresholds (§6.2); **normal bowel wall thickness** for small bowel and colon, distended and non-distended (§6.8); **small bowel calibre threshold for dilatation** (§6.10); **splenic length upper limit** (§6.5); **main pancreatic duct upper limit** (§6.1); and **current society guidance on CEUS in blunt abdominal trauma**, including pediatric recommendations, which is an actively developing area (§6.6).

Scope note. This chapter covers three organs and inevitably compresses each relative to a dedicated treatment. Pediatric intussusception and pyloric stenosis are deliberately deferred to Chapter 12 rather than duplicated here; the cross-references must be checked at layout so neither topic falls between the two chapters.

Figure count: 7 Lane A, 2 Lane B. The chapter is figure-light relative to its breadth, which is deliberate — the material is largely pattern-based and the patterns are described in tables. If one further Lane B slot is added, the highest-value candidate is a normal pancreas with and without the water-filled stomach window, which is already specified in `fig-6-4`.

Cross-reference targets to fix at layout: §6.1 retroperitoneal spaces → Chapter 3 §3.1; §6.2 biliary etiology → Chapter 5 §5.3; §6.2 pseudoaneurysm → Chapter 3 §3.8; §6.4 double duct sign → Chapter 5 §5.8; §6.6 FAST → Chapter 8; §6.6 splenomegaly in portal hypertension → Chapter 4 §4.5; §6.9 ovarian mimics → Chapter 17; §6.10 pediatric intussusception and pyloric stenosis → Chapter 12; §6.10 portal venous gas → Chapter 4 §4.9.

Word count: approximately 10,300 excluding image prompt blocks, learning objectives, registry questions, and these notes.

Chapter 7: The Urinary System and Retroperitoneum

Learning Objectives

On completing this chapter you should be able to:

1. Identify normal renal architecture, and distinguish the common pseudotumors from true masses.
2. Recognize the principal congenital variants and state the clinical consequence of each.
3. Measure renal length reproducibly and obtain a technically valid resistive index.
4. Grade hydronephrosis, determine the level of obstruction, and exclude the conditions that mimic it.
5. Optimize for stone detection, and use secondary signs when the stone itself is not seen.
6. Recognize the sonographic pattern of medical renal disease and state what ultrasound can and cannot contribute.
7. Describe a cystic lesion using the features a classification system requires.
8. Characterize solid renal masses and state where ultrasound cannot distinguish between them.
9. Measure bladder volume, assess wall pathology, and distinguish tumor from clot.
10. Locate the adrenal glands and recognize the retroperitoneal compartment of a collection or mass.

The Modality's Strongest and Weakest Suits

The urinary tract shows both extremes of what ultrasound does.

It is **excellent** at answering the questions that matter most urgently: is the kidney obstructed, is there a stone, is the bladder emptying, is this mass cystic or solid, is there a collection. These are anatomical and mechanical questions, and ultrasound answers them at the bedside, without radiation, repeatedly.

It is **poor** at the questions that require tissue characterization: what kind of medical renal disease is this, is this small mass a carcinoma or an angiomyolipoma, is this complex cyst malignant, is this adrenal nodule an adenoma. For these, ultrasound describes and directs — and the professional skill is knowing which kind of question you have been asked.

7.1 Renal Anatomy, Variants, and Congenital Anomalies

Normal architecture

The kidneys are **retroperitoneal**, within the **perirenal space** enclosed by Gerota's fascia (Chapter 3 §3.1), lying obliquely alongside the vertebral column with their upper poles more posterior and medial. **The right kidney sits lower than the left**, displaced by the liver — a normal asymmetry, not a finding.

Three zones are distinguished sonographically:

Renal sinus — the central echogenic complex, containing fat, the collecting system, and the hilar vessels. It is the brightest structure in the kidney and its fat content increases with age and obesity (renal sinus lipomatosis).

Renal medulla — the pyramids, appearing as **hypoechoic triangles** arranged around the sinus with their apices pointing toward it. They are frequently mistaken for cysts or hydronephrosis by the inexperienced; their triangular shape, regular arrangement, and position distinguish them.

Renal cortex — surrounding the pyramids and extending between them as the **columns of Bertin**.

The echogenicity hierarchy is the basis of most renal assessment and must be committed to memory:

Renal sinus > liver and spleen ≥ renal cortex > medullary pyramids

Corticomedullary differentiation — the visible contrast between cortex and pyramids — is a marker of normal architecture, and its loss is a general sign of medical renal disease (§7.5).

Measurements. Renal length is taken in the **coronal plane through the hilum, along the longest axis**. Cortical thickness and the difference in length between the two sides are also assessed; a significant discrepancy is meaningful even when both kidneys fall within the population range. [VERIFY: current reference ranges for adult renal length, cortical thickness, and the maximum acceptable inter-renal difference]

Vascular anatomy. The renal arteries arise from the aorta below the SMA, with **the right renal artery passing posterior to the IVC** (Chapter 3 §3.4). Within the kidney: segmental → **interlobar** arteries (running between pyramids) → **arcuate** arteries (arching along the corticomedullary junction) → interlobular. The arcuate and interlobar vessels are the ones interrogated for resistive index (§7.2).

Pseudotumors

Four normal appearances are regularly reported as masses. All four are identified by the same principle: **their echotexture is identical to normal cortex, and their vascular architecture is normal and undisplaced.**

Hypertrophied column of Bertin — an unusually prominent cortical column indenting the sinus. It is continuous with the adjacent cortex, contains normal interlobar vessels running through it, and does not bulge the renal contour.

Dromedary hump — a focal bulge on the **lateral border of the left kidney**, from splenic impression. Normal cortex, normal contour continuity.

Fetal lobulation — smooth surface indentations lying **between** pyramids, a persistent embryonic pattern. Distinguished from cortical scarring, which is a depression **overlying** a pyramid.

Junctional parenchymal defect — a triangular echogenic area at the **anterosuperior aspect of the right kidney**, representing the fusion plane of the embryonic renunculi. Frequently mistaken for a scar or a lesion.

Congenital variants and anomalies

Extrarenal pelvis — a renal pelvis lying outside the sinus, appearing as a central anechoic structure. **The commonest mimic of hydronephrosis** (§7.3). It is distinguished by the absence of calyceal dilatation and by decompression after voiding.

Duplex collecting system — a common variant with two collecting systems and often two ureters. The **Weigert–Meyer rule** governs the pattern and its consequences:

> The **upper** pole ureter inserts **inferomedially** and ectopically — prone to **obstruction and ureterocele**. The **lower** pole ureter inserts **superolaterally** — prone to **vesicoureteric reflux**.

The sonographic clue is a band of central echogenic sinus tissue dividing the kidney into two collecting systems, with the kidney often longer than usual. When you find a dilated upper pole moiety, **examine the bladder for a ureterocele** — the two findings go together, and the pediatric presentation is developed in Chapter 12.

Horseshoe kidney — fusion of the lower poles across the midline by an isthmus lying **anterior to the aorta and inferior to the origin of the inferior mesenteric artery**, which arrests its ascent. The kidneys are low-lying and malrotated. Clinically it matters because of an increased incidence of **obstruction, stone formation, infection, and vulnerability to trauma**. It is easily missed: the lower poles appear to fade medially on standard coronal views, and the isthmus is only seen if you deliberately scan across the midline anterior to the aorta.

Renal ectopia — most often pelvic, and **crossed fused ectopia** in which both kidneys lie on the same side. Before diagnosing renal agenesis, search the pelvis.

Renal agenesis — a genuinely absent kidney, with **compensatory hypertrophy of the contralateral kidney** as the supporting sign. An empty renal fossa alone is insufficient; look for the ectopic organ, and note that the ipsilateral adrenal adopts a flattened elongated configuration in the empty fossa.

Malrotation — the hilum facing anteriorly or posteriorly rather than medially, producing an unfamiliar appearance without pathological significance.

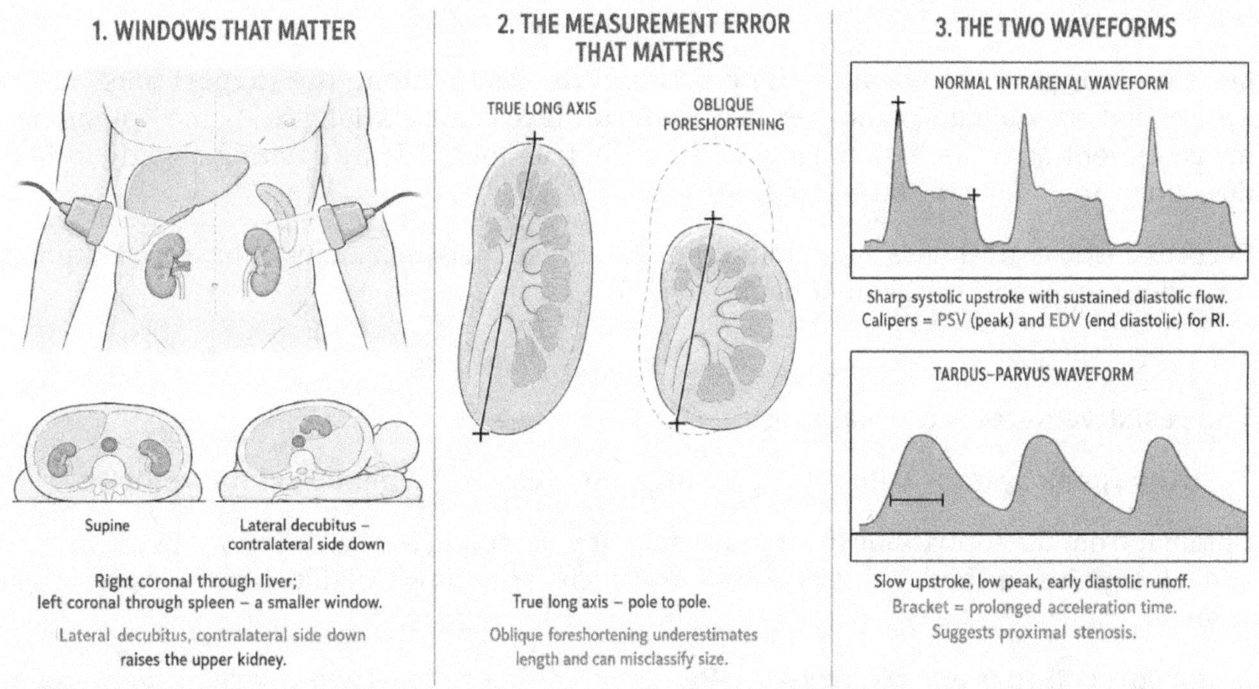

7.2 Scanning Protocol and Renal Doppler Technique

Preparation and windows

Bladder filling should be moderate — enough to assess the bladder and the ureteric jets, not so much that it distorts the pelvis or causes discomfort. Fasting is helpful for reducing bowel gas but is not essential.

Transducer. Curvilinear for the survey. A **high-frequency linear** probe adds value for a superficial kidney, in thin patients and children, and for the anterior surface of a transplant (Chapter 9).

Windows and positions:

Approach	Notes
Right coronal via the liver	The most reliable window in the body for a kidney
Left coronal via the spleen	Harder — the spleen is a smaller window and the splenic flexure interferes. Expect to work for it
Posterolateral / translumbar	Useful when anterior windows fail
Prone	For biopsy guidance and difficult windows
Lateral decubitus, contralateral side down	Brings the kidney upward and away from bowel; the standard rescue position
Erect	Occasionally helpful, and used to assess renal mobility

Deep inspiration displaces the kidneys caudally into the intercostal windows.

Measurement

Measure **length in the coronal plane through the hilum along the longest axis**, and be aware that an oblique plane systematically **underestimates** length — the commonest measurement error here. Confirm you have the true long axis by rotating slightly in both directions and taking the largest value.

Record cortical thickness, and note the difference between sides. For serial studies, reproduce the prior technique (Chapter 1 §1.5).

Doppler technique

The resistive index is calculated as:

RI = (peak systolic velocity – end-diastolic velocity) / peak systolic velocity

Obtain it from the **interlobar or arcuate arteries**, sampling several locations in upper, mid, and lower poles and both kidneys. Use a low velocity scale, low wall filter, and a small sample volume.

Angle correction is not required for RI, because it is a ratio of two velocities measured in the same vessel — the angle-dependent term cancels. This is one of the few Doppler measurements where a suboptimal angle does not invalidate the number, though a poor angle still degrades the trace quality.

What raises RI: obstruction (acute), acute tubular necrosis, transplant rejection and other transplant complications, medical renal disease, renal vein thrombosis, and hepatorenal syndrome. **It is highly non-specific.** It is also affected by age, heart rate, blood pressure, and the presence of aortic regurgitation, which makes an isolated value of limited use.

The side-to-side difference is often more informative than the absolute value, particularly in suspected unilateral obstruction. [VERIFY: current normal upper limit for renal resistive index and the threshold for a significant inter-renal difference]

Renal artery assessment

Direct interrogation of the main renal artery at its **origin, mid-portion, and hilum**, with a low insonation angle. This is technically demanding — the origins are deep, obscured by bowel gas, and the right renal artery courses behind the IVC.

Indirect intrarenal assessment looks for the **tardus–parvus waveform** distal to a stenosis: a **slow, blunted systolic upstroke** (prolonged acceleration time) with a **reduced peak** and loss of the normal early systolic peak. This is the pattern of a proximal stenosis, and it can be detected in intrarenal vessels even when the origin cannot be seen — a genuine practical advantage.

Diagnostic criteria for renal artery stenosis combine direct peak systolic velocity, the renal-to-aortic velocity ratio, acceleration time, and acceleration index. **These thresholds are laboratory- and guideline-specific and must be taken from the criteria your**

department has validated. [VERIFY: current velocity criteria for renal artery stenosis, including PSV threshold, renal-aortic ratio, and acceleration time]

Documentation

Both kidneys in **long axis and transverse**, upper pole to lower pole; length measurement on each; cortical echogenicity compared with liver on the right and spleen on the left **in the same frame**; the collecting system; the bladder before and, where indicated, after voiding; ureteric jets where obstruction is a question; and Doppler as indicated by the clinical question.

id: fig-7-2
lane: A
prompt: >-

7.3 Hydronephrosis and Obstructive Uropathy

Recognizing and grading

Hydronephrosis is dilatation of the pelvicalyceal system, appearing as anechoic branching structures within the echogenic sinus, communicating with each other and converging on the pelvis.

Grading is conventionally descriptive:

Grade	Findings
Mild	Dilated pelvis with or without major calyces; normal cortex
Moderate	Pelvis and calyces dilated with blunting of the normal calyceal cupping; cortex preserved
Severe	Marked dilatation with ballooned calyces, loss of the normal architecture, and **cortical thinning**

Formal grading systems exist and are used particularly in pediatric practice, where they drive follow-up decisions (Chapter 12). [VERIFY: current grading systems for hydronephrosis in adult and pediatric practice, including the classification used for antenatal and postnatal urinary tract dilatation]

Cortical thinning is the finding that indicates chronicity and irreversible loss, and it should always be commented on.

Determining the level

The reasoning is the same as for the biliary tree (Chapter 5 §5.8): the pattern tells you where the obstruction is, even when the cause is invisible.

Pattern	Level
Pelvicalyceal dilatation, **ureter not dilated**	**Pelviureteric junction**

Pattern	Level
Pelvicalyceal **and ureteric** dilatation to a point in mid-abdomen	Mid-ureter, often at the **pelvic brim** where the ureter crosses the iliac vessels
Dilatation to the **bladder**, with a distended distal ureter behind it	**Vesicoureteric junction** — the commonest site of stone impaction
Bilateral hydronephrosis with a distended bladder	**Bladder outlet obstruction** — prostate, urethral stricture, neurogenic bladder
Bilateral hydronephrosis with an **empty** bladder	Bilateral ureteric obstruction, or a pelvic or retroperitoneal process

Scan the ureter deliberately. A dilated ureter can often be followed from the renal pelvis inferiorly along the psoas, and the distal ureter behind a filled bladder is frequently visible when the mid-ureter is not — a stone at the VUJ is often best seen through the bladder window.

The mimics — exclude these before reporting obstruction

Extrarenal pelvis — a prominent pelvis with **no calyceal dilatation**. The commonest mimic.

Parapelvic (peripelvic) cysts — multiple cysts in the sinus that resemble a dilated system but **do not communicate with each other**, do not converge on a ureter, and do not decompress. Careful real-time observation with slow probe movement distinguishes them.

Prominent renal vessels — resolved instantly with **color Doppler**, which should be applied to any questionable "dilatation" before it is reported. This is a one-second check that prevents a recurrent error.

Overdistended bladder — produces mild bilateral pelvicalyceal fullness that resolves after voiding. **Rescan post-void** before reporting mild bilateral hydronephrosis.

High urine flow — diuretics, diabetes insipidus, high fluid intake.

Vesicoureteric reflux — dilatation without obstruction.

Pregnancy — physiological dilatation, typically **right greater than left**, from mechanical compression and hormonal effects. Common, expected, and should be described as physiological unless the clinical picture suggests otherwise.

Congenital megacalyces, and a chronically dilated system after a previously relieved obstruction.

Obstruction without dilatation

An important false-negative pattern. Dilatation may be absent or minimal in:

- **Very early (hyperacute) obstruction**, before the system has distended
- **Dehydration and volume depletion**

- **Retroperitoneal fibrosis or malignant encasement**, where the ureter is held open-walled but non-compliant and cannot dilate
- A staghorn calculus filling the system

A patient with renal colic and no hydronephrosis has not been excluded. Use **secondary signs**: absent ureteric jet on the affected side, elevated RI or an inter-renal RI difference, perinephric fluid, and a visualized stone.

Pyonephrosis

An infected obstructed system — pus under pressure. It is a **urological emergency requiring urgent decompression**, and mortality without drainage is high.

Findings: dilated collecting system containing **low-level internal echoes, debris, or a fluid–debris level**, sometimes with gas producing dirty shadowing, in a patient with fever and sepsis. Urothelial wall thickening may be present.

The echoes are the diagnosis, and they are easy to miss at low gain. In any obstructed, febrile patient, examine the dilated system carefully at adequate gain for internal content.

Suspected pyonephrosis is a critical finding requiring immediate communication (Chapter 1 §1.5).

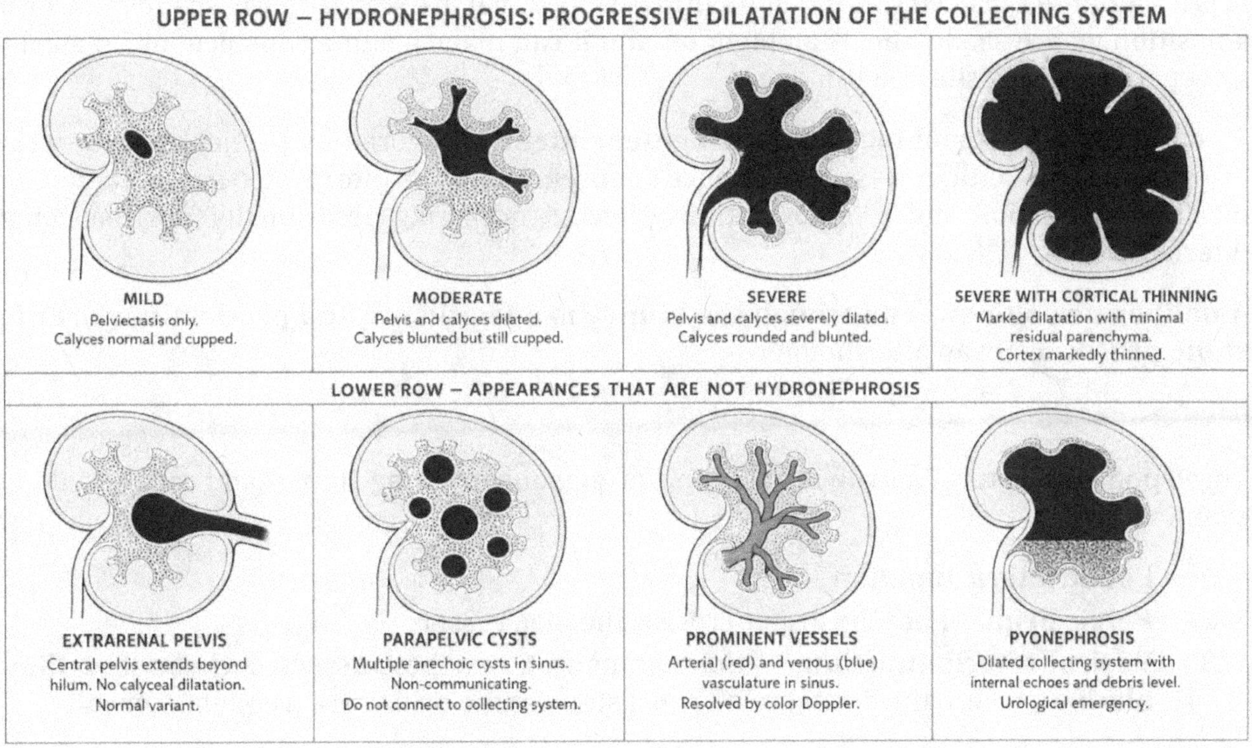

7.4 Nephrolithiasis and the Twinkling Artifact

Detection

A calculus appears as an **echogenic focus within the collecting system with clean posterior acoustic shadowing** (Chapter 2 §2.7 — the clean-versus-dirty distinction).

Optimization, applied before concluding a focus does not shadow:

1. **Disable spatial compounding** — the single most consequential setting (Chapter 2 §2.4)
2. **Place the focal zone at the stone**
3. **Raise the frequency** if penetration allows
4. **Narrow the dynamic range** to increase contrast
5. **Reposition** so the stone lies in the centre of the beam rather than at the sector edge

Twinkling artifact

Introduced in Chapter 2 §2.9, and this is its principal clinical application. A rapidly alternating color mosaic appearing **behind a rough crystalline surface**, with a disorganized spectral signal, arising from phase jitter in the returning signal rather than from motion.

It is a valuable positive finding. It identifies stones that are small, poorly shadowing, or in a position where shadowing is ambiguous, and it can make a stone conspicuous on a color sweep that was invisible on B-mode.

Two cautions: it is **machine- and setting-dependent** — favored by particular color write priority and PRF settings — so its presence or absence must be interpreted against your own machine's behavior; and it is not entirely specific, occurring occasionally at other rough interfaces.

A deliberate color sweep through the kidney is a legitimate and productive part of a stone protocol, not an afterthought.

Sites of impaction

Three points of natural narrowing account for most obstructing stones, and each should be examined:

1. **Pelviureteric junction**
2. **Pelvic brim**, where the ureter crosses the iliac vessels
3. **Vesicoureteric junction** — the commonest, and best assessed **through a filled bladder**, where the distal ureter and a stone at the orifice are frequently visible

Secondary signs

When the stone itself is not seen — which is common, since the mid-ureter is usually obscured by bowel gas — the diagnosis may rest on:

- **Hydronephrosis and hydroureter** to a level
- **Absent or abnormal ureteric jet** on the affected side (§7.8)
- **Elevated RI, or an inter-renal RI difference**
- **Perinephric or periureteric fluid**, and **urinoma** in forniceal rupture

Staghorn calculus

A large branching stone filling the collecting system. It may not look like a stone at all: rather than a discrete focus, it produces a **broad curved echogenic line following the sinus with dense shadowing behind it**, obscuring the underlying anatomy. It is associated with chronic infection and with **xanthogranulomatous pyelonephritis** (§7.5).

Nephrocalcinosis

Calcium deposition within the renal parenchyma, distinguished by its distribution:

Medullary nephrocalcinosis — echogenic pyramids, an inversion of the normal pattern in which pyramids are the darkest structure. Causes include hyperparathyroidism, distal renal tubular acidosis, medullary sponge kidney, hypervitaminosis D, and — in neonates — loop diuretic therapy (Chapter 12).

Cortical nephrocalcinosis — less common; echogenic cortex from chronic glomerulonephritis, cortical necrosis, or Alport syndrome.

Modality choice

Non-contrast CT is the reference standard for urinary calculi, with markedly higher sensitivity, particularly for ureteric stones.

Ultrasound is preferred first-line in **pregnancy**, in **children**, and in **recurrent stone-formers** in whom cumulative radiation is a real concern, and it is the appropriate bedside test where the immediate question is obstruction rather than stone.

The report should state which question was answered: absence of a visualized stone is not absence of a stone, and this should be explicit.

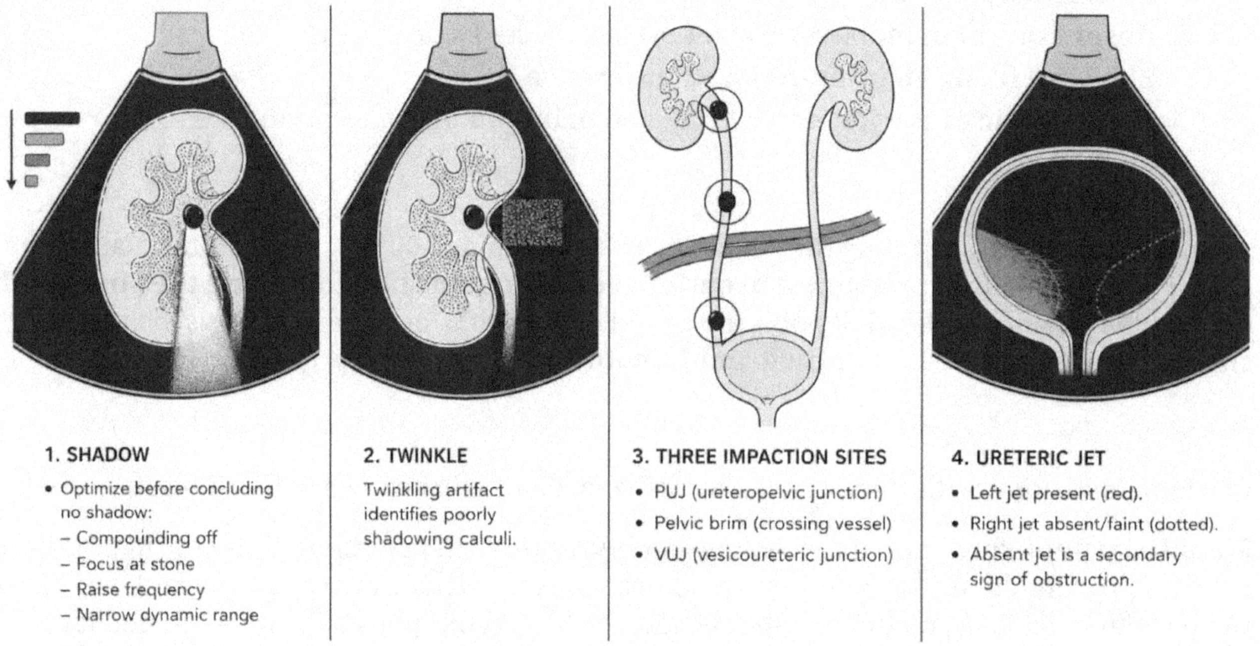

7.5 Medical Renal Disease and Correlative Laboratory Values

The sonographic pattern

Medical renal disease — parenchymal disease as opposed to obstruction or a mass — produces a limited and largely non-specific set of findings:

Increased cortical echogenicity. The key comparison is against the adjacent organ: **cortex should be equal to or less echogenic than liver on the right, and spleen on the left.** Cortex that is clearly *more* echogenic than liver is abnormal. As in Chapter 4, **acquire the comparison in a single frame at matched depth and gain**, or the assessment cannot be verified.

Loss of corticomedullary differentiation — the pyramids become less distinct from the cortex.

Reduced renal size and cortical thinning in chronic disease.

Increased or normal size in some acute and infiltrative processes.

The pattern that matters clinically is size:

> **Small, echogenic kidneys with thin cortex** → chronic, irreversible disease
> **Normal-sized or enlarged echogenic kidneys** → acute or potentially reversible process, or an infiltrative disease

This distinction is genuinely useful to the nephrologist and is one of ultrasound's real contributions here.

What ultrasound is for in renal impairment

It does not diagnose the type of parenchymal disease. Its defined roles are:

1. **Exclude obstruction** — the reversible cause that must not be missed. This is the primary indication for imaging in acute kidney injury.
2. **Assess size and cortical thickness**, informing whether the disease is acute or chronic and whether recovery is plausible.
3. **Identify structural causes** — cysts, masses, stones, scarring, asymmetry suggesting vascular disease.
4. **Guide biopsy**, which is what actually makes the diagnosis (Chapter 9).
5. **Assess for complications of chronic kidney disease**, including acquired cystic disease and its associated malignancy risk (§7.6).

Some specific patterns:

HIV-associated nephropathy — markedly echogenic kidneys that are normal-sized or enlarged, with loss of corticomedullary differentiation; the degree of echogenicity is often striking.

Acute glomerulonephritis and acute interstitial nephritis — normal or enlarged echogenic kidneys.

Acute tubular necrosis — often sonographically normal, with an elevated RI.

Diabetic nephropathy — enlarged early, small and echogenic late.

Amyloidosis and infiltrative disease — enlarged echogenic kidneys.

Correlative laboratory values

Creatinine and estimated GFR quantify function and, in serial form, distinguish acute from chronic. **Urea** rises in impairment and in volume depletion and gastrointestinal bleeding. **Proteinuria** points to glomerular disease. **Hematuria** directs toward stones, tumor, infection, or glomerular disease, and in an adult always requires exclusion of urothelial malignancy (§7.7).

A **rising creatinine** is the trigger for the study, and the question you are being asked is usually "is it obstructed" — answer that first and clearly.

Infection

Acute pyelonephritis is usually **sonographically normal**, and this must be understood rather than treated as a negative finding. When abnormal:

- Renal enlargement, focal or diffuse
- Focal areas of altered echogenicity, hypo- or hyperechoic, with loss of corticomedullary differentiation
- **Urothelial (pelvic wall) thickening**

- Reduced or absent perfusion in the affected segment on power Doppler — a useful sign requiring a sensitive setting
- Perinephric fluid

Imaging is indicated in pyelonephritis mainly to detect complications, not to make the diagnosis:

Renal or perinephric abscess — a complex collection with debris and no internal flow, with peripheral hyperemia.

Emphysematous pyelonephritis — gas within the parenchyma, producing **dirty shadowing and ring-down** (Chapter 2 §2.8). Strongly associated with diabetes, carries a high mortality, and is a **critical finding requiring immediate communication**.

Pyonephrosis — as in §7.3, and equally urgent.

Xanthogranulomatous pyelonephritis — chronic destructive infection, typically with a **staghorn calculus**, an enlarged non-functioning kidney, and dilated calyces replaced by inflammatory tissue, producing the "bear paw" appearance on cross-sectional imaging. It mimics malignancy.

Chronic pyelonephritis and reflux nephropathy — cortical scarring with focal thinning **overlying a calyx**, distinguished from fetal lobulation, which lies **between** pyramids.

Renal vein thrombosis

An enlarged, echogenic kidney with **absent venous flow**, and characteristically **reversed diastolic flow** in the arterial waveform — a distinctive and important sign. Causes include nephrotic syndrome, malignancy (particularly renal cell carcinoma with tumor thrombus, §7.7), dehydration in neonates, and prothrombotic states.

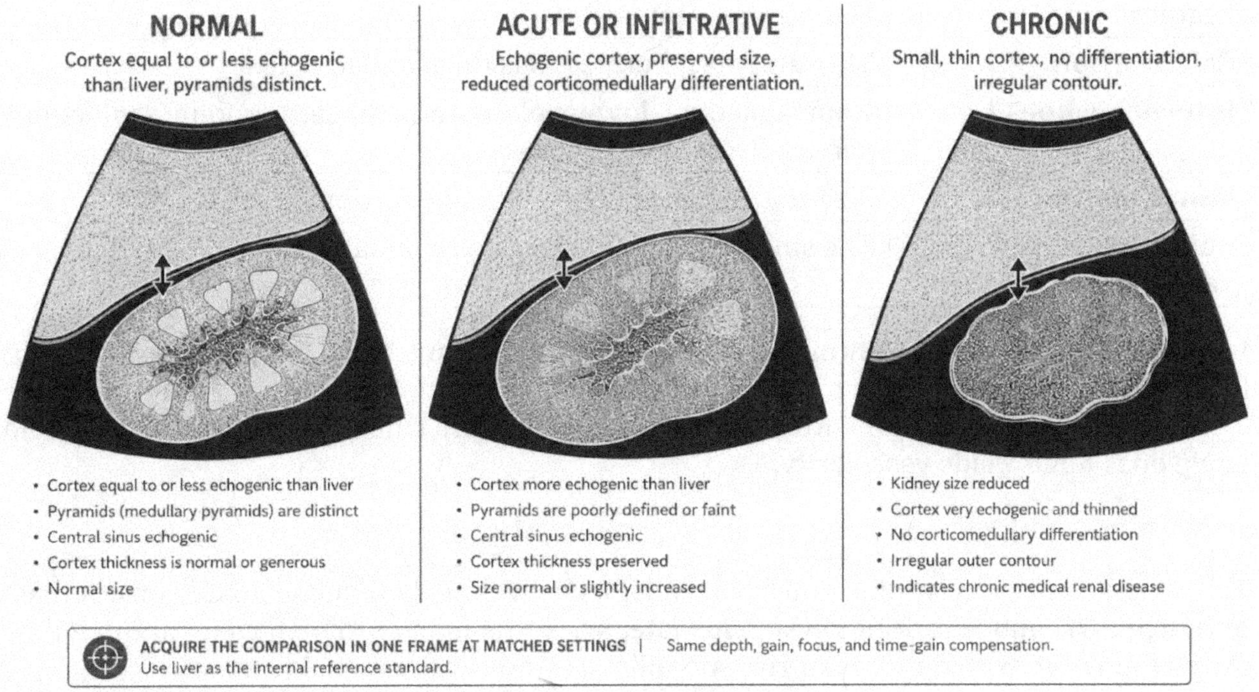

7.6 Renal Cystic Disease and Cyst Classification

The simple cyst

Extremely common, increasing in prevalence with age, and of no significance when it meets all the criteria:

- **Anechoic** throughout
- **Thin, imperceptible wall**
- **Sharply marginated**
- **Posterior acoustic enhancement**
- **No septations, no calcification, no mural nodule, no internal flow**

As established in Chapter 2, **spatial compounding suppresses posterior enhancement** and **harmonic imaging suppresses genuine low-level internal echoes**. Before calling a cyst simple, check it with compounding off and on fundamental. This matters more here than almost anywhere else, because the whole classification hinges on whether internal features are present.

Features that make a cyst complex

Each of the following moves a lesion up the risk spectrum, and each must be described specifically because the classification systems are built from them:

Feature	Description required
Septations	Number, thickness, whether they show flow
Wall thickening	Uniform or irregular

Feature	Description required
Calcification	Thin and peripheral versus thick and irregular
Internal echoes	Homogeneous low-level (hemorrhage, protein, infection) versus discrete solid material
Mural nodule	Size, and — decisively — whether it demonstrates **flow**
Enhancement / vascularity	The single most important discriminator

Vascularity within a septum or nodule is the finding that most raises concern. Interrogate any complex cyst with color Doppler at a low velocity scale, and note that conventional Doppler is insensitive to the slow flow within a small nodule — a negative color study does not exclude vascularity.

Classification

The widely used cyst classification framework was developed for and validated on **contrast-enhanced CT**, and it stratifies cysts into categories that map onto management: no follow-up, no follow-up with minor features, surveillance, and surgical consideration.

Applying it directly to ultrasound is not straightforward, because the defining criterion in the original system is **contrast enhancement**, which conventional B-mode cannot assess. Adaptations for **contrast-enhanced ultrasound** exist and are increasingly used, and CEUS is genuinely good at this application — it demonstrates septal and nodular enhancement well and avoids nephrotoxic contrast in patients who frequently have impaired renal function.

The practical position: describe the features fully, state which system (if any) you are applying and on what basis, and where classification will drive management, direct to CEUS or contrast-enhanced CT/MRI. [VERIFY: current cyst classification system, its category definitions, and the status of its adaptation for contrast-enhanced ultrasound]

Hereditary and acquired cystic disease

Autosomal dominant polycystic kidney disease — bilaterally enlarged kidneys containing innumerable cysts of varying size, progressively replacing normal parenchyma. Look for:

- **Hepatic cysts**, present in a majority
- Pancreatic and splenic cysts
- A **family history**, though a substantial minority have no known one
- Complications: hemorrhage into cysts, infection, stones, hypertension, and progressive renal failure

Diagnostic criteria are age-stratified, requiring different cyst numbers at different ages, and screening of at-risk relatives is a defined clinical activity. [VERIFY: current age-stratified ultrasound diagnostic criteria for ADPKD and current recommendations for screening at-risk family members]

Note the extrarenal association with **intracranial berry aneurysms**, which is why family and personal history matter.

Autosomal recessive polycystic kidney disease presents in infancy with enlarged, diffusely echogenic kidneys and congenital hepatic fibrosis — Chapter 12.

Acquired cystic kidney disease — multiple cysts developing in the small, end-stage kidneys of patients on long-term dialysis. **It carries an increased risk of renal cell carcinoma**, so a solid or complex lesion in a dialysis patient's cystic kidneys is significant and should not be dismissed as another cyst.

Multicystic dysplastic kidney — a congenital non-functioning kidney replaced by non-communicating cysts, distinguished from severe hydronephrosis by the absence of communication and of a dilated renal pelvis. Chapter 12.

Von Hippel–Lindau and **tuberous sclerosis** — syndromic associations with renal cysts and, respectively, with renal cell carcinoma and angiomyolipoma.

Parapelvic and peripelvic cysts — as in §7.3, mimicking hydronephrosis.

Medullary sponge kidney — tubular ectasia with medullary calcification, producing echogenic pyramids.

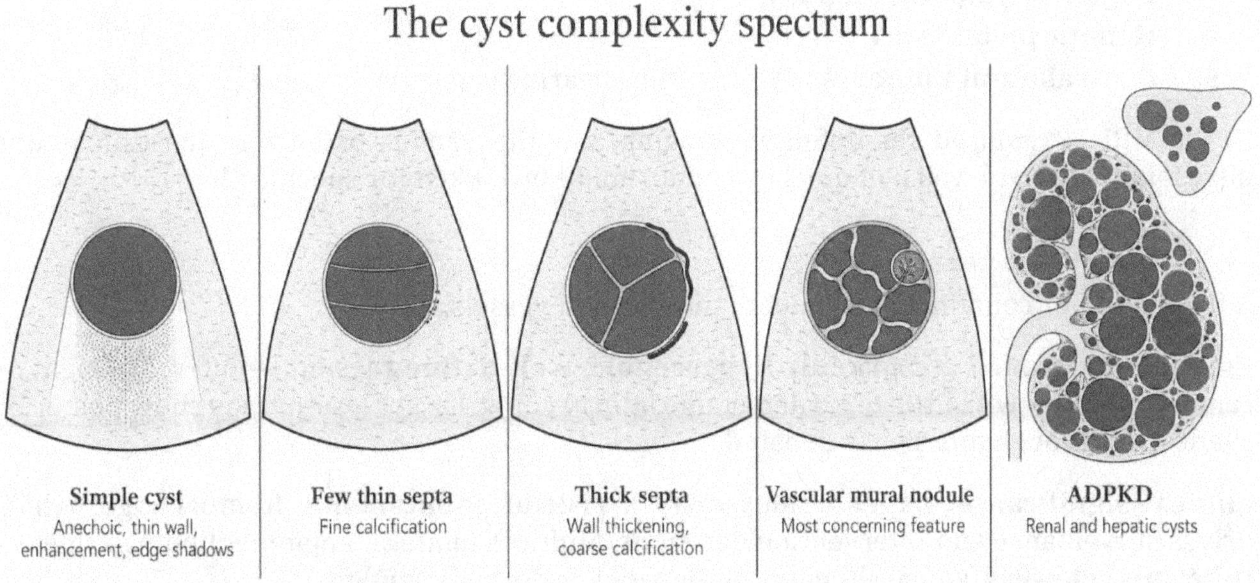

Check with compounding off and in fundamental mode before calling a cyst simple.

7.7 Renal Neoplasms

Renal cell carcinoma

The dominant renal malignancy, and increasingly detected incidentally at a small size during imaging performed for other reasons.

Appearance is variable and this is the central difficulty:

- **Small tumors are frequently hyperechoic**, closely resembling angiomyolipoma
- **Larger tumors** are typically heterogeneous, with necrosis, hemorrhage, and sometimes cystic change or calcification
- **Cystic RCC** exists and is why complex cysts are followed
- **Infiltrative forms** distort architecture without forming a discrete mass

Doppler typically shows internal vascularity, often with a peripheral vascular rim, though small tumors may show little detectable flow.

Staging assessment — what must be reported:

- **Size and location**, and whether the tumor is exophytic, endophytic, or hilar
- **Perinephric extension** and involvement of Gerota's fascia
- **Renal vein and IVC extension** — a defining behavior of RCC. Look for **echogenic material expanding the renal vein or IVC**, and apply the Chapter 3 §3.5 discriminator: **arterial flow within the thrombus indicates tumor thrombus** rather than bland thrombus. Determine the **cephalad extent** — whether it reaches the intrahepatic IVC or the right atrium — because this changes the operation profoundly
- **Regional lymphadenopathy**
- **Hepatic metastases**
- **Contralateral kidney**, and its function-bearing capacity

CT or MRI is required for definitive staging, but the venous extension question is one ultrasound answers well and quickly, and it should be looked for specifically.

Angiomyolipoma

A benign tumor containing fat, smooth muscle, and vessels.

Classic appearance: a **markedly hyperechoic, well-defined** lesion — often as bright as renal sinus fat — with little or no detectable internal flow. Larger lesions may show posterior shadowing, though this sign is debated.

Clinical significance: larger lesions carry a **risk of spontaneous hemorrhage**, which drives surveillance and intervention decisions. Multiple bilateral angiomyolipomas suggest **tuberous sclerosis**, which should prompt a look for other stigmata.

The critical limitation: a small hyperechoic renal mass cannot be reliably distinguished from renal cell carcinoma on ultrasound. A meaningful proportion of small RCCs are hyperechoic. Fat detection on CT or MRI makes the diagnosis; ultrasound cannot. This must be stated in the report rather than assumed away — describing a small echogenic lesion as "consistent with angiomyolipoma" without qualification is a real and consequential error.

Other tumors

Oncocytoma — benign, sometimes with a central stellate scar, but **indistinguishable from RCC on imaging**; it is typically a post-operative diagnosis.

Urothelial (transitional cell) carcinoma — arising in the collecting system, presenting with **hematuria**. Sonographically a **soft-tissue filling defect within the sinus or collecting system**, sometimes with hydronephrosis, and often subtle or invisible. Because urothelial tumors are frequently multifocal, **the bladder and the contralateral system must be examined**. Ultrasound is not adequate to exclude urothelial malignancy; adult hematuria requires CT urography and cystoscopy.

Lymphoma — usually secondary, producing multiple hypoechoic masses, diffuse infiltration with enlargement, or perirenal soft tissue.

Metastases — from lung, breast, melanoma, and colon; usually in a patient with known disease.

Wilms tumor — the principal pediatric renal malignancy, Chapter 12.

The pseudotumor check

Before reporting any renal "mass", confirm it is not one of the §7.1 pseudotumors. The discriminating principle again: **a pseudotumor has echotexture identical to normal cortex, and normal undisplaced vessels running through it**. A true mass has different echotexture, displaces vessels, and often distorts the contour.

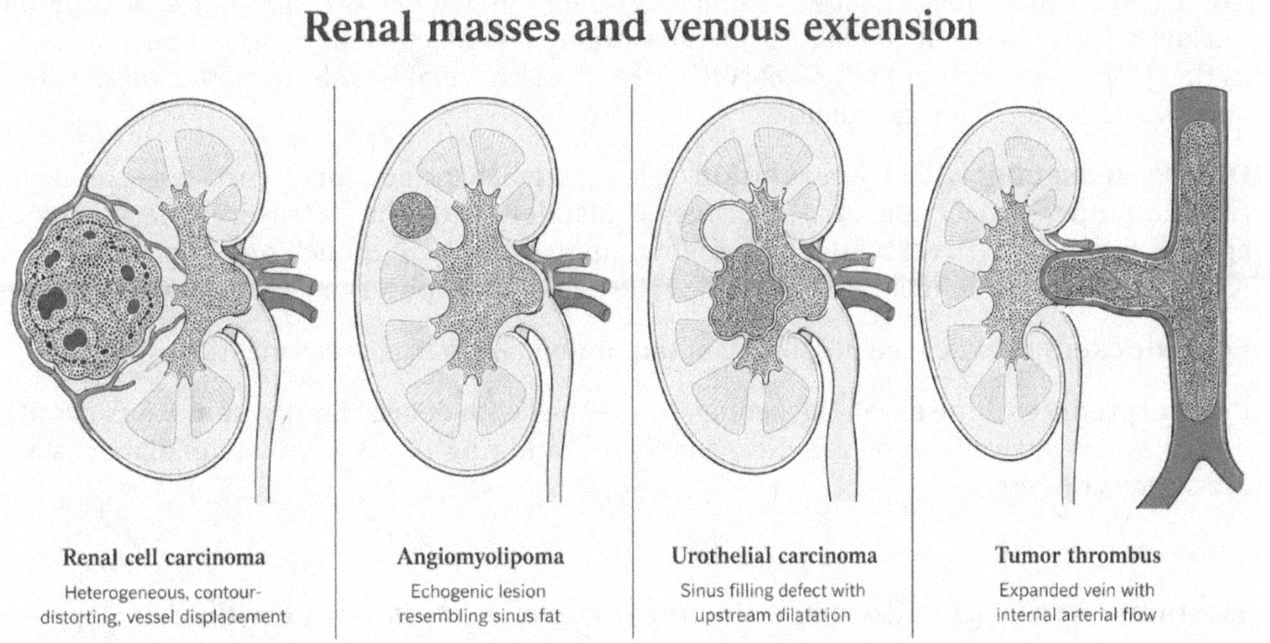

7.8 The Bladder: Volume, Wall, and Pathology

Technique and volume

The bladder must be **adequately but not excessively filled**. An empty bladder cannot be assessed; an overdistended one distorts pelvic anatomy, causes discomfort, and can produce mild bilateral upper tract fullness (§7.3).

Scan in **transverse and sagittal**, sweeping fully through the organ in both planes. The bladder is superficial and a **linear probe** improves wall assessment considerably.

Volume is estimated from three orthogonal dimensions using an ellipsoid approximation:

Volume ≈ length × width × height × 0.52

The coefficient varies between conventions and machine implementations, and the estimate degrades in an irregularly shaped or trabeculated bladder. [VERIFY: current accepted coefficient and its variants, and the reported accuracy of ultrasound bladder volume estimation]

Post-void residual volume is measured immediately after voiding — delay allows refilling and overestimates. It is a core measurement in outlet obstruction, neurogenic bladder, and retention, and its interpretation depends on thresholds that vary by clinical context. [VERIFY: current thresholds for clinically significant post-void residual volume]

The wall

Normal wall thickness is a few millimetres when the bladder is distended, and apparent thickening in an underfilled bladder is a measurement artifact — the same distension caveat as the gallbladder in Chapter 5 §5.6. [VERIFY: current normal bladder wall thickness values and the distension state assumed]

Diffuse thickening with trabeculation — an irregular, ridged inner surface — indicates chronic outlet obstruction or a neurogenic bladder, with the detrusor hypertrophying against resistance. **Diverticula** may follow, appearing as outpouchings connected by a narrow neck, best demonstrated by finding the neck and by observing changes with voiding.

Focal thickening raises the possibility of tumor and requires characterization.

Cystitis produces diffuse wall thickening, sometimes with debris. **Emphysematous cystitis** — gas within the wall, producing dirty shadowing and ring-down — occurs in diabetics and is a serious finding.

Intraluminal findings

The tumor-versus-clot discrimination is the key one, and it is made with color Doppler:

	Bladder tumor	Blood clot
Mobility	Fixed, arises from the wall	**Mobile** with position change

	Bladder tumor	Blood clot
Flow	**Internal vascularity present**	**No internal flow**
Shape	Polypoid or sessile, wall-based	Irregular, may layer dependently

Roll the patient and apply color Doppler to any intravesical mass. Both maneuvers take seconds and the distinction changes everything that follows.

Bladder calculi — mobile, echogenic, shadowing, rolling to the dependent position.

Ureterocele — a cystic structure protruding into the bladder at the ureteric orifice, with a thin wall, classically described as a **cobra-head** appearance. Associated with **duplex systems and the upper pole moiety** (§7.1), and a specific thing to look for when you find upper pole dilatation.

Foley catheter balloon — a round anechoic structure with a bright wall, easily mistaken for a lesion by the unwary, and confirmed by the tube.

Debris and pyuria — mobile low-level echoes.

Ureteric jets

Periodic **plumes of flow entering the bladder from each ureteric orifice**, demonstrable on color Doppler, and produced by the density difference between ureteric urine and bladder urine.

Their diagnostic value: in unilateral obstruction, the jet on the affected side may be **absent, continuous and low-level rather than pulsatile, or asymmetric in frequency and force**. An absent jet on the symptomatic side, with contralateral jets present, supports obstruction.

Technique: color Doppler at a low velocity scale over the trigone, observed patiently for **several minutes** — jets are intermittent and a short look proves nothing. Hydration status affects jet frequency and must be considered.

The prostate, transabdominally

Assess size, and note **intravesical protrusion** of the median lobe, which correlates with obstruction. Transabdominal assessment is a screening view only; dedicated prostatic evaluation is transrectal.

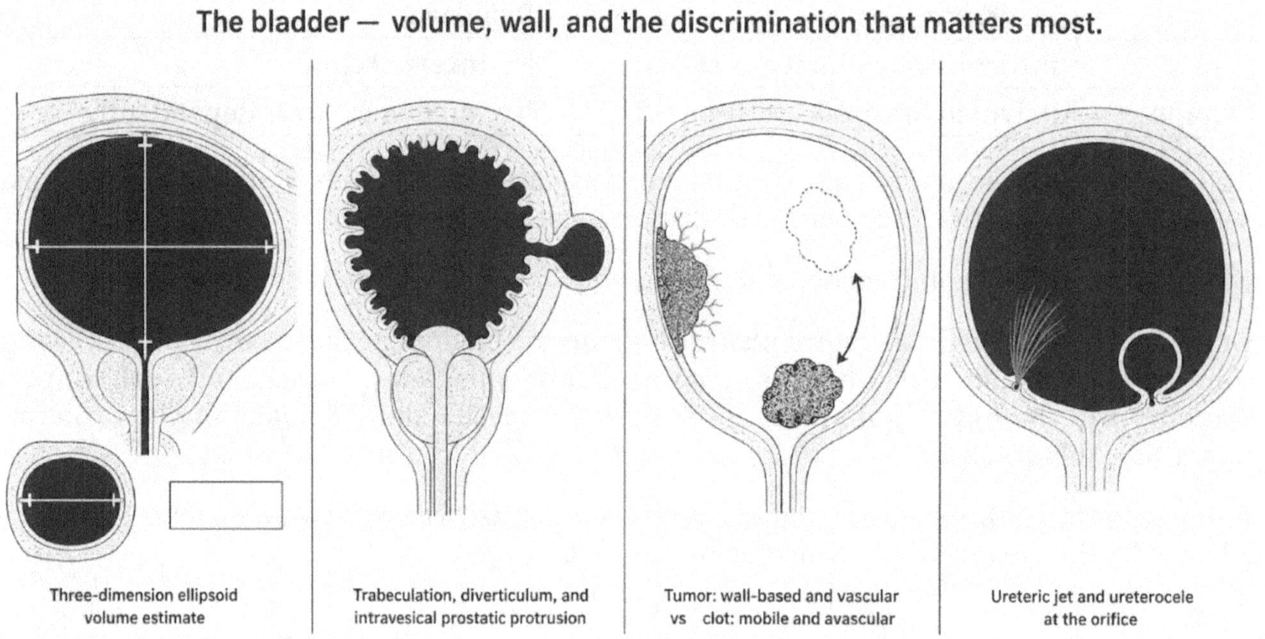

7.9 The Adrenal Glands

Anatomy and access

The adrenals are **retroperitoneal, within the perirenal space**, sitting superomedial to the upper renal poles. They are small, flat, and closely applied to surrounding structures, which makes them difficult.

Right adrenal — lies **posterior to the IVC**, between the IVC, the right crus of the diaphragm, and the upper pole of the right kidney. It is approached through the **liver** in a right coronal or subcostal view, and this is by some margin the easier of the two.

Left adrenal — lies **anteromedial to the upper pole of the left kidney**, lateral to the aorta and posterior to the splenic vessels and pancreatic tail. It is approached from a **left coronal intercostal window through the spleen**, and it is genuinely hard.

The normal adult adrenal is usually not visualized, and its non-visualization is not a finding. Non-visualization should not be reported as normality.

The neonatal adrenal is a different matter entirely — relatively much larger and readily seen, with a hypoechoic cortex and a thin echogenic central medulla. Neonatal adrenal imaging is a routine and productive study, and it is developed in Chapter 12.

Pathology

Adenoma — the commonest adrenal mass, usually a small, well-defined, homogeneous lesion. Frequently an incidental finding. **Characterization requires CT or MRI**, which assess lipid content; ultrasound cannot distinguish an adenoma from other lesions.

Myelolipoma — benign, containing macroscopic fat, appearing **markedly hyperechoic**, sometimes strikingly so. The differential with a retroperitoneal fat-containing lesion or an exophytic renal angiomyolipoma is real.

Pheochromocytoma — often larger at presentation, heterogeneous with cystic change and hemorrhage. Biochemical diagnosis; imaging localizes.

Adrenocortical carcinoma — large, heterogeneous, with necrosis and often local invasion or venous extension.

Metastases — the adrenal is a common metastatic site, particularly from lung and breast primaries. Usually bilateral or in a patient with known malignancy.

Adrenal hemorrhage — in adults, associated with trauma, anticoagulation, sepsis, and stress. In neonates it is much more common and is a routine ultrasound diagnosis (Chapter 12): an initially echogenic suprarenal mass that becomes progressively hypoechoic, cystic, and smaller on follow-up, sometimes calcifying. **Serial ultrasound is the appropriate follow-up**, and demonstrating the expected evolution distinguishes hemorrhage from neuroblastoma, which is the critical differential.

Adrenal cysts and **granulomatous disease** with calcification complete the list.

The reporting position

For adults, ultrasound's role in adrenal disease is limited: it may detect a mass incidentally, but CT and MRI characterize. A report should describe what was seen and direct onward, and should not imply that the glands were assessed if they were not visualized.

7.10 Retroperitoneal Spaces, Fluid Collections, and Masses

Localizing to the retroperitoneum

The compartments — anterior pararenal, perirenal, and posterior pararenal — are described in Chapter 3 §3.1, and localizing a collection or mass to one of them narrows the differential substantially.

The primary discrimination is retroperitoneal versus intraperitoneal, and it rests on **vessel displacement** (Chapter 3 §3.4):

> A mass that **displaces the aorta and IVC anteriorly**, away from the vertebral bodies, arises **behind** them and is retroperitoneal. A mass that **encases** them without displacing them suggests **infiltrative retroperitoneal disease** — lymphoma or fibrosis. A mass that indents them from the front is anterior retroperitoneal or intraperitoneal.

Additional localizing features: a retroperitoneal mass **does not move with respiration** to the degree an intraperitoneal one does, displaces retroperitoneal structures such as the kidney and pancreas, and is not surrounded by bowel.

Collections

Collection	Features and context
Urinoma	Anechoic, perirenal or periureteric; follows obstruction with forniceal rupture, trauma, or surgery
Lymphocele	Anechoic, often septated; follows pelvic or retroperitoneal lymph node dissection and renal transplantation (Chapter 9)
Hematoma	Echogenicity evolving with age — initially echogenic, becoming complex and then hypoechoic; anticoagulation, trauma, post-procedural
Abscess	Complex with debris, irregular wall, possible gas with dirty shadowing or ring-down; peripheral hyperemia, no internal flow
Psoas collection	Within the psoas muscle, enlarging and distorting it; abscess (including tuberculous, tracking from the spine) or hematoma

Aspiration under ultrasound guidance frequently distinguishes them, and the guidance technique is in Chapter 9.

Masses

Lymphadenopathy is the commonest retroperitoneal mass. Nodes appear as hypoechoic rounded structures, typically para-aortic and paracaval. When confluent, they **encase the vessels**, and when they lift the aorta forward off the spine the appearance is described as the **"floating aorta"** sign. Assess: distribution, size, whether the vessels are encased or displaced, and whether the ureters are obstructed.

Retroperitoneal sarcoma — most commonly liposarcoma and leiomyosarcoma. Typically large at presentation, heterogeneous, displacing rather than encasing. Well-differentiated liposarcoma may be echogenic from its fat content and can be surprisingly inconspicuous despite great size.

Germ cell tumor metastases — para-aortic nodal masses in a young male patient; **always examine the testes** when these are found, since the primary may be clinically occult (Chapter 11).

Retroperitoneal fibrosis — a **periaortic soft-tissue mantle**, typically hypoechoic, enveloping the aorta and IVC and often the ureters, producing **hydronephrosis with medial deviation of the ureters**. It may be idiopathic, IgG4-related, drug-associated, or malignant, and it characteristically does not lift the aorta off the spine — a discriminator from lymphoma.

Neurogenic tumors — arising in the paraspinal region.

Primary and metastatic disease of the psoas and posterior abdominal wall.

Technique

Retroperitoneal assessment is technically limited by depth and bowel gas, and **CT is the appropriate modality** for a suspected retroperitoneal mass. Ultrasound's contributions are: detecting hydronephrosis, characterizing a collection as simple or complex, guiding aspiration or drainage, and demonstrating vascular displacement or encasement. State the limitation where the retroperitoneum was incompletely assessed.

Key Points

1. The echogenicity hierarchy — sinus > liver/spleen ≥ cortex > pyramids — underlies most renal assessment. Acquire the organ comparison in one frame at matched settings.
2. Pseudotumors have cortical echotexture and normal undisplaced vessels running through them. True masses displace vessels and distort the contour.
3. When you find a dilated upper pole moiety, look in the bladder for a ureterocele. The Weigert–Meyer pattern links them.
4. Measure renal length in the true coronal long axis. An oblique plane systematically underestimates it.
5. Resistive index needs no angle correction, because the angle term cancels in the ratio. The side-to-side difference is often more useful than the absolute value.
6. Tardus–parvus in intrarenal vessels indicates proximal stenosis, and can be detected when the artery origin cannot be seen.
7. Put color Doppler on any questionable "collecting system dilatation" before reporting it. Prominent vessels are a one-second exclusion.
8. Rescan post-void before reporting mild bilateral hydronephrosis in a patient with a full bladder.
9. A patient with colic and no hydronephrosis has not been excluded. Use secondary signs — absent jet, RI difference, perinephric fluid.
10. Internal echoes within an obstructed system in a febrile patient mean pyonephrosis, a urological emergency. They are easy to miss at low gain.
11. Twinkling artifact is a positive finding for calculus. A deliberate color sweep belongs in every stone protocol.
12. Echogenic pyramids invert the normal pattern and indicate medullary nephrocalcinosis.
13. Small echogenic kidneys mean chronic irreversible disease; normal-sized or enlarged echogenic kidneys leave the door open. That distinction is one of ultrasound's real contributions in renal impairment.
14. Acute pyelonephritis is usually sonographically normal. Imaging is for complications, not diagnosis.
15. Check a cyst with compounding off and on fundamental before calling it simple — the whole classification depends on whether internal features are present.
16. A small hyperechoic renal mass cannot be reliably distinguished from renal cell carcinoma on ultrasound. Say so rather than calling it an angiomyolipoma.
17. Arterial flow within material expanding the renal vein or IVC indicates tumor thrombus. Determine the cephalad extent — it changes the operation.
18. Roll the patient and apply color Doppler to any intravesical mass. Tumor is fixed and vascular; clot is mobile and avascular.

19. A mass that lifts the aorta and IVC forward off the spine is retroperitoneal. One that encases without displacing suggests lymphoma or fibrosis.

Registry Check

1. A rounded region of tissue indents the renal sinus. It has the same echogenicity as the cortex, is continuous with it, contains normal interlobar vessels running through it, and does not distort the renal contour. This represents:

A. Renal cell carcinoma **B.** Hypertrophied column of Bertin **C.** Angiomyolipoma **D.** Oncocytoma

> **Answer: B.** Identical cortical echotexture, continuity with the cortex, normal undisplaced vasculature, and an undistorted contour define a pseudotumor. A true mass differs in echotexture, displaces vessels, and commonly bulges the capsule.

2. In a duplex collecting system, the upper pole moiety ureter characteristically:

A. Inserts superolaterally and is prone to reflux **B.** Inserts inferomedially and is prone to obstruction and ureterocele **C.** Inserts normally with the lower pole ureter **D.** Is absent

> **Answer: B.** The Weigert–Meyer rule states that the upper pole ureter inserts inferomedially and ectopically, predisposing to obstruction and ureterocele formation, while the lower pole ureter inserts superolaterally and is prone to vesicoureteric reflux. Finding a dilated upper pole should prompt examination of the bladder.

3. Angle correction is not required when measuring renal resistive index because:

A. The intrarenal vessels are always insonated at 0 degrees **B.** RI is a ratio of two velocities in the same vessel, so the angle term cancels **C.** Resistive index does not depend on velocity **D.** Angle correction is applied automatically by the machine

> **Answer: B.** RI equals (PSV – EDV)/PSV. Because both velocities are measured in the same vessel at the same insonation angle, the cosine term appears in every measured value and cancels in the ratio. A poor angle still degrades trace quality but does not invalidate the index.

4. Multiple anechoic structures are seen within the renal sinus. They do not communicate with one another, do not converge on a ureter, and show no flow on color Doppler. These most likely represent:

A. Hydronephrosis **B.** Parapelvic cysts **C.** Prominent renal vessels **D.** Pyonephrosis

> **Answer: B.** Parapelvic cysts mimic a dilated collecting system but are separate non-communicating structures that do not converge on a ureter. Hydronephrotic calyces communicate and converge on the pelvis; prominent vessels fill with color.

5. A febrile patient has a dilated collecting system containing low-level internal echoes with a dependent debris level. The appropriate response is:

A. Routine reporting with outpatient urology follow-up **B.** Immediate communication, as this suggests pyonephrosis requiring urgent decompression **C.** Repeat the scan after hydration **D.** Proceed to contrast-enhanced ultrasound

> **Answer: B.** Internal echoes within an obstructed system in a febrile patient indicate an infected obstructed kidney. Pyonephrosis is a urological emergency with high mortality if decompression is delayed, and it is a critical finding requiring immediate direct communication.

6. A 1.5 cm markedly hyperechoic, well-defined mass is found in the renal cortex of an adult. The correct report:

A. States that this is an angiomyolipoma **B.** States that this is a benign lesion requiring no follow-up **C.** Describes the lesion and states that a small hyperechoic mass cannot be reliably distinguished from renal cell carcinoma on ultrasound, recommending CT or MRI **D.** States that this is a renal cell carcinoma

> **Answer: C.** Although angiomyolipoma is the commonest cause of a markedly echogenic small renal lesion, a meaningful proportion of small renal cell carcinomas are also hyperechoic, and ultrasound cannot detect the macroscopic fat that makes the diagnosis. Definitive characterization requires CT or MRI.

7. A mass is seen within the bladder lumen. It does not move when the patient is repositioned, arises from the wall, and demonstrates internal vascularity on color Doppler. This represents:

A. Blood clot **B.** Bladder calculus **C.** Bladder tumor **D.** Ureterocele

> **Answer: C.** Fixed position, wall attachment, and internal vascularity identify a tumor. Clot is mobile and avascular, a calculus is mobile and shadows, and a ureterocele is a thin-walled cystic structure at the ureteric orifice.

8. A retroperitoneal soft-tissue process envelops the aorta and inferior vena cava without displacing them anteriorly, and is associated with bilateral hydronephrosis and medial deviation of the ureters. This suggests:

A. Retroperitoneal sarcoma **B.** Retroperitoneal fibrosis **C.** Lymphoma with the floating aorta sign **D.** Psoas abscess

> **Answer: B.** A periaortic mantle that encases without lifting the vessels off the spine, with ureteric obstruction and medial ureteric deviation, is characteristic of retroperitoneal fibrosis. Confluent lymphoma also encases but classically lifts the aorta anteriorly, producing the floating aorta sign; sarcoma displaces rather than encases.

Chapter Notes for the Editorial Pass

Verification queue. In priority order: the **renal cyst classification system**, its category definitions, and the status of its contrast-enhanced ultrasound adaptation (§7.6) — this drives surveillance versus surgery and the CT-derived original does not transfer cleanly to B-mode; **renal artery stenosis velocity criteria**, which are laboratory-validated rather than universal (§7.2); **resistive index thresholds** and the significant inter-renal difference (§7.2); **ADPKD age-stratified diagnostic criteria and family screening recommendations** (§7.6); **hydronephrosis grading systems**, adult and pediatric, including the antenatal/postnatal dilatation classification (§7.3); **post-void residual thresholds** (§7.8); **bladder volume coefficient and accuracy** (§7.8); **adult renal length and cortical thickness reference ranges** (§7.1); and **bladder wall thickness values with their assumed distension state** (§7.8).

Deliberate omission. Renal transplant assessment is not covered here despite its close relationship to §7.2 Doppler technique — it is developed in Chapter 9 alongside the other transplants, where the vascular, collection, and rejection findings can be treated as a set. The cross-reference must be checked at layout so the tardus–parvus and RI material is not orphaned.

Figure count: 8 Lane A, 0 Lane B. This chapter is specified without Lane B slots because the two highest-value real-image demands — twinkling artifact and the hepatorenal echogenicity comparison — are already specified as `fig-2-13` and `fig-4-3` respectively. Reusing those images with new captions here is more efficient than acquiring duplicates, and the layout should plan for it. If one Lane B slot is added, the strongest candidate is a hydronephrosis series showing mild, moderate, and severe grades from the same department.

Cross-reference targets to fix at layout: §7.1 retroperitoneal spaces → Chapter 3 §3.1; §7.1 right renal artery behind IVC → Chapter 3 §3.4; §7.2 tardus–parvus → Chapter 3 §3.7 and Chapter 9; §7.4 twinkling → Chapter 2 §2.9; §7.4 clean shadowing → Chapter 2 §2.7; §7.5 emphysematous infection → Chapter 2 §2.8; §7.6 compounding and enhancement → Chapter 2 §2.4; §7.7 tumor thrombus → Chapter 3 §3.5 and Chapter 4 §4.9; §7.7 Wilms tumor → Chapter 12; §7.9 neonatal adrenal → Chapter 12; §7.10 lymphocele → Chapter 9; §7.10 germ cell primary → Chapter 11.

Word count: approximately 10,400 excluding image prompt blocks, learning objectives, registry questions, and these notes.

Chapter 8: The Peritoneum, Abdominal Wall, and Emergent Abdomen

Learning Objectives

On completing this chapter you should be able to:

1. Predict where peritoneal fluid will collect from the patient's position and the site of origin.
2. Distinguish simple from complex ascites and recognize the features of malignant, infective, and hemorrhagic collections.
3. Select a safe paracentesis site using the abdominal wall anatomy.
4. Name the layers of the abdominal wall and explain the surgical significance of the arcuate line.
5. Classify abdominal wall hernias, and use the inferior epigastric vessels to distinguish direct from indirect inguinal hernias.
6. Perform dynamic hernia assessment and recognize the findings of incarceration and strangulation.
7. Perform the FAST and extended FAST examinations, naming what each window interrogates.
8. Recognize pneumothorax, hemothorax, and pericardial tamponade sonographically.
9. Conduct an emergent aortic assessment and state why absence of visible rupture does not exclude it.
10. State the documented limits of focused protocols and report a focused examination as focused.

The Chapter Where the Question Changes

Every previous chapter has asked what a structure looks like. This one mostly asks **whether something is present, right now, in a patient who may be dying**.

That difference reorganizes everything. Sensitivity for a binary finding matters more than characterization. Speed matters. Knowing the false negatives matters more than knowing the fine detail, because the cost of a missed positive is measured in minutes. And the discipline of reporting a **focused** examination as focused — rather than allowing it to be read as a complete one — becomes a patient safety issue rather than a documentation preference.

The first half of this chapter is anatomy and elective pathology. The second half is emergency medicine. They belong together because the anatomy of the first half is what makes the emergency examinations of the second half interpretable.

8.1 Peritoneal Compartments and Fluid Distribution

The architecture

The peritoneal cavity is a single continuous potential space, but its ligaments and mesenteries divide it into compartments that determine how fluid and disease travel. The **transverse mesocolon** divides it into supramesocolic and inframesocolic compartments; the **small bowel mesentery**, running obliquely from the duodenojejunal flexure to the ileocecal region, divides the inframesocolic compartment into right and left infracolic spaces.

Supramesocolic spaces:

- **Right subphrenic** — between the diaphragm and the liver dome
- **Right subhepatic (Morison's pouch, hepatorenal recess)** — between the right hepatic lobe and the right kidney, communicating freely with the right subphrenic space
- **Left subphrenic (perisplenic)** — over the spleen and left hepatic lobe
- **Lesser sac (omental bursa)** — behind the stomach, communicating with the greater sac only through the narrow **epiploic foramen**

Inframesocolic and pelvic:

- **Right and left infracolic spaces**
- **Right paracolic gutter** — deep and continuous, the principal vertical conduit between the upper abdomen and the pelvis
- **Left paracolic gutter** — shallower and interrupted superiorly by the **phrenicocolic ligament**, which limits upward flow
- **Pelvic recesses** — the **rectouterine pouch (of Douglas)** in women and the **rectovesical pouch** in men, with the paravesical spaces laterally

Where fluid goes

Two rules cover most of practice:

> **In the supine patient, the most dependent part of the upper abdomen is Morison's pouch. In any position, the most dependent part of the whole peritoneal cavity is the pelvis.**

This is why the FAST examination (§8.6) interrogates precisely those locations, and why a small volume of free fluid appears in the pelvis before anywhere else.

Two asymmetries are worth holding:

On the right, fluid tracks from the subphrenic space into Morison's pouch and down the right paracolic gutter to the pelvis — a continuous pathway.

On the left, the phrenicocolic ligament impedes flow, and fluid tends to accumulate in the **subphrenic space above the spleen** rather than in the splenorenal recess. This has a direct technical consequence: **in the left upper quadrant FAST view, look above the spleen**

first, not between spleen and kidney. Positioning the probe too anteriorly and too caudally is why the LUQ view is the most commonly failed one.

Loculation and why the compartment matters

Fluid confined to a compartment tells you where it came from:

- **Lesser sac only** — locally generated, because the epiploic foramen restricts communication. Pancreatitis, gastric or duodenal perforation.
- **Perihepatic and right gutter** — upper abdominal source, or generalized ascites.
- **Pelvic only** — small volume from any source, or a pelvic origin.
- **Interloop, wedge-shaped, non-mobile** — loculated, suggesting an exudative or infective process rather than simple ascites.

Mobility is the discriminator. Free fluid changes shape and position with patient movement, forms **sharp acute angles** where it meets bowel and organ surfaces, and allows gas-filled bowel to float. Loculated fluid retains its shape, has convex margins, and does not shift.

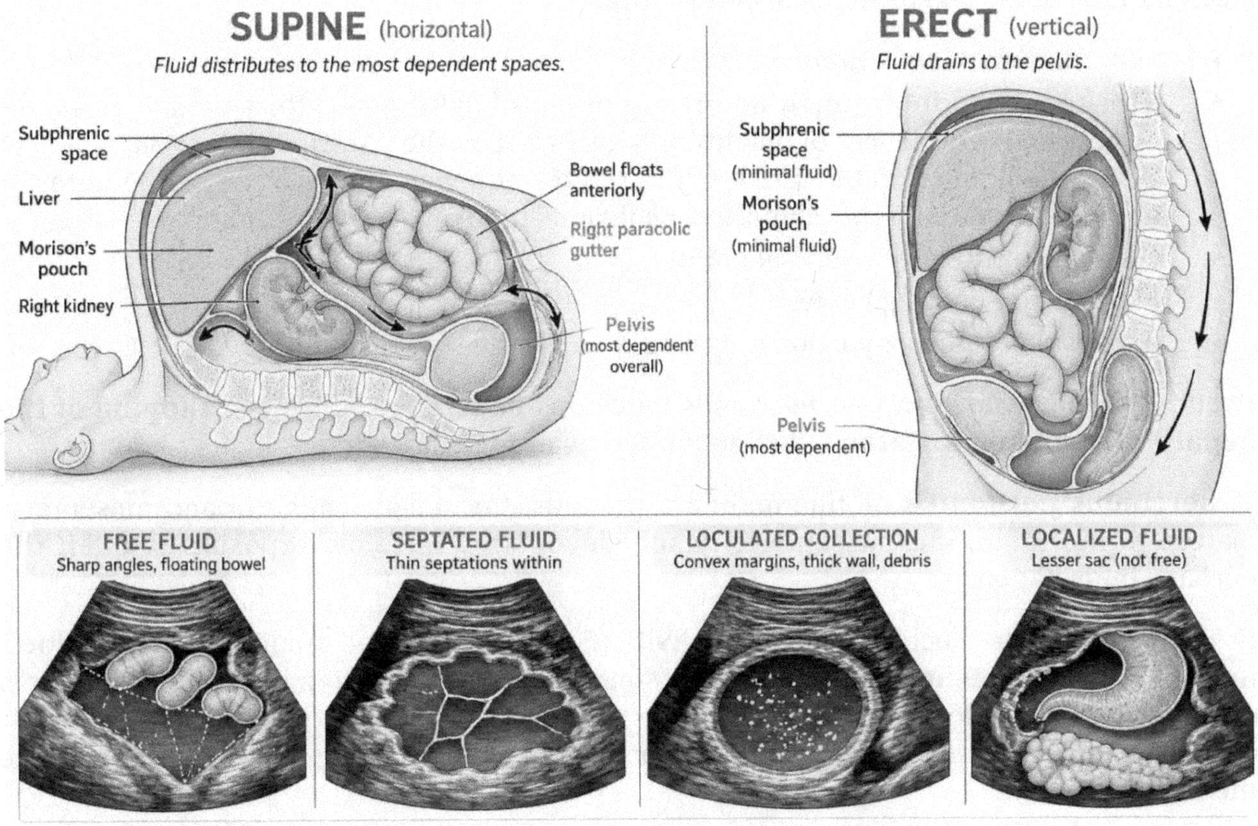

8.2 Ascites, Loculated Collections, and Abscess

Simple versus complex

Simple (transudative) ascites is anechoic, freely mobile, conforms to the shape of the space it occupies, meets structures at **sharp acute angles**, and allows bowel loops to float and move freely within it. Causes: cirrhosis and portal hypertension (much the commonest — Chapter 4 §4.5), congestive heart failure, nephrotic syndrome, and hypoalbuminemia.

Complex (exudative) ascites contains internal echoes, septations, or debris; loculates; and is associated with matted, tethered bowel that does not float freely. Causes: malignancy, infection including tuberculous peritonitis, pancreatitis, and chylous ascites.

The sonographic distinction is suggestive, not diagnostic — the diagnosis is made by aspirating and analyzing the fluid. But the appearance directs the workup and the report should describe it specifically rather than writing "ascites" alone.

Characteristic patterns

Malignant ascites / peritoneal carcinomatosis:

- Septations and loculations
- **Thickened, nodular peritoneum** and **omental caking** — a thickened, hypoechoic or heterogeneous sheet of omentum lying between the anterior abdominal wall and bowel. Look for it deliberately with a high-frequency linear probe in the anterior abdomen, where it is often more conspicuous than on a curvilinear survey
- Discrete peritoneal or serosal nodules
- Matted, non-floating bowel
- Ascites that is disproportionately loculated relative to its volume

Pseudomyxoma peritonei — gelatinous mucinous material producing **scalloping of the hepatic and splenic surfaces**, a distinctive and near-specific finding.

Tuberculous peritonitis — fine mobile septations, thickened omentum and mesentery, matted bowel loops, and mesenteric lymphadenopathy. Endemic exposure is often the decisive information.

Hemoperitoneum — echogenicity varies with the age of the blood. **Acute unclotted blood may be entirely anechoic**, which is why a "simple-looking" collection in a trauma patient is not reassuring. As clot forms it becomes echogenic, and the **sentinel clot** — the most echogenic, most organized collection, lying adjacent to the bleeding source — can localize the injury.

Bile (bile peritonitis) and **urine (bladder or collecting system rupture)** are typically anechoic and indistinguishable from simple ascites on appearance alone; the clinical context and aspiration decide.

Abscess

An intraperitoneal abscess is a walled collection of infected material, and its appearance is variable enough that the diagnosis is often made on context and evolution rather than a single look.

Findings:

- **Complex collection** with internal debris, septations, and sometimes a fluid–debris level
- **Thick, irregular wall**
- **Gas** producing **dirty shadowing or ring-down** (Chapter 2 §2.8) — highly suggestive
- **No internal flow** on color Doppler, with **peripheral hyperemia**
- Adjacent inflammatory change in fat

Characteristic sites, and the reason for each: **subphrenic** and **subhepatic** (from upper abdominal sources or postoperative), **pelvic** (the most dependent space, so a common destination for infected fluid from anywhere), **paracolic**, and **interloop** — the last being the hardest to see and the one most often missed, because it is small, surrounded by gas, and irregular.

Ultrasound-guided **aspiration or drainage** frequently follows, and the technique is in Chapter 9.

Paracentesis site selection

Where ultrasound marks or guides paracentesis, the site selection is a specific skill with specific hazards.

The preferred site is the left lower quadrant, lateral to the rectus sheath, roughly a third of the way along a line from the umbilicus to the anterior superior iliac spine — chosen because the abdominal wall is thinner there, the cecum is not in the way, and the site is lateral to the rectus.

What must be avoided:

- **The inferior epigastric artery**, which runs within the rectus sheath. Staying **lateral to the rectus muscle** avoids it, and **color Doppler over the intended site** confirms it. Puncturing this vessel is the classic serious complication of paracentesis
- **Surgical scars**, where adherent bowel may be tethered directly beneath the wall
- **Distended bladder and bowel** — confirm an adequate fluid pocket free of interposed bowel
- Visible collateral veins in a patient with portal hypertension

Real-time guidance is preferable to skin marking, because the fluid pocket and bowel position change when the patient moves between the marking and the procedure.

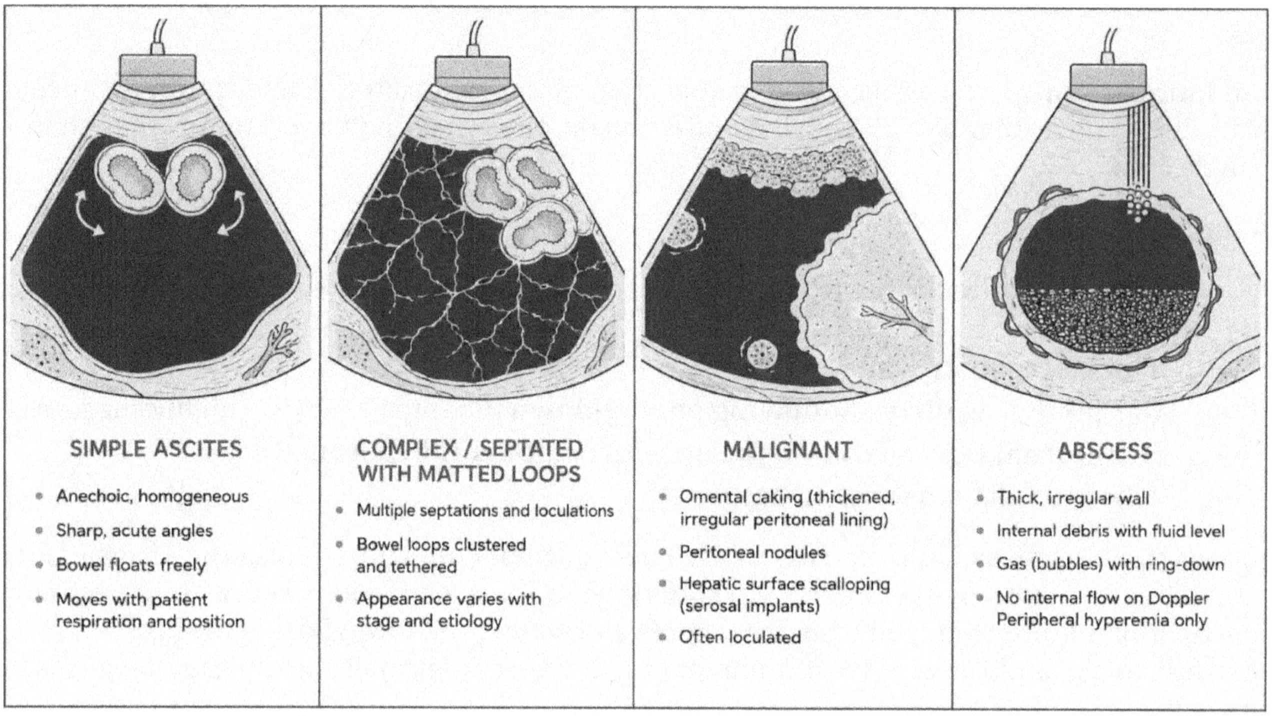

8.3 Abdominal Wall Layers and Scanning Technique

The layers

From superficial to deep, resolvable with a high-frequency linear probe:

1. **Skin** — a thin echogenic line
2. **Subcutaneous fat** — hypoechoic, traversed by echogenic fibrous septa; divided into the superficial fatty layer and the deeper membranous fascia
3. **Muscle layer** — hypoechoic muscle with echogenic fascial planes and internal perimysial striations
4. **Transversalis fascia** — an echogenic line
5. **Preperitoneal fat**
6. **Peritoneum** — a thin echogenic line, with the abdominal contents beyond

Laterally, the muscle layer is three distinct sheets: **external oblique, internal oblique, and transversus abdominis**, separated by echogenic fascial planes. Counting them is the standard way to confirm you are in the lateral wall.

Anteriorly, the **rectus abdominis** muscles lie within the **rectus sheath**, separated in the midline by the **linea alba** and bounded laterally by the **linea semilunaris**.

The arcuate line

Approximately midway between the umbilicus and the pubic symphysis, the composition of the rectus sheath changes:

Above the arcuate line, aponeuroses pass both anterior and posterior to the rectus muscle — there is a **complete posterior rectus sheath**. **Below the arcuate line**, all the aponeuroses pass **anterior** to the muscle — there is **no posterior sheath**, only transversalis fascia.

This single anatomical fact explains two distinct clinical phenomena, and it is why it earns its own subsection:

1. **Rectus sheath hematoma below the arcuate line is unconstrained** posteriorly and can become large, cross the midline, and extend into the prevesical space to present as a pelvic mass (§8.5).
2. **Spigelian hernias** occur characteristically at the level of the arcuate line, where the linea semilunaris is weakest (§8.4).

The inferior epigastric vessels

The **inferior epigastric artery** arises from the external iliac artery just above the inguinal ligament, runs superomedially, and enters the rectus sheath to ascend deep to the rectus muscle.

It matters three times in this chapter:

- It is the vessel at risk in **paracentesis** (§8.2)
- It is the vessel injured in **rectus sheath hematoma** (§8.5)
- Its position is the landmark that distinguishes **direct from indirect inguinal hernia** (§8.4)

Identify it routinely with color Doppler when working on the lower abdominal wall.

Technique

High-frequency linear transducer, always. The wall is superficial and abdominal-frequency imaging cannot resolve the layers.

Copious gel and light pressure. Pressing hard on the abdominal wall obliterates the very structures you are assessing — it reduces a hernia, collapses a fluid collection, and compresses a superficial mass out of view. Where the target is extremely superficial, use additional gel as a standoff.

Extended field-of-view imaging, where available, is genuinely useful for demonstrating the relationship of a wall lesion or a hernia defect to landmarks such as the umbilicus and the midline.

Compare with the contralateral side, which is the fastest way to establish whether an appearance is a variant or a lesion.

Dynamic maneuvers — Valsalva, coughing, standing, straining — are the essential addition and are covered in §8.4.

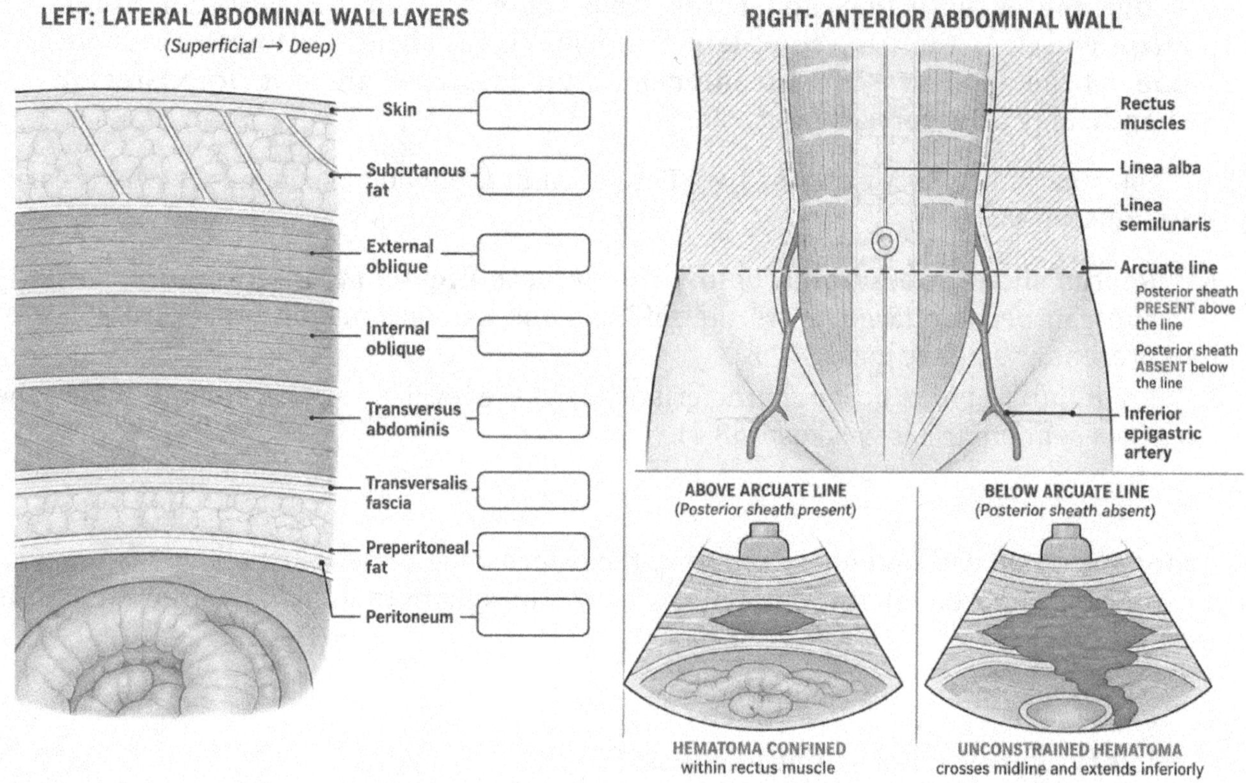

8.4 Hernias: Classification, Technique, and Dynamic Maneuvers

Why ultrasound is the right modality

A hernia is a **dynamic** phenomenon: contents pass through a defect under raised intra-abdominal pressure and reduce when the pressure falls. A supine CT frequently shows nothing, because the patient is relaxed and horizontal.

Ultrasound can watch the hernia happen. Real-time imaging during Valsalva, coughing, or standing demonstrates the defect, the contents entering and leaving, and the reducibility. This is a genuine advantage over cross-sectional imaging and it is the reason ultrasound is often the definitive study for a clinically suspected but non-palpable hernia.

Classification

Hernia	Location and landmark
Indirect inguinal	Through the deep inguinal ring, **lateral to the inferior epigastric vessels**; follows the inguinal canal and the spermatic cord; may extend into the scrotum
Direct inguinal	Through the posterior wall of the inguinal canal (Hesselbach's triangle), **medial to the inferior epigastric vessels**; protrudes anteriorly rather than travelling along the canal

Hernia	Location and landmark
Femoral	**Below the inguinal ligament**, medial to the femoral vein, which it may compress; more common in women; **high risk of strangulation**
Umbilical / paraumbilical	Through or adjacent to the umbilical ring
Epigastric	Through the linea alba above the umbilicus; often small and fat-containing
Spigelian	Through the **linea semilunaris at the level of the arcuate line**; **interparietal** — lying between muscle layers rather than subcutaneously, so often not palpable and easily missed; high strangulation risk
Incisional / port-site	At a previous surgical wound
Lumbar	Through the superior or inferior lumbar triangles
Obturator	Through the obturator canal; rare, typically in thin elderly women; presents with bowel obstruction
Parastomal	Adjacent to a stoma

The inferior epigastric vessel landmark is the key discriminator in the groin and should be identified with color Doppler before the hernia is classified. Trace the vessels from their origin at the external iliac artery, and determine whether the neck of the hernia lies medial or lateral to them.

Femoral hernias must be distinguished from inguinal, because their strangulation risk is substantially higher and management is more urgent. The relationship to the **inguinal ligament** and to the **femoral vein** settles it: a femoral hernia lies below the ligament and medial to the vein, often compressing it.

Technique

1. **High-frequency linear probe**, light pressure, ample gel.
2. **Scan at rest first** to establish baseline anatomy and identify the landmarks — the inferior epigastric vessels, the inguinal ligament, the femoral vessels, the linea semilunaris and arcuate line as relevant.
3. **Identify the defect** in the fascial or muscular layer, and **measure its width**. The defect size is what the surgeon needs, and a narrow neck is associated with higher strangulation risk.
4. **Apply dynamic maneuvers** — Valsalva, cough, and, where a hernia is not demonstrated supine, **stand the patient up** and repeat. **Standing is essential and it is the step most often omitted.** A hernia that only appears on standing is still a hernia.
5. **Identify the contents**: fat is echogenic and homogeneous; **bowel is identified by its wall layers, its content, and — decisively — by peristalsis**; bladder, ovary, and other structures occasionally.

6. **Assess reducibility** by observing whether the contents return with relaxation or gentle pressure.
7. **Examine the contralateral side and the other common sites** — hernias are frequently multiple, and finding a second one changes the operation.

Incarceration and strangulation

Incarceration is irreducibility. **Strangulation** is vascular compromise of the contents, and it is a surgical emergency.

Findings suggesting strangulation:

- **Non-reducible** contents that do not change with maneuvers
- **Absent peristalsis** in herniated bowel
- **Wall thickening** of the herniated loop
- **Absent flow** in the bowel wall on color Doppler — set a low velocity scale, and interpret cautiously because absence of detectable flow in a small vessel is not the same as absence of flow
- **Fluid within the hernia sac**
- **Echogenic, inflamed surrounding fat**
- **Proximal bowel dilatation** indicating obstruction
- Marked focal tenderness

Suspected strangulation is a critical finding requiring immediate communication (Chapter 1 §1.5).

Mesh and recurrence

Surgical mesh appears as a **thin, echogenic, often gently curved layer** within the wall, sometimes with reverberation. In post-repair assessment, look for recurrence **at the mesh margins**, mesh folding or migration, and associated seroma or collection.

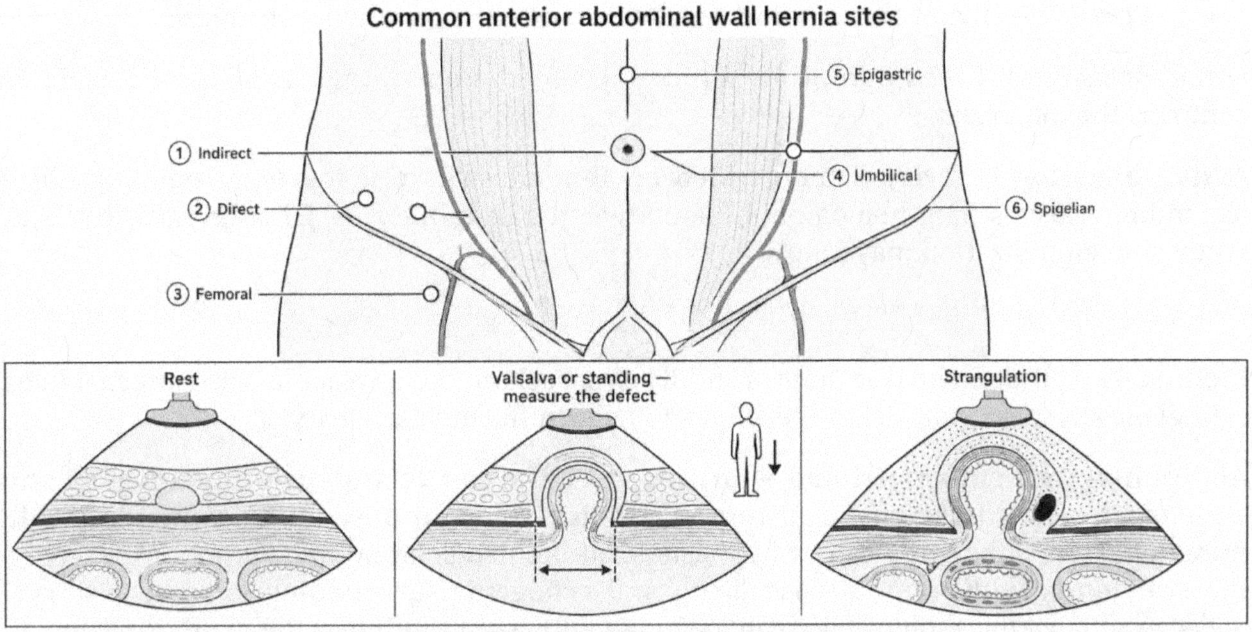

Hernia sites, and the dynamic assessment only ultrasound can perform.
Indirect lateral to inferior epigastric vessels; direct medial; femoral below the inguinal ligament; umbilical, epigastric, and Spigelian hernias.
Dynamic assessment shows rest, provocation, and signs of strangulation.

8.5 Rectus Sheath Hematoma and Wall Masses

Rectus sheath hematoma

Bleeding into the rectus sheath, usually from **injury to the inferior epigastric artery or its branches**, or from tearing of muscle fibres.

Precipitants: anticoagulation (the commonest context), vigorous coughing or straining, direct trauma, abdominal wall injection including anticoagulant injections, and recent surgery. It presents with acute abdominal pain and a palpable mass, and it is frequently mistaken for an intra-abdominal emergency, which is why recognizing it matters — the management is usually conservative.

The arcuate line determines the appearance, as set out in §8.3:

Above the arcuate line — the complete rectus sheath confines the hematoma, producing a **spindle-shaped (fusiform) collection within the muscle** that **does not cross the midline** and remains within the sheath boundaries.

Below the arcuate line — no posterior sheath. The hematoma is unconstrained posteriorly and may become **large, cross the midline, and extend inferiorly into the prevesical (Retzius) space**, presenting as a pelvic mass and occasionally causing hemodynamic compromise.

Evolution of appearance:

- **Acute** — echogenic or heterogeneous, sometimes similar to muscle
- **Subacute** — increasingly complex, with heterogeneous and cystic areas

- **Chronic** — hypoechoic or anechoic with septations, gradually shrinking

Serial ultrasound is the appropriate follow-up, and demonstrating the expected evolution confirms the diagnosis.

Active bleeding is rarely demonstrated on B-mode; where it is suspected clinically — expanding mass, falling hemoglobin, hemodynamic instability — **CT angiography** is the study, and embolization may follow.

Other wall masses

Lipoma — well-defined, isoechoic or mildly hyperechoic, compressible, with internal linear echogenic striations parallel to the skin, and no significant vascularity.

Abdominal wall endometrioma — arising in a **cesarean section or other surgical scar**, with the highly characteristic history of **cyclical pain and swelling coinciding with menstruation**. Sonographically a hypoechoic, ill-defined solid nodule within or adjacent to the scar, often with internal vascularity and echogenic surrounding fat. The history is decisive, and asking about cyclicity in a woman with a scar nodule is the diagnostic step.

Desmoid tumor — a locally aggressive fibromatosis, often in the rectus or oblique muscles, associated with prior surgery, pregnancy, and **familial adenomatous polyposis**. Typically a well-defined hypoechoic mass.

Metastasis — including the **umbilical nodule (Sister Mary Joseph nodule)**, which signifies intra-abdominal malignancy and should prompt a full abdominal and pelvic assessment.

Seroma and abscess at surgical sites, distinguished by wall thickening, debris, gas, and hyperemia.

Foreign body and retained surgical material — echogenic with shadowing or reverberation, often with surrounding hypoechoic granulation.

Neuroma, particularly at scars and after hernia repair, presenting with focal neuropathic pain reproducible with transducer pressure.

Hernia — always in the differential of a wall mass, and excluded by the dynamic assessment of §8.4.

Sarcoma — uncommon, but a rapidly enlarging deep wall mass warrants cross-sectional imaging and biopsy rather than reassurance.

The examination

For any wall mass: high-frequency linear probe, light pressure; determine **which layer** it occupies — subcutaneous, intramuscular, or deep to the wall — because layer localization narrows the differential immediately; assess **compressibility**, **vascularity**, **relationship to scars**, and **change with Valsalva**; and compare with the contralateral side.

Ultrasound-guided aspiration or biopsy is often the next step and is straightforward given the superficial location (Chapter 9).

8.6 The FAST and Extended FAST Examination

What FAST is, and what it is not

FAST — Focused Assessment with Sonography for Trauma — answers **one binary question**: is there free fluid in the peritoneal cavity or pericardium, in a patient with blunt or penetrating torso trauma?

It is **not** an assessment of solid organ injury. It is **not** a complete abdominal examination. It does not evaluate the retroperitoneum, and it does not evaluate the bowel. Understanding this is not pedantry — it is the difference between using the test correctly and being misled by it, and §8.9 is devoted to the consequences.

Its value is speed and location: performed at the bedside in the resuscitation bay in under two minutes, it can convert an unstable patient with an uncertain diagnosis into a patient going directly to theatre.

The four windows

Transducer: curvilinear or phased array. Depth set to see the far side of the recess being interrogated.

1. Right upper quadrant (perihepatic). Probe in the right mid-to-posterior axillary line, around the 8th–11th intercostal spaces, coronal, marker cephalad.

Interrogate, and sweep through each: the **hepatorenal recess (Morison's pouch)**, the **right subphrenic space** above the liver, the **caudal tip of the liver** at the inferior edge, and the **right pleural space** above the diaphragm.

The caudal liver tip and the inferior pole region are frequently the most sensitive locations in this window, more so than the hepatorenal interface itself — a point often missed in training, where the probe is placed once at Morison's pouch and not swept. [VERIFY: comparative sensitivity of sub-locations within the right upper quadrant FAST window]

2. Left upper quadrant (perisplenic). Probe in the left posterior axillary line, higher and more posterior than most operators expect — the common instruction is to get the knuckles to the bed.

Interrogate the **subphrenic space above the spleen first** — because the phrenicocolic ligament directs fluid there rather than into the splenorenal recess (§8.1) — then the **splenorenal recess**, the **inferior splenic pole**, and the **left pleural space**.

This is the most commonly failed view, and the failure is almost always positional: too anterior and too caudal.

3. Pelvic (suprapubic). Probe just above the pubic symphysis, in **both transverse and sagittal**. A **full bladder** provides the acoustic window and dramatically improves the view; an empty bladder degrades it.

Interrogate the **rectovesical pouch** in men and the **rectouterine pouch (of Douglas)** in women, sweeping posterior and lateral to the bladder.

This is where **small volumes appear first**, so it is the most sensitive window for a small hemoperitoneum.

4. Subxiphoid / pericardial. Probe below the xiphoid, angled steeply cephalad and toward the left shoulder, using the liver as a window, to obtain a four-chamber view.

Interrogate for **pericardial effusion** — an anechoic rim surrounding the heart within the pericardium — and for **tamponade physiology**: **right ventricular diastolic collapse**, right atrial systolic collapse, and a **dilated, non-collapsing IVC**.

Where the subxiphoid view fails — common in the tense or obese abdomen — a **parasternal** view substitutes.

Extended FAST (eFAST)

Adds thoracic assessment, which changes management in the resuscitation bay as often as the abdominal views do.

Pneumothorax — high-frequency linear probe, anterior chest, patient supine, at the most non-dependent point (typically the 2nd–4th intercostal spaces mid-clavicular line, since air rises).

Finding	Normal	Pneumothorax
Lung sliding	Present — shimmering movement at the pleural line with respiration	**Absent**
B-lines	May be present	**Absent** (a single B-line excludes pneumothorax at that spot)
Lung pulse	Present — subtle pleural movement with cardiac pulsation	Absent
M-mode	**"Seashore" sign** — motionless linear layers above, granular sand-like pattern below the pleural line	**"Barcode" or "stratosphere" sign** — uniform horizontal lines throughout, no granular pattern
Lung point	Absent	**Present** — the transition point where sliding reappears; **highly specific** for pneumothorax and locates its extent

Absent lung sliding is sensitive but not specific — it also occurs in mainstem intubation, pleural adhesions, apnea, severe consolidation, and ARDS. **The lung point is the specific finding**, and where it can be demonstrated the diagnosis is secure.

Hemothorax — probe above the diaphragm in the RUQ and LUQ views. Blood appears as an **anechoic or complex region above the diaphragm**. The **"spine sign"** is the useful confirmatory finding: the thoracic **vertebral bodies become visible above the diaphragm**, because fluid transmits sound where aerated lung would have blocked it. Normal aerated lung makes the spine disappear at the diaphragm; if you can see it above, there is fluid.

Interpretation and integration

Positive FAST = anechoic fluid in a dependent recess. In blunt trauma, this is presumed to be blood until proven otherwise.

The decision logic:

	Positive FAST	Negative FAST
Hemodynamically unstable	**Laparotomy** — the diagnosis is made, do not delay for CT	Look elsewhere: chest, pelvis, retroperitoneum, external hemorrhage, non-hemorrhagic shock. Consider repeat FAST
Hemodynamically stable	**CT** for characterization and grading	**CT** if mechanism or examination warrants; observation and **repeat FAST** are reasonable in selected cases

Serial FAST is valuable and underused. A negative early scan in a patient who is bleeding slowly becomes positive with time, and repeating the examination costs nothing.

8.7 Emergent Aortic Assessment

The clinical question

An older patient presents with **abdominal or back pain, syncope, or unexplained hypotension**. The question is not "characterize this aneurysm" — it is **"does this patient have an abdominal aortic aneurysm?"**, because in the right clinical context that single fact redirects the patient to theatre.

Ruptured AAA is frequently misdiagnosed as renal colic, diverticulitis, or musculoskeletal back pain. A ninety-second bedside aortic scan in any older patient with these presentations is among the highest-yield uses of ultrasound in medicine.

The rapid protocol

Transducer: curvilinear or phased. Depth adequate to reach the vertebral bodies, which are the posterior landmark.

Technique: transverse plane, starting at the subxiphoid region and sweeping continuously caudally to the bifurcation, applying **firm steady pressure** to displace bowel gas. Measure at three levels: **proximal (subxiphoid), mid (at or near the renal arteries), and distal (just above the bifurcation)**, then continue into the proximal common iliac arteries.

Measurement, as established in Chapter 3 §3.8 and restated because the errors are so consequential:

- **Outer wall to outer wall**, including mural thrombus
- **Anteroposterior diameter on a true transverse image**, with the plane **perpendicular to the vessel axis** — a tortuous aorta cut obliquely yields an ellipse and overestimates
- Confirm on longitudinal that you measured at the maximum

Threshold: 3.0 cm defines an aneurysm. In a symptomatic hypotensive patient, an aneurysm of any significant size is presumed to be the cause until proven otherwise.

Rescue technique when bowel gas defeats the anterior approach: **left lateral decubitus with a left coronal flank window**, using the same approach as for the left kidney. This works frequently and is the standard fallback.

Rupture — and the crucial limitation

Ultrasound is excellent at detecting the aneurysm and poor at detecting the rupture. Rupture is usually **retroperitoneal**, and retroperitoneal blood is difficult to distinguish from surrounding tissue at the depths involved, in a patient who is often obese, gas-filled, and unable to cooperate.

Findings that suggest rupture when present:

- **Periaortic or retroperitoneal hypoechoic or heterogeneous material** displacing normal structures
- **Loss of definition of the aortic wall** or a discontinuity
- **Free intraperitoneal fluid** — usually a late finding, since most ruptures are retroperitoneal first
- Rapid interval enlargement on comparison with prior imaging

The essential teaching point: absence of visible rupture does not exclude it. In an unstable patient with a demonstrated aneurysm and a compatible presentation, the sonographic diagnosis is sufficient to act on, and waiting for CT confirmation may cost the patient their life. **This is a critical finding requiring immediate direct communication and, usually, direct transfer** (Chapter 1 §1.5).

The corollary: the examination should be **abbreviated the moment the question is answered**. Completeness is not the goal here.

Mimics and technical traps

A tortuous aorta cut obliquely appears wider than it is — the commonest false positive. **Retroperitoneal lymphadenopathy** surrounding the aorta may be mistaken for aneurysmal wall. **A horseshoe kidney isthmus** crossing anterior to the aorta can confuse the anatomy. **Measuring the lumen rather than the outer wall** underestimates, sometimes grossly, in a thrombus-filled sac. **Failing to reach the bifurcation** misses distal aneurysms, which are common — the sweep must continue to the iliac origins.

Post-repair surveillance

Patients with endovascular repair undergo lifelong surveillance for **endoleak** — persistent perfusion of the aneurysm sac outside the graft — and for **sac enlargement**, which is the finding that matters most. **Contrast-enhanced ultrasound performs well** for endoleak detection and avoids repeated CT radiation and nephrotoxic contrast in a population that frequently has renal impairment. Sac diameter measured with the same technique and compared with the prior study is the core surveillance measurement. [VERIFY: current surveillance protocols and imaging modality recommendations after endovascular aneurysm repair, including the role of CEUS]

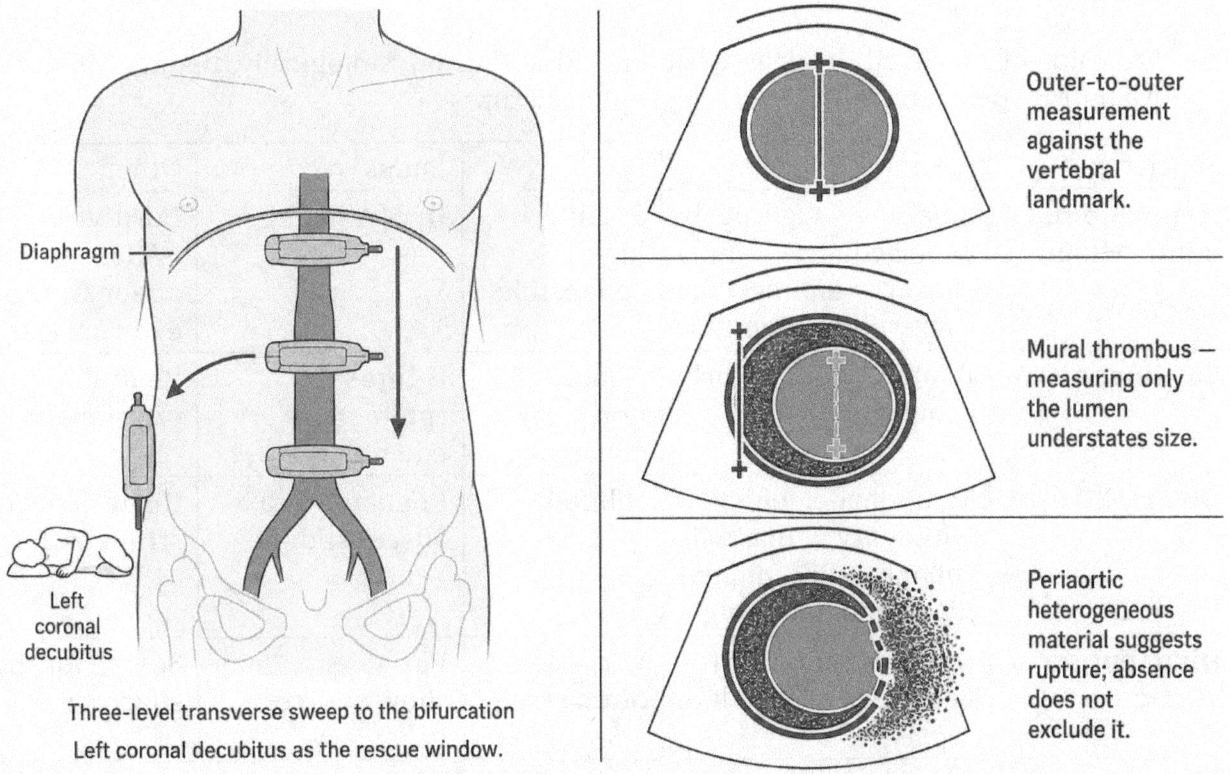

The ninety-second aortic scan
Detection is reliable; exclusion of rupture is not.

8.8 Point-of-Care Protocols and Their Documented Limits

The protocol family

Point-of-care ultrasound has produced a set of structured protocols, each designed to answer a defined question at a decision point:

Protocol	Question
FAST / eFAST	Free intraperitoneal or pericardial fluid; pneumothorax; hemothorax

Protocol	Question
Shock protocols (e.g. RUSH and similar)	Which category of shock is this?
Lung protocols (e.g. BLUE and similar)	What is causing this dyspnea?
Focused cardiac assessment	Global function, effusion, right heart strain, volume status
Aortic screening	Is there an aneurysm?

Differentiating shock

The core value of a focused shock assessment is that four physiologically distinct categories produce four recognizably different sonographic pictures:

Shock type	Cardiac	IVC	Lungs	Other
Hypovolemic / hemorrhagic	Small, vigorously contracting, may show end-systolic cavity obliteration	Small, highly collapsible	Dry (A-lines)	Positive FAST, aneurysm, or external loss
Cardiogenic	Dilated, poorly contracting	Dilated, non-collapsing	**B-lines** (pulmonary edema)	Pleural effusions
Obstructive	Tamponade: effusion with RV diastolic collapse. PE: dilated RV, septal flattening	Dilated	Pneumothorax: absent sliding	Right heart strain pattern
Distributive / septic	Hyperdynamic (or depressed in late sepsis)	Variable, often small	Variable; may show source	Search for the source

This is genuinely powerful at the bedside, and it is also where over-confidence does the most damage — which brings us to the limits.

The documented limits

1. Focused is not complete, and must be reported as focused. A focused negative study excludes only what the protocol was designed to detect. Recording "ultrasound normal" after a FAST is a serious documentation error, because it will be read later as a complete abdominal examination. The record must state which examination was performed and what it was capable of excluding.

2. Volume and location thresholds. FAST requires a detectable volume of fluid in an interrogated recess. Below that threshold, and in locations not interrogated, it is blind. [VERIFY: current published minimum detectable free fluid volumes for FAST by window and by operator experience]

3. Anchoring bias. A positive finding is not necessarily *the* cause. A patient with chronic ascites and shock has ascites and shock, not necessarily hemoperitoneum. A pericardial effusion may be incidental. The finding must be integrated with the clinical picture, not substituted for it.

4. Operator dependence and training volume. Performance in focused ultrasound correlates strongly with training and scan volume, and it degrades in the difficult patient — obese, gas-filled, uncooperative, or with subcutaneous emphysema, which abolishes the acoustic window entirely.

5. Credentialing heterogeneity. Standards for who may perform and interpret focused ultrasound vary widely between specialties and institutions (Chapter 1 §1.2).

6. Archiving and quality assurance. Focused examinations are frequently not archived, which prevents review, prevents audit, prevents comparison with later studies, and removes the record that would demonstrate what was actually seen. **Any diagnostic ultrasound that informs a clinical decision should be archived and auditable.** This is a professional position worth holding.

7. Incidental findings still require action. Finding an unexpected mass, aneurysm, or hydronephrosis on a focused scan creates the same obligation to document and communicate as it would on a formal study (Chapter 1 §1.8). Scope does not limit responsibility for what has been seen.

The integration principle

Focused ultrasound answers a **binary question at a decision point**. A formal complete examination characterizes. They are complementary and neither replaces the other — and the record must never allow one to be mistaken for the other.

8.9 Trauma Pitfalls and Escalation to Cross-Sectional Imaging

Free fluid is not always blood

In the trauma bay, anechoic fluid is presumed to be blood — but the alternatives are real and each has been mistaken for hemoperitoneum:

- **Pre-existing ascites** — cirrhosis, heart failure, malignancy
- **Physiological pelvic fluid** in women of reproductive age — a small volume in the pouch of Douglas is normal
- **Urine** from bladder rupture, which typically follows pelvic fracture with a full bladder
- **Peritoneal dialysis fluid**
- **Ruptured ovarian cyst**
- **Bowel content** from hollow viscus perforation
- **Bile**

Conversely, in the non-trauma setting, unexpected free fluid may be the first sign of a ruptured ectopic pregnancy, a ruptured aneurysm, or perforation — and in a woman of reproductive age with abdominal pain and free fluid, **ectopic pregnancy must be actively excluded** (Chapter 18).

Blood is not always free

This is the most consequential limitation of FAST. Significant injury frequently produces no free intraperitoneal fluid:

- **Retroperitoneal hemorrhage** — renal, duodenal, pancreatic, aortic, and pelvic fracture bleeding, all outside the peritoneal cavity
- **Contained subcapsular hematoma** of liver, spleen, or kidney, with an intact capsule
- **Isolated solid organ injury** without capsular breach
- **Hollow viscus and mesenteric injury**, which is notoriously difficult and may present late

A meaningful proportion of solid organ injuries have no detectable free fluid on initial FAST, and **a negative FAST in a patient with a concerning mechanism does not exclude injury**. [VERIFY: current published sensitivity and negative predictive value of FAST for solid organ injury in blunt abdominal trauma]

Specific false positives

Each of these has been reported as free fluid:

- **Perinephric fat**, hypoechoic and crescentic in the hepatorenal recess
- **Fluid-filled bowel**, distinguished by wall layers and by watching for peristalsis
- **The gallbladder or a renal cyst** at the edge of a window
- **Seminal vesicles** behind the bladder
- **An ovarian cyst** mistaken for pelvic free fluid
- **The epicardial fat pad** mistaken for pericardial effusion — it is echogenic rather than anechoic, moves with the myocardium, and is typically anterior only
- **Pleural versus pericardial fluid** in the subxiphoid or parasternal view — the relationship to the **descending thoracic aorta** distinguishes them: pericardial fluid tracks anterior to it, pleural fluid posterior

Escalation

The decision framework from §8.6, extended:

Hemodynamically unstable with positive FAST → laparotomy. Do not delay for CT.

Hemodynamically unstable with negative FAST → the bleeding is elsewhere. Assess chest, pelvis, retroperitoneum, long bones, and external sources; consider non-hemorrhagic causes of shock; **repeat the FAST**.

Hemodynamically stable, any FAST result → contrast-enhanced CT where the mechanism or examination warrants it. CT grades solid organ injury, detects retroperitoneal and hollow viscus injury, and enables non-operative management decisions.

Children → the same logic, with additional weight given to radiation avoidance. **Serial ultrasound and contrast-enhanced ultrasound have a growing role** in stable pediatric blunt trauma, and CEUS performs substantially better than B-mode for parenchymal injury (Chapter 6 §6.6). [VERIFY: current society guidance on imaging pathways in pediatric blunt abdominal trauma, including the role of CEUS]

Pregnancy → FAST is applicable and radiation avoidance is a priority; the gravid uterus alters fluid distribution and the windows, and fetal assessment is a separate concurrent obligation.

The reporting obligation

A trauma ultrasound report should state: which examination was performed (FAST or eFAST, and which windows), what was found, **which windows were inadequate and why**, and that the study does not exclude solid organ, retroperitoneal, or hollow viscus injury.

Free fluid in a trauma patient is a critical finding, communicated immediately and directly, not left in a report (Chapter 1 §1.5).

Key Points

1. Morison's pouch is the most dependent upper abdominal space supine; the pelvis is the most dependent space overall and shows small volumes first.
2. On the left, the phrenicocolic ligament directs fluid **above** the spleen. Look subphrenic first, and place the probe higher and more posterior than feels natural.
3. Free fluid is mobile, meets structures at sharp angles, and lets bowel float. Loculated fluid keeps its shape and has convex margins.
4. Acute unclotted blood may be entirely anechoic. A simple-looking collection in a trauma patient is not reassuring.
5. Look for omental caking with a linear probe in the anterior abdomen — it is often more conspicuous there than on the curvilinear survey.
6. Paracentesis goes lateral to the rectus, and color Doppler over the site confirms you are clear of the inferior epigastric artery.
7. Below the arcuate line there is no posterior rectus sheath. That single fact explains why a low rectus sheath hematoma can be large, cross the midline, and present as a pelvic mass.
8. The inferior epigastric vessels distinguish direct from indirect inguinal hernia. Identify them with color Doppler before classifying.
9. Femoral hernias lie below the inguinal ligament and medial to the femoral vein, and carry a higher strangulation risk than inguinal hernias.
10. Stand the patient up. A hernia that appears only on standing is still a hernia, and standing is the step most often omitted.
11. Absent peristalsis, wall thickening, absent mural flow, and fluid in the sac suggest strangulation — a critical finding.
12. Ask about cyclical pain in any woman with a nodule in a cesarean scar. The history makes the diagnosis of endometrioma.

13. The caudal liver tip is frequently more sensitive than the hepatorenal interface itself. Sweep the RUQ window, do not place the probe once.
14. Absent lung sliding is sensitive but not specific. The **lung point** is the specific finding for pneumothorax.
15. The spine sign — vertebral bodies visible above the diaphragm — indicates pleural fluid, because aerated lung would have blocked the sound.
16. Unstable plus positive FAST means laparotomy. Do not wait for CT.
17. Ultrasound detects aortic aneurysm reliably and detects rupture unreliably. In an unstable patient with an aneurysm, the absence of visible rupture excludes nothing.
18. Report a focused examination as focused. "Ultrasound normal" after a FAST will be read later as a complete abdominal study, and that is a documentation failure with clinical consequences.
19. A negative FAST does not exclude solid organ, retroperitoneal, or hollow viscus injury. Repeat it, and escalate to CT in the stable patient.

Registry Check

1. In the left upper quadrant FAST view, free fluid most characteristically collects:

A. In the splenorenal recess **B.** In the subphrenic space above the spleen **C.** Along the left paracolic gutter **D.** In the lesser sac

> **Answer: B.** The phrenicocolic ligament limits flow along the left paracolic gutter and directs fluid into the subphrenic space above the spleen. This is why the left probe position must be higher and more posterior than the right, and why placing it too anteriorly and caudally is the commonest cause of a missed positive.

2. A hernia neck in the groin lies medial to the inferior epigastric vessels. This is:

A. An indirect inguinal hernia **B.** A direct inguinal hernia **C.** A femoral hernia **D.** A Spigelian hernia

> **Answer: B.** Direct inguinal hernias pass through the posterior wall of the inguinal canal medial to the inferior epigastric vessels. Indirect hernias pass through the deep ring lateral to them and travel along the canal. Femoral hernias lie below the inguinal ligament.

3. A large hematoma within the abdominal wall crosses the midline and extends inferiorly toward the bladder. This location indicates the bleed occurred:

A. Above the arcuate line **B.** Below the arcuate line **C.** Within the linea alba **D.** In the external oblique

> **Answer: B.** Below the arcuate line there is no posterior rectus sheath, so a hematoma is unconstrained posteriorly and can enlarge, cross the midline, and extend into the prevesical space. Above the arcuate line the intact sheath confines it to a spindle shape that does not cross the midline.

4. M-mode over the anterior chest shows uniform horizontal parallel lines both above and below the pleural line, with no granular pattern. This is:

A. The seashore sign, indicating normal lung sliding **B.** The barcode sign, indicating absent lung sliding **C.** The lung point **D.** The spine sign

> **Answer: B.** The granular "sand" below the pleural line in the normal seashore pattern is produced by lung sliding. Its replacement by uniform horizontal lines is the barcode or stratosphere sign, indicating absent sliding — sensitive for pneumothorax but not specific, since mainstem intubation, adhesions, apnea, and consolidation also abolish sliding.

5. Which sonographic finding is most specific for pneumothorax?

A. Absent lung sliding **B.** Absent B-lines **C.** The lung point **D.** The barcode sign

> **Answer: C.** The lung point is the transition where sliding resumes at the edge of the pneumothorax. It is highly specific and additionally defines the extent. Absent sliding, absent B-lines, and the barcode sign are all sensitive but occur in other conditions.

6. A hypotensive 74-year-old with back pain has a 6.2 cm infrarenal abdominal aortic aneurysm on bedside ultrasound. No periaortic hematoma is visible. The appropriate action is:

A. Reassure, since no rupture is demonstrated **B.** Proceed to CT for confirmation before surgical referral **C.** Immediate direct communication and surgical involvement, since ultrasound cannot exclude rupture **D.** Repeat the ultrasound in one hour

> **Answer: C.** Ultrasound detects aneurysms reliably but detects retroperitoneal rupture poorly. In a hemodynamically unstable patient with a compatible presentation and a demonstrated aneurysm, the absence of visible rupture excludes nothing, and delay for CT confirmation may be fatal.

7. In the subxiphoid view, an anechoic collection is seen. It lies posterior to the descending thoracic aorta. This represents:

A. Pericardial effusion **B.** Pleural effusion **C.** Epicardial fat pad **D.** Ascites

> **Answer: B.** The relationship to the descending thoracic aorta distinguishes the two: pericardial fluid tracks anterior to it, while pleural fluid lies posterior. The epicardial fat pad is echogenic rather than anechoic and moves with the myocardium.

8. A hemodynamically stable patient after blunt abdominal trauma has a negative FAST. The correct interpretation is:

A. Abdominal injury is excluded **B.** The examination excludes free intraperitoneal fluid above its detection threshold in the interrogated windows, but does not exclude solid organ, retroperitoneal, or hollow viscus injury **C.** No further imaging is required **D.** The patient may be discharged

> **Answer: B.** FAST detects free fluid in specific recesses above a volume threshold. Solid organ injury without capsular breach, retroperitoneal hemorrhage, and hollow viscus or mesenteric injury may all produce no free fluid. In a stable patient with a concerning mechanism, CT is the appropriate next study, and serial FAST is a reasonable adjunct.

Chapter Notes for the Editorial Pass

Verification queue. In priority order: **FAST sensitivity, negative predictive value, and minimum detectable fluid volumes** (§8.6, §8.8, §8.9) — these figures are quoted constantly, vary widely between studies by window and operator experience, and a single stale number printed here would be repeated indefinitely; **current society guidance on imaging pathways in pediatric blunt abdominal trauma including CEUS** (§8.9), an actively developing area; **comparative sensitivity of sub-locations within the RUQ window** (§8.6), where the caudal liver tip claim is well supported in the literature but should be cited rather than asserted; and **post-EVAR surveillance protocols and the role of CEUS in endoleak detection** (§8.7).

Structural note. This chapter contains the book's only sustained thoracic content — the eFAST lung and pleural material in §8.6. It sits here rather than in the cardiac part because it belongs to the trauma protocol, but the layout should carry a clear cross-reference from Chapter 14, and the index must catch lung sliding, B-lines, lung point, and spine sign under both trauma and thoracic headings.

Deliberate overlap. Aortic measurement technique appears in both Chapter 3 §3.8 and §8.7 here. This is intentional rather than redundant: the first is the elective surveillance context, the second is the ninety-second emergency scan, and the emphasis differs. At layout, confirm the two read as complementary and that §8.7 explicitly refers back rather than restating from scratch.

Figure count: 6 Lane A, 1 Lane B. Lower than the chapter's breadth might suggest, because the FAST windows figure and the eFAST thoracic figure each carry a great deal. The single Lane B slot combines a positive FAST with the M-mode pair; if a second is added, the strongest candidate is a dynamic hernia sequence showing rest and Valsalva, which is difficult to convey in a still figure and would benefit from real images.

Cross-reference targets to fix at layout: §8.1 recesses → Chapter 3 §3.1; §8.2 portal hypertension → Chapter 4 §4.5; §8.2 abscess gas → Chapter 2 §2.8; §8.2 drainage technique → Chapter 9; §8.5 endometrioma → Chapter 17; §8.6 pericardial and cardiac findings → Chapters 14 and 15; §8.7 aortic measurement → Chapter 3 §3.8; §8.9 splenic and hepatic trauma → Chapters 4 and 6; §8.9 ectopic pregnancy → Chapter 18; §8.9 pediatric trauma → Chapter 12.

Word count: approximately 10,300 excluding image prompt blocks, learning objectives, registry questions, and these notes.

Chapter 9: Contrast-Enhanced, Interventional, and Transplant Sonography

Learning Objectives

On completing this chapter you should be able to:

1. Describe microbubble composition and clearance, and explain why ultrasound contrast is a pure blood-pool agent.
2. State the safety profile and contraindications of ultrasound contrast agents, and administer one correctly.
3. Set the machine for contrast imaging and interpret the vascular phases against a timer.
4. Select appropriate abdominal applications for contrast-enhanced ultrasound, including the non-hepatic ones.
5. Plan a guided procedure: consent, coagulation, sterility, path selection, and respiratory control.
6. Distinguish fine-needle aspiration from core biopsy, and describe the coaxial technique and its advantages.
7. Explain why needle conspicuity depends on the angle of insonation, and apply the maneuvers that improve it.
8. Perform a complete renal transplant protocol and interpret the resistive index correctly.
9. Assess a liver transplant and recognize hepatic artery thrombosis as a critical finding.
10. Categorize transplant complications by type and timing, and report them without over-claiming a diagnosis of rejection.

What Unites This Chapter

These three subjects sit together because each represents ultrasound doing something the other cross-sectional modalities cannot.

Contrast makes ultrasound a real-time perfusion technique, with a purely intravascular tracer, at the bedside, in patients whose kidneys cannot tolerate CT contrast.

Intervention exploits the modality's defining advantage — you watch the needle move while it moves.

Transplant surveillance requires frequent, repeated, radiation-free vascular assessment in patients who will be imaged for the rest of their lives.

All three also share a professional characteristic: they involve **doing something to the patient**, or generating a finding that will trigger someone else to. The reporting discipline, the consent discipline, and the escalation discipline from Chapter 1 apply here more directly than anywhere else in the book.

9.1 Ultrasound Contrast Agents: Composition, Safety, and Administration

What a microbubble is

Ultrasound contrast agents are suspensions of **gas-filled microbubbles**, typically a few micrometres in diameter — comparable to or smaller than a red blood cell, which is what allows them to pass freely through the pulmonary capillary bed and reach the systemic circulation.

Each bubble has two components:

A gas core — a high-molecular-weight, low-solubility gas such as sulphur hexafluoride or a perfluorocarbon, chosen because it diffuses out of the bubble slowly and so persists long enough to image.

A stabilising shell — most commonly a phospholipid monolayer, thin and flexible enough to allow the bubble to oscillate.

That oscillation is the whole point. When insonated at low acoustic pressure, microbubbles resonate and produce a **strongly non-linear** acoustic signal, quite unlike the largely linear echo from tissue. Contrast-specific imaging exploits this difference to display bubbles and suppress everything else (§9.2).

The property that distinguishes it from CT and MRI contrast

Ultrasound contrast is a pure blood-pool agent. The bubbles are too large to cross the vascular endothelium and do **not** diffuse into the interstitium.

Iodinated CT contrast and gadolinium do diffuse into the extracellular space, so their enhancement reflects a mixture of perfusion and interstitial distribution. Microbubbles reflect **perfusion only**, continuously, in real time.

Three consequences follow, and they define the technique's clinical niche:

1. **True real-time perfusion imaging** — you watch enhancement arrive and leave, at frame rates no other modality achieves. Washout *timing* becomes measurable, which is the basis of hepatic lesion characterization (Chapter 4 §4.7).
2. **Repeatable within a session** — the agent clears quickly, so a second bolus can be given to examine a second lesion or repeat an equivocal observation.
3. **Not nephrotoxic**, which matters enormously in the populations where it is most useful.

Clearance and safety

The gas is **exhaled through the lungs** within minutes; the phospholipid shell is metabolised and cleared, largely hepatically.

There is no nephrotoxicity, no thyroid effect, and no ionising radiation. This is the practical basis for using CEUS in patients with renal impairment — including the renal transplant population and patients with complex cystic renal lesions in chronic kidney disease (§9.3) — for whom CT and MRI contrast carry real risk.

The safety profile is favourable, with serious hypersensitivity reactions rare. That rarity is not zero, and the practical requirements follow from it rather than from the numbers: resuscitation equipment and trained personnel must be immediately available, the patient must be observed after administration, and the operator must be prepared to manage anaphylaxis. [VERIFY: current published incidence of serious adverse reactions to ultrasound contrast agents, and current observation-period recommendations]

Contraindications and cautions vary by agent and by regulatory jurisdiction, and the product's current labelling governs. Those commonly listed include known hypersensitivity to the agent or its components; **right-to-left cardiac shunt**; severe pulmonary hypertension; acute coronary syndrome or clinically unstable ischaemic cardiac disease; and severe respiratory failure. Pregnancy and lactation are generally areas of limited data. [VERIFY: current contraindications, warnings, and licensed indications for the specific agents in use, which differ between agents and between jurisdictions]

Much clinical CEUS use is off-label relative to the licensed indications in a given country. Where that is the case, institutional policy and the consent conversation must reflect it (Chapter 1 §1.5).

Administration

Access. A peripheral intravenous cannula, preferably of reasonable bore, with a three-way tap. Very small cannulae and high injection pressures **destroy microbubbles mechanically**, which is a common cause of an apparently failed study.

Handling. Reconstitute strictly per the manufacturer's instructions, agitate as directed, and use within the stated stability window. Handle gently — vigorous handling destroys bubbles. Draw up immediately before use.

Injection. Give the bolus **at a controlled, moderate rate**, immediately followed by a saline flush to clear the line and deliver the residual bubbles. Injecting forcefully does not improve enhancement and reduces it.

Start the timer at the moment of injection. Not at the moment enhancement appears. The timing of washout relative to injection is the diagnosis (§9.2), and a study without a timer running is substantially less interpretable.

Dose varies by agent, by application, and by the equipment's sensitivity, and is taken from the product information and local protocol. Renal and cardiac applications typically use different doses from hepatic ones. [VERIFY: current dosing for each agent by application]

Infusion rather than bolus administration is used where prolonged or whole-organ assessment is required, giving a steady-state concentration.

9.2 Contrast Imaging Technique and Phase Interpretation

Low mechanical index imaging

The central technical requirement: **the acoustic pressure must be low enough to make bubbles oscillate without destroying them.**

Contrast studies are therefore performed at **low mechanical index** — well below the settings used for conventional B-mode (Chapter 1 §1.7). At higher MI, bubbles undergo inertial collapse, producing a bright transient signal followed by loss of contrast in the insonated region. A study performed at conventional MI destroys its own signal, and this is one of the commonest reasons a CEUS study fails.

Contrast-specific pulse sequences — such as pulse inversion and amplitude modulation, and combinations of the two — transmit sequences of pulses whose linear echoes cancel on summation, leaving only the non-linear bubble signal. The result is a display in which **tissue is nearly black and bubbles are bright**.

Most systems present a **dual display**: the contrast image alongside a simultaneous low-MI B-mode image, so the lesion can be kept in view even before enhancement arrives.

Setting up before the injection

The single most important practical point in this section: **the study is set up completely before any contrast is given**, because the arterial phase lasts seconds and cannot be repeated without another bolus.

1. **Find the lesion on B-mode** and establish the window and patient position that hold it steadily in view.
2. **Fix the probe position** and, where possible, brace your hand against the patient so the lesion cannot drift.
3. **Set depth and a single focal zone at or just below the lesion.** Multiple focal zones increase acoustic exposure and destroy bubbles.
4. **Switch to the contrast preset**, confirm low MI, and set contrast gain so that **the pre-injection image is almost entirely black** with only the faintest tissue outline.
5. **Rehearse respiration** with the patient — quiet shallow breathing is usually better than repeated breath-holds for a study lasting minutes.
6. **Start recording a continuous clip**, not still frames. The dynamics are the diagnosis.
7. **Inject, flush, and start the timer.**

The phases

In the liver, which has a dual blood supply, the phases are distinct and are the basis of lesion characterization:

Phase	Approximate timing after injection	Supplied by
Arterial	From roughly 10 seconds to 30–45 seconds	Hepatic artery

Phase	Approximate timing after injection	Supplied by
Portal venous	From roughly 30–45 seconds to about 2 minutes	Portal vein predominates
Late	From about 2 minutes to agent clearance, often 4–6 minutes	Residual circulating bubbles

[VERIFY: current consensus phase timings for hepatic contrast-enhanced ultrasound]

Some agents additionally show a **post-vascular (Kupffer) phase**, with retention in reticuloendothelial cells, which improves lesion detection.

Observe continuously through the arterial phase — the enhancement pattern here suggests the diagnosis — **and then through to the late phase**, because **washout timing and degree confirm it** (Chapter 4 §4.7: HCC washes out late and mildly, metastasis early and markedly).

In the kidney, there is no dual supply and no reticuloendothelial uptake, so the pattern differs: rapid **cortical** enhancement followed by **medullary** filling, with no true late phase. Renal CEUS therefore assesses presence or absence of perfusion rather than washout kinetics.

Destruction–replenishment

A deliberate **high-MI "flash"** destroys all bubbles within the imaged plane; returning to low MI then allows the refill to be observed. The **rate of replenishment** reflects perfusion, and this technique underlies quantitative perfusion assessment and time–intensity curve analysis.

Pitfalls

- **MI too high** — bubbles destroyed, study fails
- **Probe drift** — the lesion leaves the plane during the arterial phase and cannot be recovered in time
- **Depth and attenuation** — deep lesions in large patients enhance poorly, because the low acoustic pressure that preserves bubbles also limits penetration
- **One region per bolus** — CEUS interrogates the plane you are holding. It is not a whole-organ or whole-body survey, which is its principal limitation against CT
- **Late arrival mistaken for absent enhancement** — keep watching
- **No timer** — the study becomes qualitative and loses its main advantage

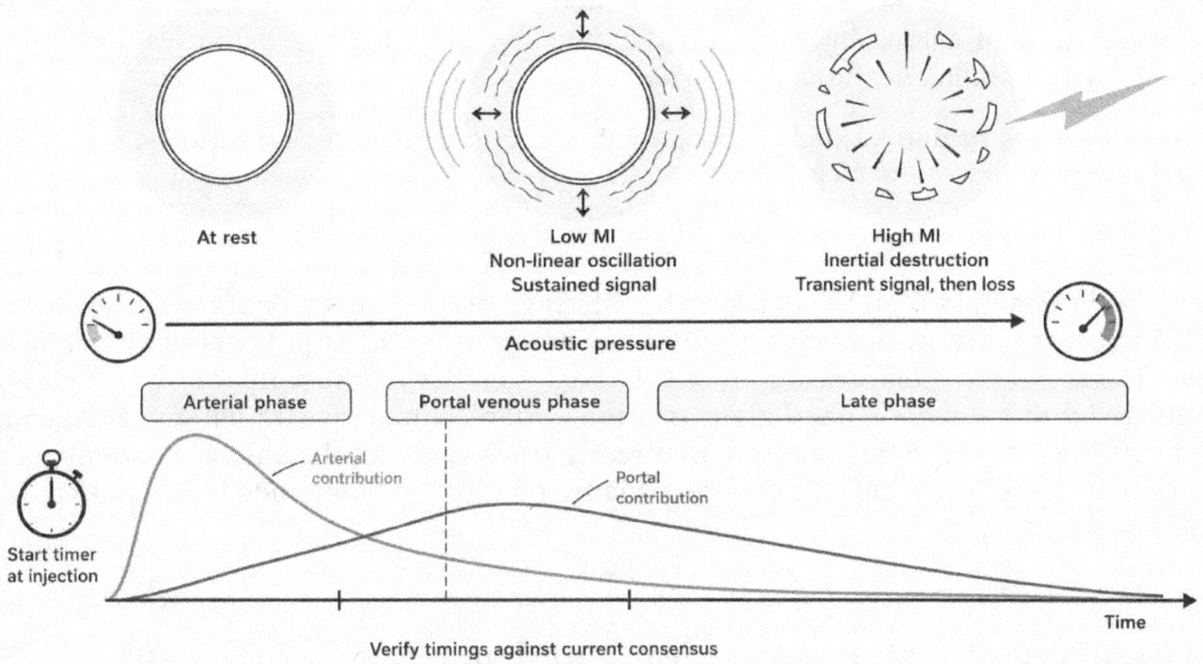

9.3 Abdominal Applications of Contrast-Enhanced Ultrasound

Liver

The dominant application, developed fully in **Chapter 4 §4.6–4.7**: characterization of focal lesions by arterial pattern and washout timing, and improved detection of additional lesions in the late phase. Not repeated here.

Two additional hepatic uses belong in this chapter: **pre-ablation targeting** and **post-ablation assessment of residual viable tumour**, both covered in §9.5.

Kidney

This is CEUS's most under-used strong application, and the reason is worth stating: **the population that needs renal lesion characterization frequently has impaired renal function**, which restricts CT and MRI contrast. CEUS has no nephrotoxicity.

Complex cystic lesion characterization. The features that determine management are **septal and nodular enhancement** (Chapter 7 §7.6), and conventional colour Doppler is insensitive to the slow flow within a thin septum or a small nodule. CEUS demonstrates it directly and is genuinely superior to Doppler for this question.

Infarct versus mass. A renal infarct appears as a **sharply demarcated, wedge-shaped, non-enhancing region in all phases**, with its base at the capsule (Chapter 6 §6.6 for the splenic equivalent). This resolves the frequent B-mode ambiguity of a subtle acute infarct.

Pseudotumour confirmation. A hypertrophied column of Bertin enhances **identically to adjacent normal cortex** in all phases (Chapter 7 §7.1). This is a definitive, inexpensive answer to a common question.

Abscess versus tumour, extent of pyelonephritis, and **post-ablation follow-up** of treated renal tumours.

Trauma

Covered in Chapters 6 and 8, and worth restating because the evidence base has moved: **CEUS substantially outperforms B-mode for detecting solid organ parenchymal injury**, demonstrates active extravasation, and is well suited to **follow-up of conservatively managed injury** and to **paediatric trauma**, where cumulative radiation is a genuine concern. It is applied in the **haemodynamically stable** patient; the unstable patient goes to CT or theatre. [VERIFY: current society guidance on CEUS in blunt abdominal trauma, adult and paediatric]

Vascular

Endoleak detection after endovascular aneurysm repair (Chapter 8 §8.7) — CEUS performs well, avoids repeated CT radiation and iodinated contrast in a population with frequent renal impairment, and can characterize the leak.

TIPS patency assessment where Doppler is equivocal (Chapter 4 §4.5).

Carotid plaque neovascularisation as a marker of plaque instability (Chapter 16).

Pancreas and bowel

Pancreatic cystic lesions — demonstrating whether a suspected mural nodule enhances, which is the feature that most changes management (Chapter 6 §6.4).

Pancreatic necrosis extent, and confirmation of a suspected **pseudoaneurysm** (Chapter 6 §6.2).

Crohn disease — quantifying mural enhancement as a marker of inflammatory activity, and distinguishing an **inflammatory phlegmon** (which enhances) from an **abscess** (which does not enhance centrally), a distinction that determines whether drainage is appropriate.

Intracavitary CEUS

A distinct technique in which diluted contrast is instilled **into a cavity rather than a vein**:

- **Contrast-enhanced voiding urosonography** for vesicoureteric reflux, instilled into the bladder — a radiation-free alternative to fluoroscopic cystography, and a significant paediatric application (Chapter 12)
- **Confirming drain position** and demonstrating the extent of a drained cavity
- **Delineating fistulae and sinus tracts**
- Demonstrating whether a collection communicates with the biliary tree, bowel, or another cavity

Limitations

One region per bolus — CEUS examines the plane you are holding, so it cannot stage disease or survey a whole organ the way CT does. **Depth and attenuation** limit it in large patients. **Motion** degrades it. And it requires a trained operator holding a fixed plane for several minutes, which is a real resource commitment

9.4 Principles of Ultrasound-Guided Intervention

Why ultrasound

Real-time visualization of a moving needle is the decisive advantage, and no other cross-sectional modality offers it as readily. Add: no ionising radiation, any imaging plane rather than fixed axial sections, portability to the bedside or theatre, colour Doppler to identify and avoid vessels in the path, and low cost.

The limitation is the same as everywhere else — targets obscured by gas or bone are not accessible, and **fusion imaging** with previously acquired CT or MRI exists partly to address it (§9.6).

Before the procedure

Confirm the indication and that the result will change management. A biopsy that will not alter treatment is a complication risk with no benefit.

Consent — explicit, informed, documented, covering the procedure, the alternatives, and the specific risks: bleeding, infection, pain, damage to adjacent structures, pneumothorax where relevant, and the possibility of a non-diagnostic sample. Chapter 1 §1.5.

Coagulation status. Platelet count, INR, and the patient's anticoagulant and antiplatelet medications, with a documented plan for withholding and restarting them. Thresholds and withholding intervals are procedure-specific and institution-specific and must be taken from local policy. [VERIFY: current society guidance on periprocedural coagulation thresholds and anticoagulant management for image-guided procedures, stratified by bleeding risk]

Allergies, antibiotic prophylaxis where indicated, **intravenous access**, **monitoring**, and **fasting** where sedation is planned.

The time-out — correct patient, correct site, correct side, correct procedure, consent verified, relevant results available (Chapter 1 §1.5). Laterality errors in guided procedures are catastrophic and entirely preventable.

Relative contraindications: uncorrectable coagulopathy, absence of a safe acoustic window and path, an uncooperative patient who cannot hold still or suspend respiration, and haemodynamic instability.

Sterility

Under the Spaulding framework (Chapter 1 §1.4), a transducer used within a sterile field or in contact with sterile tissue falls into the **critical** category. In practice this means:

- **Skin antisepsis** per local protocol, allowed to dry
- **Sterile probe cover** and **sterile gel** — sterile gel inside the cover as the coupling medium and sterile gel outside as the skin coupling medium
- **Sterile field, sterile gloves, and appropriate personal protective equipment**
- **Needle guides** either single-use disposable or sterilised between uses
- The transducer itself reprocessed to the level appropriate to its use afterwards

Planning the path

Choose the shortest safe path, not simply the shortest.

Avoid: bowel, large vessels (use colour Doppler over the intended path, every time), the gallbladder, the pleura where possible, dilated ducts, and the pancreas when it is not the target.

Traverse normal parenchyma where possible in liver and kidney biopsy. A tract through normal tissue tamponades better than a direct subcapsular puncture, and the risk of bleeding is lower.

Respect the intercostal neurovascular bundle — it runs along the *inferior* margin of each rib, so an intercostal needle passes **just above the superior margin of the lower rib**.

Avoid crossing the pleura. A subcostal approach is preferable to an intercostal one where anatomy allows, and the **lung base position changes with respiration**, so a path that is clear in expiration may not be in inspiration.

Rehearse respiration. The patient must be able to suspend respiration reproducibly at the same point in the cycle, because the target moves several centimetres between inspiration and expiration. Practise it before the needle is anywhere near the skin, and choose the respiratory position in which the target is best placed.

After the procedure

Observation for an appropriate interval with monitoring; post-procedure imaging where a complication is suspected; documentation of the approach, the number of passes, the specimens obtained and where they were sent; and clear discharge instructions covering symptoms that should prompt return.

9.5 Biopsy, Aspiration, and Drainage Technique

Fine-needle aspiration versus core biopsy

	Fine-needle aspiration	Core biopsy
Needle	Fine gauge	Larger gauge, spring-loaded cutting device
Yields	**Cytology** — cells	**Histology** — tissue architecture
Answers	Is this malignant? Is this the known primary?	What type is it, what grade, what receptor status, is the architecture diagnostic
Risk	Lower	Higher, though still low

	Fine-needle aspiration	Core biopsy
Use	Lymph nodes, thyroid, cyst fluid, confirming recurrence	Most solid organ and mass biopsies where subtyping matters

Core biopsy has become the default for most solid lesions because modern pathology increasingly requires architecture and ancillary studies rather than cell morphology alone.

Know the throw length of your biopsy device, and account for it. The device fires forward by a fixed distance, and **the far end of that throw must be clear of any structure you are avoiding**. Firing a device whose throw extends into a vessel or bowel loop that was safely beyond the needle tip is a specific and avoidable error.

The coaxial technique

An outer introducer needle is positioned once, up to the edge of the target, and multiple biopsy passes are then taken through it without re-puncturing the capsule.

Advantages: a single capsular pass rather than several, reducing bleeding risk; multiple cores from slightly different angles improving sampling; the ability to **embolise the tract** with gelatin or another agent on withdrawal in higher-risk cases; and a theoretical reduction in tumour seeding along the tract.

This is the standard approach for most organ biopsies where more than one core is needed.

Targeting

Sample the viable tissue, not the necrotic centre. Large tumours frequently have a necrotic core that yields non-diagnostic material. Target the **enhancing periphery**, and where the viable component is not apparent on B-mode, **CEUS can be used to identify it immediately before the procedure** — a genuinely useful application (§9.3).

For diffuse disease — a liver biopsy for suspected cirrhosis, a renal biopsy for glomerular disease — the goal is adequate representative parenchyma rather than a target, and the sampling site is chosen for safety.

Organ-specific points

Liver. Traverse normal parenchyma. Avoid the gallbladder, large vessels, and dilated ducts. A subcostal approach in deep inspiration often brings the lesion into a safe window and avoids the pleura. **Do not biopsy a lesion with features of haemangioma** without careful consideration.

Native kidney. The **lower pole cortex** is the standard target for medical renal biopsy — it maximises glomeruli and avoids the hilar vessels. Prone or oblique positioning; deep inspiration and breath-hold.

Transplant kidney. Superficial and accessible in the iliac fossa; the **lower pole** is again the target, avoiding the hilum and the collecting system.

Pancreas, retroperitoneum, and deep targets — assess whether endoscopic ultrasound offers a shorter, safer path; for many pancreatic lesions it does.

Superficial targets — thyroid, lymph node, abdominal wall — are straightforward, and a linear probe with a shallow approach gives excellent needle visibility.

Aspiration and drainage

Diagnostic aspiration — a small sample for microbiology, cytology, or biochemistry, distinguishing an abscess from a sterile collection, a biloma from a urinoma, or exudate from transudate.

Therapeutic aspiration — of a symptomatic simple collection, ascites, or pleural fluid. Paracentesis site selection is in Chapter 8 §8.2.

Catheter drainage for collections that will re-accumulate:

- **Seldinger technique** — needle, guidewire, serial dilatation, catheter over the wire. More steps, greater control, preferred for deeper or more difficult collections.
- **Trocar technique** — catheter mounted on a stylet placed in a single pass. Faster, suited to large superficial collections.
- **Catheter size** is chosen for the viscosity of the contents: thin fluid drains through a small catheter, thick pus and debris require a larger one. Under-sizing is the commonest cause of a failed drainage.
- **Secure fixation**, a documented **flushing regimen**, and **output monitoring**.
- **Contrast injection through the catheter** (a sinogram, or intracavitary CEUS per §9.3) confirms position and demonstrates whether the cavity communicates elsewhere.

A crucial cross-reference: a pancreatic collection containing solid necrotic debris will not drain through a percutaneous catheter (Chapter 6 §6.2). Assess the contents before recommending the route.

Complications

Bleeding is the commonest significant complication, and its risk rises with lesion vascularity, needle gauge, number of passes, and coagulopathy. **Pneumothorax** with upper abdominal and thoracic approaches. **Infection. Injury to bowel, gallbladder, or vessels. Pancreatitis** after pancreatic biopsy. **Vasovagal reactions. Tumour seeding** — rare, but the reason tract embolisation and coaxial technique are used in selected cases.

Post-procedure imaging where bleeding is suspected: look for a new perihepatic or perinephric collection, subcapsular haematoma, or free fluid, and consider CEUS or CT angiography for active extravasation.

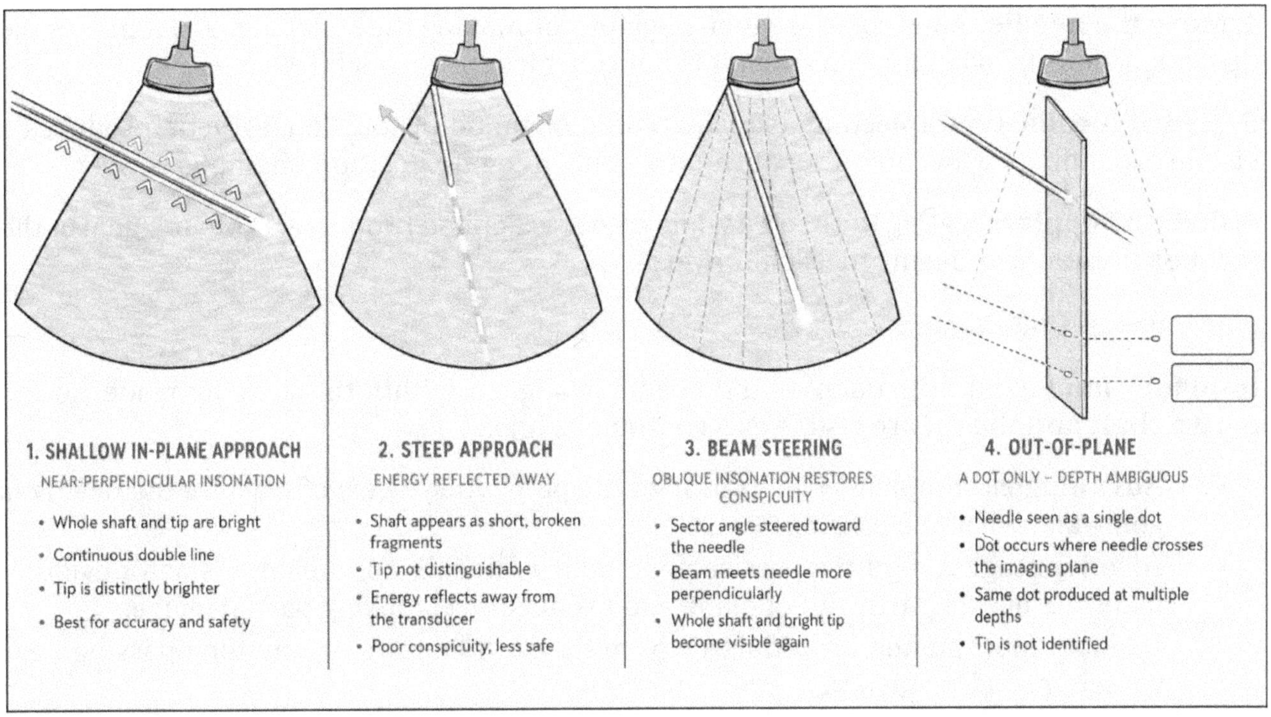

9.6 Needle Visualization and Guidance Systems

The physics of the problem

A needle is a **smooth, highly reflective, specular reflector** (Chapter 2 §2.1). Specular reflectors return energy along the angle of reflection, so a needle is brilliantly visible when the beam strikes it **perpendicularly** and progressively invisible as the angle steepens, because the reflected energy travels away from the transducer rather than back to it.

This single fact governs everything about needle visualization. A needle that has "disappeared" has almost always not moved — the geometry has changed.

Improving conspicuity

In order of usefulness:

1. Choose a shallow angle of approach. The most effective measure by a wide margin. A needle entering at a shallow angle relative to the skin is closer to perpendicular to the beam and is far more visible. For deep targets a shallow approach means a longer path, which is a genuine trade-off, but the visibility gain usually justifies it.

2. Beam steering. Most modern systems offer needle-enhancement software that steers the transmit beam to strike the needle more squarely, restoring conspicuity at steep angles. On a linear array this is highly effective. Know whether your machine has it and where the control is.

3. Echogenic needles. Needles with a dimpled, etched, or coated surface at the tip scatter energy back from a wider range of angles. Genuinely helpful for deep or steep approaches.

4. Move the needle. Small rotation, gentle jiggling, or moving the stylet in and out makes the tip conspicuous through motion when it is not conspicuous through reflection.

5. Hydro-localisation. Injecting a small volume of saline or local anaesthetic produces a visible expanding hypoechoic area **at the tip**, confirming tip position unambiguously.

6. Colour Doppler. Jiggling the needle while colour is applied produces a colour signal at the point of vibration, localising the shaft or tip.

In-plane versus out-of-plane

In-plane (long-axis) approach — the needle is aligned within the imaging plane, so the **entire shaft and the tip** are visible as a continuous line.

- **Advantages:** complete visualization of the path; you see exactly where the needle is going and what it is passing.
- **Disadvantages:** requires precise alignment of needle and beam; a small deviation takes the needle partly out of plane and produces a confusing partial image.
- **Use for:** most guided procedures where the path matters — anything passing near vessels, bowel, or pleura.

Out-of-plane (short-axis) approach — the needle crosses the imaging plane, appearing as a **single bright dot**.

- **Advantage:** easier alignment, and the surrounding structures are seen in cross-section.
- **The critical disadvantage: a dot does not tell you which part of the needle you are seeing.** The same dot is produced by the shaft crossing the plane as by the tip crossing it, so **the needle may be considerably deeper than you think**. This is the mechanism behind a substantial proportion of guided-procedure complications.

The rule that follows: in out-of-plane technique, **track the tip continuously** by advancing the probe slightly ahead of the needle and following the tip as it appears, or use hydro-localisation to confirm. Never assume a bright dot is the tip.

Freehand versus needle guide

Needle guide — a bracket attached to the transducer that fixes the needle at a defined angle, with the predicted path displayed on screen.

- **Advantages:** reliable alignment, needle stays in plane, shorter learning curve, useful for deep or small targets.
- **Disadvantages:** the angle is fixed, so the path cannot be adjusted mid-procedure without withdrawing; the entry site is determined by the probe position; sterility requires a single-use or sterilisable guide.

Freehand — needle and transducer manipulated independently.

- **Advantages:** complete flexibility of angle and entry point, the ability to adjust the path continuously, and no additional equipment.
- **Disadvantages:** a genuinely difficult psychomotor skill requiring sustained practice, with a real learning curve.

Both are legitimate. Most experienced operators use freehand for accessible targets and a guide for deep, small, or angulated ones.

Fusion and tracking

Electromagnetic or optical tracking registers the transducer position in space and displays a **previously acquired CT or MRI dataset reformatted in the same plane as the live ultrasound**, side by side or overlaid.

Its main application is targeting **lesions that are visible on CT or MRI but not on ultrasound** — a small liver lesion in a fatty or cirrhotic liver, an ablation target after previous treatment, a lesion obscured by ribs. It converts a procedure that could not be done under ultrasound into one that can, and it retains ultrasound's real-time needle visualization.

The single most important habit

Confirm the tip, not just a bright line. Operators see a bright linear echo, assume it is the needle in its entirety, and advance. The bright line may be the shaft with the tip beyond the plane; it may be a different needle-like reflector; it may be a partial-volume artefact. Before advancing, and before firing a biopsy device, establish where the tip actually is — by continuity in plane, by hydro-localisation, or by motion.

9.7 Renal Transplant Evaluation

Anatomy and access

The transplanted kidney is placed **extraperitoneally in the iliac fossa**, most often the right, which makes it **superficial and unusually accessible** — a high-frequency linear probe can often be used in addition to the curvilinear, and image quality is typically far better than for a native kidney.

Anastomoses:

- **Arterial** — donor renal artery to the **external iliac artery** end-to-side, or to the internal iliac artery end-to-end. Deceased donor grafts often include an aortic (Carrel) patch.
- **Venous** — donor renal vein to the **external iliac vein**.
- **Ureteric** — implanted directly into the bladder (ureteroneocystostomy), usually with an antireflux tunnel.

Knowing which configuration was used matters, because it determines where you interrogate.

The protocol

Greyscale:

- Graft **length and volume**, compared with prior studies
- **Cortical echogenicity** and **corticomedullary differentiation**
- **Collecting system** — any dilatation, and whether it is new
- **Perinephric and pelvic collections** — location, size, and relationship to the graft and its vessels
- **Bladder**, including volume and any distension that might itself obstruct the graft
- **Urothelial thickening**

Colour Doppler:

- Perfusion **throughout the cortex to the capsule**. A regional or global perfusion defect is a significant finding, and a graft that does not perfuse to the capsule is abnormal.

Spectral Doppler — sample systematically:

- **Main renal artery** at the anastomosis, and proximal, mid, and distal segments
- **Segmental, interlobar, and arcuate arteries** at **upper, mid, and lower poles**, recording **resistive index** at each
- **Renal vein**, confirming flow and its direction
- **External iliac artery** above and below the anastomosis, to establish a reference velocity and detect inflow disease

The baseline study performed in the early postoperative period is the reference against which everything later is compared. Serial change matters far more than any single absolute value, which makes the comparison discipline of Chapter 1 §1.5 central to transplant work.

Normal findings and interpreting the resistive index

A normal graft shows a **low-resistance arterial waveform** with abundant continuous diastolic flow, **continuous venous flow**, and perfusion extending to the capsule.

Resistive index is the most requested and most misinterpreted measurement in transplant sonography. Stated plainly:

> **An elevated RI is non-specific. It does not diagnose rejection.**

Elevated RI occurs in: acute tubular necrosis, acute and chronic rejection, obstruction, **extrinsic compression by a perinephric collection**, calcineurin inhibitor toxicity, renal vein thrombosis, pyelonephritis, and from systemic factors including bradycardia, hypertension, and older donor age.

What RI is actually useful for is trend. A rising RI on serial studies in a graft with deteriorating function is a meaningful signal that something has changed and warrants investigation — most often biopsy. A single elevated value in isolation is a finding, not a diagnosis. [VERIFY: current normal resistive index range in renal transplants and the significance attached to serial change]

Absent or reversed diastolic flow is a much more serious finding, indicating severely elevated intrarenal resistance. Causes include **renal vein thrombosis** (classically **reversed diastolic arterial flow with absent venous flow** — a near-specific combination), severe rejection, severe acute tubular necrosis, and acute compression by a collection. It warrants urgent communication.

The report

Describe: graft size and echogenicity, collecting system, collections and their relationship to the graft, arterial and venous patency and waveforms, RI values by pole with comparison to prior, and any focal perfusion abnormality.

Do not report "rejection." Rejection is a histological diagnosis made on biopsy. Report the findings, note the change from baseline, and let the transplant team integrate them.

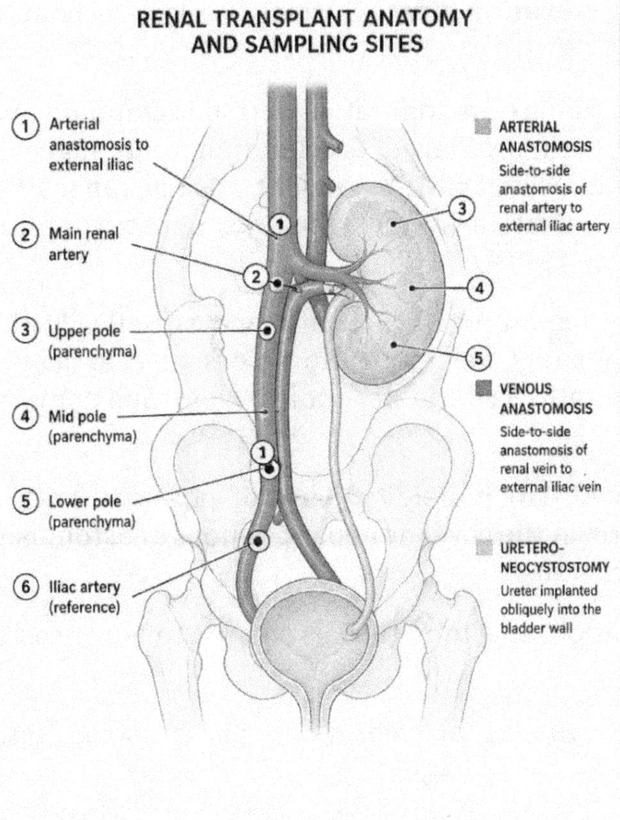

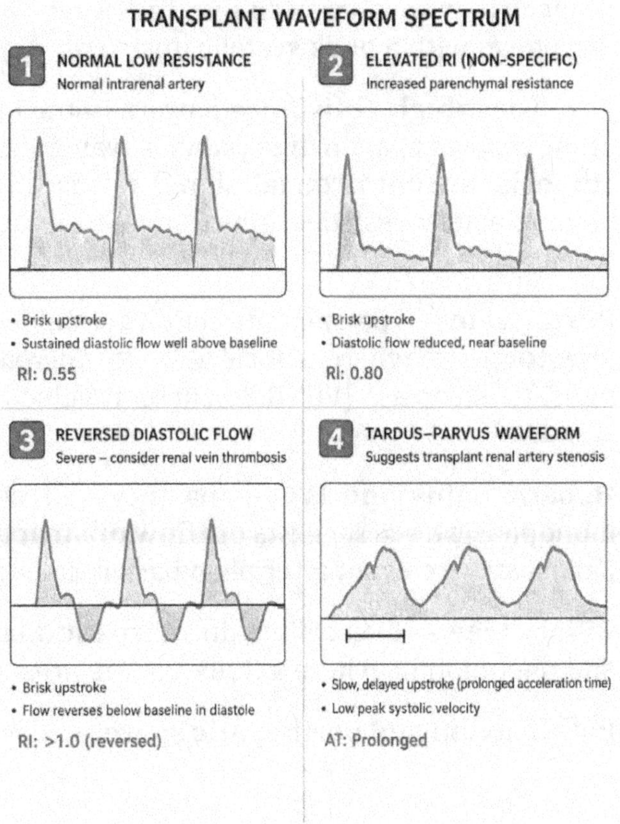

9.8 Liver and Pancreas Transplant Evaluation

Liver transplant anatomy

Four anastomoses, and the assessment is organised around them:

Hepatic artery — donor to recipient hepatic artery, frequently with reconstruction because of the common arterial variants noted in Chapter 4 §4.1. This is the anastomosis that matters most.

Portal vein — end-to-end.

Inferior vena cava — either the classic interposition (donor IVC replacing a segment of recipient IVC, with two anastomoses) or the **piggyback** technique (donor IVC anastomosed to the confluence of the recipient hepatic veins, with one anastomosis).

Biliary — either **duct-to-duct** (choledochocholedochostomy) or a **Roux-en-Y hepaticojejunostomy**, the latter used in living donor grafts, in re-transplantation, and in primary sclerosing cholangitis. Knowing which is present is essential, because a Roux-en-Y produces **expected pneumobilia** (Chapter 5 §5.10) that would be alarming in a duct-to-duct graft.

The protocol

Hepatic artery — the priority. Interrogate at the porta and within the liver (right and left branches), recording **resistive index** and **acceleration time**. Normal is a low-resistance waveform with a brisk systolic upstroke.

A transient **high-resistance** pattern in the immediate postoperative period is common and often resolves; a **tardus–parvus** waveform with prolonged acceleration time suggests **stenosis**; **absent arterial signal** raises thrombosis. [VERIFY: current normal ranges for hepatic artery resistive index and acceleration time in liver transplants, and criteria for stenosis]

Portal vein — patency, direction (should be hepatopetal), velocity, and specifically the **anastomosis**, where a focal velocity increase and a velocity ratio across the narrowing indicate stenosis. [VERIFY: current velocity ratio criteria for portal vein anastomotic stenosis]

Hepatic veins and IVC — patency and **waveform phasicity**. Loss of phasicity with a monophasic trace suggests **outflow obstruction** at the caval or hepatic venous anastomosis, particularly relevant after piggyback reconstruction.

Biliary tree — duct calibre, intrahepatic dilatation, anastomotic narrowing, stones or casts, and pneumobilia where a Roux-en-Y is present.

Parenchyma and perihepatic space — echotexture, focal lesions, collections, and ascites.

Hepatic artery thrombosis

The most feared early complication of liver transplantation. The graft's biliary tree is supplied **exclusively by the hepatic artery** — unlike the parenchyma, which also receives portal flow — so arterial occlusion causes **biliary ischaemia and necrosis**, leading to bile leaks, ischaemic cholangiopathy, abscess, and frequently graft loss or re-transplantation.

Sonographic findings: absent hepatic arterial signal at the porta and intrahepatically, despite careful interrogation with a low velocity scale, low wall filter, and adequate time spent searching. In partial or evolving cases, a tardus–parvus waveform may be found in intrahepatic branches.

The examination is technically demanding and false negatives occur — a small or slow arterial signal is easy to miss, and postoperative dressings, drains, and patient factors make it harder. Where the artery cannot be demonstrated:

- Search deliberately in multiple windows with optimised settings
- **CEUS is excellent for this question** and can rapidly confirm or exclude arterial perfusion (§9.3)
- **CT angiography** is the confirmatory study

Suspected hepatic artery thrombosis is a critical finding requiring immediate direct communication (Chapter 1 §1.5). Time to revascularisation determines graft survival.

Other liver transplant complications

Portal vein stenosis or thrombosis — focal velocity elevation with turbulence, or absent flow.

Outflow obstruction — monophasic hepatic vein waveform, hepatomegaly, ascites.

Biliary complications — the second major category. Anastomotic stricture (dilatation above the anastomosis), leak with biloma formation, **ischaemic cholangiopathy** from arterial compromise with intrahepatic strictures and casts, and stones.

Collections — haematoma, biloma, seroma, abscess.

Recurrent disease — hepatitis C or B, autoimmune disease, and recurrent hepatocellular carcinoma in patients transplanted for it.

Post-transplant lymphoproliferative disorder — hypoechoic masses in the graft, porta, bowel, or elsewhere, in a chronically immunosuppressed patient.

Pancreas transplant

Usually performed **simultaneously with a kidney (SPK)** in type 1 diabetes with renal failure. The graft is placed intraperitoneally or extraperitoneally with arterial inflow via a donor iliac **Y-graft** and venous drainage either systemic (to the iliac vein) or portal (to the SMV); exocrine drainage is enteric or, less commonly now, to the bladder.

Assessment is technically difficult — the graft is deep, often surrounded by bowel gas, and its vasculature is complex.

Graft thrombosis is the principal early complication and the leading cause of early graft loss. Assess arterial and venous flow throughout the graft; absent venous flow with an oedematous graft is the characteristic picture.

Also assess for: peripancreatic collections, pancreatitis of the graft, ductal dilatation, and pseudoaneurysm.

In SPK recipients, rejection frequently manifests in the kidney first and is diagnosed there, since the renal graft is far more accessible to biopsy — a useful practical point.

9.9 Transplant Complications: Vascular, Collections, and Rejection

Vascular complications

Complication	Findings
Arterial thrombosis	Absent arterial signal despite optimised settings; confirm with CEUS or CT angiography. Catastrophic in liver, graft-threatening in kidney and pancreas
Arterial stenosis	Focal peak systolic velocity elevation at the anastomosis, elevated ratio against the adjacent native artery, post-stenotic turbulence, and **tardus–parvus** distally
Venous thrombosis	Absent venous flow; in the kidney, the near-specific combination of **reversed diastolic arterial flow with absent venous flow**
Venous or outflow stenosis	Focal velocity increase; loss of phasicity in hepatic veins after liver transplant
Pseudoaneurysm	Yin-yang swirling flow with a to-and-fro neck waveform (Chapter 3 §3.8); most often post-biopsy or at an anastomosis, and at risk of rupture
Arteriovenous fistula	Post-biopsy; focal colour mosaic with perivascular tissue vibration, a high-velocity low-resistance feeding artery and arterialised draining vein
Kinking or extrinsic compression	Velocity change at a fixed point, often positional; consider a compressing collection

Collections — categorised by timing

The timing of a collection is often more informative than its appearance, because most collections look broadly similar:

Collection	Typical timing	Features
Haematoma	Immediate to early	Initially echogenic, becoming complex then hypoechoic; usually decreases over time
Urinoma (renal graft)	Days to weeks	Anechoic, perigraft or near the ureteric implantation; associated with ureteric leak; may increase rapidly
Biloma (liver graft)	Days to weeks	Anechoic or minimally complex, perihepatic or intrahepatic; associated with biliary leak and often with arterial compromise

Collection	Typical timing	Features
Lymphocele (renal graft)	Weeks to months	Anechoic, often **septated**, perigraft; may **compress the ureter or the vessels**, causing hydronephrosis or a rising RI
Abscess	Any time	Complex, thick-walled, debris, possible gas, peripheral hyperemia
Seroma	Early to intermediate	Simple, usually asymptomatic

The essential point: the appearance alone rarely distinguishes them, and **aspiration under ultrasound guidance frequently does** (§9.5). Report the size, location, and — decisively — the **relationship to the vessels, ureter, and graft**, because compression is what makes a collection clinically significant rather than incidental.

Rejection

There is no specific sonographic sign of rejection. This deserves stating unambiguously, because it is the question the requesting team most wants answered and the one ultrasound cannot answer.

Findings **associated** with rejection — none of them specific:

- Graft enlargement and swelling
- Increased cortical echogenicity and **loss of corticomedullary differentiation** (renal)
- **Urothelial and pelvic wall thickening** (renal)
- Prominent hypoechoic pyramids (renal)
- **Elevated resistive index**, particularly a rising trend
- Reduced or heterogeneous perfusion

Every one of these also occurs in acute tubular necrosis, drug toxicity, infection, obstruction, and compression.

Biopsy makes the diagnosis. Ultrasound's contributions are to **exclude the alternatives** — obstruction, a compressing collection, vascular occlusion — which is genuinely valuable, and to **guide the biopsy** that will settle it.

Infection and malignancy

Infection — graft pyelonephritis, abscess, and opportunistic infection in an immunosuppressed patient. Cytomegalovirus and fungal disease may produce nonspecific findings.

Post-transplant lymphoproliferative disorder — a lymphoid proliferation driven by immunosuppression and Epstein–Barr virus, appearing as hypoechoic masses in the graft, at the hilum, in nodes, in bowel, or elsewhere in the abdomen. It is an important diagnosis in this population and should be considered whenever new hypoechoic masses appear.

Recurrent and de novo malignancy, with a raised overall incidence under long-term immunosuppression.

The reporting principle for all transplant work

Compare with the baseline and prior studies; describe findings rather than assigning a diagnosis that requires histology; state which vessels were and were not adequately interrogated; and communicate vascular occlusion immediately rather than by report.

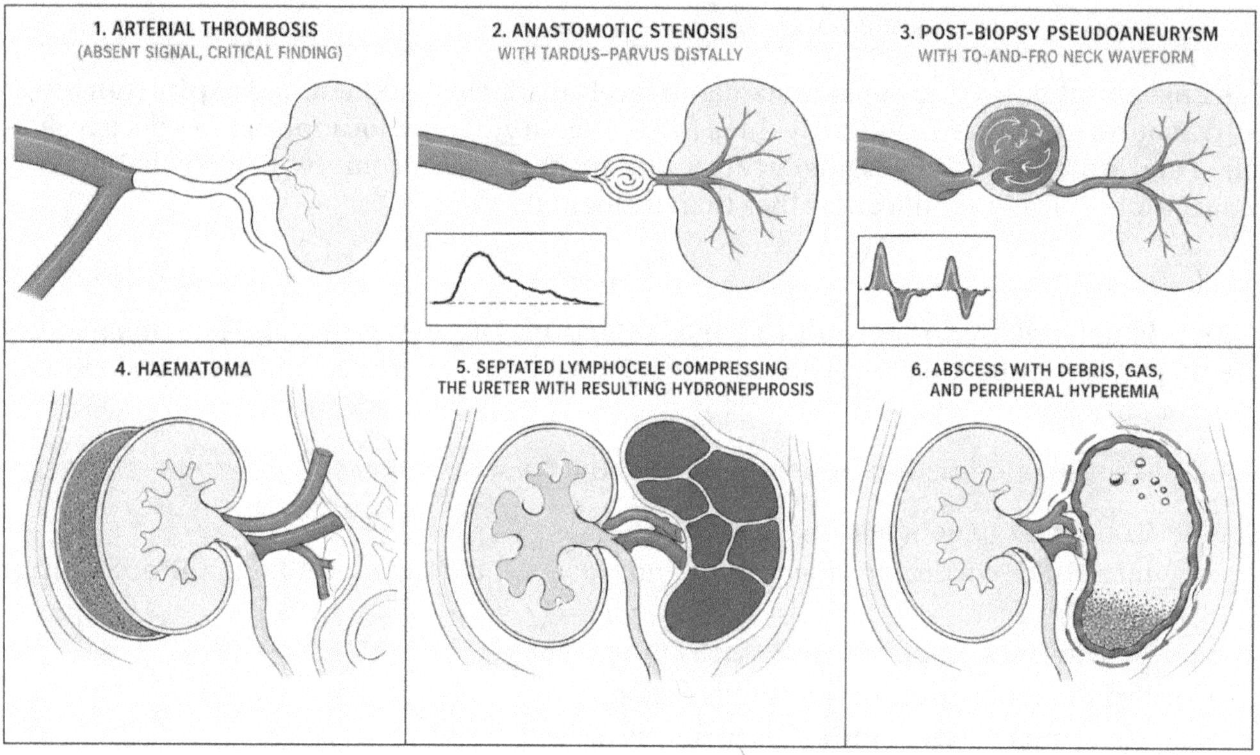

Key Points

1. Ultrasound contrast is a pure blood-pool agent — bubbles do not cross the endothelium. That is why it images perfusion in real time and why washout timing is measurable.
2. It is not nephrotoxic. This is the basis of its use in renal impairment, including complex renal cyst characterization and transplant assessment.
3. Small cannulae and forceful injection destroy microbubbles. A "failed" contrast study is frequently an administration problem.
4. Start the timer at injection, not at the appearance of enhancement. The timing is the diagnosis.
5. Set the entire study up before injecting. The arterial phase lasts seconds and cannot be repeated without another bolus.
6. Imaging at conventional mechanical index destroys the bubbles you are trying to image.
7. CEUS interrogates one plane per bolus. It characterizes; it does not stage.
8. Confirm that the result of a biopsy will change management before accepting its risk.

9. Colour Doppler over the intended needle path, every time.
10. The intercostal neurovascular bundle runs along the inferior rib margin, so pass just above the superior margin of the lower rib.
11. Traverse normal parenchyma in liver and kidney biopsy — the tract tamponades better than a direct subcapsular puncture.
12. Know your device's throw length and clear the far end of it before firing.
13. Sample the enhancing periphery, not the necrotic centre. CEUS can identify the viable component immediately beforehand.
14. A collection containing solid debris will not drain through a percutaneous catheter. Under-sized catheters are the commonest cause of failed drainage.
15. Needle conspicuity is a specular reflection problem. A shallow approach is the single most effective fix; beam steering is the second.
16. Out-of-plane, a bright dot may be the shaft rather than the tip, and the needle may be deeper than you think. Track the tip; never assume.
17. An elevated transplant resistive index is non-specific and does not diagnose rejection. The trend across serial studies is what carries information.
18. Reversed diastolic arterial flow with absent venous flow in a renal graft is near-specific for renal vein thrombosis.
19. The transplanted liver's biliary tree depends entirely on the hepatic artery. Hepatic artery thrombosis causes biliary necrosis and is a critical finding.
20. There is no specific sonographic sign of rejection. Report the findings, exclude the alternatives, guide the biopsy — and do not write "rejection."

Registry Check

1. Ultrasound contrast agents differ fundamentally from iodinated CT contrast in that microbubbles:

A. Are excreted by the kidneys **B.** Remain entirely within the vascular space and do not diffuse into the interstitium **C.** Accumulate in the extracellular space over several minutes **D.** Require a delay before imaging

> **Answer: B.** Microbubbles are too large to cross the vascular endothelium, making ultrasound contrast a pure blood-pool agent that reflects perfusion alone. CT and MR agents diffuse into the extracellular space, so their enhancement mixes perfusion with interstitial distribution. The gas is exhaled and there is no renal excretion or nephrotoxicity.

2. A contrast study shows brief bright enhancement followed by rapid loss of signal throughout the imaged region. The most likely cause is:

A. Inadequate contrast dose **B.** Mechanical index set too high, destroying the microbubbles **C.** Portal vein thrombosis **D.** A malfunctioning cannula

> **Answer: B.** Bubbles undergo inertial destruction at high acoustic pressure, producing a bright transient signal followed by loss of contrast. Contrast imaging

requires low MI to allow non-linear oscillation without destruction, and imaging at conventional B-mode settings is a common cause of a failed study.

3. During an intercostal biopsy approach, the needle should pass:

A. Along the inferior margin of the upper rib **B.** Just above the superior margin of the lower rib **C.** Through the centre of the intercostal space **D.** Directly over a rib

Answer: B. The intercostal neurovascular bundle runs along the inferior margin of each rib, so the safe path is immediately superior to the lower rib of the space, keeping the needle away from the bundle above.

4. In an out-of-plane guided procedure, a bright dot is seen within the target. The correct interpretation is:

A. The needle tip is at that location **B.** The dot may represent the shaft crossing the plane, and the tip may be deeper **C.** The needle has passed beyond the target **D.** The needle is not in the imaging plane

Answer: B. Out-of-plane technique produces a single dot wherever the needle crosses the imaging plane, and that dot cannot distinguish shaft from tip. The tip may lie considerably deeper. Tracking the tip by advancing the probe ahead of the needle, or confirming with hydro-localisation, is required.

5. The most effective single measure for improving needle visibility at a steep angle of approach is:

A. Increasing overall gain **B.** Using a lower-frequency transducer **C.** Beam steering toward the needle **D.** Increasing the dynamic range

Answer: C. Needle conspicuity is a specular reflection problem — at steep angles the reflected energy travels away from the transducer. Beam steering directs the transmit beam to strike the needle more perpendicularly and restores conspicuity. A shallower approach angle is the most effective measure overall, but where a steep angle is unavoidable, steering is the answer.

6. A renal transplant shows an intrarenal resistive index of 0.85. This finding indicates:

A. Acute rejection **B.** Acute tubular necrosis **C.** A non-specific elevation with many possible causes, requiring correlation with the trend and exclusion of obstruction and compression **D.** Renal artery stenosis

Answer: C. Elevated RI occurs in rejection, acute tubular necrosis, obstruction, extrinsic compression by a collection, drug toxicity, venous thrombosis, and from systemic factors. It is not diagnostic of any of them. Its value lies in serial trend, and the sonographer's contribution is to exclude the mechanical causes.

7. A renal transplant demonstrates reversed diastolic arterial flow with no detectable venous signal. This combination most specifically suggests:

A. Acute rejection **B.** Renal vein thrombosis **C.** Transplant renal artery stenosis **D.** Lymphocele compression

> **Answer: B.** Reversed diastolic arterial flow with absent venous flow is the near-specific sonographic combination of renal vein thrombosis. Arterial stenosis produces tardus–parvus distally rather than diastolic reversal, and compression typically elevates RI without reversing diastolic flow unless very severe.

8. Hepatic artery thrombosis after liver transplantation is particularly catastrophic because:

A. The parenchyma has no alternative blood supply **B.** The biliary tree is supplied exclusively by the hepatic artery and undergoes ischaemic necrosis **C.** It always causes portal vein thrombosis **D.** It cannot be detected sonographically

> **Answer: B.** Hepatic parenchyma retains portal inflow, but the biliary epithelium depends entirely on arterial supply. Arterial occlusion therefore produces biliary ischaemia and necrosis, with leaks, ischaemic cholangiopathy, abscess, and frequently graft loss. It is a critical finding requiring immediate communication and confirmation by CEUS or CT angiography.

Chapter Notes for the Editorial Pass

Verification queue. In priority order: **contrast agent contraindications, licensed indications, and dosing** (§9.1) — these differ between agents and between regulatory jurisdictions, and a single generic statement would be wrong somewhere; **periprocedural coagulation thresholds and anticoagulant management stratified by bleeding risk** (§9.4), which directly govern whether a procedure proceeds; **hepatic CEUS phase timings** (§9.2), which underpin the Chapter 4 washout discriminator; **normal hepatic artery RI and acceleration time in transplants, and stenosis criteria** (§9.8); **portal vein anastomotic stenosis velocity ratio criteria** (§9.8); **normal transplant renal RI range and the significance of serial change** (§9.7); **incidence of serious adverse reactions to contrast and observation-period recommendations** (§9.1); and **current society guidance on CEUS in trauma** (§9.3).

Off-label note. §9.1 states that much clinical CEUS use is off-label relative to licensed indications. This is jurisdiction-dependent and should be checked against the intended market before publication, since the consent implications differ.

Figure count: 5 Lane A, 2 Lane B. `fig-9-3` deliberately commissions the CEUS phase sequence that the Chapter 4 editorial notes identified as a gap — one acquisition serving two chapters, and the cross-reference should be set at layout so it is not duplicated. `fig-9-6` is the transplant waveform set, which should be sourced from a single transplant unit for consistency of annotation.

Scope note. Endoscopic ultrasound is referred to repeatedly across Chapters 5, 6, and 9 as the onward pathway, but is nowhere described. If the book is to cover it, this chapter is the natural home and it would add roughly a section; if not, the references should be checked at layout to ensure they read as signposts to another service rather than to an absent section of this book.

Word count: approximately 10,300 excluding image prompt blocks, learning objectives, registry questions, and these notes.

Chapter 10: Breast Sonography

Learning Objectives

On completing this chapter you should be able to:

1. Identify the zonal architecture of the breast and explain why most pathology arises in the terminal ductal lobular unit.
2. Perform a breast protocol using radial and antiradial planes, with appropriate positioning and pressure.
3. Localize a lesion unambiguously using side, clock position, distance from nipple, depth, and probe orientation.
4. Apply the standardized descriptor set — shape, orientation, margin, echo pattern, posterior features — and explain why one suspicious feature outweighs several benign ones.
5. Recognize simple cysts, fibroadenoma, and fat necrosis, and state where each can mimic malignancy.
6. Identify the sonographic features of malignancy and name the histological types that violate them.
7. Assess axillary nodes, recognizing focal eccentric cortical thickening as an early sign.
8. Evaluate the male breast, implants, and the postoperative breast.
9. Perform breast intervention safely, keeping the needle parallel to the chest wall, and assess radiologic–pathologic concordance.
10. Position ultrasound correctly relative to mammography and MRI.

A Modality Working Inside a System

Breast sonography is rarely a standalone examination. It sits inside **triple assessment** — clinical examination, imaging, and pathology — and its findings are read alongside a mammogram, sometimes an MRI, and often a biopsy result that must be reconciled with them.

That has two consequences that shape this whole chapter.

Standardized language is mandatory. A lesion described in idiosyncratic terms cannot be matched to a mammographic finding, cannot be compared with a prior study, and cannot be relocated for biopsy. The descriptor set in §10.3 and the localization convention in §10.2 are not stylistic preferences; they are the interface between you and everyone else who touches the case.

Concordance is a formal step, not an impression. When a biopsy result comes back, someone must ask whether the pathology explains the imaging. If it does not, the workup continues. This is covered in §10.8 and it is one of the genuine safety mechanisms of breast practice.

10.1 Anatomy and Zonal Architecture

Structure

The breast is a modified apocrine gland lying on the anterior chest wall, extending roughly from the second to the sixth ribs and from the sternal edge to the mid-axillary line, with the **axillary tail (of Spence)** projecting superolaterally toward the axilla.

It contains **15–20 lobes**, each drained by a lactiferous duct converging on the nipple. Each lobe subdivides into lobules, and the functional unit is the **terminal ductal lobular unit (TDLU)** — the terminal duct together with its cluster of acini.

The TDLU is where almost all breast pathology originates, benign and malignant alike: fibrocystic change, fibroadenoma, and the great majority of carcinomas. This is not an anatomical footnote — it is the reason **radial scanning along the ductal axis** is a productive technique (§10.2), and it explains why disease so often extends along duct lines.

The zones, superficial to deep

The breast is imaged as a layered structure, and naming the layer a lesion occupies is part of describing it:

Layer	Sonographic appearance
Skin	Thin echogenic band, a few millimetres
Premammary (subcutaneous) fat zone	Hypoechoic fat lobules separated by echogenic septa
Mammary zone	The fibroglandular tissue — **echogenic** background containing ducts, TDLUs, and hypoechoic fat interspersed
Retromammary fat zone	A thin hypoechoic layer
Pectoralis major	Hypoechoic muscle with echogenic fascial planes and internal striations
Ribs and intercostal muscles	Ribs shadow; costal cartilage is hypoechoic and can mimic a mass
Pleura	The bright line beyond which the needle must never go

Cooper's ligaments are fibrous septa running from the deep fascia through the parenchyma to the skin, appearing as thin echogenic lines. They matter clinically: **malignant infiltration retracts them**, producing the skin dimpling seen on examination, and their straightening or retraction on ultrasound is an associated feature of malignancy.

Costal cartilage deserves specific mention as a recurrent pseudolesion — hypoechoic, oval, and located deep, it is identified by its segmental arrangement in a line and its continuity with the rib.

The nipple–areolar complex

Dense fibrous tissue beneath the nipple produces **marked posterior shadowing**, and the retroareolar region is consequently one of the hardest areas to assess — and a common site for papillomas and for carcinoma.

Technique to see behind the nipple: angle the transducer from the periphery of the areola beneath the nipple rather than scanning directly through it; use the "rolled nipple" or peripheral compression technique; and use generous gel with light pressure. This region must be deliberately worked at, not scanned past.

Vascular and lymphatic anatomy

Arterial supply comes from the internal mammary (internal thoracic) artery medially, the lateral thoracic artery laterally, and intercostal perforators.

Lymphatic drainage is predominantly to the **axilla**, which is why axillary assessment is part of every diagnostic breast examination (§10.6). Axillary nodes are described by level relative to pectoralis minor: **level I** lateral to it, **level II** behind it, **level III** medial to it. Additional pathways drain to the **internal mammary chain**, the **supraclavicular** nodes, and the **interpectoral (Rotter's)** nodes.

Normal variation

Age and hormonal state change the background dramatically. Young breasts are densely fibroglandular and echogenic; with age, progressive fatty replacement produces a predominantly hypoechoic background. **A hypoechoic mass is far more conspicuous against fatty tissue than against dense fibroglandular tissue**, and this is one reason ultrasound adds most in dense breasts (§10.9).

Lactation produces glandular hypertrophy, dilated ducts, and a diffusely hypoechoic, heterogeneous background that makes lesion detection harder.

Accessory breast tissue occurs anywhere along the embryonic milk line, most often in the axilla, and can develop the same pathology as the breast proper.

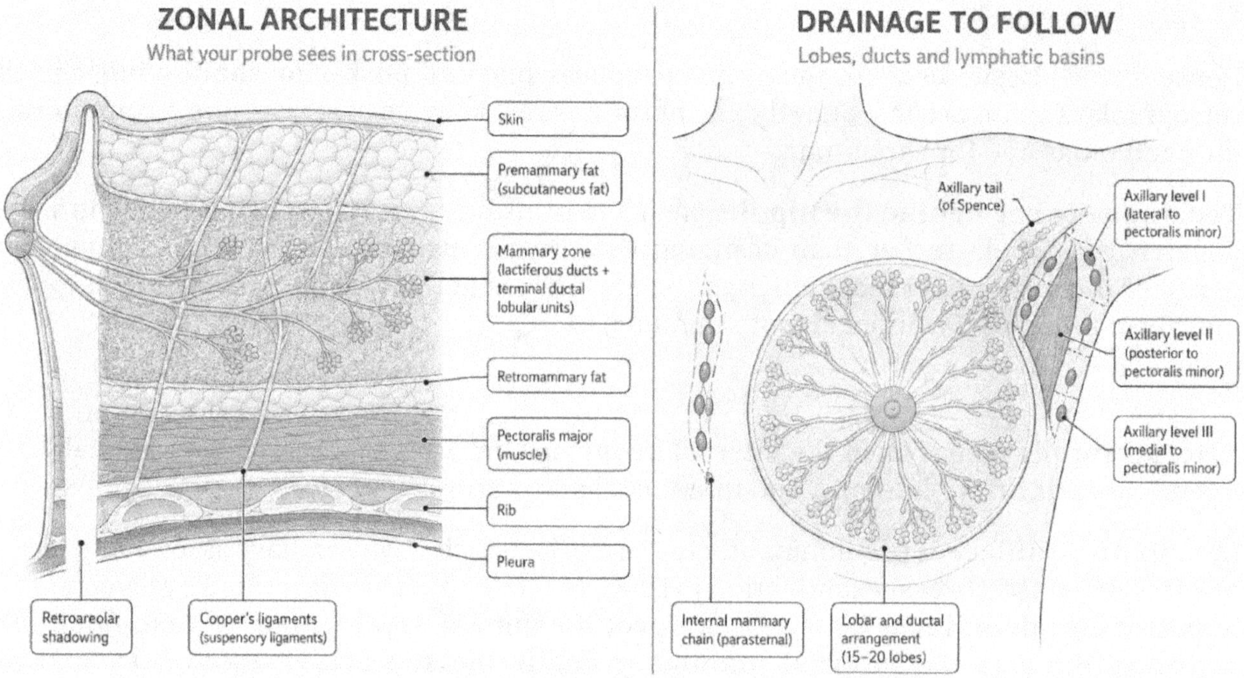

10.2 Scanning Protocol, Documentation, and Lesion Localization

Equipment and settings

A high-frequency linear transducer is mandatory — the highest frequency that penetrates to the chest wall. Breast work is superficial work, and imaging at abdominal frequencies is not breast sonography. [VERIFY: current recommended minimum transducer frequency for diagnostic breast ultrasound]

Focal zone at the depth of interest, moved as you change depth. A single focal zone at the lesion gives the best lateral resolution.

Light pressure. Excessive compression flattens lesions, obliterates cysts, distorts shape and orientation — which are diagnostic features — and can push a lesion out of the imaging plane. Where deeper tissue in a large breast needs to be reached, use **graded** compression deliberately and note that measurements taken under compression are not comparable with uncompressed ones.

Compounding and harmonics — the Chapter 2 §2.4 rules apply directly here. **Turn compounding off** when assessing posterior features, because it suppresses both shadowing and enhancement, and those are diagnostic descriptors. Check questionable low-level internal echoes in a possible cyst on **fundamental** as well as harmonics.

Positioning

The aim is to **flatten the breast tissue** so that it lies in a thin, even layer over the chest wall, reducing the depth to be imaged and minimizing shadowing.

- **Supine with the ipsilateral arm above the head** for the medial quadrants
- **Contralateral posterior oblique** — the patient rolled partly onto the opposite side, arm above head — for the **lateral quadrants**, which otherwise fall laterally and become thick
- Adjust as needed for large or pendulous breasts

Scanning planes

Two systems are used, and breast practice favours the first:

Radial and antiradial. Radial planes run along the ductal axis, outward from the nipple like spokes; **antiradial** planes are perpendicular to them. Because ducts and the disease that travels along them are aligned this way, radial/antiradial imaging demonstrates **ductal extension, intraductal lesions, and the true long axis of a lesion** better than a rectilinear system.

Transverse and sagittal. Simpler and adequate for a survey, and still widely used.

Whichever is used, **document the orientation** in the image annotation (§ below), because a measurement without a plane is not reproducible.

Coverage

Targeted examination — for a palpable lump, a mammographic finding, or focal symptoms. **Ask the patient to point to the area of concern with one finger and scan there first**, then extend outward. This exploits ultrasound's unique ability to correlate imaging directly with symptoms, and it is the same principle as in Chapter 6 §6.8.

Whole-breast survey — overlapping sweeps covering all quadrants, the retroareolar region, and the axillary tail, plus the axilla.

Both breasts where the clinical question requires comparison, and the **axilla** in any diagnostic examination for a suspicious finding.

The localization convention

This is the most practically important part of the section. A lesion must be described so that another operator, on another day, can find exactly the same lesion.

Five elements, always:

1. **Side** — right or left
2. **Clock position** — 1 to 12 o'clock, as viewed facing the patient
3. **Distance from the nipple** — in centimetres, measured from the edge of the areola or from the nipple per local convention (state which)
4. **Depth** — anterior, middle, or posterior third of the breast thickness
5. **Probe orientation** at the time of the image — radial/antiradial or transverse/longitudinal

The mirror-image trap: clock positions are mirrored between the breasts. **3 o'clock is lateral on the right breast and medial on the left.** Confusing this sends a surgeon to the wrong quadrant, and it is the commonest localization error.

Also document: lesion measurements in **three dimensions**, images **with and without calipers** (calipers obscure the margin, which is a diagnostic feature), at least **two orthogonal planes**, and a **colour Doppler** image.

Record the technical limitations — a very dense breast, an inaccessible retroareolar region, an implant restricting access — explicitly (Chapter 1 §1.5).

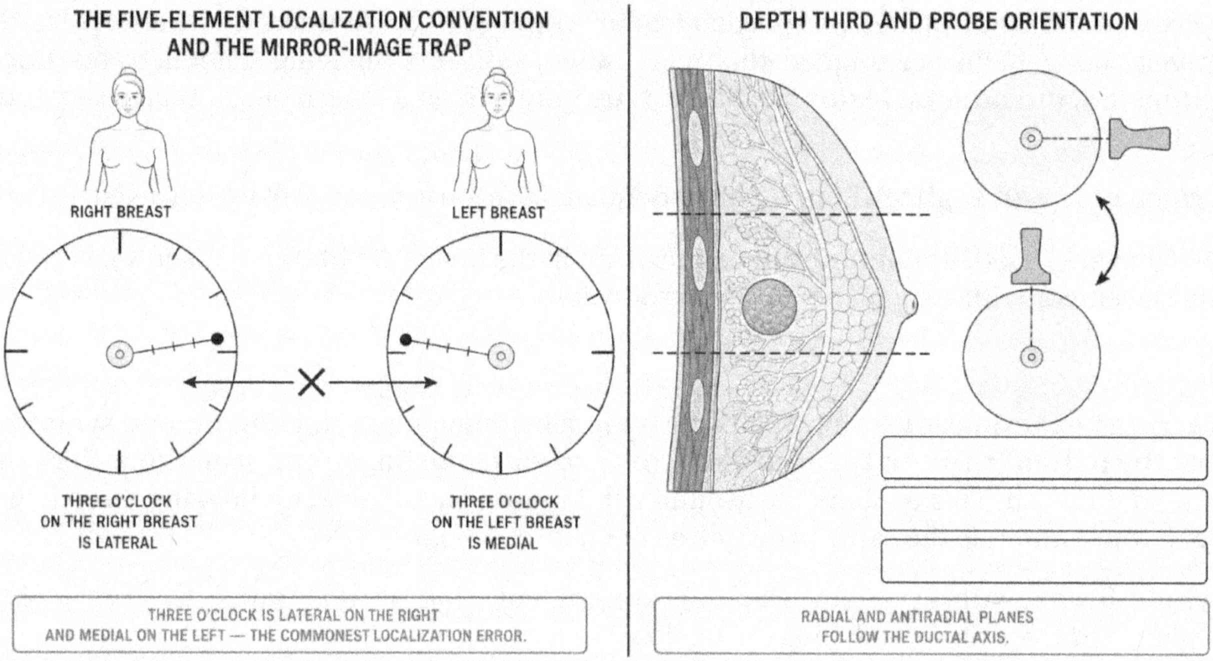

10.3 Lesion Characterization and Standardized Descriptors

Why a fixed lexicon

Breast reporting uses a **standardized descriptor lexicon** with defined terms and a numbered **assessment category** that carries an explicit management recommendation. The system exists so that "probably benign" means the same interval follow-up in every department, and so that audit is possible.

The categories, their definitions, and the management attached to each are specified by the current edition of the lexicon and are periodically revised. They must be taken from that document rather than from memory or a textbook. [VERIFY: current edition of the breast imaging lexicon and assessment categories, their definitions, and the management recommendation attached to each]

What follows is the descriptor set itself — the observations from which the category is derived.

Shape

Oval (including gently lobulated with two or three smooth undulations), **round**, or **irregular**.

Irregular shape is suspicious. Round is less reassuring than oval — many circumscribed carcinomas are round.

Orientation — the ultrasound-specific feature

Parallel ("wider than tall") — the long axis lies parallel to the skin. **Not parallel** ("taller than wide") — the long axis is perpendicular to the skin.

Not-parallel orientation is suspicious, because it indicates growth **across** the normal tissue planes rather than along them. This descriptor has no mammographic equivalent and is one of ultrasound's genuine contributions to lesion assessment.

Caveat: very small lesions may appear not-parallel without significance, and a lesion within a duct may follow the duct's own orientation.

Margin

Circumscribed — a sharp, abrupt transition to surrounding tissue for the entire perimeter. **The whole perimeter must qualify**; a lesion that is circumscribed for most of its border and indistinct in one segment is **not circumscribed.**

Not circumscribed, subdivided into:

- **Indistinct** — no clear demarcation
- **Angular** — sharp corners, often acute
- **Microlobulated** — many small undulations, distinct from the two or three gentle lobulations of a fibroadenoma
- **Spiculated** — radiating lines from the margin

Margin is the single most important descriptor, and it is why an image without calipers must always be acquired — calipers sit exactly where the margin needs to be assessed.

Echo pattern

Anechoic, **hypoechoic**, **isoechoic**, **hyperechoic**, **complex cystic and solid**, or **heterogeneous**.

Marked hypoechogenicity relative to fat is suspicious. **Hyperechogenicity** relative to fat is uncommon and usually — though not invariably — benign.

Posterior acoustic features

No posterior features, enhancement, shadowing, or a **combined pattern**.

Shadowing suggests a desmoplastic reaction and is suspicious. **Enhancement** is typical of cysts but also occurs behind some malignancies, notably mucinous and highly cellular tumours — so enhancement is supportive of a cyst only when every other cyst criterion is also met.

Both descriptors are abolished by spatial compounding. Turn it off before assessing them (Chapter 2 §2.4).

Calcifications

Ultrasound is **poor at detecting microcalcifications** — mammography is far superior, and this is one of the clearest divisions of labour between the modalities. Calcifications may be described as within a mass, outside a mass, or intraductal, but **absence on ultrasound means nothing**, and a mammographic calcification cluster is not excluded by a normal ultrasound.

Associated features

Architectural distortion, **duct changes** (dilatation or an intraductal mass), **skin thickening or retraction**, **nipple retraction**, **oedema**, **Cooper's ligament straightening or retraction**, and **vascularity** — increased, disorganised, or penetrating rather than displaced.

Elastography (Chapter 2 §2.10) adds specificity as an adjunct: malignant lesions are typically stiffer. It refines, but does not override, the B-mode descriptors, and the strain ratio thresholds are platform-dependent. [VERIFY: current evidence and platform-specific thresholds for breast elastography]

The governing rule

> **One suspicious feature outweighs several benign ones.**

A lesion that is oval, parallel, and homogeneous but has one **spiculated segment of margin** is a suspicious lesion. The descriptors are not scored and averaged. This is the single most important interpretive principle in the chapter.

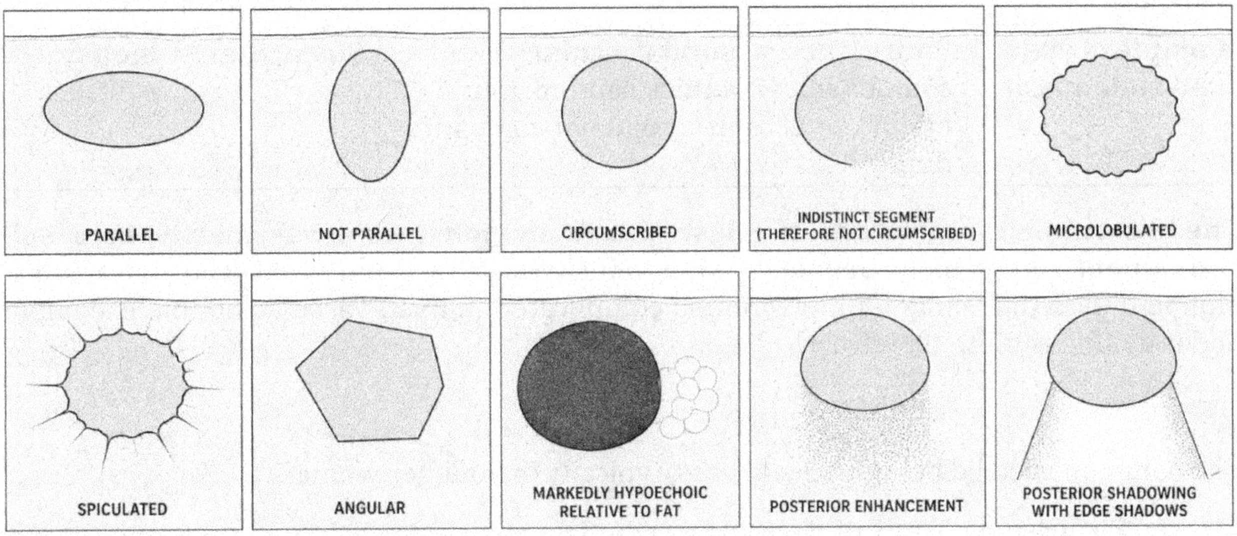

10.4 Benign Findings: Cysts, Fibroadenoma, Fat Necrosis

Simple cyst

Criteria — all must be met: anechoic, circumscribed, oval or round, imperceptible thin wall, **posterior enhancement**, and **no internal vascularity**. Edge refractive shadows are commonly present.

A lesion meeting all criteria is essentially always benign and requires no intervention unless symptomatic.

Before calling a cyst simple, apply the Chapter 2 rules: **compounding off** (it suppresses the enhancement you are relying on) and **check on fundamental** (harmonics suppress genuine low-level internal echoes). This matters more here than almost anywhere, because the entire management decision rests on whether internal content is present.

The cystic spectrum

Category	Findings	Significance
Simple cyst	All criteria met	Benign
Clustered microcysts	A cluster of tiny anechoic foci separated by thin (under about 0.5 mm) septations, **no solid component**	Almost always benign
Complicated cyst	Low-level internal echoes, debris, or a fluid–fluid level; **no solid vascular component**; may show mobile echoes on repositioning	Usually benign; aspiration if symptomatic or diagnostically uncertain

Category	Findings	Significance
Complex cystic and solid mass	Both cystic and **solid vascular** components — a thick septum, mural nodule, or eccentric solid portion with flow	**Suspicious — biopsy**

The discriminator between the last two is demonstrable vascularity in a solid component. Apply colour Doppler at a low velocity scale to any internal echogenic material. Mobile debris that shifts with position is complicated; a fixed vascular nodule is complex, and is a different lesion entirely.

Fibroadenoma

The commonest solid benign breast mass, typically in younger women.

Classic features: oval, parallel, circumscribed, homogeneously **hypoechoic**, with at most **two or three gentle lobulations**, no posterior features or mild enhancement, and minimal internal vascularity.

They may grow, may involute and calcify with age (producing the coarse calcification recognizable on mammography), and are frequently multiple and bilateral.

The important caveat: these are also the features of some circumscribed carcinomas, particularly mucinous, medullary, and papillary types (§10.5). A circumscribed oval parallel mass is **probably** a fibroadenoma, and the management pathway for such lesions — short-interval follow-up or biopsy — is defined by the assessment category system, not by assumption.

Phyllodes tumour cannot be reliably distinguished from fibroadenoma sonographically. Features raising the possibility include **larger size, rapid growth, heterogeneity, and internal cystic clefts**. Because phyllodes tumours require wide excision and can recur or behave malignantly, a large or rapidly enlarging "fibroadenoma" warrants biopsy rather than reassurance.

Juvenile and giant fibroadenomas occur in adolescents and can be very large.

Fat necrosis

The great mimic, and the reason the history is decisive.

It follows **trauma, surgery, biopsy, radiotherapy, or reconstruction** — including seat-belt injury — and its appearance is extremely variable and evolves over time:

- **Oil cyst** — a round anechoic or complex mass, sometimes with mural calcification. On mammography a radiolucent oil cyst is **effectively diagnostic**, which is why correlation resolves this lesion so efficiently
- **Echogenic mass** or focal echogenic area
- **Irregular hypoechoic mass with posterior shadowing** — indistinguishable from carcinoma on ultrasound alone

- **Architectural distortion**
- Evolving to a calcified, stable scar

The approach: establish the history and the site of prior injury or surgery; correlate with mammography, which frequently settles it; and where the appearance is suspicious and the history does not clearly explain it, **biopsy**. Attributing a suspicious mass to fat necrosis on history alone, without imaging correlation, is a recognised route to a delayed cancer diagnosis.

Other benign entities

Fibrocystic change — the commonest of all findings: cysts, fibrosis, and heterogeneous parenchyma, generally a background rather than a lesion.

Lipoma — circumscribed, isoechoic or mildly hyperechoic, compressible, with fine internal echogenic striations.

Hamartoma — a circumscribed mass containing fat and fibroglandular tissue, producing the "breast within a breast" appearance.

Galactocele — in a lactating or recently lactating woman; may show a **fat–fluid level**.

Mastitis and abscess — lactational or non-lactational (including periductal mastitis in smokers). Abscess appears as a complex collection with debris, an irregular wall, peripheral hyperemia and no internal flow. **Inflammatory carcinoma must be considered in any "mastitis" that does not resolve with treatment** (§10.5).

Duct ectasia — dilated retroareolar ducts, often with inspissated content.

Intraductal papilloma — a solid intraductal mass with a **vascular stalk** within a dilated duct, presenting with **nipple discharge**, often bloody. It requires excision because it may harbour atypia or malignancy, and because sampling error is a real risk.

Granulomatous mastitis, diabetic mastopathy, and pseudoangiomatous stromal hyperplasia (PASH) — benign entities that can mimic malignancy and usually require biopsy.

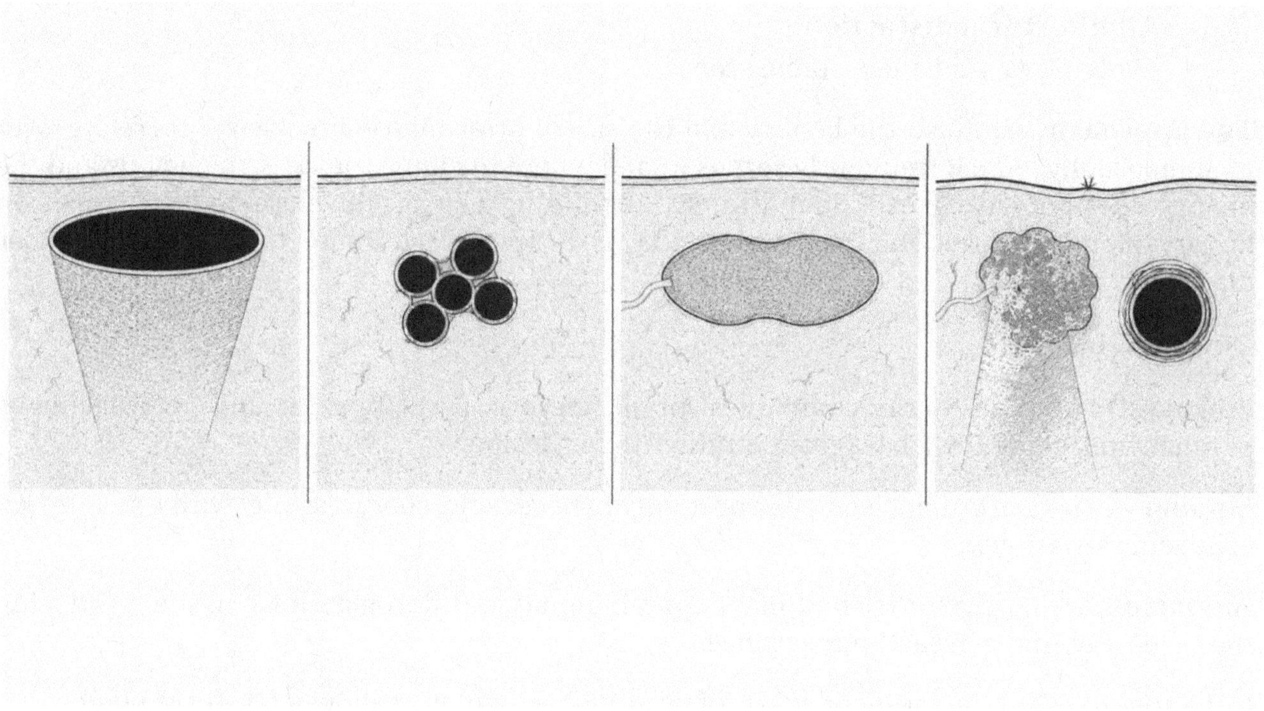

10.5 Malignant Features and Growth Patterns

The suspicious feature set

Drawn from §10.3 and assembled here:

Primary features:

- **Irregular shape**
- **Not-parallel orientation** (taller than wide)
- **Non-circumscribed margin** — spiculated, angular, microlobulated, or indistinct
- **Marked hypoechogenicity**
- **Posterior acoustic shadowing**
- **Echogenic halo or rim** surrounding the lesion

Associated features:

- **Architectural distortion** and disruption of tissue planes
- **Duct extension** — the lesion tracking along a duct toward the nipple
- **Skin thickening, retraction, or invasion**
- **Nipple retraction**
- **Cooper's ligament straightening or retraction**
- **Increased, disorganised, or penetrating internal vascularity**
- **Increased stiffness** on elastography
- **Associated microcalcifications** — insensitive on ultrasound, but significant when seen

Restate the governing rule: one suspicious feature is enough. A well-behaved lesion with a single spiculated margin segment is a suspicious lesion.

The histological types and how they behave

Invasive ductal carcinoma of no special type — much the commonest, and the source of the classic description: an irregular, markedly hypoechoic, non-circumscribed, taller-than-wide mass with posterior shadowing and an echogenic halo.

Invasive lobular carcinoma — the important exception. It grows by **single-file infiltration** through tissue rather than forming a discrete mass, so it may produce only **subtle architectural distortion or shadowing without a definable lesion**, or may be sonographically occult. It is also **frequently underestimated in extent** and is more often multifocal and bilateral. **MRI is substantially better for extent in lobular carcinoma**, and this is one of the clearest indications for it (§10.9).

Ductal carcinoma in situ — often **sonographically occult**. When visible, it may appear as non-mass hypoechoic areas, ductal changes, or associated microcalcifications. **Mammography is the modality for DCIS**, principally through calcification detection, and a normal ultrasound does not address it.

Circumscribed malignancies — mucinous (colloid), medullary, and papillary carcinomas can be oval, circumscribed, and even show posterior enhancement, closely mimicking a fibroadenoma or a complicated cyst. **Circumscribed does not mean benign**, and this is why the assessment category system routes even probably-benign solid masses to follow-up or biopsy rather than dismissal.

Inflammatory breast carcinoma — diffuse skin thickening, subcutaneous oedema with dilated lymphatics producing a reticular pattern, diffusely increased parenchymal echogenicity or heterogeneity, and often no discrete mass. It presents as a red, swollen, painful breast and is **routinely mistaken for mastitis**. The rule: **any presumed mastitis failing to resolve on appropriate treatment requires imaging and skin biopsy**.

Paget disease of the nipple, **lymphoma, metastases** (typically circumscribed and multiple), **angiosarcoma** (including post-radiation), and **phyllodes** complete the differential.

Assessing extent

Once malignancy is suspected, the examination changes purpose from detection to **staging**, and specific questions must be answered:

Size — measured in three dimensions. Note that ultrasound tends to underestimate the extent of infiltrative and in-situ disease relative to MRI.

Multifocality (additional lesions in the same quadrant) versus **multicentricity** (lesions in different quadrants) — this affects candidacy for breast-conserving surgery, so the **whole ipsilateral breast must be surveyed**, not just the index lesion.

Contralateral breast survey.

Skin involvement — thickening, retraction, or direct invasion.

Chest wall and pectoralis involvement — assessed by loss of the retromammary fat plane and, dynamically, by **observing whether the lesion moves independently of the pectoralis during respiration or with gentle compression**. This real-time assessment is something only ultrasound offers.

Nipple and retroareolar involvement, and duct extension toward the nipple.

The axilla and other nodal basins (§10.6).

Neoadjuvant therapy

Where chemotherapy precedes surgery, ultrasound is used to measure response — and this creates a specific obligation: **a marker clip must be placed in the lesion before treatment begins**, because a complete response can render the tumour invisible and unlocalizable at surgery (§10.8). Assessing response requires reproducing the prior technique and comparing like with like (Chapter 1 §1.5).

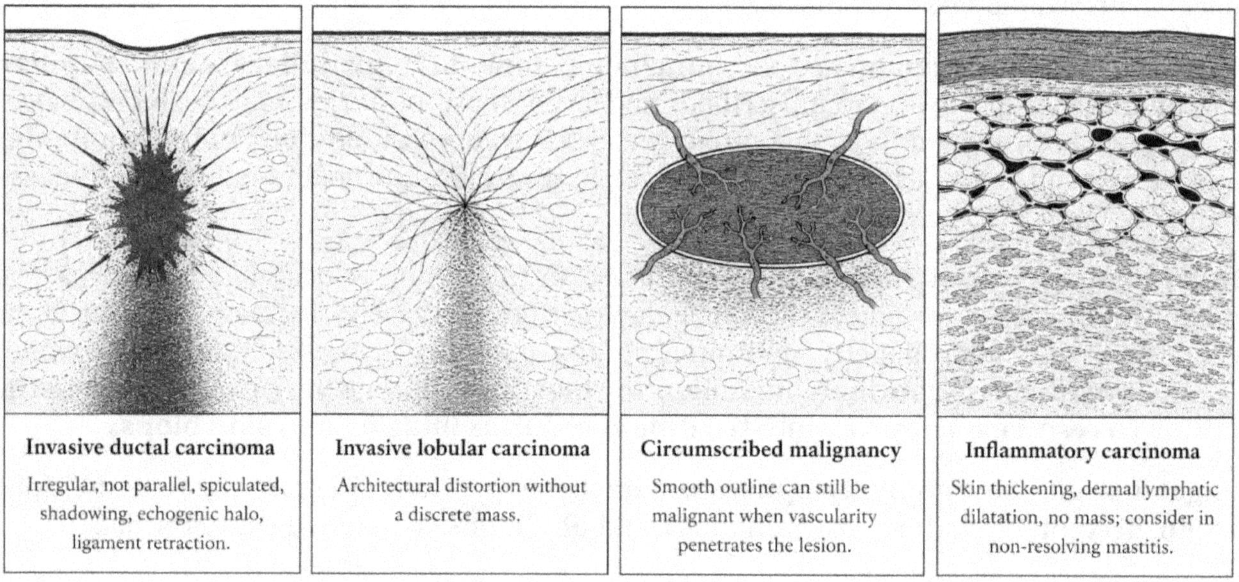

Malignant patterns, including the two that break the rules.

10.6 The Axilla and Nodal Assessment

Why and when

Axillary nodal status is among the strongest determinants of prognosis and of surgical planning in breast cancer. **Axillary assessment is part of every diagnostic breast examination performed for a suspicious finding**, and it is not an optional add-on.

Anatomy of the assessment

Sweep systematically through:

- **Level I** — lateral to pectoralis minor, the commonest site of disease and the most accessible
- **Level II** — deep to pectoralis minor
- **Level III** — medial to pectoralis minor, extending toward the infraclavicular region
- **Interpectoral (Rotter's)** nodes, between the pectoral muscles
- **Supraclavicular fossa**
- **Internal mammary chain**, in the parasternal intercostal spaces — small, easily overlooked, and relevant particularly in medial tumours

The normal node

A normal lymph node has a specific and recognisable architecture:

- **Oval or reniform** shape
- A **thin, uniform, hypoechoic cortex**
- A **central echogenic fatty hilum**, often with a hilar notch
- **Hilar vascularity** — flow entering at the hilum and branching centrally

Nodes vary greatly in size, and **size alone is an unreliable criterion**. A large node with normal architecture is usually reactive; a small node with an effaced hilum is not.

The abnormal node

In descending order of usefulness:

1. Cortical thickening. The earliest and most useful sign. **Focal, eccentric cortical bulging is more suspicious than uniform concentric thickening**, because metastatic deposits arrive in the subcapsular sinus and expand the cortex locally. **This focal eccentric bulge is the finding to look for deliberately**, and it is easy to overlook if you are scanning for enlarged nodes.

Cortical thickness thresholds are used, and they vary between practices and are the subject of ongoing refinement. [VERIFY: current cortical thickness thresholds for suspicious axillary nodes and their reported performance]

2. Loss or effacement of the fatty hilum — as metastatic tissue replaces the node, the hilum becomes compressed, displaced, or invisible. Complete effacement is a strong sign.

3. Rounded shape — loss of the normal oval configuration.

4. Non-hilar (peripheral or capsular) vascularity — flow entering through the capsule rather than the hilum, reflecting neovascularity, and displacement of the normal hilar vessels.

5. Matting, irregular margins, or extracapsular extension — advanced disease.

Differential and pitfalls

Reactive nodes show uniform concentric cortical thickening with a **preserved hilum** and preserved hilar vascularity, and are common in infection, inflammatory skin conditions, recent vaccination in the ipsilateral arm, and after biopsy.

Lymphoma produces markedly hypoechoic nodes, sometimes so hypoechoic as to resemble cysts, often with a preserved though displaced hilum.

Silicone-laden nodes in patients with silicone implants show the "snowstorm" echogenic pattern (§10.7).

Intramammary lymph nodes are normal structures with the same architecture, typically in the upper outer quadrant, and are frequently misreported as masses. The **fatty hilum identifies them**.

Sampling

Suspicious nodes are sampled — **fine-needle aspiration** for cytology or **core biopsy** for histology — and a positive result can change the surgical plan substantially, in many pathways diverting a patient from sentinel node biopsy to axillary dissection or to a targeted approach.

Where a node is biopsied before neoadjuvant therapy, **a marker clip is placed in it**, so that the same node can be retrieved and assessed after treatment. The protocols governing this vary and are evolving. [VERIFY: current pathways for axillary staging, including the role of preoperative ultrasound-guided nodal biopsy and targeted axillary dissection]

Nodal architecture

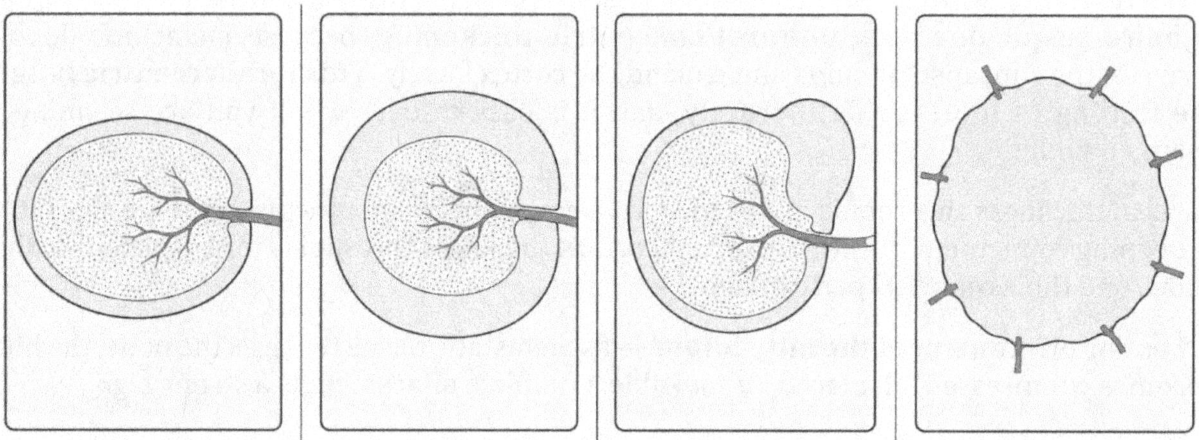

Normal	**Reactive**	**Suspicious early change**	**Advanced involvement**
Thin uniform cortex, fatty hilum, hilar vascularity	Concentric cortical thickening with preserved hilum	Focal eccentric cortical bulge	Effaced hilum, peripheral non-hilar vascularity

10.7 The Male Breast, Implants, and the Postoperative Breast

Gynaecomastia

Proliferation of male ductal and stromal tissue, presenting as a palpable subareolar lump or diffuse enlargement.

Sonographic appearance: hypoechoic fibroglandular tissue in a **subareolar, retroareolar location, radiating outward from the nipple** — described as flame-shaped or triangular with its apex at the nipple. Three patterns are recognised: **nodular** (early), **dendritic** (branching, later), and **diffuse** (glandular, resembling a female breast).

It is frequently **bilateral but asymmetric**, and unilateral presentation is common.

Causes are worth knowing because the imaging prompts the search: physiological (neonatal, pubertal, senescent), **drugs** (a long list including spironolactone, digoxin, cimetidine, antiretrovirals, antipsychotics, and anabolic steroids), **chronic liver disease**, **hypogonadism**, **renal failure**, thyroid disease, and **hormone-secreting tumours — including testicular tumours**.

That last point has a practical consequence: new gynaecomastia in a young adult male warrants consideration of testicular examination and imaging (Chapter 11).

Pseudogynaecomastia is fat alone, without a fibroglandular component.

Male breast carcinoma

Uncommon, but it presents at a more advanced stage, partly because it is not expected.

The single most useful discriminator is position. Gynaecomastia is **centred on and radiates from the nipple**; male breast carcinoma is characteristically **eccentric to the nipple**. Add the standard suspicious descriptors — irregular shape, non-circumscribed margins, not-parallel orientation — plus skin or nipple retraction and axillary nodes.

Any eccentric solid mass in the male breast should be treated as suspicious until proven otherwise, and biopsied rather than followed.

Implants

Types and planes. Saline or silicone filled; single or double lumen; placed **subglandular** (in front of pectoralis major) or **subpectoral/retropectoral** (behind it). Establish which before interpreting anything.

Normal appearance: an anechoic lumen bounded by a thin echogenic shell, with near-field reverberation artefact within the anterior lumen (Chapter 2 §2.8). The body forms a fibrous capsule around the implant.

Radial folds — infoldings of the shell producing echogenic lines extending into the lumen from the periphery — are **normal** and must be distinguished from rupture.

Intracapsular rupture — the shell fails but the fibrous capsule contains the silicone. The sonographic sign is the **"stepladder" appearance**: multiple discontinuous parallel echogenic lines running across the lumen, representing the collapsed shell floating in the silicone. (The MRI equivalent is the "linguine" sign.)

Extracapsular rupture — silicone escapes beyond the fibrous capsule into the surrounding tissue. The sign is the **"snowstorm" appearance**: an intensely echogenic region with dirty posterior shadowing, obscuring underlying detail. Free silicone may form **silicone granulomas**, and may travel to **axillary lymph nodes**, producing the same snowstorm appearance within a node — a specific and easily recognised finding.

Saline implant rupture produces deflation and is usually clinically apparent.

Other implant complications: capsular contracture, seroma, haematoma, infection, and **late peri-implant seroma or mass**, which requires consideration of implant-associated lymphoma and sampling of the fluid rather than simple drainage. [VERIFY: current guidance on evaluation and sampling of late peri-implant seroma, including implant-associated anaplastic large cell lymphoma]

MRI is the reference standard for implant integrity, and ultrasound is a reasonable first-line and follow-up tool. Scanning a patient with implants also requires care: **light pressure, awareness that the implant restricts access to posterior tissue**, and explicit documentation of any region that could not be assessed.

The postoperative and irradiated breast

Expected findings: a **seroma** in the surgical cavity, which shrinks over months; **skin thickening and parenchymal oedema** after radiotherapy, maximal in the first year and gradually improving; **architectural distortion and shadowing at the scar**; and **fat necrosis**, which is common after both surgery and reconstruction (§10.4).

The critical principle: a scar should stabilise or regress; a recurrence grows. Serial comparison is therefore the diagnostic tool, and reproducing the prior technique and site is what makes the comparison valid (Chapter 1 §1.5).

Features suggesting recurrence: a new or enlarging hypoechoic mass at or near the surgical site, **internal vascularity** (a mature scar is avascular), irregular margins, and new nodal abnormality.

Reconstruction — implant-based, or autologous flaps such as TRAM and DIEP — brings its own findings, of which **fat necrosis is by far the commonest**, and requires knowing what was done before interpreting the images.

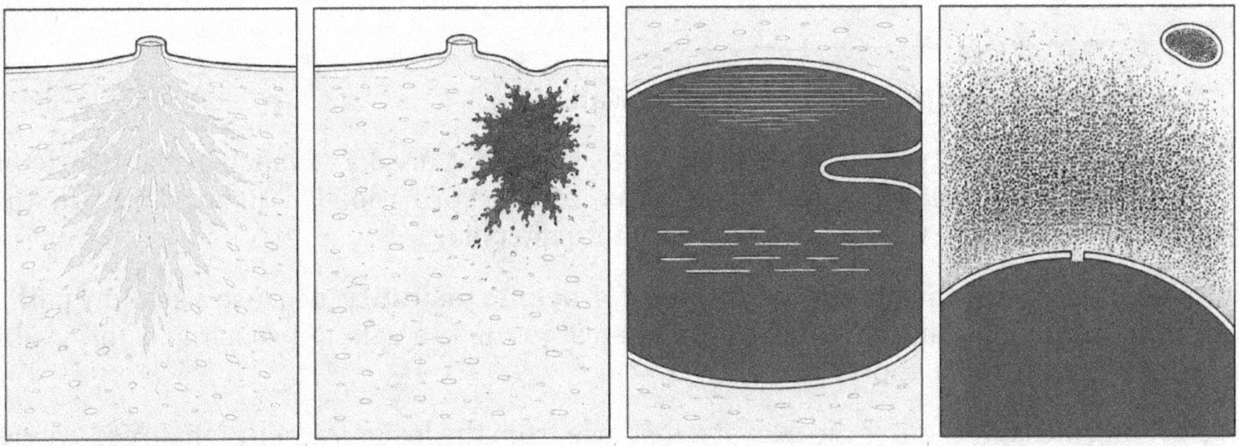

Key sonographic patterns of the male breast and breast implant complications.

10.8 Interventional Breast Procedures

Why ultrasound is the default guidance modality

Any lesion visible on ultrasound should be biopsied under ultrasound. It is faster than stereotactic or MRI guidance, involves no radiation, allows real-time confirmation of needle position within the lesion, is more comfortable, and requires no compression. Stereotactic guidance is reserved for lesions visible only on mammography — principally calcification clusters — and MRI guidance for lesions visible only on MRI.

The general principles of guided intervention — consent, coagulation, sterility, path planning, and needle visualization — are in **Chapter 9 §9.4–9.6** and apply in full. What follows is breast-specific.

The procedures

Fine-needle aspiration — for cyst aspiration (symptomatic or diagnostically uncertain complicated cysts), and for **axillary node sampling**, where cytology is often sufficient to establish metastatic involvement.

Core needle biopsy — the standard for solid masses. Multiple cores are taken, sampling different parts of the lesion, and the **periphery rather than any necrotic centre** (Chapter 9 §9.5).

Vacuum-assisted biopsy — retrieves a larger tissue volume through a single insertion. Used for small lesions where sampling error is a concern, for complex or heterogeneous lesions, for some papillary lesions, and where an earlier core biopsy was discordant or yielded atypia.

Abscess drainage — aspiration or catheter drainage, frequently repeated, with microbiological sampling.

The rule that matters most

Keep the needle parallel to the chest wall.

This is the central safety principle of breast intervention. A needle advancing at a steep angle toward the chest wall risks **pneumothorax**, and a spring-loaded device fired in that orientation carries the throw length forward into the pleura.

It also happens to be the optimal orientation for **needle visibility**, because a shallow path is closer to perpendicular to the beam (Chapter 9 §9.6). The safe approach and the visible approach are the same approach.

Supporting measures: enter the skin at a distance from the lesion rather than directly above it, so the path is long and shallow; use local anaesthetic to raise a wheal and, where useful, to **hydrodissect** the lesion away from the chest wall; and **know the throw length of the device and confirm the far end of the throw is clear** before firing.

Documentation

- **Pre-fire image** showing the needle tip at the edge of the lesion, in plane
- **Post-fire image** showing the needle traversing the lesion — this is the image that proves the lesion was sampled
- Number of cores, needle gauge, approach
- The specimen destination and the clinical details supplied

Marker clips

A **marker clip is placed at the biopsy site** in most core biopsies, and this is not optional in two situations:

1. **Before neoadjuvant chemotherapy**, in both the tumour and any biopsied node — because a complete response can render the lesion invisible, and the surgeon must still be able to find and excise the site.
2. Where the lesion is small enough that the biopsy itself may remove or obscure it.

Confirm clip position after deployment, and be aware that clips can migrate.

Preoperative localization

Where a non-palpable lesion is to be excised, its position must be marked for the surgeon. **Wire localization** places a hooked wire under ultrasound guidance on the morning of surgery. **Non-wire techniques** — radioactive seeds, magnetic markers, radar reflectors, and radiofrequency tags — can be placed days or weeks in advance, decoupling radiology and theatre scheduling, and are increasingly used.

Concordance — a formal step

When the histology returns, someone must ask whether it explains the imaging.

- **Concordant benign** — a fibroadenoma reported on a circumscribed oval parallel mass. Proceed to routine or short-interval follow-up.
- **Discordant benign** — "fibrocystic change" reported on a spiculated shadowing mass. **The workup does not stop.** Repeat biopsy, vacuum-assisted sampling, or surgical excision follows.
- **Benign but high-risk lesion** — atypical ductal hyperplasia, lobular neoplasia, radial scar, papillary lesion. These carry an upgrade risk at excision and are managed by defined pathways. [VERIFY: current management recommendations for high-risk lesions diagnosed on core biopsy, including upgrade rates and excision criteria]

Concordance assessment is a genuine safety mechanism, and its failure is a recognised route to delayed diagnosis. It is normally performed in a multidisciplinary meeting, and the imaging description must be detailed enough to support it — another reason the descriptor discipline of §10.3 matters.

Complications

Bleeding and haematoma — the commonest, usually controlled by firm compression for several minutes after the procedure. **Infection. Vasovagal reaction. Pneumothorax** — rare and essentially avoidable by the parallel approach. **Implant puncture** in a patient with implants, requiring a deliberately planned path.

10.9 Correlation with Mammography and MRI

The division of labour

Modality	Strengths	Limitations
Mammography	Population screening; **microcalcifications**; whole-breast architectural overview; DCIS detection	Sensitivity falls markedly in **dense breasts**; ionising radiation; compression discomfort
Ultrasound	Cystic versus solid; dense breasts; young, pregnant, and lactating patients; palpable lump assessment; **axilla**; real-time guidance; no radiation	Operator dependent; poor for microcalcification; no whole-breast overview; limited for DCIS
MRI	Highest sensitivity; **extent of disease**, especially lobular carcinoma; high-risk screening; implant integrity; neoadjuvant response; occult primary with nodal metastasis	Cost, access, contrast; lower specificity, generating findings that require second-look ultrasound

Triple assessment

The organising framework of breast practice: **clinical examination, imaging, and pathology**, with the requirement that all three be **concordant** before a benign conclusion is accepted.

The corollary that must be internalised: a **negative ultrasound does not exclude carcinoma in a patient with a clinically suspicious lump**. Sonographically occult cancers exist — invasive lobular carcinoma above all — and the pathway continues on clinical grounds regardless of the imaging.

Age-based pathways

Broadly, and subject to local protocol:

Younger patients with a palpable lump are assessed with **ultrasound first**, because the breasts are dense, mammographic sensitivity is reduced, and radiation avoidance matters in a young population.

Older patients are assessed with **mammography and ultrasound together**, since mammographic sensitivity is higher in fattier breasts and calcification detection matters.

Pregnant and lactating patients are assessed with ultrasound first; mammography can be performed with shielding where indicated, and pregnancy-associated breast cancer is a real entity that should not be dismissed as lactational change.

[VERIFY: current age thresholds and imaging pathways for symptomatic breast assessment in the relevant jurisdiction]

Supplemental ultrasound screening in dense breasts

Adding whole-breast ultrasound to mammographic screening in women with dense breasts **increases cancer detection**, at the cost of an **increase in false positives and consequent benign biopsies**. Automated breast ultrasound systems exist to make this practical at scale.

Whether and how this is offered varies by jurisdiction and by density notification legislation, and the balance of benefit and harm is an active area. [VERIFY: current evidence and recommendations for supplemental ultrasound screening in dense breasts, including incremental cancer detection rate and false positive rate]

Second-look ultrasound

An MRI-detected lesion with no mammographic or sonographic correlate presents a practical problem: MRI-guided biopsy is slower, costlier, and less available.

Second-look (targeted) ultrasound is performed with the MRI in front of you, scanning the specific location the MRI describes. Where a correlate is found, biopsy proceeds under ultrasound guidance — faster, cheaper, and more comfortable.

Success depends on **precise correlation of position**, which requires translating the MRI's coordinates into the clock-position and distance-from-nipple convention of §10.2, and accounting for the different patient positions between the two examinations — **prone for MRI, supine for ultrasound** — which shifts tissue substantially. This is a specific skill, and it is where the localization discipline of this chapter earns its keep.

The report

A breast ultrasound report should carry: the indication; the technique and any limitation; the findings, described in the standardized lexicon; **the full five-element localization** for any lesion; measurements; the axillary assessment; correlation with prior imaging and other modalities; an **assessment category**; and an explicit **management recommendation**.

Key Points

1. Almost all breast pathology arises in the terminal ductal lobular unit, which is why radial and antiradial scanning along the ductal axis is productive.
2. Scan the retroareolar region deliberately — angle beneath the nipple from the periphery. Dense fibrous tissue shadows it, and both papillomas and carcinomas occur there.
3. Use light pressure. Compression flattens lesions and distorts shape and orientation, which are diagnostic features.
4. Turn compounding off before assessing posterior features, and check questionable cyst contents on fundamental. Both descriptors depend on it.
5. Localize with all five elements: side, clock position, distance from nipple, depth third, and probe orientation.
6. Three o'clock is lateral on the right breast and medial on the left. This mirror-image error sends surgeons to the wrong quadrant.
7. Acquire images with and without calipers — calipers sit exactly where the margin must be assessed, and margin is the most important descriptor.
8. Not-parallel orientation indicates growth across tissue planes and is a genuinely ultrasound-specific suspicious feature.
9. One suspicious feature outweighs several benign ones. The descriptors are not averaged.
10. Vascularity in a solid component distinguishes a complex cystic and solid mass, which requires biopsy, from a complicated cyst, which usually does not.
11. A large or rapidly enlarging "fibroadenoma" warrants biopsy, because phyllodes tumour cannot be excluded sonographically.
12. Fat necrosis mimics carcinoma freely. The history and mammographic correlation resolve it; history alone does not.
13. Invasive lobular carcinoma may produce only architectural distortion without a mass, and its extent is underestimated. MRI is better for it.
14. Circumscribed does not mean benign — mucinous, medullary, and papillary carcinomas can look reassuring.
15. Any presumed mastitis that fails to resolve on treatment requires imaging and skin biopsy for inflammatory carcinoma.
16. In nodes, size is unreliable. Focal eccentric cortical bulging is the earliest useful sign, and hilar effacement is a strong one.
17. Gynaecomastia radiates from and is centred on the nipple; male carcinoma is eccentric to it. Any eccentric male breast mass is suspicious.

18. Keep the biopsy needle parallel to the chest wall. It is the safe approach and also the most visible one.
19. Place a marker clip before neoadjuvant therapy, in both tumour and biopsied node, because a complete response can make the site unfindable.
20. Concordance is a formal step. A benign result on a suspicious lesion does not end the workup.
21. A negative ultrasound does not exclude carcinoma in a clinically suspicious lump.

Registry Check

1. A breast lesion is described as taller than it is wide. This orientation is significant because it indicates:

A. The lesion is cystic **B.** Growth across normal tissue planes rather than along them, which is suspicious **C.** The lesion is superficial **D.** Excessive transducer compression was applied

> **Answer: B.** Not-parallel orientation reflects growth that crosses tissue planes and is a suspicious feature. It has no mammographic equivalent and is one of ultrasound's specific contributions to lesion characterization, though very small lesions and intraductal lesions can appear not-parallel without significance.

2. A mass is circumscribed and oval over most of its perimeter but has one segment of indistinct margin. It should be classified as:

A. Circumscribed, since most of the margin qualifies **B.** Not circumscribed **C.** Microlobulated **D.** Circumscribed with an artefact

> **Answer: B.** Circumscription requires a sharp abrupt transition around the **entire** perimeter. A single non-circumscribed segment makes the lesion not circumscribed, and under the governing rule a single suspicious feature outweighs the several benign ones present.

3. A lesion in the right breast is described as being at 3 o'clock. This position is:

A. Medial **B.** Lateral **C.** Superior **D.** Inferior

> **Answer: B.** Clock positions are mirrored between the breasts as viewed facing the patient. Three o'clock is lateral on the right breast and medial on the left. Confusing this is the commonest localization error and can direct surgery to the wrong quadrant.

4. A cystic lesion contains internal echoes. The feature that distinguishes a complex cystic and solid mass requiring biopsy from a complicated cyst is:

A. The presence of posterior enhancement **B.** Demonstrable vascularity within a solid component **C.** The size of the lesion **D.** A fluid–fluid level

> **Answer: B.** Mobile debris that shifts with repositioning and shows no flow indicates a complicated cyst, usually benign. A fixed solid component with

demonstrable internal vascularity — a mural nodule, thick septum, or eccentric solid portion — defines a complex cystic and solid mass, which requires biopsy.

5. An axillary lymph node measures within normal limits for size but shows a focal eccentric bulge of the cortex on one side. The correct interpretation is:

A. Normal, since the node is not enlarged **B.** Reactive change **C.** Suspicious — focal eccentric cortical thickening is an early sign of metastatic involvement **D.** A silicone-laden node

Answer: C. Metastatic deposits arrive in the subcapsular sinus and expand the cortex locally, so a focal eccentric bulge is an early and useful sign. Nodal size alone is unreliable, and reactive nodes typically show uniform concentric cortical thickening with a preserved hilum.

6. Multiple discontinuous parallel echogenic lines are seen floating within the lumen of a silicone implant. This represents:

A. A normal radial fold **B.** Intracapsular rupture — the stepladder sign **C.** Extracapsular rupture **D.** Capsular contracture

Answer: B. The collapsed implant shell floating within contained silicone produces the stepladder appearance of intracapsular rupture. A radial fold is continuous with the shell at its periphery; extracapsular rupture produces the echogenic snowstorm appearance in tissue outside the fibrous capsule.

7. During ultrasound-guided core biopsy of a deep breast lesion, the needle should be oriented:

A. Perpendicular to the skin for the shortest path **B.** Parallel to the chest wall **C.** At 45 degrees to the chest wall **D.** Whichever orientation the needle guide permits

Answer: B. A path parallel to the chest wall avoids directing the needle and the device's throw toward the pleura, and it is also the shallow orientation that maximises needle conspicuity by keeping the beam more nearly perpendicular to the shaft. The safe approach and the visible approach coincide.

8. Core biopsy of a spiculated, shadowing, not-parallel mass returns a histological diagnosis of fibrocystic change. The correct next step is:

A. Routine annual follow-up **B.** Six-month follow-up ultrasound **C.** Recognise the result as discordant and proceed to repeat sampling or surgical excision **D.** Accept the benign result and reassure the patient

Answer: C. The pathology does not explain the imaging appearance, making the result discordant. Concordance assessment is a formal safety step, and a benign result on an imaging-suspicious lesion requires repeat biopsy, vacuum-assisted sampling, or excision rather than surveillance.

Chapter Notes for the Editorial Pass

Verification queue. In priority order: **the current edition of the breast imaging lexicon, its assessment categories, and the management recommendation attached to each** (§10.3) — this is the single most consequential verification in the chapter, since the categories drive every management decision and the lexicon is periodically revised; **management of high-risk lesions diagnosed on core biopsy, including upgrade rates and excision criteria** (§10.8); **axillary staging pathways, including preoperative nodal biopsy and targeted axillary dissection** (§10.6), an actively changing area; **cortical thickness thresholds for suspicious nodes** (§10.6); **supplemental ultrasound screening in dense breasts — incremental detection and false-positive rates** (§10.9); **guidance on late peri-implant seroma and implant-associated lymphoma** (§10.7); **minimum transducer frequency for diagnostic breast ultrasound** (§10.2); **elastography thresholds** (§10.3); and **age-based symptomatic imaging pathways for the intended jurisdiction** (§10.9).

Jurisdiction note. More than any preceding chapter, this one describes practice that is organised differently between health systems — screening intervals, density notification, symptomatic pathways, and axillary management all vary. The text has been written to describe principles rather than a single national protocol, but §10.9 in particular should be reviewed against the intended market before publication.

Figure count: 7 Lane A, 0 Lane B. Breast is unusually well served by schematic figures because the descriptors are geometric rather than textural, and `fig-10-3` in particular does the work a photographic panel would. If Lane B slots are added, the two strongest candidates are a simple cyst and a spiculated carcinoma imaged at matched settings for direct comparison, and an axillary node series showing normal, reactive, and focally thickened cortex.

Cross-reference targets to fix at layout: §10.2 compounding and posterior features → Chapter 2 §2.4; §10.3 elastography → Chapter 2 §2.10; §10.7 testicular cause of gynaecomastia → Chapter 11; §10.8 guided intervention principles and needle visualization → Chapter 9 §9.4–9.6; §10.8 comparison discipline → Chapter 1 §1.5; §10.9 concordance and multidisciplinary governance → Chapter 1 §1.8.

Word count: approximately 10,400 excluding image prompt blocks, learning objectives, registry questions, and these notes.

Chapter 11: Thyroid, Parathyroid, Scrotum, and Musculoskeletal

Learning Objectives

On completing this chapter you should be able to:

1. Perform a thyroid protocol using the strap muscles as the echogenicity reference, and recognize the structures that mimic nodules.
2. Distinguish the diffuse thyroid diseases, and use vascularity to separate Graves disease from destructive thyroiditis.
3. Apply the nodule feature set that drives risk stratification, and name the benign features that permit reassurance.
4. Locate a parathyroid adenoma and state why imaging is performed for localization rather than diagnosis.
5. Recognize the nodal patterns specific to papillary thyroid carcinoma and lymphoma.
6. Perform a scrotal examination with comparative bilateral imaging at matched settings.
7. Distinguish testicular torsion from epididymo-orchitis, and recognize the whirlpool sign and testicular rupture.
8. Apply the intratesticular-versus-extratesticular rule, and assess a varicocele including the finding that mandates abdominal imaging.
9. Recognize and defeat anisotropy, and use dynamic maneuvers that no other modality offers.
10. Identify the principal tendon, muscle, ligament, nerve, and joint pathologies.

Four Regions, One Transducer

The subjects in this chapter share no anatomy and no physiology. What they share is a technical situation: **all are superficial, all are imaged with a high-frequency linear transducer, and in all of them ultrasound is the first-line modality rather than a supplement**.

That gives ultrasound an unusual position here. In the abdomen it competes with CT; in these regions it frequently *is* the definitive imaging test, and the referring clinician acts directly on the report. Two chapters' worth of consequence follows: the technical standard must be high, and the reporting must be decisive rather than deferential.

11.1 Thyroid Anatomy and Scanning Protocol

Anatomy

Two lobes joined across the midline by the **isthmus**, lying anterior and lateral to the trachea, below the cricoid cartilage. A **pyramidal lobe** ascends from the isthmus in a substantial minority — a remnant of the thyroglossal duct, and worth identifying because it is resected in total thyroidectomy.

Echotexture is homogeneous and fine, and characteristically hyperechoic relative to the adjacent strap muscles. That comparison is the reference standard for the gland, exactly as liver-to-kidney is for the abdomen, and it must be acquired in a single frame at matched settings.

Relations that matter at the machine:

Structure	Position	Why it matters
Strap muscles (sternohyoid, sternothyroid)	Anterior	The echogenicity reference
Sternocleidomastoid	Anterolateral	Landmark
Common carotid artery and internal jugular vein	Lateral	Landmarks; the IJV compresses with pressure
Trachea	Medial	Air, so a bright interface with reverberation
Oesophagus	Posterolateral, usually on the **left**	**A recurrent pseudonodule** — identified by its gut signature (Chapter 6 §6.8) and by watching it move on swallowing
Longus colli	Posterior	Hypoechoic muscle, mistaken for a mass or a parathyroid
Recurrent laryngeal nerve	Tracheo-oesophageal groove	Rarely seen; surgically critical
Parathyroid glands	Posterior	§11.4

Vascular supply is from the superior thyroid artery (from the external carotid) and the inferior thyroid artery (from the thyrocervical trunk).

Measurements. Each lobe in three dimensions plus isthmus thickness; volume by the ellipsoid approximation where required. [VERIFY: current reference values for thyroid lobe dimensions, isthmus thickness, and volume]

Protocol

Position supine with the neck extended, a pillow or roll beneath the shoulders. This is uncomfortable for some patients and impossible for a few — note it if the study is limited.

Transducer: high-frequency linear, the highest that reaches the posterior gland. A small-footprint or hockey-stick probe helps in the suprasternal region and in children.

Sweeps: complete transverse and longitudinal coverage of both lobes and the isthmus, extending superiorly to the upper pole and **inferiorly toward the sternal notch**.

The swallowing maneuver is specific and useful: ask the patient to swallow and watch the gland rise. It brings a **retrosternal extension** up into view, and it demonstrates whether a mass moves with the thyroid — which distinguishes a thyroid lesion from an adjacent one.

Assess the cervical nodes routinely (§11.5), particularly levels III, IV, and VI, in any patient with a suspicious nodule or known thyroid malignancy.

Document: both lobes and isthmus with measurements, background echotexture and vascularity, every nodule with full characterization and precise location, and the nodal survey.

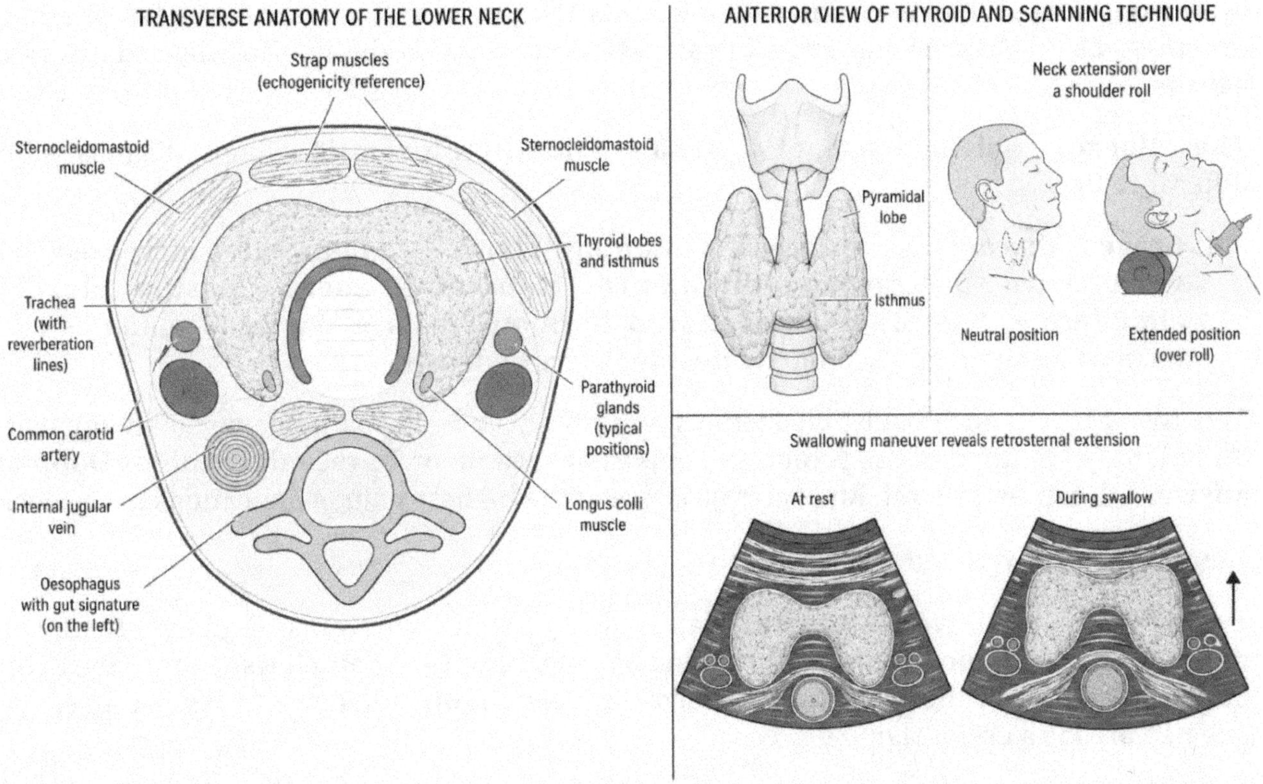

11.2 Diffuse Thyroid Disease

Hashimoto (chronic lymphocytic) thyroiditis

The commonest cause of hypothyroidism in iodine-replete populations.

Findings: a **heterogeneous, coarsened, diffusely hypoechoic** gland with **micronodulation** — innumerable small hypoechoic areas separated by echogenic fibrous septa, an appearance sometimes likened to a giraffe-skin pattern. The gland is often **enlarged early** and becomes **atrophic and fibrotic late**. Vascularity is variable — increased in active disease, reduced in the atrophic phase.

Associated findings: reactive nodes in the central compartment, and **"white knight" nodules** — small hyperechoic regions of spared or regenerative tissue against the hypoechoic background, which are benign and must not be reported as suspicious nodules.

Clinical significance: a modestly increased risk of papillary carcinoma, and a small but real association with **primary thyroid lymphoma** — which should be considered when a gland with Hashimoto disease enlarges rapidly.

Graves disease

Findings: a **diffusely enlarged, hypoechoic, heterogeneous** gland with **markedly increased vascularity** — colour Doppler fills the gland with flow, an appearance long described as the **"thyroid inferno."** Peak systolic velocity in the inferior thyroid artery is elevated.

The clinically valuable use of ultrasound in thyrotoxicosis is not diagnosis but differentiation:

> **Graves disease is a hyperfunctioning gland — markedly increased vascularity. Destructive thyroiditis (subacute, silent, postpartum, amiodarone type 2) releases stored hormone from a damaged gland — normal or reduced vascularity despite thyrotoxicosis.**

The two present identically biochemically at first, and they are managed in opposite directions — antithyroid drugs for one, supportive treatment for the other. **Colour Doppler answers the question quickly**, and this is one of the highest-value applications in the neck.

Subacute (de Quervain) granulomatous thyroiditis

Typically post-viral, with a **painful** gland and systemic symptoms. Findings: **focal, ill-defined, hypoechoic areas** with **reduced vascularity**, characteristically **migrating** between regions of the gland over weeks. Tenderness on transducer pressure over the affected area is a useful sign.

Multinodular goitre

An enlarged gland containing multiple nodules of varying appearance. The tasks are: assess **overall size and any retrosternal extension**; document **tracheal deviation or compression**; and — most importantly — **identify any nodule with suspicious features** rather than treating the whole gland as benign because it is nodular. A dominant or discordant nodule in a multinodular gland requires the same assessment as a solitary nodule (§11.3).

Other diffuse conditions

Acute suppurative thyroiditis — rare; abscess formation, and in children an underlying pyriform sinus fistula should be considered.

Riedel thyroiditis — a fibrosing process producing a hard, hypoechoic gland that **extends beyond the capsule and encases adjacent structures**, related to IgG4 disease and mimicking malignancy.

Amiodarone-induced thyroid dysfunction, **postpartum thyroiditis**, and **iodine deficiency goitre** complete the list.

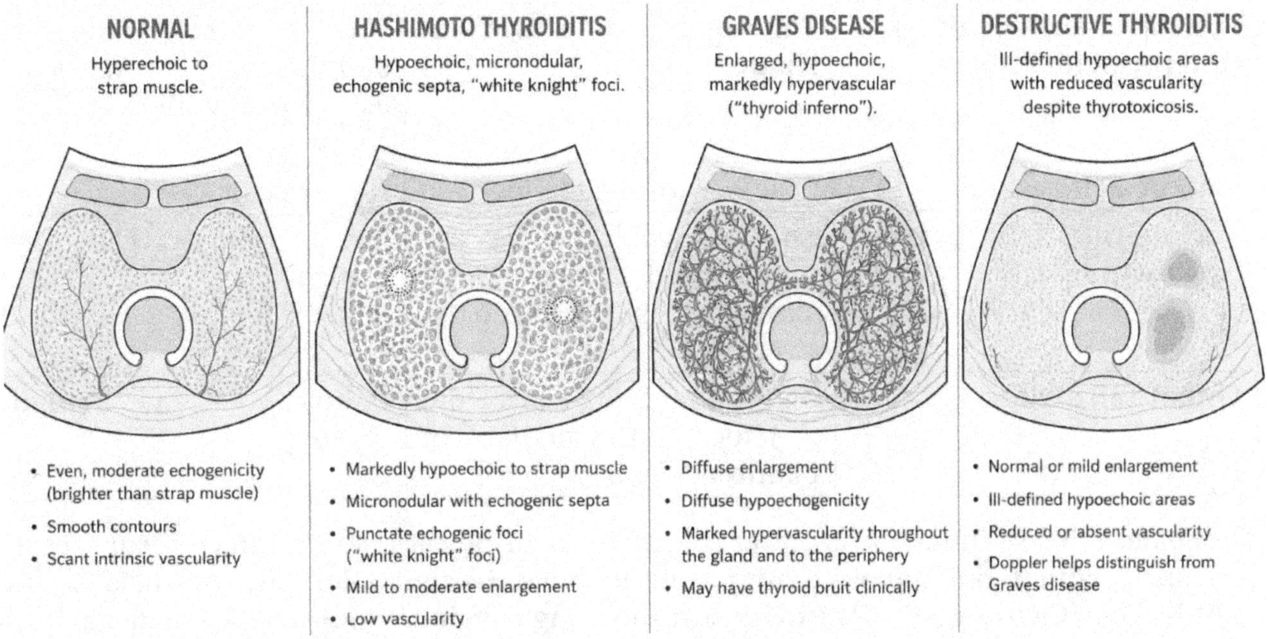

11.3 Thyroid Nodules and Risk Stratification

The actual problem

Thyroid nodules are extremely common and **the great majority are benign**. The clinical task is not to detect nodules — that is easy — but to **select which nodules warrant fine-needle aspiration**, avoiding both missed malignancy and a cascade of unnecessary biopsies, indeterminate cytology, and surgery for benign disease.

Every element of this section serves that selection.

The suspicious feature set

Composition — solid is more suspicious than cystic or predominantly cystic.

Echogenicity — marked hypoechogenicity (darker than the strap muscles) is the most suspicious level; mild hypoechogenicity less so; iso- and hyperechoic nodules less again.

Shape — taller than wide (not parallel), the same principle as in the breast (Chapter 10 §10.3): growth across tissue planes.

Margin — irregular, lobulated, or infiltrative, and above all **extrathyroidal extension**, where the nodule breaches the capsule into adjacent tissue. Extrathyroidal extension is a strongly suspicious sign and changes staging.

Echogenic foci — this is where careful discrimination matters most:

Focus type	Appearance	Significance
Punctate echogenic foci (microcalcifications)	Tiny bright dots **without shadowing**	**The most specific suspicious feature,** associated with papillary carcinoma
Macrocalcification	Coarse, with shadowing	Non-specific
Peripheral (rim) calcification	An echogenic rim; an **interrupted rim with extrusive soft tissue** is suspicious	Intact rim is generally benign
Comet-tail artifact	Discrete tapering trails from tiny foci — **the artifact of Chapter 2 §2.8**	**Colloid — a benign finding**

The comet-tail discrimination is a direct payoff from the physics chapter, and it recurs across this book: **comet tail means benign colloid here, benign adenomyomatosis in the gallbladder (Chapter 5 §5.7), and its non-tapering cousin ring-down means gas in both regions.**

Vascularity — intranodular chaotic flow was historically weighted heavily and is now regarded as **less reliable** than the morphological features. It should not override them.

Benign feature set

- **Pure cyst** — anechoic, thin-walled
- **Spongiform** — an aggregation of numerous microcystic spaces occupying the majority of the nodule; a reassuring pattern
- **Colloid nodules with comet-tail artifact**
- **"White knight"** hyperechoic foci in Hashimoto disease (§11.2)

Risk stratification systems

Several formal systems exist that combine these features into risk categories and pair each category with a **size threshold above which fine-needle aspiration is recommended**. They differ from one another in feature weighting, in category structure, and in size thresholds, and each is periodically revised.

A department must select one system and apply it consistently, and the report should state which is being used. Applying features from one system to the thresholds of another produces incoherent recommendations. [VERIFY: the risk stratification system to be adopted for this text, its current edition, its category definitions, and its size thresholds for fine-needle aspiration — and note that competing systems exist and differ]

Cytology reporting likewise uses a standardized category system with associated malignancy risks and management implications, and **molecular testing** is increasingly used to refine indeterminate categories. [VERIFY: current cytology reporting categories, associated risk of malignancy, and the role of molecular testing]

Thyroid malignancies

Papillary carcinoma — much the commonest. Typically solid, hypoechoic, with **punctate echogenic foci**, and it metastasises to **cervical nodes** with a distinctive appearance (§11.5). Generally excellent prognosis.

Follicular carcinoma — cannot be diagnosed by fine-needle aspiration, because the distinction from follicular adenoma rests on capsular and vascular invasion, which requires the whole lesion. This is an important limitation to understand: a follicular neoplasm on cytology means diagnostic surgery, not a diagnosis.

Medullary carcinoma — arising from C cells, marked by elevated calcitonin, associated with **MEN 2**; often with coarse calcification.

Anaplastic carcinoma — elderly patients, rapidly enlarging, invasive, encasing vessels; a grave prognosis.

Lymphoma — arising on a background of Hashimoto disease; markedly hypoechoic.

Incidental nodules

Nodules found incidentally on carotid ultrasound, CT, or MRI are common. Whether they require dedicated assessment depends on size, appearance, patient age, and risk factors, and is governed by the same stratification pathways. The report should apply the system rather than either ignoring the finding or escalating it reflexively.

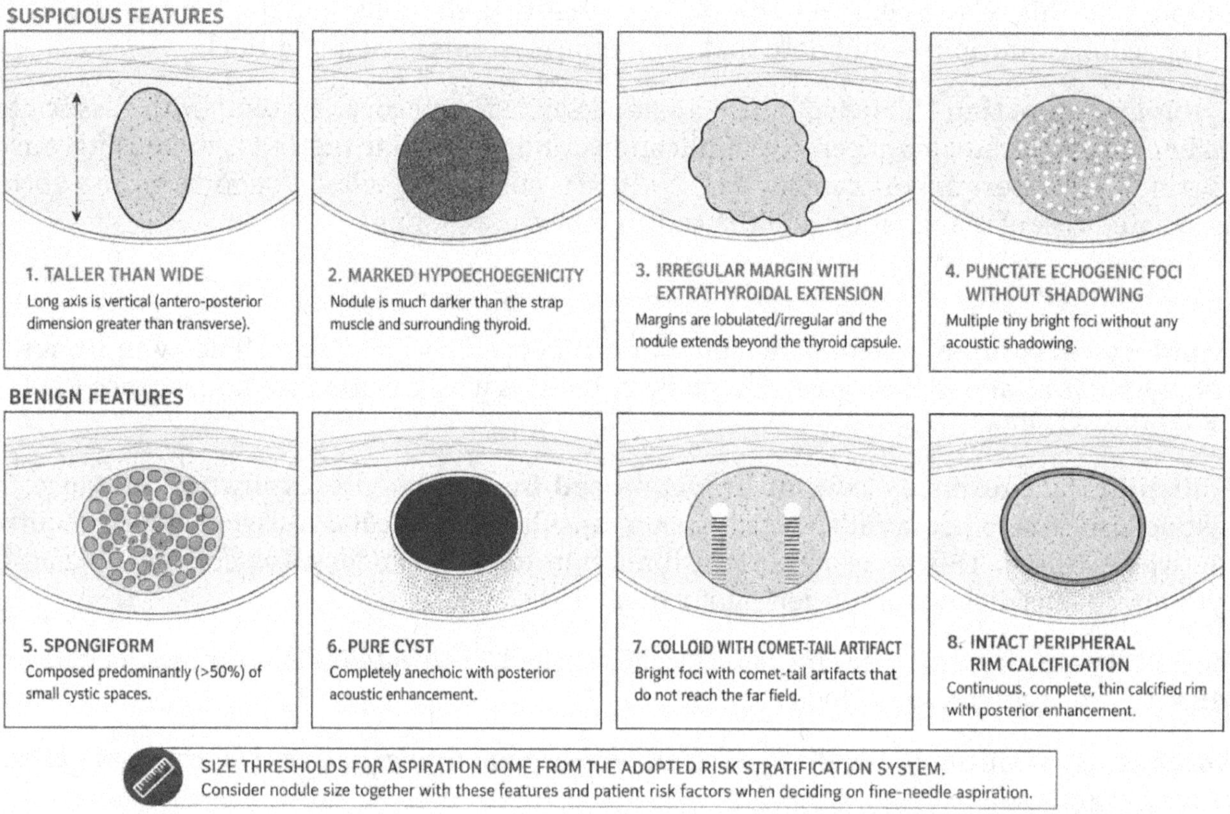

11.4 Parathyroid Anatomy, Adenoma, and Preoperative Localization

Anatomy and embryology

Usually four glands, and their embryological origin explains their positions:

Superior parathyroids derive from the **fourth** pharyngeal pouch. They are **relatively constant in position**, lying posterior to the upper or middle third of the thyroid lobe near the cricothyroid junction, and deep to the plane of the recurrent laryngeal nerve.

Inferior parathyroids derive from the **third** pouch, descending with the thymus. They are consequently **far more variable**, lying anywhere from the angle of the mandible to the mediastinum, and anterior to the plane of the recurrent laryngeal nerve.

Supernumerary glands occur, and **ectopic locations** — intrathyroidal, within the carotid sheath, retro-oesophageal, and mediastinal — account for a meaningful proportion of failed explorations.

Normal parathyroid glands are not usually visible on ultrasound.

The role of imaging — an important framing

Primary hyperparathyroidism is a biochemical diagnosis, established by hypercalcaemia with an inappropriately elevated parathyroid hormone level. **Imaging does**

not make the diagnosis; imaging localizes the culprit gland so that a focused, minimally invasive parathyroidectomy can replace a four-gland exploration.

This matters for reporting. A negative ultrasound does not exclude hyperparathyroidism — it means the gland has not been localized by this modality, and the pathway continues.

The adenoma

Appearance: an **oval or bean-shaped, markedly hypoechoic, homogeneous, well-defined** mass, lying **posterior to the thyroid** and **separated from it by an echogenic capsular plane**. That separating plane is the finding that distinguishes an adenoma from a posterior thyroid nodule, and it should be sought specifically.

Vascularity: a characteristic **polar feeding vessel** entering at one pole, often with an arc of vascularity curving around the gland — the "polar vessel" or "vascular arc" sign, which is a genuinely useful confirmatory finding.

Larger adenomas may become heterogeneous or contain cystic change.

Mimics

Mimic	Discriminator
Lymph node	Has a **fatty hilum** and hilar vascularity
Thyroid nodule	Lies **within** the gland; no separating capsular plane; moves entirely with the thyroid
Oesophagus	Gut signature; moves on swallowing
Longus colli	Muscle striations; continuous along the length of the neck
Thymic remnant	Inferior, in children and young adults

Multiglandular disease and carcinoma

Hyperplasia affecting all four glands occurs in **MEN syndromes** and in **secondary and tertiary hyperparathyroidism** of chronic renal failure. Ultrasound may show several enlarged glands, and the surgical approach differs entirely — this is a case where finding one adenoma and stopping is a mistake, and all four sites should be examined.

Parathyroid carcinoma is rare, and suggested by a **large, irregular, heterogeneous, locally invasive** gland in a patient with markedly elevated calcium.

Combining modalities

Ultrasound's sensitivity is real but limited, particularly for ectopic and mediastinal glands and in multiglandular disease. It is routinely paired with **sestamibi scintigraphy (with SPECT-CT)** or **four-dimensional CT**.

Concordance between ultrasound and a functional study substantially increases confidence and is what typically permits a focused unilateral operation. Discordant or negative studies push toward bilateral exploration or further imaging. [VERIFY: current sensitivity figures and recommended preoperative localization algorithms for primary hyperparathyroidism]

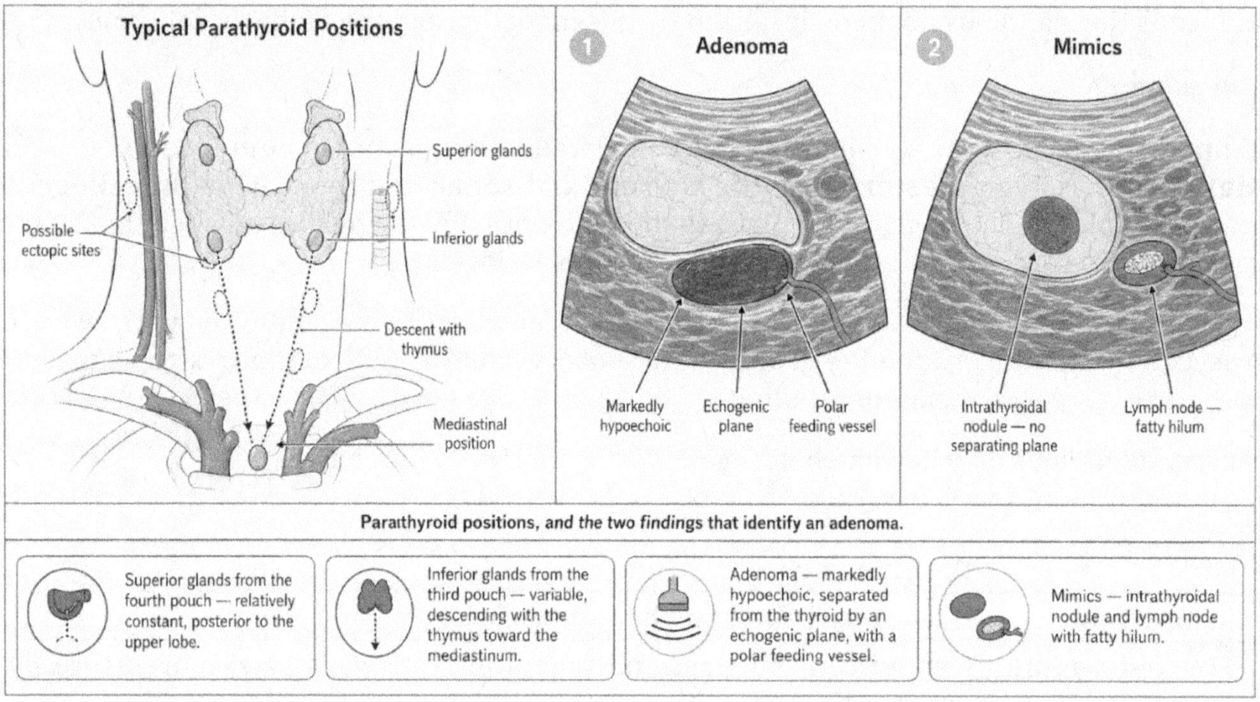

Parathyroid positions, and the two findings that identify an adenoma.

11.5 Cervical Lymph Nodes

The level map

Cervical nodes are described by a standardized level system, and using it is what makes reports comparable between radiology, surgery, and oncology:

Level	Location
I	Submental and submandibular
II	Upper jugular, from skull base to the hyoid
III	Mid jugular, hyoid to the cricoid
IV	Lower jugular, cricoid to the clavicle
V	Posterior triangle
VI	Central compartment — pretracheal, paratracheal, prelaryngeal
VII	Superior mediastinal

For thyroid disease, levels VI, III, and IV are the priority, and level VI is the first station for papillary carcinoma.

Normal and abnormal architecture

The general architecture — oval shape, thin uniform cortex, echogenic fatty hilum, hilar vascularity — and the abnormal features — focal eccentric cortical thickening, hilar effacement, rounding, and peripheral non-hilar vascularity — are set out in **Chapter 10 §10.6** and apply identically here.

The patterns specific to the neck

What distinguishes cervical nodal assessment is that several diseases produce **characteristic** appearances:

Metastatic papillary thyroid carcinoma — a distinctive and highly useful pattern:

- **Cystic change** within the node
- **Punctate echogenic foci** (microcalcifications), mirroring the primary tumour
- **Hyperechoic content**, attributed to thyroglobulin
- **Peripheral vascularity**
- Rounded shape with hilar loss

Any of these in a level VI, III, or IV node in a patient with thyroid disease is significant, and cystic or echogenic nodal change is close to specific.

Lymphoma — markedly hypoechoic, sometimes so profoundly that a node appears almost anechoic and can be mistaken for a cyst; posterior enhancement may be present despite the node being solid (Chapter 2 §2.7). Often multiple, in clusters, with a reticular internal pattern.

Squamous cell carcinoma metastasis — rounded, with **central necrosis**, typically at levels II and III, in a patient with a head and neck primary.

Tuberculous adenitis — matted nodes with necrosis, surrounding soft-tissue oedema, and sometimes a sinus tract to the skin.

Reactive nodes — preserved architecture, uniform cortical thickening, preserved hilar flow.

Sampling and surveillance

Suspicious nodes are sampled by fine-needle aspiration. In suspected metastatic thyroid carcinoma, **measurement of thyroglobulin in the needle washout** substantially increases sensitivity over cytology alone and is a standard adjunct.

Post-thyroidectomy surveillance is a major part of neck ultrasound practice: systematic mapping of all levels, comparison with prior studies, and assessment of the thyroid bed for recurrence. The comparison discipline of Chapter 1 §1.5 governs, and reporting by level is what makes serial comparison possible.

11.6 Scrotal Anatomy and Scanning Technique

Anatomy

Testis — an ovoid organ with **homogeneous mid-level echogenicity**, surrounded by the **tunica albuginea**, a thin echogenic capsule. The **mediastinum testis** appears as an echogenic band running craniocaudally where the tunica invaginates, carrying vessels and ducts; the **rete testis** lies adjacent to it as a subtle hypoechoic tubular region.

Epididymis — the **head (globus major)** superiorly and posteriorly, slightly larger and coarser than the testis; the **body** running along the posterior surface; and the **tail** inferiorly, continuing as the vas deferens.

Appendix testis and appendix epididymis — small pedunculated embryological remnants at the upper pole, of no significance except that they can undergo torsion (§11.7).

Tunica vaginalis — the potential space around the testis; **a small volume of fluid is normal**.

Vascular anatomy:

- **Testicular (gonadal) artery** from the aorta → **capsular arteries** running beneath the tunica → **centripetal branches** running toward the mediastinum
- A **transmediastinal artery** is present in a substantial proportion — a prominent vessel crossing the testis with an accompanying vein, which must not be mistaken for a lesion or a fracture line
- **Deferential and cremasteric arteries** supply the epididymis and scrotal wall, which is why **epididymal flow may persist in testicular torsion**
- **Pampiniform plexus** draining to the gonadal vein: **right into the IVC, left into the left renal vein** — the asymmetry from Chapter 3 §3.5, and the anatomical basis of §11.8

Technique

Position: supine, penis retracted onto the abdomen and covered, a towel supporting the scrotum between the thighs. Warm gel. Explain the examination and offer a chaperone (Chapter 1 §1.3).

Transducer: high-frequency linear.

The single most important technical rule:

> **Image both testes together in a single transverse view — the "buddy view" — and compare echogenicity, size, and flow at identical settings.**

Almost every scrotal diagnosis is comparative. A testis is hypoechoic *relative to its fellow*; flow is reduced *relative to the other side*. Changing gain, PRF, or wall filter between sides destroys the comparison, and a colour Doppler study of one testis alone cannot answer the torsion question.

Doppler settings: low velocity scale, low wall filter, high colour sensitivity — testicular flow is slow and easily missed with abdominal settings. Establish the settings on the normal side and **do not alter them** when moving across.

Additional maneuvers: Valsalva and **upright positioning** for varicocele; gentle compression to assess a mass; and assessment of the inguinal canal where a hernia or undescended testis is in question.

Document: both testes in three dimensions, comparative transverse greyscale and colour views, each epididymis, any focal lesion in two planes with colour, the tunica and any hydrocele, the scrotal wall, and the spermatic cord.

11.7 The Acute Scrotum: Torsion, Epididymo-orchitis, Trauma

Testicular torsion

A surgical emergency in which salvage falls steeply with time. The examination must be immediate, focused, and communicated directly.

Findings, in order of usefulness:

1. Absent or markedly reduced intratesticular flow compared with the contralateral testis, at identical Doppler settings. This is the central finding and the reason the comparative technique of §11.6 exists.

2. The whirlpool sign — a spiral or snail-shell twist of the spermatic cord above the testis, best sought in transverse just superior to the upper pole and traced up toward the external ring. **It is highly specific, and crucially it can be present even when intratesticular flow is preserved**, as in incomplete or intermittent torsion. **Look for it in every suspected torsion**, and do not be reassured by residual flow without examining the cord.

3. Greyscale changes — normal early, which is the trap; later an **enlarged, heterogeneous, hypoechoic** testis indicating infarction, which carries a poor prognosis for salvage.

4. Secondary findings — reactive hydrocele, scrotal wall thickening, an enlarged hypoechoic epididymis.

Important caveats:

- **Epididymal and scrotal wall flow may persist** because they are supplied by the deferential and cremasteric arteries — peripheral flow does not exclude torsion.
- **Partial or intermittent torsion** may show preserved but abnormal flow with a high-resistance waveform and reduced diastolic flow, and the whirlpool sign may be the only positive finding.
- **Torsion–detorsion** produces reactive **hyperaemia**, which can be mistaken for epididymo-orchitis in a patient whose testis has just untwisted.
- **A bell-clapper deformity** — a high, horizontal testicular lie from a redundant tunica vaginalis — predisposes and is **bilateral**, which is why the contralateral testis is usually fixed at surgery.

- **Neonatal (extravaginal) torsion** differs and is covered in Chapter 12.

Suspected torsion is a critical finding. Communicate directly and immediately, and do not prolong the examination for completeness (Chapter 1 §1.5).

Torsion of a testicular appendage

The commonest cause of acute scrotal pain in prepubertal boys, and the diagnosis matters because it is **self-limiting and does not require surgery**.

Findings: a small, rounded, **avascular paratesticular nodule** at the upper pole between testis and epididymal head, with **normal intratesticular flow**, often with reactive epididymal hyperaemia, hydrocele, and skin thickening. The clinical "blue dot sign" may be visible.

Making this diagnosis confidently spares an operation, which makes it one of the more valuable calls in scrotal ultrasound.

Epididymo-orchitis

Findings: an **enlarged, hypoechoic, markedly hyperaemic epididymis** — usually the **tail first**, then extending — with **increased flow** being the defining feature. Orchitis follows in a proportion, producing an enlarged hyperaemic testis. Reactive hydrocele and scrotal wall thickening are common.

The discrimination from torsion is flow direction of change: increased in inflammation, absent or reduced in torsion. That distinction is usually straightforward, with the caveats above.

Complications to seek: abscess (a complex avascular collection within testis or epididymis), **pyocele**, **venous infarction** from inflammatory compression (producing hypoechoic avascular segments — a serious finding), and chronic changes.

Trauma

Testicular rupture is a surgical emergency with time-dependent salvage, and the examination must specifically address it.

Injury	Findings
Contusion / haematoma	Focal heterogeneous area, contour and tunica intact
Fracture	A hypoechoic linear defect crossing the parenchyma with **intact tunica albuginea and preserved contour**
Rupture	**Disruption of the tunica albuginea**, contour irregularity, and heterogeneous extruded parenchyma — the defining findings
Haematocele	Complex fluid in the tunica vaginalis, evolving with time
Devascularised segment	Absent flow in part or all of the testis on colour Doppler

Assess and report specifically: tunical integrity, contour, parenchymal heterogeneity, and vascularity. **Contour irregularity with tunical disruption is the finding that takes the patient to theatre**, and it should be looked for deliberately rather than described in passing.

Fournier gangrene — necrotising fasciitis of the perineum and scrotum, showing **gas within the scrotal wall** producing dirty shadowing and ring-down (Chapter 2 §2.8), with wall thickening. A surgical emergency with high mortality, and a critical finding.

The Acute Scrotum

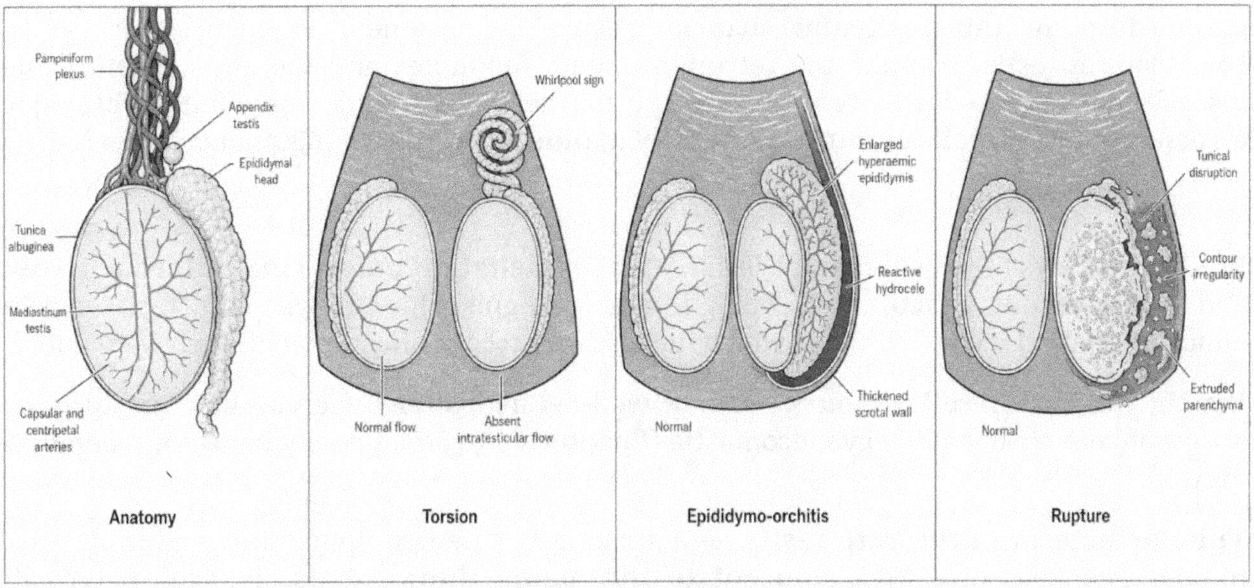

Every diagnosis here is comparative — image both testes together at identical settings.

11.8 Scrotal Masses, Varicocele, and Male Infertility Assessment

The organizing rule

> **A solid intratesticular mass is malignant until proven otherwise. An extratesticular mass is usually benign.**

This single distinction does more work than any other in scrotal imaging, and the first task with any scrotal mass is to establish which side of it the lesion falls on — by identifying the tunica albuginea and determining whether the lesion lies within or outside it.

Intratesticular malignancy

Germ cell tumours account for the great majority in young and middle-aged men:

Seminoma — typically **homogeneous, hypoechoic, well-defined**, sometimes lobulated, confined within the tunica. The commonest single type.

Non-seminomatous germ cell tumours — embryonal carcinoma, teratoma, yolk sac tumour, choriocarcinoma, and mixed forms. Typically **heterogeneous**, with **cystic areas, calcification, and irregular margins**.

"Burnt-out" tumour — a regressed primary appearing only as a scar or a calcified focus, in a patient presenting with retroperitoneal nodal disease. **Any young man with a retroperitoneal mass should have his testes examined** (Chapter 3 §3.10).

Lymphoma and leukaemia — the **commonest testicular malignancy over the age of about 60**, often **bilateral**, and characteristically producing **diffuse hypoechoic infiltration** rather than a discrete mass, with preserved testicular shape and increased vascularity.

Metastases to the testis are rare.

On finding an intratesticular mass: measure it, document vascularity, assess the contralateral testis, examine the retroperitoneum for nodes and the abdomen for other disease, and communicate promptly. Tumour markers and orchidectomy follow; **biopsy of a suspected germ cell tumour is generally avoided** in favour of inguinal orchidectomy.

Benign intratesticular lesions

Epidermoid cyst — a well-defined lesion with a **lamellated "onion-ring" internal pattern** and **no internal vascularity**. Benign, and recognisable enough that testis-sparing enucleation can be considered — which makes correct identification genuinely valuable.

Leydig and Sertoli cell tumours — small, well-defined, often hypervascular; may produce hormonal effects including gynaecomastia (Chapter 10 §10.7). Usually benign but generally excised.

Tubular ectasia of the rete testis — a striking but benign appearance: multiple small tubular anechoic structures **adjacent to the mediastinum testis**, **avascular**, typically bilateral, and associated with epididymal obstruction and spermatoceles. Recognising it prevents a mistaken diagnosis of a cystic tumour.

Simple intratesticular cyst, **segmental infarction** (a wedge-shaped avascular area), **sarcoidosis**, and **tuberculosis**.

Testicular microlithiasis — multiple tiny echogenic foci without shadowing scattered through the parenchyma. Its association with germ cell tumour, and therefore whether surveillance is warranted, has been substantially reassessed and depends on the presence of other risk factors. [VERIFY: current guidance on the significance and management of testicular microlithiasis]

Extratesticular lesions

Spermatocele and epididymal cyst — anechoic, thin-walled, at the epididymal head; extremely common.

Adenomatoid tumour — the **commonest solid extratesticular tumour**, benign, usually at the epididymal tail.

Hydrocele — fluid in the tunica vaginalis; simple, or complex where inflammatory or haemorrhagic.

Inguinoscrotal hernia — bowel or omentum within the scrotum; **identified by peristalsis and bowel wall layers** (Chapter 6 §6.8), and by tracing continuity through the inguinal canal.

Sperm granuloma, fibrous pseudotumour, scrotal wall lesions, and rarely **liposarcoma** of the cord.

Varicocele

Dilatation of the pampiniform plexus veins, with reflux.

Findings: multiple **serpiginous anechoic tubular structures** adjacent to the testis, typically posterosuperior, **increasing in size with Valsalva and on standing**, with demonstrable **reflux on colour Doppler during Valsalva**. Diameter thresholds and grading systems are used. [VERIFY: current diameter threshold and grading system for varicocele, and the criteria for reflux duration]

Technique matters: examine **supine and then standing**, and perform **Valsalva in both positions**. A varicocele that is not demonstrable supine may be obvious upright, and a study performed only supine understates the finding.

Left-sided predominance is expected and explained by the anatomy of Chapter 3 §3.5 — the left gonadal vein drains into the left renal vein at a right angle, producing a longer, higher-pressure column, with the additional contribution of left renal vein compression in some patients.

The finding that changes the examination:

> **An isolated right-sided varicocele, or a new varicocele that does not decompress when the patient lies down, requires abdominal and retroperitoneal imaging** to exclude a mass obstructing the gonadal vein or the IVC.

This is a small point that occasionally finds a renal or retroperitoneal tumour, and it should be a reflex.

Infertility assessment

Ultrasound contributes:

- **Testicular volume** — reduced volume correlates with impaired spermatogenesis; measure in three dimensions and calculate
- **Echotexture** — heterogeneity or reduced echogenicity in impaired spermatogenesis
- **Varicocele**, with its recognised association with impaired parameters and testicular atrophy
- **Signs of obstruction** — dilated rete testis, enlarged epididymis, spermatoceles
- **Absent vas deferens** — congenital bilateral absence, associated with cystic fibrosis mutations, requiring genetic counselling
- **Undescended or atrophic testis**, and any history of cryptorchidism

- **Transrectal ultrasound** where ejaculatory duct obstruction is suspected, assessing the seminal vesicles and ejaculatory ducts

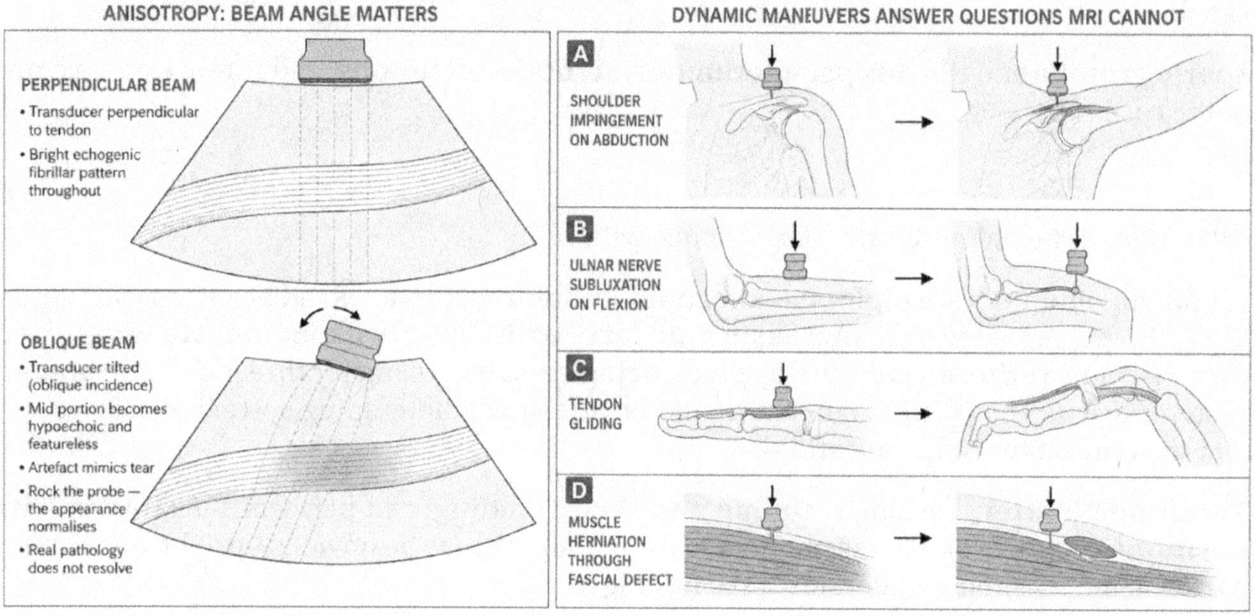

11.9 Musculoskeletal Technique, Anisotropy, and Dynamic Maneuvers

Anisotropy — the defining artifact

Tendons are highly ordered parallel collagen bundles, which makes them **strongly specular reflectors** (Chapter 2 §2.1). They return echoes brightly **only when the beam strikes them perpendicularly**. A deviation of a few degrees causes the reflected energy to travel away from the transducer, and the tendon appears **artificially hypoechoic**.

This is the single most important technical fact in musculoskeletal ultrasound, because an anisotropic tendon looks exactly like tendinopathy or a tear.

How to defeat it:

- **Keep the beam perpendicular to the structure at all times** — heel-toe and angle continuously as you follow a curving tendon. This is a constant active adjustment, not a setup step.
- **Test any hypoechoic area by changing the angle. Anisotropy resolves; real pathology persists.** This is the definitive manoeuvre and it takes one second.
- Beam steering, where available, helps for structures that cannot be approached perpendicularly.
- Anisotropy affects tendons most, then ligaments and nerves, and muscle least.

Equipment and settings

The highest-frequency linear transducer available — superficial musculoskeletal work benefits from frequencies well above those used elsewhere in this book, and a **small-footprint or hockey-stick probe** is needed for small joints, digits, and around bony prominences. [VERIFY: current recommended frequency ranges for musculoskeletal ultrasound by depth and application]

Copious gel, and a standoff for very superficial structures.

Light pressure — pressure obliterates small effusions, collapses veins and bursae, and abolishes the low-velocity flow of neovascularity that you may be trying to demonstrate. **This is particularly important when applying Doppler for synovitis or tendinopathy**: a heavy hand produces a false-negative Doppler study.

Core discipline

Image every structure in both long and short axis. Short axis assesses the **full width** of a tendon and detects partial-width tears that a long-axis image passes beside; long axis assesses **extent, retraction, and gap**. A tear reported from one plane only is inadequately assessed.

Compare with the contralateral side routinely — variation between individuals is wide, variation within an individual is small.

Sonopalpate. Place the probe on the point the patient identifies as most painful and correlate what you see with what they feel. As in Chapters 6 and 10, this exploits the modality's unique real-time correlation with symptoms.

Dynamic maneuvers

This is where ultrasound is not merely an alternative to MRI but superior to it. MRI images a still patient in one position; ultrasound watches structures move.

Maneuver	What it demonstrates
Shoulder abduction	Subacromial impingement; supraspinatus and bursa gathering beneath the acromion
Elbow flexion	Ulnar nerve subluxation or dislocation from the cubital tunnel
Ankle eversion / dorsiflexion	Peroneal tendon subluxation
Muscle contraction	Tear gap and retraction; tendon continuity; muscle herniation through a fascial defect
Valgus or varus stress	Ligament laxity — ulnar collateral, medial collateral
Anterior drawer	Ankle ligament integrity
Finger flexion and extension	Tendon gliding, triggering, pulley integrity

Maneuver	What it demonstrates
Standing / Valsalva	Hernia (Chapter 8 §8.4), varicocele (§11.8)

Record dynamic findings as cine clips, not still frames — a still image cannot demonstrate movement, and the finding will not be reproducible for the next reader.

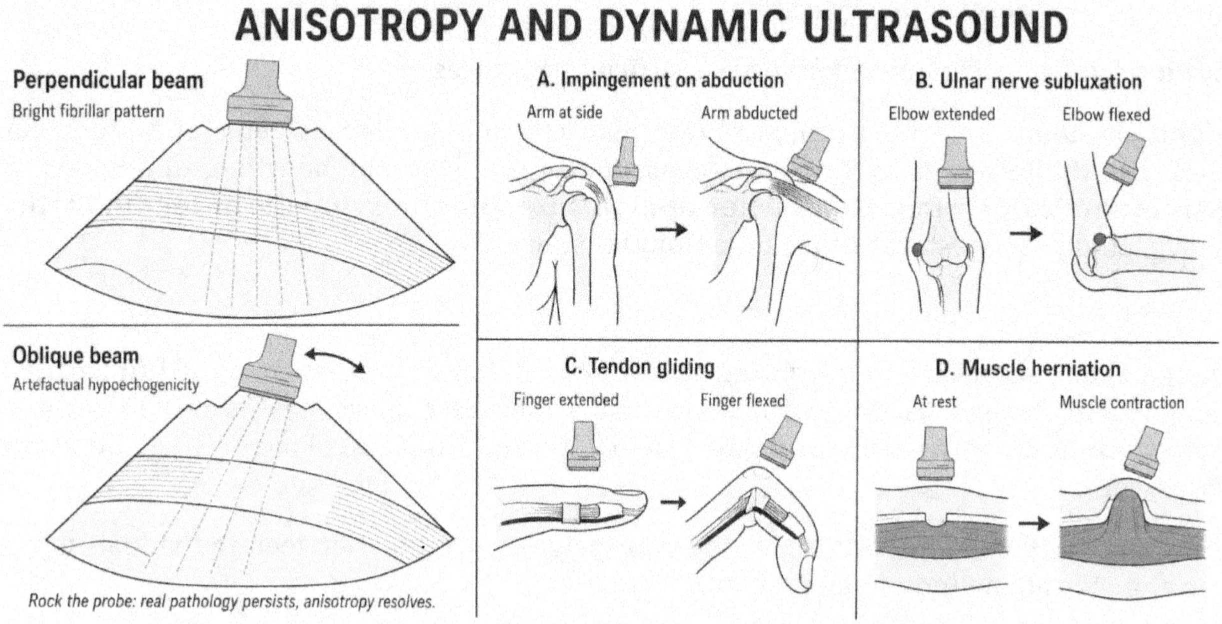

The same tendon can appear normal or artefactually hypoechoic depending on beam angle.
Dynamic maneuvers reveal impingement, nerve subluxation, tendon motion, and muscle herniation.

11.10 Tendon, Muscle, Ligament, Nerve, and Joint Pathology

Tendon

Normal: a compact band with a **fibrillar pattern** — fine parallel echogenic lines in long axis, a stippled pattern in short axis. Sheathed tendons have a thin surrounding synovial sheath; unsheathed tendons such as the Achilles have a paratenon instead.

Tendinopathy — the correct term for what was historically called tendinitis, since the process is largely **degenerative rather than inflammatory**. Findings: **thickening, hypoechogenicity, loss of the fibrillar pattern**, sometimes **intrasubstance calcification**, and **neovascularity** on Doppler, which correlates with symptoms.

Partial-thickness tear — a focal hypoechoic or anechoic defect that **does not span the full thickness**. In the rotator cuff, specify **articular-sided, bursal-sided, or intrasubstance**, because management differs.

Full-thickness tear — a defect spanning the tendon from one surface to the other, with:

- **Fluid filling the gap**, which is compressible
- **Retraction** of the torn end, with the gap measured
- **"Naked tuberosity"** — bare bone where the tendon should insert

- **Cartilage interface sign** — a bright line at the cartilage surface where fluid replaces tendon above it

Measure the gap and describe retraction, since these determine reparability.

Tenosynovitis — fluid and synovial thickening **within a tendon sheath**, with hyperaemia. Only possible in sheathed tendons.

Calcific tendinopathy — echogenic deposits, most familiar in the rotator cuff, with variable shadowing depending on maturity. Ultrasound-guided **barbotage** (lavage and aspiration) is a treatment.

Enthesopathy — abnormality at the tendon insertion: hypoechoic thickening, cortical erosion, enthesophyte, and Doppler signal. A cardinal feature of the **spondyloarthropathies** and a specific reason for referral.

Muscle

Normal: hypoechoic fascicles separated by echogenic perimysial septa, producing a "veined marble" appearance.

Strain — most often at the **myotendinous junction**. Graded from oedema and fibre disruption without architectural loss, through partial disruption with haematoma, to complete rupture with retraction and a gap. **Dynamic assessment during contraction defines the gap** better than static imaging.

Haematoma — evolving echogenicity as elsewhere in the body.

Myositis ossificans — heterotopic bone after trauma, showing **peripheral calcification with central lucency** (zoning), maturing over weeks. Recognising the zoning pattern prevents a mistaken diagnosis of sarcoma.

Muscle hernia — a fascial defect through which muscle bulges **on contraction**, a purely dynamic diagnosis.

Denervation atrophy — reduced bulk with increased echogenicity, prompting a search for the responsible nerve lesion.

Ligament

Normal: a compact fibrillar band bridging a joint.

Injury graded from sprain with thickening and hypoechogenicity, through partial tear, to complete disruption with a gap and abnormal laxity on **stress testing** — again, the dynamic advantage.

Commonly assessed: the **anterior talofibular ligament**, the **ulnar collateral ligament** of the elbow and thumb, and the **medial collateral ligament** of the knee.

Nerve

Normal: in short axis a **fascicular "honeycomb"** pattern — hypoechoic fascicles within an echogenic epineurium; in long axis, parallel hypoechoic bands.

Entrapment neuropathy — the pattern is consistent wherever it occurs: **swelling proximal to the compression, flattening at the point of compression, and loss of the fascicular pattern**, with increased **cross-sectional area** measured at a defined site. The median nerve at the carpal tunnel is the archetype, and cross-sectional area thresholds are used. [VERIFY: current cross-sectional area thresholds for median nerve at the carpal tunnel and for other common entrapment sites]

Ulnar nerve at the cubital tunnel — with dynamic assessment for **subluxation** on elbow flexion (§11.9).

Morton neuroma — an interdigital hypoechoic mass in the intermetatarsal space, with the **Mulder click** demonstrable by transverse compression of the forefoot while scanning from the plantar side.

Peripheral nerve sheath tumours — **schwannoma** typically eccentric, with the nerve **entering and exiting** the mass, sometimes with a target appearance; neurofibroma more central.

Traumatic neuroma — at a nerve end after injury or surgery, reproducing symptoms on sonopalpation.

Joint and bursa

Effusion — anechoic, **compressible and displaceable**, without Doppler signal.

Synovitis — hypoechoic intra-articular tissue that is **non-compressible and non-displaceable**, with **Doppler signal** indicating activity. The compressibility test distinguishes it from effusion and is essential.

Erosion — a cortical break that must be **confirmed in two perpendicular planes** to be reported, since a single-plane appearance is often a normal vascular channel or an artifact.

Crystal disease — two distinctive signs:

- **Gout** — the **"double contour" sign**, a hyperechoic band of urate deposited **on the surface of the articular cartilage**, parallel to and separate from the subchondral bone line; plus **tophi** (heterogeneous echogenic material, sometimes shadowing) and erosions
- **Calcium pyrophosphate deposition** — hyperechoic deposits **within the substance of the cartilage** and in fibrocartilage such as the meniscus and triangular fibrocartilage

The location of the deposit relative to the cartilage separates the two, which is a neat and reliable discrimination.

Septic arthritis — an effusion, often with debris and synovial thickening, but **ultrasound can neither confirm nor exclude infection**. Its role is to detect the effusion and to **guide aspiration**, which makes the diagnosis (Chapter 9 §9.5).

Bursitis — distension of a bursa with fluid or synovial thickening: subacromial–subdeltoid, olecranon, trochanteric, prepatellar, retrocalcaneal.

Baker (popliteal) cyst — fluid distending the gastrocnemius–semimembranosus bursa, identified by its characteristic **neck between the medial head of gastrocnemius and semimembranosus tendon**. **A ruptured Baker cyst mimics deep vein thrombosis clinically**, and finding it — while also excluding DVT (Chapter 16) — is a common and useful call.

Ganglion — anechoic or minimally complex, lobulated, avascular, adjacent to a joint or tendon sheath, sometimes with a demonstrable neck.

Soft tissue and bone

Foreign body — echogenic with shadowing or reverberation, surrounded by a **hypoechoic halo of granulation tissue** if longstanding. **Ultrasound is superior to radiography for radiolucent foreign bodies** — wood, plastic, thorns — which is a genuinely valuable indication.

Fracture — a **cortical step or discontinuity**, with adjacent haematoma; useful in ribs, sternum, and in children.

Periosteal reaction and stress injury — periosteal elevation and cortical irregularity.

Soft-tissue masses — lipoma, vascular malformation, and sarcoma. **A deep, enlarging, or vascular soft-tissue mass warrants MRI and specialist referral rather than reassurance**, and ultrasound's role is to identify that it requires further assessment.

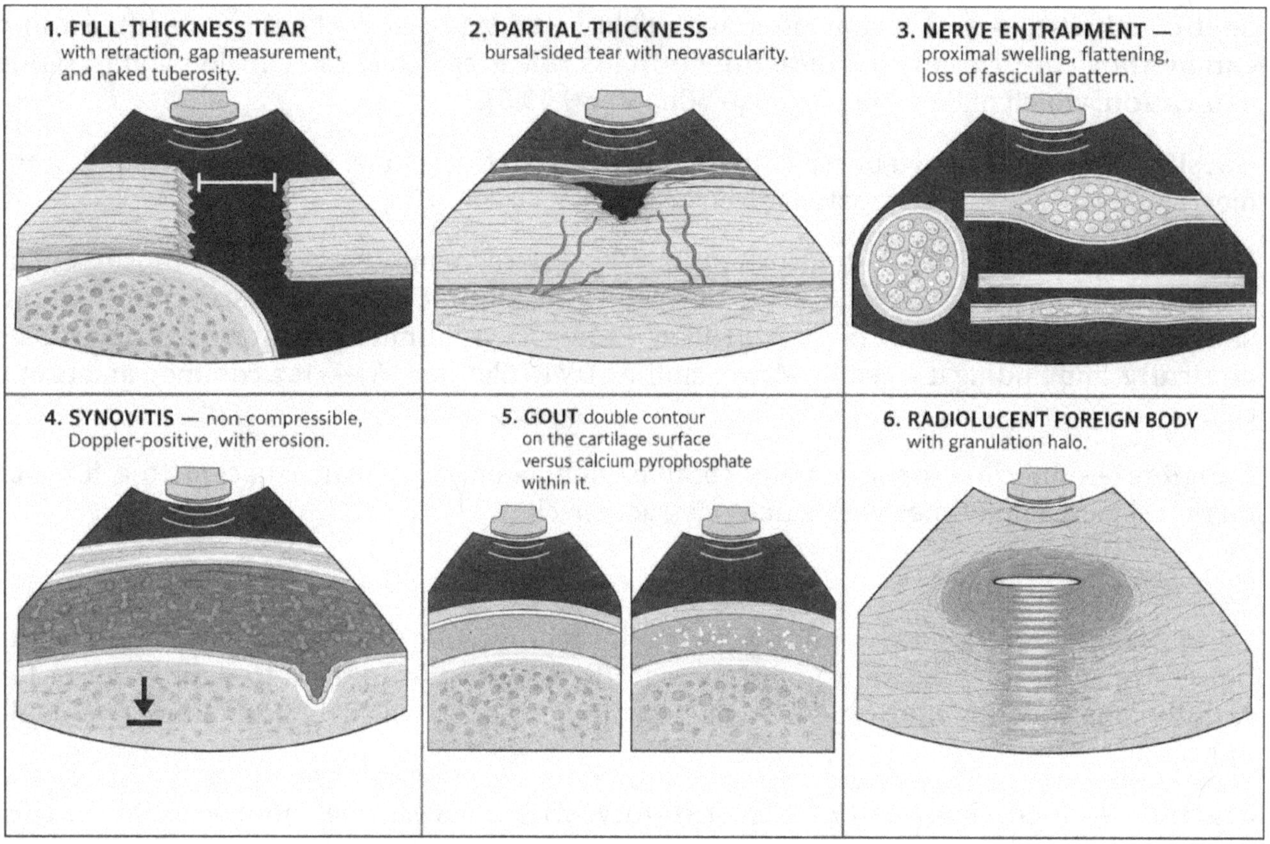

Key Points

1. The strap muscles are the thyroid's echogenicity reference; normal thyroid is hyperechoic to them.
2. The oesophagus mimics a left-sided thyroid nodule. It has a gut signature and moves on swallowing.
3. In thyrotoxicosis, colour Doppler separates Graves disease (markedly hypervascular) from destructive thyroiditis (reduced vascularity) — and they are managed in opposite directions.
4. Punctate echogenic foci without shadowing are the most specific suspicious nodule feature. Comet-tail artifact means benign colloid.
5. Follicular carcinoma cannot be diagnosed by fine-needle aspiration, because the diagnosis requires capsular and vascular invasion.
6. Adopt one nodule risk stratification system and apply it consistently. Mixing features from one with thresholds from another produces incoherent recommendations.
7. Parathyroid imaging localizes; it does not diagnose. A negative study does not exclude hyperparathyroidism.
8. An adenoma is separated from the thyroid by an echogenic plane and has a polar feeding vessel. A lymph node has a fatty hilum.
9. Cystic or echogenic change in a level VI, III, or IV node is close to specific for metastatic papillary thyroid carcinoma.

10. Image both testes in one transverse view at identical settings. Almost every scrotal diagnosis is comparative.
11. Epididymal and scrotal wall flow persist in torsion because they come from different arteries. Peripheral flow does not exclude it.
12. Look for the whirlpool sign in every suspected torsion. It is highly specific and may be positive when intratesticular flow is preserved.
13. Torsion of a testicular appendage is self-limiting; confidently diagnosing it — avascular paratesticular nodule with normal testicular flow — spares an operation.
14. Tunical disruption with contour irregularity is testicular rupture and takes the patient to theatre.
15. A solid intratesticular mass is malignant until proven otherwise; an extratesticular mass is usually benign.
16. Lymphoma is the commonest testicular malignancy over about 60, is often bilateral, and infiltrates diffusely rather than forming a mass.
17. Examine for varicocele supine and standing, with Valsalva in both. An isolated right-sided varicocele requires abdominal imaging.
18. Anisotropy resolves when you change the beam angle; real pathology does not. That one-second test is the most important skill in musculoskeletal ultrasound.
19. Image every musculoskeletal structure in both long and short axis. Short axis finds partial-width tears that long axis passes beside.
20. Use light pressure when applying Doppler — a heavy hand abolishes the neovascularity you are looking for.
21. Effusion compresses and displaces; synovitis does not and shows Doppler signal.
22. Gout deposits urate on the cartilage surface (double contour); calcium pyrophosphate deposits within the cartilage.
23. Ultrasound cannot confirm or exclude septic arthritis. It detects the effusion and guides the aspiration that makes the diagnosis.

Registry Check

1. A thyrotoxic patient has a diffusely enlarged hypoechoic thyroid with markedly increased colour Doppler flow throughout. This favours:

A. Subacute granulomatous thyroiditis **B.** Graves disease **C.** Silent thyroiditis **D.** Multinodular goitre

> **Answer: B.** Graves disease is a hyperfunctioning gland with markedly increased vascularity. Destructive thyroiditides release stored hormone from a damaged gland and show normal or reduced vascularity despite thyrotoxicosis. The distinction is clinically decisive because treatment differs entirely.

2. Which nodule feature is the most specific for malignancy?

A. Coarse macrocalcification with shadowing **B.** Punctate echogenic foci without shadowing **C.** Comet-tail artifact within the nodule **D.** Intranodular vascularity

Answer: B. Punctate echogenic foci without posterior shadowing represent microcalcification and are the most specific suspicious feature, associated with papillary carcinoma. Comet-tail artifact indicates benign colloid, macrocalcification is non-specific, and intranodular vascularity is now regarded as less reliable than morphological features.

3. A markedly hypoechoic oval mass lies posterior to the lower thyroid lobe, separated from it by a thin echogenic line, with a single vessel entering at one pole. This most likely represents:

A. A posterior thyroid nodule **B.** A cervical lymph node **C.** A parathyroid adenoma **D.** The longus colli muscle

Answer: C. The separating echogenic capsular plane establishes that the lesion is extrathyroidal, and the polar feeding vessel is characteristic of a parathyroid adenoma. A thyroid nodule lies within the gland with no separating plane, and a lymph node has a fatty hilum with hilar vascularity.

4. In suspected testicular torsion, intratesticular flow appears present but reduced. The most useful additional finding to seek is:

A. Reactive hydrocele **B.** Scrotal wall thickening **C.** The whirlpool sign in the spermatic cord **D.** Epididymal hyperaemia

Answer: C. Partial or intermittent torsion may preserve some intratesticular flow, and the spiral twist of the cord above the testis is highly specific and can be present despite residual flow. Failing to examine the cord is a recognised route to a missed torsion. The other findings are non-specific reactive changes.

5. An avascular paratesticular nodule is seen at the upper pole between the testis and epididymal head, with normal intratesticular flow and a reactive hydrocele, in a 10-year-old with acute scrotal pain. This represents:

A. Testicular torsion **B.** Torsion of the appendix testis **C.** Epididymo-orchitis **D.** Testicular tumour

Answer: B. Torsion of a testicular appendage is the commonest cause of acute scrotal pain in prepubertal boys and is self-limiting. Preserved intratesticular flow excludes torsion of the testis, and confidently making this diagnosis spares an unnecessary operation.

6. A newly identified isolated right-sided varicocele should prompt:

A. Reassurance, since varicoceles are common **B.** Semen analysis alone **C.** Abdominal and retroperitoneal imaging to exclude an obstructing mass **D.** Repeat scrotal ultrasound in six months

Answer: C. Varicoceles are predominantly left-sided because of the left gonadal vein's drainage into the left renal vein. An isolated right-sided varicocele, or one that fails to decompress when supine, raises the possibility of a retroperitoneal or renal mass obstructing the right gonadal vein or IVC.

7. A tendon appears focally hypoechoic with loss of the fibrillar pattern. The first step before reporting a tear is to:

A. Increase the overall gain **B.** Apply colour Doppler **C.** Change the beam angle by rocking the transducer **D.** Image the contralateral side

Answer: C. Anisotropy makes a normal tendon appear hypoechoic when the beam is not perpendicular, and it mimics tendinopathy and tear. Rocking the probe resolves anisotropy while genuine pathology persists — a one-second test that must precede any tendon abnormality report.

8. A hyperechoic band is seen lying on the surface of the articular cartilage, parallel to and separate from the subchondral bone line. This represents:

A. Calcium pyrophosphate deposition **B.** The double contour sign of gout **C.** An osteophyte **D.** Synovitis

Answer: B. Urate crystals deposit on the cartilage surface, producing a second bright line parallel to the subchondral bone — the double contour sign of gout. Calcium pyrophosphate deposits within the substance of the cartilage rather than on its surface, and the location of the deposit relative to the cartilage separates the two conditions.

Chapter Notes for the Editorial Pass

Verification queue. In priority order: **the thyroid nodule risk stratification system to be adopted**, its current edition, category definitions, and size thresholds for aspiration (§11.3) — this is the chapter's most consequential decision, because several competing systems exist, they differ materially, and the book must commit to one and apply it consistently rather than describing the concept generically; **cytology reporting categories and their associated malignancy risks** (§11.3); **guidance on testicular microlithiasis**, where the historical association with germ cell tumour has been substantially reassessed (§11.8); **varicocele diameter thresholds, grading, and reflux duration criteria** (§11.8); **median nerve cross-sectional area thresholds and other entrapment criteria** (§11.10); **preoperative parathyroid localization algorithms and reported sensitivities** (§11.4); **thyroid dimension and volume reference values** (§11.1); and **recommended transducer frequency ranges for musculoskeletal work** (§11.9).

Scope note. This chapter covers four unrelated regions and compresses each relative to a dedicated treatment — musculoskeletal ultrasound in particular is a subspecialty that supports whole textbooks, and §11.9–11.10 provide a framework rather than a joint-by-joint protocol. If a second edition expands the book, splitting musculoskeletal into its own chapter is the most defensible growth point in the current structure.

Figure count: 8 Lane A, 2 Lane B. `fig-11-9` — the paired anisotropy images — is the single highest-value real acquisition in the chapter and possibly in Part III, because the phenomenon is dynamic and a schematic conveys it only partially. It should be acquired as a matched pair on one machine, seconds apart.

Cross-reference targets to fix at layout: §11.1 gut signature → Chapter 6 §6.8; §11.3 comet tail and ring-down → Chapter 2 §2.8 and Chapter 5 §5.7; §11.5 nodal architecture → Chapter 10 §10.6; §11.6 gonadal vein asymmetry → Chapter 3 §3.5; §11.7 gas and dirty shadowing → Chapter 2 §2.8; §11.8 retroperitoneal nodes and testicular primary → Chapter 3 §3.10; §11.8 gynaecomastia → Chapter 10 §10.7; §11.9 specular reflection and anisotropy → Chapter 2 §2.1; §11.9 dynamic hernia assessment → Chapter 8 §8.4; §11.10 aspiration guidance → Chapter 9 §9.5; §11.10 Baker cyst and DVT → Chapter 16.

Word count: approximately 10,400 excluding image prompt blocks, learning objectives, registry questions, and these notes.

Chapter 12: The Neonatal and Pediatric Abdomen and Urinary Tract

Learning Objectives

On completing this chapter you should be able to:

1. Adapt transducer selection, thermal management, and behavioural technique to the paediatric patient, and explain why paediatric scanning uses higher frequencies than the adult equivalent.
2. Perform and measure a pyloric ultrasound, and distinguish hypertrophic pyloric stenosis from pylorospasm.
3. Recognise intussusception and identify the features predicting failed reduction.
4. Identify the sonographic signs of malrotation and midgut volvulus, and state why bilious vomiting in a neonate is a surgical emergency.
5. Apply the paediatric modifications to appendiceal assessment and name the principal mimics.
6. Recognise the paediatric hepatic, biliary and splenic conditions that differ from adult practice.
7. Assess an infant with conjugated hyperbilirubinaemia for biliary atresia, and describe the choledochal cyst spectrum.
8. Distinguish neonatal adrenal haemorrhage from neuroblastoma using serial imaging.
9. Grade urinary tract dilatation, recognise the major congenital anomalies, and identify posterior urethral valves.
10. Differentiate Wilms tumour from neuroblastoma on imaging features.
11. Describe contrast-enhanced voiding urosonography and its advantages over fluoroscopic cystography.

Why Paediatric Sonography Is Different

Three things change when the patient is a child, and they change more than the size of the probe.

Ultrasound is usually the definitive test, not the first of several. In adults, ultrasound frequently triages toward CT. In children, radiation avoidance is a genuine clinical priority, body habitus is favourable, and ultrasound answers the question outright. Pyloric stenosis, intussusception, biliary atresia, hydronephrosis, and vesicoureteric reflux are all conditions where ultrasound either makes the diagnosis or directs the definitive intervention. The report carries more weight.

The pathology is different. Almost nothing in this chapter appears in adult practice, and the adult conditions that dominate earlier chapters — gallstones, diverticulitis, aneurysm — are rare or absent here.

The patient cannot cooperate, and may deteriorate quickly. Technique becomes partly behavioural, and thermal and handling considerations in a neonate are part of the examination rather than courtesies.

12.1 The Paediatric Patient: Technical and Behavioural Adaptations

Transducer selection — the routinely missed point

Children permit far higher frequencies than adults, and the resolution gain is dramatic. A neonatal abdomen can be scanned in its entirety with a high-frequency linear transducer, producing detail that no adult abdominal study achieves.

The commonest technical failure in paediatric sonography is **scanning a child with adult settings**: a low-frequency curvilinear probe selected out of habit, at a depth appropriate for an adult, discarding most of the available resolution.

Patient	Typical approach
Neonate and small infant	High-frequency linear for most structures; small-footprint curvilinear or microconvex for deeper or wider fields and for intercostal work
Toddler and young child	Mid-to-high-frequency linear for superficial and focused work; small curvilinear for the general survey
Older child and adolescent	Approaching adult selection, but still favouring higher frequencies than an adult of the same request

Hockey-stick and small-footprint probes are valuable for the neonatal spine, hips, and small joints, and for fitting between ribs.

Set **depth and focal zone to the actual target**, which in an infant may be only two or three centimetres.

Thermal management and handling

Neonates lose heat rapidly and have limited reserve.

- **Warm the gel and the room.** Cold gel causes crying, abdominal wall tensing, and heat loss — all three degrade the study.
- **Expose the minimum area for the minimum time**, and cover the rest.
- **Scan within the incubator or under a radiant warmer** where the infant is unstable, rather than moving them.
- **Minimal handling** in a sick or preterm neonate is a clinical instruction, not a preference. Cluster the examination with other care where possible.

ALARA applies with particular force (Chapter 1 §1.7). Keep exposure short, use the correct preset, freeze before measuring, and use spectral Doppler only where a waveform is genuinely needed.

Infection control in the neonatal unit follows the same framework as everywhere (Chapter 1 §1.4), with added attention to hand hygiene between infants, probe and cable cleaning between every patient, and single-use gel sachets.

Behavioural technique

Explain to the child at their level and to the caregiver fully. Let a young child hold the probe and feel the gel.

Keep the caregiver in view and involved — a parent holding the child's hand or maintaining eye contact is a legitimate clinical tool.

Distraction works: a screen, a phone, a toy, a story, a caregiver's voice. For neonates, a **pacifier, sucrose solution, or a feed** during the examination is often decisive.

Feeding is both distraction and technique. An infant sucking is an infant lying still, and in pyloric assessment the feed also fills the stomach (§12.2).

Scan the least tolerable part last where the protocol allows, so that a distressing manoeuvre does not end the study before the essential images are obtained.

Warm hands, a quiet voice, and unhurried movement are worth more than any machine setting.

Practical points

Bladder filling in a child who is not toilet-trained cannot be requested. Feed and wait, and reassess. Scanning the upper tracts first while the bladder fills is efficient sequencing.

Reference values are age- and size-dependent. Renal length, splenic length, and organ dimensions must be compared against **paediatric normal ranges indexed to age or body size**, never adult values. [VERIFY: source of paediatric organ size reference ranges to be adopted, indexed to age, height, or body surface area]

Consent and assent follow Chapter 1 §1.5: the guardian consents, and a child capable of assent should be asked. Sustained refusal warrants reassessment rather than restraint.

Dignity matters increasingly with age; offer a chaperone and appropriate draping for older children and adolescents exactly as for adults.

Safeguarding. Unexplained injury, findings inconsistent with the given history, or incidental findings suggesting non-accidental injury must be escalated through the local child protection pathway. This obligation sits alongside the clinical one and is not discretionary.

12.2 Hypertrophic Pyloric Stenosis

Clinical context

Progressive hypertrophy of the pyloric muscle producing gastric outlet obstruction, typically presenting between about two and twelve weeks of age with **projectile, non-bilious vomiting** in an infant who remains hungry. More common in males and in first-born infants, with a familial tendency. The metabolic consequence is a hypochloraemic, hypokalaemic metabolic alkalosis, and **correction of that precedes surgery** — this is a condition where the diagnosis is urgent but the operation is not.

The single most important discrimination is the character of the vomit.

> **Non-bilious vomiting — consider pyloric stenosis. Bilious vomiting — think malrotation with volvulus and other obstruction distal to the ampulla. That is a surgical emergency (§12.3).**

Technique

Position: supine initially, then **right posterior oblique** — the infant rolled partly onto the right side — which brings gastric fluid into the antrum and the pylorus into a favourable position.

Transducer: high-frequency linear.

Finding the pylorus: identify the gallbladder as a landmark, then move the probe inferomedially. The pylorus lies between the antrum and the duodenal bulb, anterior to the right kidney and adjacent to the pancreatic head.

Gastric contents matter:

- **An empty stomach** makes the pylorus hard to find. **Give clear fluid or allow a feed** — this both fills the antrum and settles the infant.
- **An overdistended stomach** displaces the pylorus posteriorly and away from the transducer. Turning the infant right side down, or decompressing via a nasogastric tube where one is in place, restores the view.

Measurements

Two measurements, taken with the pylorus in its **long axis** and the wall measured **perpendicular to it**:

- **Muscle wall thickness** — a **single wall**, measured on the anterior wall, from the outer edge of the muscle to the mucosal interface
- **Pyloric channel length**

Both must exceed defined thresholds, and those thresholds vary slightly between departments and are age- and size-influenced. [VERIFY: current thresholds for pyloric muscle wall thickness and channel length, including any adjustment for age or weight]

Measure repeatedly across several minutes rather than accepting a single measurement, because a transiently contracted pylorus can meet the criteria momentarily.

Signs

In transverse section: a **target or doughnut** appearance — a hypoechoic muscle ring around an echogenic mucosal centre.

In long axis:

- **Cervix sign** — the appearance of the pyloric canal projecting into the antrum
- **Antral nipple sign** — redundant mucosa protruding back into the antrum
- **Shoulder sign** — the hypertrophied muscle indenting the fluid-filled antrum
- **Double-track sign** — two thin parallel channels of fluid between compressed, redundant mucosal folds

Absent gastric emptying observed in real time is as important as any measurement.

Dynamic observation — the discriminator

Watch the pylorus for several minutes. This separates the two diagnoses that share the numbers:

Pylorospasm is transient. The muscle is usually less thickened, and — decisively — **the channel opens intermittently and fluid passes through**.

Hypertrophic pyloric stenosis does not relax. The channel remains closed, no significant fluid passes, and vigorous antral peristalsis is seen ending against a closed pylorus.

A static image cannot make this distinction, and reporting from one is the commonest error in the examination.

Differential

Malrotation with volvulus — bilious vomiting, and the priority diagnosis to exclude (§12.3). **Antral web**, **gastro-oesophageal reflux**, **cow's milk protein allergy**, **overfeeding**, and **sepsis** account for most of the remainder.

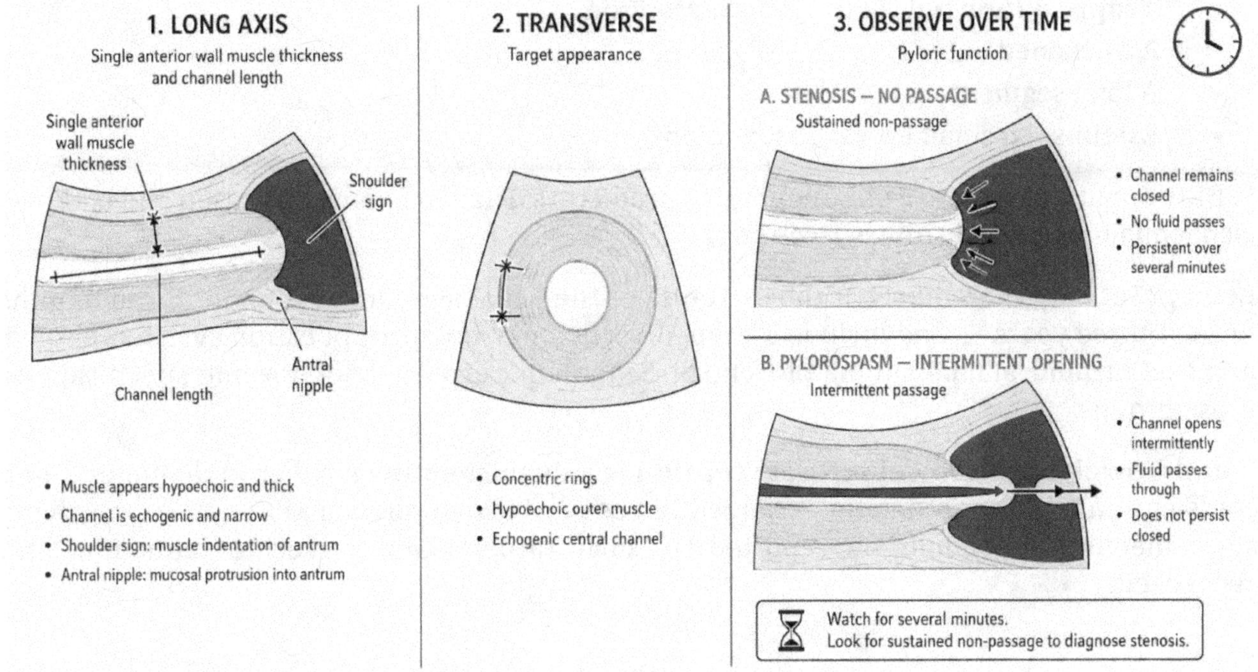

12.3 Intussusception and Malrotation

Intussusception

Telescoping of one bowel segment into the next. In children it is typically **ileocolic**, peaks between about three months and three years, and is usually **idiopathic** — attributed to lymphoid hyperplasia following a viral illness.

The classic triad of colicky pain, vomiting, and red-currant-jelly stool is frequently incomplete; a lethargic infant with intermittent screaming episodes is a common presentation.

Ultrasound is the first-line test and is highly sensitive, which makes it effectively diagnostic in experienced hands.

Findings (also Chapter 6 §6.10):

- **Transverse: the target or doughnut sign** — multiple concentric alternating hypoechoic and echogenic rings
- **Longitudinal: the pseudokidney or sandwich sign**
- Typically located in the **right upper quadrant or along the course of the colon**
- **Trapped mesenteric fat drawn in between the layers**, frequently containing **entrapped lymph nodes** — a specific and useful finding
- **Free fluid**, and fluid trapped within the intussusceptum

Features associated with failed reduction or ischaemia, which should be sought and reported because they influence management:

- **Absent flow in the wall of the intussusceptum** on colour Doppler
- **Trapped fluid** within the intussusception
- A thickened outer rim
- A long segment
- Established small bowel obstruction

[VERIFY: current evidence on sonographic predictors of failed enema reduction and of bowel ischaemia in paediatric intussusception]

Lead points are more likely at the extremes of the usual age range — under three months or over three years — and include Meckel diverticulum, polyp, duplication cyst, lymphoma, and the intramural haematoma of Henoch–Schönlein purpura. Look for one specifically in those groups.

Small-bowel–small-bowel intussusception is a distinct entity: smaller in diameter, often transient and asymptomatic, frequently seen incidentally, and usually resolving spontaneously. It should be reported as such rather than triggering reduction, and rechecked.

Management is **pneumatic or hydrostatic reduction** under fluoroscopic or ultrasound guidance, contraindicated by peritonitis, perforation, or shock. Recurrence occurs in a minority.

Malrotation and midgut volvulus

The clinical rule that governs this section:

> **Bilious vomiting in a neonate is malrotation with midgut volvulus until proven otherwise. It is a surgical emergency, and the bowel can infarct within hours.**

Normal anatomy: during rotation the duodenojejunal junction comes to lie to the left of the midline at the level of the pylorus, and the caecum in the right lower quadrant, giving a **broad mesenteric base**. In malrotation this base is narrow, allowing the midgut to twist around the superior mesenteric artery.

Sonographic signs:

1. Superior mesenteric vessel relationship. Normally the **SMV lies to the right of the SMA**. In malrotation this may be **inverted or the vein may lie directly anterior**. It is a useful screening observation but is **neither perfectly sensitive nor perfectly specific**, and normal vessel orientation does not exclude malrotation.

2. The whirlpool sign. The SMV and mesentery wrapping around the SMA in a spiral, best appreciated on a transverse sweep with colour Doppler. **This is the specific sign of volvulus** and its presence should prompt immediate surgical communication.

3. The third part of the duodenum. Normally it crosses the midline **between the SMA and the aorta**, retroperitoneally. Failure to demonstrate this normal course supports malrotation, and a fluid-filled duodenum can be traced to establish it.

4. Secondary findings: a dilated fluid-filled proximal duodenum with a tapering "beak", thickened bowel loops, and free fluid — the last suggesting compromise.

Upper gastrointestinal contrast study has been the traditional reference standard, and ultrasound is increasingly used as a first or expediting test. Local pathways differ, and the sonographer's obligation is to escalate immediately rather than to complete a survey. [VERIFY: current evidence and recommendations on ultrasound versus upper gastrointestinal contrast study for suspected malrotation]

Suspected volvulus is a critical finding requiring direct, immediate communication (Chapter 1 §1.5).

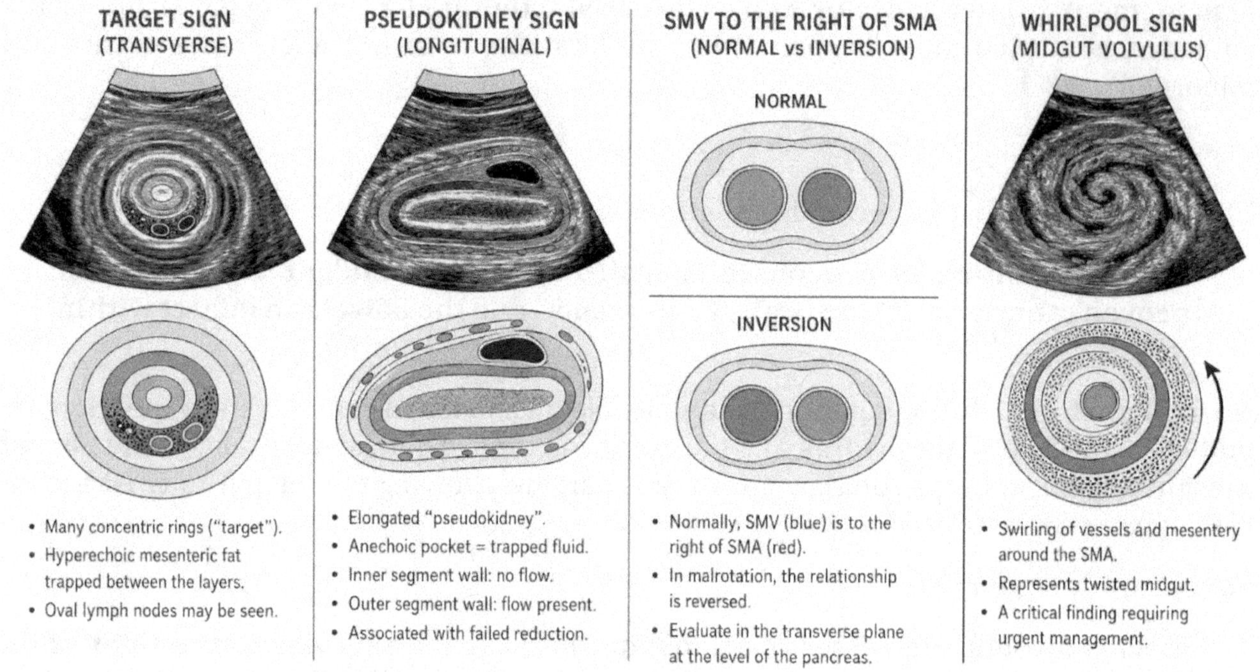

12.4 Paediatric Appendicitis

The paediatric position

Ultrasound is first-line in children, because radiation avoidance matters most in this population and because the thin abdominal wall makes the examination technically favourable.

The technique — point-of-tenderness graded compression with a high-frequency linear transducer, identification of the blind-ending non-compressible tubular structure, and the diagnostic criteria — is set out in **Chapter 6 §6.9** and is not repeated here. What follows are the paediatric modifications.

Modifications

Graded compression is well tolerated with distraction. A child who is talked through the examination, given something to watch, and has a caregiver present will usually permit adequate compression. Rushing it produces guarding and a failed study.

The appendix is smaller, and higher-frequency imaging is both possible and necessary.

Non-visualisation remains common, and the reporting obligation from Chapter 6 applies with full force: state that the appendix was not identified, describe the secondary signs present or absent — free fluid, inflamed fat, tenderness, nodes — and state the limiting factors. **"No appendicitis" from a study in which the appendix was never seen is not an acceptable report in any age group.**

Perforation is more common in younger children, who present later and localise poorly. Look for a periappendiceal collection, phlegmon, loculated fluid, and marked surrounding fat inflammation.

The paediatric mimics

Several are far more common in children than adults, and identifying one is a positive result rather than a failure:

Mesenteric adenitis — clustered enlarged mesenteric nodes with a **normal appendix**, often following a viral illness. The commonest alternative diagnosis.

Terminal ileitis — infectious or inflammatory wall thickening of the terminal ileum.

Intussusception (§12.3), particularly in the younger child.

Ovarian pathology — torsion, haemorrhagic cyst, or a complication of a cyst. **In any girl with right lower quadrant pain the pelvis must be examined**, and ovarian torsion is a diagnosis with a narrow window for salvage.

Meckel diverticulitis, **constipation**, **Henoch–Schönlein purpura** with bowel wall haematoma, **urinary tract infection**, and **pneumonia** with referred pain.

Escalation

Where ultrasound is non-diagnostic and clinical concern persists, **MRI is increasingly the second-line study in children** because it avoids radiation, with CT reserved for situations where MRI is unavailable or the child is unstable. Local pathways vary. [VERIFY: current imaging pathway recommendations for suspected paediatric appendicitis, including the role of MRI as second-line]

12.5 Paediatric Hepatic, Biliary, and Splenic Disease

The neonatal jaundice question

Jaundice is common in newborns and usually physiological. **The finding that changes everything is conjugated (direct) hyperbilirubinaemia**, which is never physiological and demands urgent assessment — principally to exclude **biliary atresia**, where the window for effective surgery is narrow (§12.6).

The sonographer's role is to perform a technically adequate hepatobiliary study, ideally with the infant fasted and then re-examined after a feed, and to escalate rather than to reassure.

Hepatic masses

Infantile hepatic haemangioma — the commonest hepatic tumour of infancy, presenting as focal, multifocal, or diffuse lesions. Sonographically, well-defined lesions with **high-velocity, low-resistance flow** and prominent vessels. Two associated observations are worth seeking:

- **Enlargement of the coeliac axis and hepatic artery**, with **reduced calibre of the aorta below the coeliac origin**, reflecting shunting
- Clinical associations with **high-output cardiac failure** and, in the diffuse form, **consumptive hypothyroidism**

Hepatoblastoma — the commonest primary hepatic malignancy of childhood, typically under five years, presenting as a large heterogeneous mass, often with calcification, with elevated alpha-fetoprotein. Assess **vascular involvement and the number of involved sectors**, since these determine the surgical approach.

Hepatocellular carcinoma occurs in older children, usually on a background of chronic liver disease.

Mesenchymal hamartoma — a benign multicystic mass in infancy.

Metastatic disease — most importantly **neuroblastoma**, which in infants may produce massive hepatic infiltration as part of a specific pattern of metastatic disease with a distinctive prognosis (§12.9).

Portal hypertension in children

The causes differ substantially from adult practice:

Extrahepatic portal vein obstruction with cavernous transformation is a leading cause of variceal bleeding in children worldwide, often following neonatal umbilical vein catheterisation or sepsis. The liver is normal; the porta contains a tangle of collaterals (Chapter 4 §4.9).

Congenital hepatic fibrosis, frequently with autosomal recessive polycystic kidney disease (§12.8).

Biliary atresia after portoenterostomy, and **cystic fibrosis liver disease**.

The sonographic complex is the same as in adults (Chapter 4 §4.5) — splenomegaly, collaterals, portal flow direction — but the **liver may look entirely normal**, which is the key difference.

Gallbladder and biliary

Gallstones in children are not rare and have specific causes: **haemolytic disease** (sickle cell disease, spherocytosis, thalassaemia), **prolonged parenteral nutrition**, **ileal disease or resection**, **cystic fibrosis**, obesity, and **ceftriaxone**, which produces a reversible biliary pseudolithiasis that resolves on stopping the drug — worth knowing before a cholecystectomy is contemplated.

Hydrops of the gallbladder occurs in Kawasaki disease and other systemic illnesses.

Choledochal cyst — §12.6.

Spleen

Splenomegaly in children most often reflects **haemolytic anaemia**, **infection**, **portal hypertension**, **storage disease**, or **malignancy**.

Sickle cell disease produces a characteristic natural history: splenic enlargement and **acute splenic sequestration crisis** in early childhood — a rapidly enlarging spleen with falling haemoglobin, a paediatric emergency — followed by progressive infarction and **autosplenectomy**, leaving a small, calcified, functionally absent spleen.

Polysplenia and asplenia occur as part of **heterotaxy syndromes** and should prompt assessment of situs and of associated cardiac anomalies (Chapter 15).

Accessory spleens are common and identified as in adults (Chapter 6 §6.5).

12.6 Biliary Atresia and Choledochal Cysts

Biliary atresia — a time-critical diagnosis

A progressive obliterative cholangiopathy of unknown cause, producing complete biliary obstruction and, untreated, cirrhosis and death in early childhood.

It presents with conjugated hyperbilirubinaemia, pale stools, and dark urine in the first weeks of life — often in an otherwise well-appearing, thriving infant, which contributes to delayed referral.

The reason urgency matters: the **Kasai portoenterostomy** re-establishes bile drainage, and its success falls markedly with increasing age at operation. Every week of diagnostic delay reduces the chance of native liver survival. [VERIFY: current evidence on age thresholds for Kasai portoenterostomy outcome]

This makes an ultrasound requested for neonatal conjugated jaundice one of the more consequential studies in this book, and it should be expedited rather than booked routinely.

Sonographic findings

The triangular cord sign — an echogenic triangular or tubular band of fibrous tissue lying **immediately anterior to the portal vein bifurcation** at the porta hepatis, representing the fibrous remnant of the extrahepatic duct. It is **highly specific** when present, and thickness criteria are applied. [VERIFY: current thickness threshold for the triangular cord sign and its reported sensitivity and specificity]

Look for it deliberately, in a **transverse or oblique view at the porta**, with a high-frequency linear probe, and measure it.

Gallbladder abnormalities — assessed **fasting and again after a feed**:

- **Absent or very small gallbladder**

- **Irregular, indistinct, or lobular wall** rather than a smooth one — the "ghost gallbladder"
- **Failure to contract after feeding** (a normal gallbladder contracts)
- Length below defined thresholds [VERIFY: current gallbladder length criteria in suspected biliary atresia]

A normal, well-formed, contracting gallbladder makes biliary atresia less likely but does **not** exclude it.

Other findings: non-visualisation of the common bile duct; **hepatic artery enlargement**; increased **hepatic subcapsular flow**; hepatomegaly with coarsened echotexture; and later, features of portal hypertension.

Associated anomalies — the **biliary atresia splenic malformation** association: polysplenia, situs anomalies, preduodenal portal vein, absent IVC, and cardiac defects. Finding polysplenia in a jaundiced infant is a significant observation.

Crucially: a normal-appearing ultrasound does not exclude biliary atresia. The pathway continues with hepatobiliary scintigraphy, liver biopsy, and operative cholangiography as locally determined. The report should state this rather than imply reassurance.

Differential diagnosis

Neonatal hepatitis (idiopathic and infective), **Alagille syndrome**, **parenteral-nutrition-associated cholestasis**, **inspissated bile syndrome**, **choledochal cyst**, and metabolic disease.

Choledochal cysts

Congenital cystic dilatation of the biliary tree, frequently associated with an **anomalous pancreaticobiliary junction** allowing pancreatic reflux into the bile duct.

Presentation: increasingly **antenatal detection**; otherwise jaundice, an abdominal mass, and pain — the classical triad rarely complete. It may present in adulthood.

A formal classification system divides them into types, of which fusiform dilatation of the common bile duct is much the commonest, with intrahepatic-only disease representing a distinct entity. [VERIFY: current choledochal cyst classification, its type definitions, and the management implications of each]

The diagnostic requirement: demonstrate communication with the biliary tree. This is what distinguishes a choledochal cyst from the other cystic right upper quadrant lesions of infancy — duplication cyst, hepatic cyst, pancreatic pseudocyst, mesenteric cyst, and ovarian cyst in girls.

A critical differential in the neonate: cystic biliary atresia can present as a cystic structure at the porta and is easily mistaken for a choledochal cyst. The distinction matters because the operations and the urgency differ, and any cystic biliary structure in a jaundiced neonate should be assessed with biliary atresia explicitly in mind.

Management is surgical excision rather than drainage, because of the **long-term risk of cholangiocarcinoma** in retained cyst epithelium.

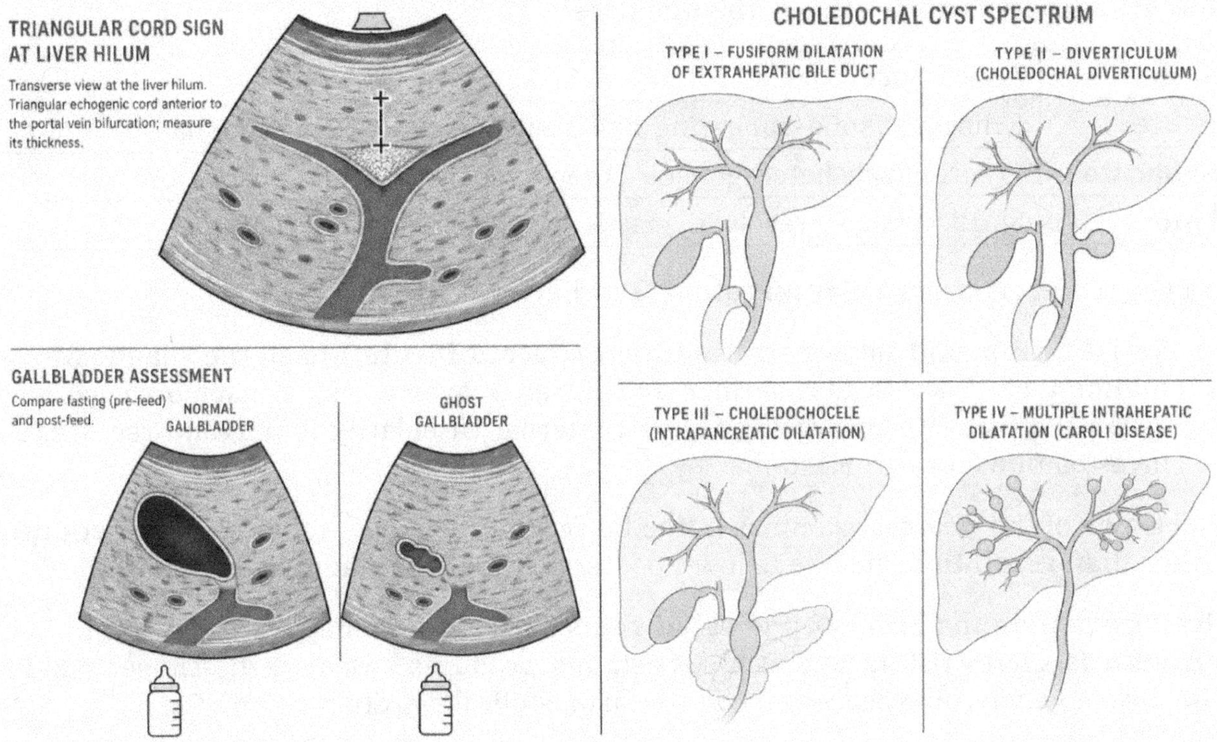

12.7 Neonatal Adrenal Haemorrhage and Masses

The normal neonatal adrenal

Unlike the adult adrenal, which is usually invisible (Chapter 7 §7.9), **the neonatal adrenal gland is relatively large and readily seen**, and its assessment is a routine and productive part of neonatal abdominal imaging.

Appearance: a **Y-, V-, or Z-shaped** structure sitting superomedial to the upper renal pole, with a **hypoechoic cortex** and a **thin echogenic central medulla**. It is proportionally much larger than in adults and involutes over the first weeks of life.

The right gland is imaged through the liver; the left through the spleen or from a posterolateral approach.

Adrenal haemorrhage

Common in neonates and usually of no long-term consequence, but its recognition matters because of what it must be distinguished from.

Risk factors: birth trauma and difficult delivery, macrosomia, perinatal hypoxia, sepsis, and coagulopathy. It is **more common on the right**, and is bilateral in a minority.

Presentation: often asymptomatic and found incidentally; otherwise a flank mass, prolonged or worsening jaundice, or anaemia.

Sonographic evolution — this is the diagnosis:

Stage	Appearance
Acute	Echogenic, solid-appearing, and easily mistaken for a solid mass
Subacute	Progressively heterogeneous, then hypoechoic with liquefaction
Late	Small, cystic, or resolved; may leave peripheral calcification

At every stage, it is avascular on colour Doppler.

> **Serial ultrasound demonstrating the expected involution is the diagnostic manoeuvre.** A lesion that shrinks and liquefies over weeks is haemorrhage; a lesion that persists, enlarges, or shows internal vascularity is not, and requires investigation for neuroblastoma.

This is one of the clearest examples in the book of ultrasound's value being in **repetition rather than resolution**, and the follow-up interval should be stated in the report.

Always examine the kidneys and renal veins at the same time — **neonatal renal vein thrombosis** shares risk factors, can coexist, and produces an enlarged echogenic kidney with absent venous flow and reversed arterial diastolic flow (Chapter 7 §7.5).

The differential

Neuroblastoma (§12.9) — solid, **vascular**, frequently calcified, does not involute, and may show local extension or metastases. Urinary catecholamine metabolites support the diagnosis.

Adrenal abscess — complex with debris, in a septic infant.

Congenital adrenal hyperplasia — bilaterally enlarged glands with a characteristic **cerebriform** surface pattern, in an infant with ambiguous genitalia or salt-wasting.

Adrenal cyst, and **extralobar pulmonary sequestration**, which sits in the suprarenal region and can closely mimic an adrenal mass — identified by its **systemic arterial supply** on colour Doppler, which is a decisive finding.

Wolman disease — bilateral adrenal enlargement with dense calcification.

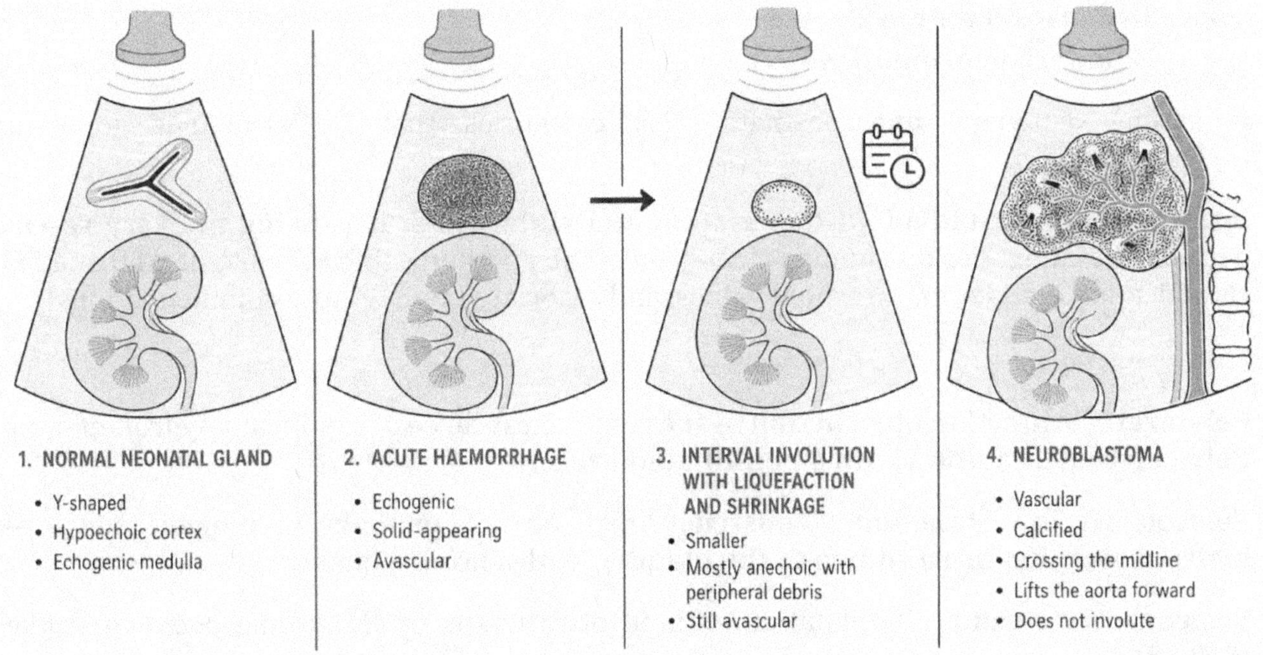

12.8 Congenital Urinary Tract Anomalies and Hydronephrosis Grading

Antenatally detected dilatation

Urinary tract dilatation is the commonest antenatally detected abnormality, and postnatal ultrasound is the follow-up pathway.

Timing matters. Scanning in the **first day or two of life underestimates dilatation**, because the neonate is relatively dehydrated and urine output is low. Postnatal imaging is therefore deferred beyond that window unless there is a reason for urgency — bilateral severe dilatation, a suspected posterior urethral valve, a solitary kidney, or oligohydramnios — in which case it is performed immediately. [VERIFY: current recommended timing of postnatal ultrasound after antenatally detected urinary tract dilatation, and the criteria for urgent early imaging]

Grading

Two systems are in common use and they are not interchangeable:

The Society for Fetal Urology grading system, based on the degree of pelvicalyceal dilatation and parenchymal thinning.

The urinary tract dilatation (UTD) classification, which is more comprehensive and is increasingly the preferred system. It stratifies risk using several parameters together:

- **Anteroposterior renal pelvic diameter**, measured in the transverse plane
- **Calyceal dilatation**, and whether it involves central or peripheral calyces
- **Parenchymal thickness and appearance**

- **Ureteric dilatation**
- **Bladder abnormalities**

It assigns antenatal and postnatal risk categories that carry defined follow-up recommendations.

A department should adopt one system and state which it is using in every report, because the categories do not map cleanly onto one another. [VERIFY: current UTD and SFU classification definitions, threshold values, and associated follow-up recommendations]

The causes

Pelviureteric junction obstruction — the commonest cause of significant hydronephrosis. **Pelvicalyceal dilatation with a non-dilated ureter.**

Vesicoureteric junction obstruction and primary megaureter — hydroureteronephrosis down to the bladder, with a normal bladder.

Vesicoureteric reflux — dilatation without obstruction, often varying between studies (§12.10).

Posterior urethral valves — the diagnosis not to miss:

> **Male infant. Bilateral hydroureteronephrosis. Thick-walled, trabeculated bladder. A dilated posterior urethra producing the "keyhole" sign.**

Associated findings include renal dysplasia (echogenic kidneys with cortical cysts), urinoma or urinary ascites from forniceal rupture, and antenatal oligohydramnios with its pulmonary consequences. **This requires urgent bladder drainage and urological referral**, and a male infant with bilateral dilatation and a thick-walled bladder should be escalated rather than reported routinely.

Duplex system with an obstructed upper pole moiety and a **ureterocele** in the bladder, and a refluxing lower pole — the Weigert–Meyer arrangement described in Chapter 7 §7.1. **When you find upper pole dilatation, examine the bladder for a ureterocele**, and vice versa.

Ectopic ureter — inserting below the bladder neck; in girls this produces continuous incontinence in a child who is otherwise toilet-trained, and the ureter may be traceable to the vagina or urethra.

Other congenital anomalies

Multicystic dysplastic kidney — a non-functioning kidney replaced by **multiple non-communicating cysts of varying size with no identifiable renal pelvis and no normal parenchyma**. It is distinguished from severe hydronephrosis by the **absence of communication between the cysts** and the absence of a dilated central pelvis. It typically involutes. **The contralateral kidney must be examined carefully**, since associated anomalies — including reflux and pelviureteric junction obstruction — are common and determine long-term function.

Renal agenesis — with contralateral compensatory hypertrophy; search the pelvis before concluding absence (Chapter 7 §7.1).

Horseshoe, ectopic, and crossed fused kidneys — as in Chapter 7 §7.1, with the same increased susceptibility to obstruction, stones, and trauma.

Autosomal recessive polycystic kidney disease — bilaterally enlarged, diffusely echogenic kidneys with loss of corticomedullary differentiation, the cysts often too small to resolve individually. Invariably associated with **congenital hepatic fibrosis**, so the liver must be assessed for periportal fibrosis and portal hypertension, and this hepatic component increasingly dominates the clinical picture with age.

Autosomal dominant polycystic kidney disease may present in childhood with discrete cysts and a family history.

Renal dysplasia — a small, echogenic kidney with loss of corticomedullary differentiation and cortical cysts.

Neonatal renal vein thrombosis — an enlarged echogenic kidney with loss of corticomedullary differentiation, absent venous flow, and **reversed arterial diastolic flow**, in an infant with dehydration, sepsis, a diabetic mother, or a central line.

Grading dilatation, and the congenital anomalies behind it.

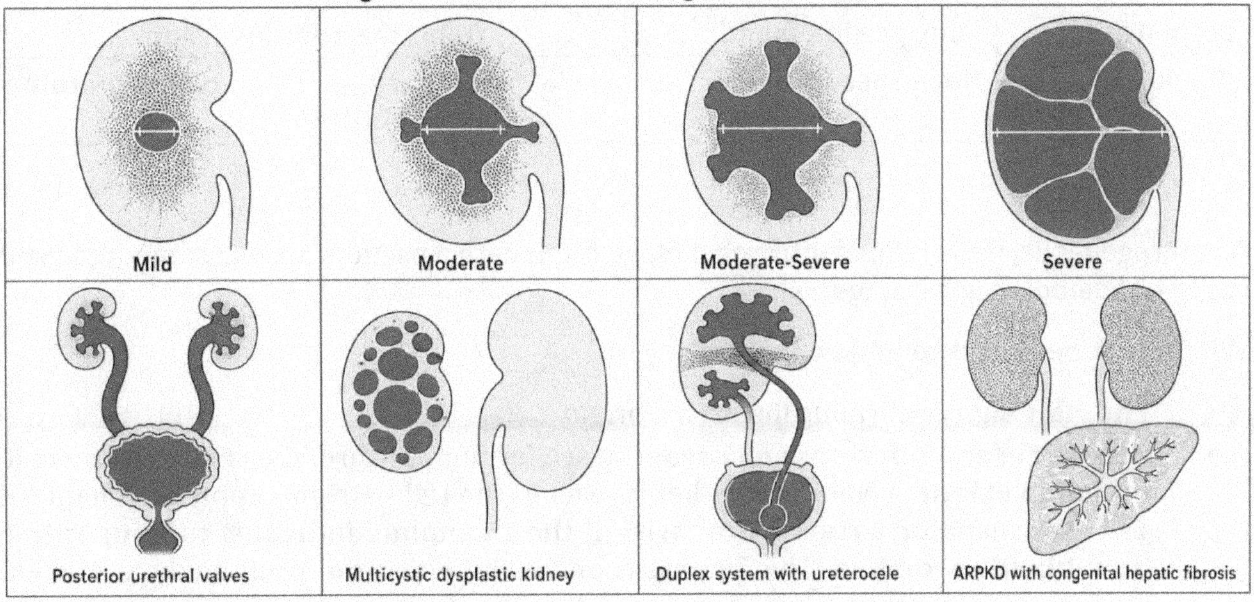

Upper: increasing grades with anteroposterior renal pelvic diameter measured; note calyceal involvement and parenchymal thickness.
Lower: common congenital anomalies associated with dilatation.

12.9 Paediatric Renal Masses: Wilms Tumour and Neuroblastoma

The central discrimination

An abdominal mass in a young child is most often one of these two, and **distinguishing them on imaging is a genuinely achievable and clinically decisive task**, because the staging pathways, the surgical approach, and the prognosis all differ.

The distinction rests on one anatomical question — **is the mass arising from the kidney or from outside it** — and on a set of behavioural differences that follow from it.

	Wilms tumour	**Neuroblastoma**
Origin	**Intrarenal** — arising from the kidney	**Extrarenal** — adrenal medulla or sympathetic chain
Typical age	Around three to four years	Younger; frequently under two years
Relationship to kidney	Arises within it, producing the **"claw sign"** of splayed residual renal parenchyma at its margin	**Displaces** the kidney downward and laterally; the kidney remains identifiable and separate
Vessel behaviour	**Displaces** vessels without encasing them	**Encases** the aorta, IVC, coeliac axis and SMA; may **lift the aorta forward off the spine**
Calcification	Uncommon	**Common**
Crosses the midline	Uncommon	**Common**
Vascular invasion	**Renal vein and IVC tumour thrombus** is characteristic	Encasement rather than intraluminal extension
Metastases	Lung predominantly	Bone, marrow, liver, and skin
Markers	None specific	**Urinary catecholamine metabolites**

Wilms tumour

A heterogeneous, well-defined intrarenal mass, often with a pseudocapsule, sometimes with cystic or haemorrhagic change.

What must be assessed and reported:

- **The claw sign** confirming intrarenal origin
- **Renal vein and inferior vena cava** — trace for tumour thrombus and determine its **cephalad extent**, including whether it reaches the right atrium. Apply the Chapter 3 §3.5 discriminator: **arterial flow within the thrombus indicates tumour rather than bland thrombus.** This finding changes the operation profoundly and is one ultrasound answers well
- **The contralateral kidney** — bilateral disease occurs in a minority and alters management entirely
- **The liver** for metastases
- **Nephrogenic rests / nephroblastomatosis** — homogeneous peripheral subcapsular lesions representing precursor tissue, which warrant surveillance

Syndromic associations — Beckwith–Wiedemann, WAGR, hemihypertrophy, Denys–Drash — place children in surveillance programmes, and knowing that a child is under surveillance changes the threshold for concern.

A note on biopsy: management protocols differ internationally in whether preoperative biopsy is performed or avoided, because in some staging systems biopsy upstages the tumour. **Do not assume a biopsy pathway.** [VERIFY: current protocol position on preoperative biopsy of suspected Wilms tumour in the relevant jurisdiction]

Neuroblastoma

A heterogeneous, often poorly marginated suprarenal or paraspinal mass, **frequently containing calcification** and characteristically **encasing rather than displacing** the great vessels.

What must be assessed:

- **Vessel encasement** — which vessels, and whether the aorta is lifted anteriorly off the vertebral bodies
- **Midline crossing**
- **Liver** — infantile metastatic disease may produce massive hepatic infiltration as part of a specific pattern with a distinctive natural history and prognosis
- **Paraspinal extension** — a "dumbbell" configuration through the neural foramina, which requires MRI and has neurological implications
- The **kidney**, confirming it is displaced rather than invaded

The other paediatric renal masses

Mesoblastic nephroma — the **commonest renal tumour of the neonate**, benign, typically presenting under three months as a solid intrarenal mass. Age is the strongest discriminator from Wilms tumour.

Rhabdoid tumour and **clear cell sarcoma** — aggressive, and not reliably distinguishable from Wilms on imaging.

Multilocular cystic nephroma — a well-defined multiseptated cystic mass.

Renal cell carcinoma — occurs in older children and adolescents.

Lymphoma and leukaemic infiltration — bilateral, producing enlarged kidneys with multiple hypoechoic masses or diffuse infiltration.

Adrenal haemorrhage (§12.7) — the benign mimic, distinguished by avascularity and involution.

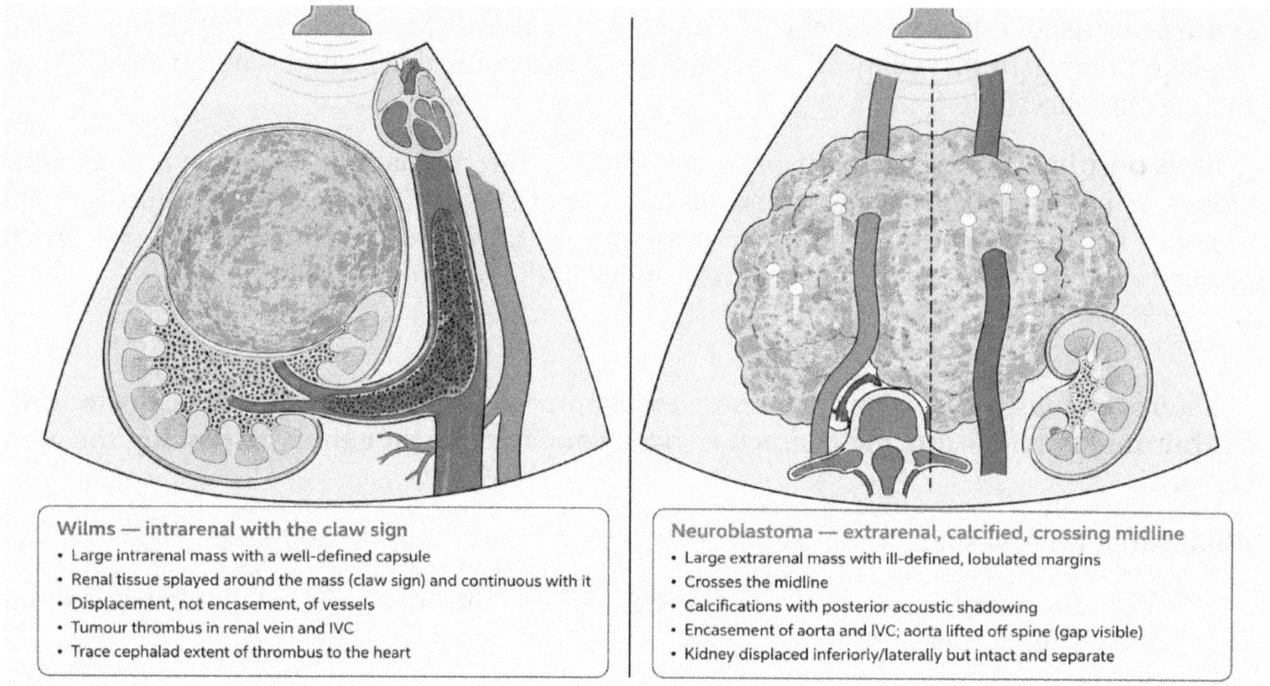

12.10 Vesicoureteric Reflux and Contrast-Enhanced Voiding Urosonography

Why reflux matters

Vesicoureteric reflux is retrograde flow of urine from the bladder into the upper tract, resulting from a short or abnormal intramural ureteric tunnel (**primary**) or from raised bladder pressure in outlet obstruction or neurogenic bladder (**secondary**).

Its significance is not the reflux itself but its consequences: **recurrent urinary infection, acute pyelonephritis, renal scarring (reflux nephropathy), hypertension, and in severe cases chronic kidney disease.**

Standard greyscale ultrasound cannot diagnose or exclude reflux. It may show hydronephrosis that varies between studies, a dilated ureter, urothelial thickening, or scarring — all suggestive, none diagnostic. A dedicated cystographic study is required.

The investigations

Study	What it provides	Cost
Fluoroscopic voiding cystourethrography (VCUG/MCUG)	The traditional reference standard; grades reflux; **images the urethra**, which is essential in boys to exclude posterior urethral valves	**Ionising radiation** to the pelvis and gonads in a young child

Study	What it provides	Cost
Contrast-enhanced voiding urosonography (ceVUS)	Detects and grades reflux; **no ionising radiation**; allows prolonged and repeated observation	Requires catheterisation; urethral assessment needs specific technique; availability and regulatory status vary
DMSA scintigraphy	Cortical scarring and differential function	Radiation; does not assess reflux

Contrast-enhanced voiding urosonography

An application of **intracavitary contrast** (Chapter 9 §9.3): ultrasound contrast agent is instilled into the bladder rather than injected intravenously, and reflux is detected as **microbubbles appearing in the ureter and pelvicalyceal system**.

Technique:

1. **Confirm the child is free of active urinary infection**, and follow local policy on antibiotic prophylaxis. Obtain **informed consent** for catheterisation and contrast (Chapter 1 §1.5).
2. **Baseline greyscale ultrasound** of both kidneys, ureters, and bladder.
3. **Aseptic urethral catheterisation** — the least pleasant part of the study, and the point at which the child's cooperation is most at risk. Distraction and a calm unhurried approach matter.
4. **Instil saline mixed with ultrasound contrast agent** by gravity, with the bladder filled to age-appropriate capacity.
5. **Scan continuously and alternately** — right kidney, left kidney, bladder, and the retrovesical ureters — **during filling, during voiding, and after voiding**. Reflux is frequently intermittent, and voiding is when it most often occurs.
6. **Grade** the reflux by the extent of contrast in the ureter and collecting system and the degree of dilatation, using the categories analogous to the fluoroscopic grading scale.
7. Assess **post-void residual**, bladder wall thickness, and any ureterocele or duplication.

[VERIFY: current reflux grading definitions, and current recommendations, contrast dosing, and regulatory status for contrast-enhanced voiding urosonography, which is off-label in some jurisdictions]

Advantages over fluoroscopy:

- **No ionising radiation** in a young child undergoing a study that is frequently repeated
- **Prolonged and repeated observation** is possible without a radiation penalty, which increases detection of **intermittent** reflux
- Excellent simultaneous assessment of renal parenchyma and the collecting system
- Well suited to **follow-up** of known reflux

Limitations:

- **The urethra is not assessed** in the standard technique. **In a boy in whom posterior urethral valves must be excluded, the urethral study is the point of the examination**, and a transperineal technique or fluoroscopic VCUG is required. This is the single most important limitation to understand.
- Catheterisation is still required — ceVUS avoids radiation, not instrumentation
- Operator time and expertise
- Regulatory and licensing status varies

Associated assessment

Bladder–bowel dysfunction is common in children with reflux and recurrent infection, and ultrasound contributes by measuring **post-void residual**, **bladder wall thickness**, and **rectal diameter** as a marker of constipation. Addressing it is often as important as addressing the reflux itself.

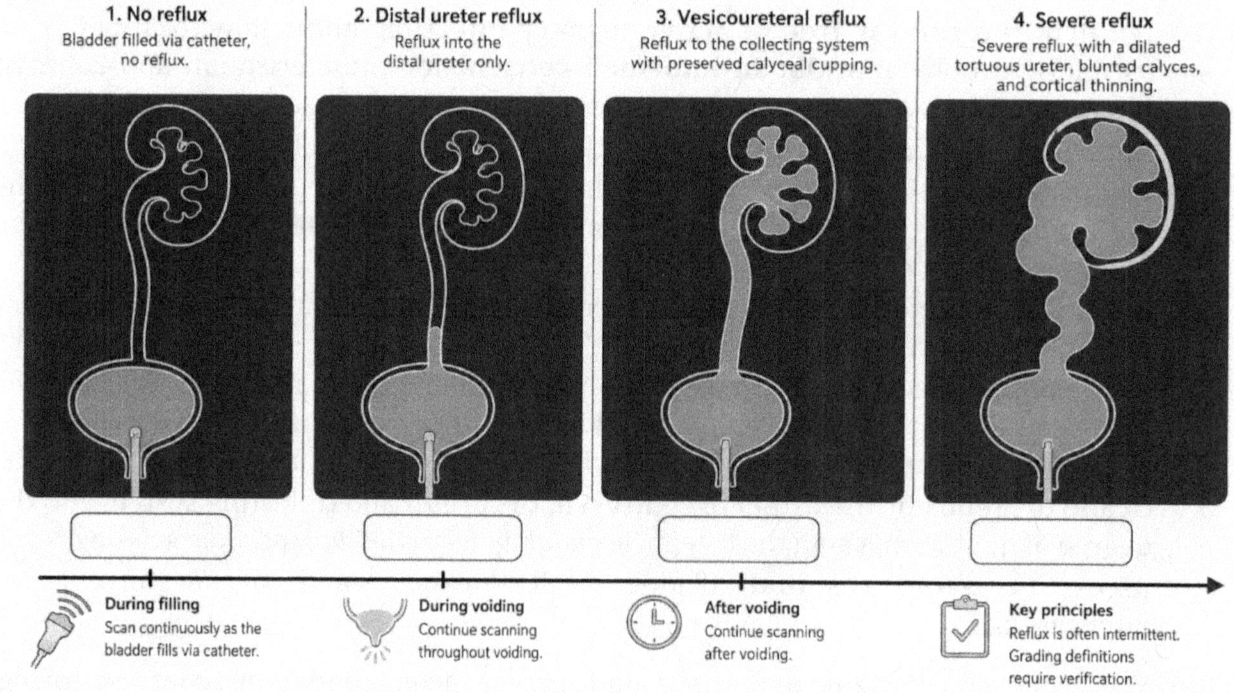

Key Points

1. Children permit far higher frequencies than adults. Scanning a child with adult settings discards most of the available resolution, and it is the commonest technical failure in paediatric practice.
2. Warm the gel and the room, expose the minimum area, and scan an unstable neonate in the incubator. Thermal management is part of the examination.
3. Feeding is both distraction and technique — an infant sucking is an infant lying still.
4. Non-bilious vomiting suggests pyloric stenosis. **Bilious vomiting in a neonate is malrotation with volvulus until proven otherwise.**

5. Pyloric stenosis is diagnosed by watching, not by a still frame. Pylorospasm opens intermittently; stenosis does not.
6. Entrapped mesenteric fat and lymph nodes within an intussusception are a specific finding; absent flow in the intussusceptum wall predicts difficulty with reduction.
7. Small-bowel–small-bowel intussusception is usually transient and self-limiting. Report it as such rather than triggering reduction.
8. Inverted superior mesenteric vessels are suggestive but imperfect. The **whirlpool sign** is the specific sign of volvulus and warrants immediate surgical contact.
9. In any girl with right lower quadrant pain, examine the pelvis — ovarian torsion has a narrow salvage window.
10. Conjugated hyperbilirubinaemia in an infant is never physiological, and the biliary atresia pathway is time-critical.
11. Assess the gallbladder fasting and after a feed, and look deliberately for the triangular cord sign at the porta. A normal ultrasound does not exclude biliary atresia.
12. Demonstrating communication with the biliary tree is what identifies a choledochal cyst — and cystic biliary atresia is the differential that must not be missed.
13. The neonatal adrenal is large and readily seen. Adrenal haemorrhage is avascular and involutes; neuroblastoma is vascular, calcifies, and does not. Serial ultrasound is the diagnostic manoeuvre.
14. Defer postnatal imaging of antenatal dilatation beyond the first day or two, unless there is a reason for urgency — and a male infant with bilateral dilatation and a thick-walled bladder is such a reason.
15. Posterior urethral valves: male, bilateral hydroureteronephrosis, trabeculated bladder, keyhole posterior urethra. Escalate.
16. When you find a dilated upper pole moiety, look in the bladder for a ureterocele.
17. Multicystic dysplastic kidney has non-communicating cysts and no renal pelvis — and the contralateral kidney must be examined, because that is where function resides.
18. Wilms tumour is intrarenal with a claw sign and displaces vessels; neuroblastoma is extrarenal, calcifies, crosses the midline, and encases them.
19. Trace the renal vein and IVC to the atrium in suspected Wilms tumour. Arterial flow within thrombus means tumour thrombus, and the cephalad extent changes the operation.
20. Standard ultrasound cannot exclude vesicoureteric reflux.
21. Contrast-enhanced voiding urosonography detects reflux without radiation and permits prolonged observation — but it does not image the urethra in the standard technique, and in a boy with suspected posterior urethral valves the urethra is the point of the study.

Registry Check

1. A four-week-old infant presents with projectile non-bilious vomiting. Pyloric muscle measurements are borderline. The most important additional assessment is:

A. Measuring the pylorus in a second plane **B.** Observing the pyloric channel in real time for several minutes to determine whether fluid passes **C.** Applying colour Doppler to the pyloric muscle **D.** Repeating the measurements after a feed

> **Answer: B.** Pylorospasm and hypertrophic pyloric stenosis can produce overlapping measurements. Pylorospasm relaxes intermittently and allows fluid through; stenosis does not. Sustained non-passage observed dynamically is what distinguishes them, and a static image cannot make the distinction.

2. A neonate presents with bilious vomiting. The priority diagnosis to exclude is:

A. Hypertrophic pyloric stenosis **B.** Gastro-oesophageal reflux **C.** Malrotation with midgut volvulus **D.** Intussusception

> **Answer: C.** Bile in the vomit indicates obstruction distal to the ampulla, and malrotation with volvulus is the diagnosis that can infarct the entire midgut within hours. Pyloric stenosis produces non-bilious vomiting because the obstruction is proximal to the ampulla.

3. On transverse imaging of the upper abdomen in an infant, the superior mesenteric vein and surrounding mesentery are seen wrapping in a spiral around the superior mesenteric artery. This represents:

A. Normal variant vessel orientation **B.** The whirlpool sign of midgut volvulus **C.** Superior mesenteric artery syndrome **D.** Intussusception

> **Answer: B.** The spiral wrapping of the vein and mesentery around the artery is the whirlpool sign, specific for midgut volvulus, and is a critical finding requiring immediate surgical communication. Simple inversion of the vessel positions is suggestive of malrotation but is neither perfectly sensitive nor specific.

4. A six-week-old infant has conjugated hyperbilirubinaemia and pale stools. Ultrasound shows a small, irregular gallbladder that does not contract after a feed, and an echogenic triangular structure anterior to the portal vein bifurcation. These findings suggest:

A. Neonatal hepatitis **B.** Choledochal cyst **C.** Biliary atresia **D.** Inspissated bile syndrome

> **Answer: C.** The triangular cord sign and an abnormal, non-contracting "ghost" gallbladder are the characteristic sonographic features of biliary atresia. The diagnosis is time-critical because the success of portoenterostomy declines with increasing age at surgery, so these findings require urgent escalation.

5. A well neonate has an echogenic suprarenal mass found incidentally. It shows no internal flow on colour Doppler. The most appropriate next step is:

A. Urgent biopsy **B.** CT of the abdomen **C.** Interval ultrasound to demonstrate expected involution **D.** Immediate surgical referral

> **Answer: C.** Acute adrenal haemorrhage is echogenic and solid-appearing, and is distinguished from neuroblastoma by being avascular and by shrinking and

liquefying over subsequent weeks. Serial ultrasound demonstrating that expected evolution is the diagnostic manoeuvre; a lesion that persists, enlarges, or shows vascularity requires further investigation.

6. A male neonate has bilateral hydroureteronephrosis, a thick-walled trabeculated bladder, and a dilated posterior urethra. This indicates:

A. Vesicoureteric reflux **B.** Posterior urethral valves **C.** Pelviureteric junction obstruction **D.** Multicystic dysplastic kidney

Answer: B. The combination of male sex, bilateral upper tract dilatation, a thick-walled trabeculated bladder, and the dilated posterior urethra producing the keyhole appearance is characteristic of posterior urethral valves. It requires urgent bladder drainage and urological referral.

7. A large abdominal mass in a two-year-old encases the aorta, lifts it forward off the vertebral bodies, crosses the midline, and contains calcification. The kidney is displaced but intact. This favours:

A. Wilms tumour **B.** Neuroblastoma **C.** Mesoblastic nephroma **D.** Multilocular cystic nephroma

Answer: B. Vessel encasement rather than displacement, anterior displacement of the aorta off the spine, midline crossing, and calcification are all characteristic of neuroblastoma. Wilms tumour arises within the kidney, produces the claw sign of splayed renal parenchyma, displaces rather than encases vessels, and calcifies uncommonly.

8. Contrast-enhanced voiding urosonography is being considered in a male infant with recurrent urinary infection and suspected posterior urethral valves. The principal limitation of the standard technique is that it:

A. Cannot detect vesicoureteric reflux **B.** Requires ionising radiation **C.** Does not image the urethra **D.** Cannot be repeated

Answer: C. ceVUS detects and grades reflux without radiation and permits prolonged observation, but the standard technique does not assess the urethra. Where posterior urethral valves must be excluded, urethral imaging is the point of the study, requiring either a dedicated transperineal technique or fluoroscopic voiding cystourethrography.

Chapter Notes for the Editorial Pass

Verification queue. In priority order: **urinary tract dilatation classification definitions, thresholds, and follow-up recommendations** (§12.8) — the book must adopt one system and apply it consistently, because the SFU and UTD categories do not map onto one another; **pyloric muscle thickness and channel length thresholds**, including any age or weight adjustment (§12.2); **age thresholds for Kasai portoenterostomy outcome, and the triangular cord thickness criterion with its reported performance** (§12.6);

choledochal cyst classification and the management implications of each type (§12.6); **reflux grading definitions and the current recommendations, dosing, and regulatory status of ceVUS**, which is off-label in some jurisdictions (§12.10); **timing of postnatal imaging after antenatally detected dilatation and the criteria for urgent early imaging** (§12.8); **protocol position on preoperative biopsy of suspected Wilms tumour**, which differs internationally (§12.9); **sonographic predictors of failed intussusception reduction** (§12.3); **imaging pathway for suspected paediatric appendicitis including the role of MRI** (§12.4); and **the paediatric organ size reference source to be adopted**, indexed to age or body size (§12.1).

Structural note. This chapter deliberately defers appendiceal technique to Chapter 6 §6.9 rather than duplicating it, covering only the paediatric modifications and mimics. Confirm at layout that the cross-reference is prominent, so a reader coming to Chapter 12 for paediatric appendicitis is directed to the technique rather than concluding it is absent.

Figure count: 7 Lane A, 2 Lane B. Lane B demand is modest because paediatric pathology is largely pattern-based and the patterns are geometric. The pyloric measurement pair is the higher-value acquisition of the two, and a short cine clip demonstrating absent channel opening would teach the §12.2 dynamic point far better than any still image — worth capturing if the archive permits video.

Cross-reference targets to fix at layout: §12.1 ALARA → Chapter 1 §1.7; §12.1 infection control → Chapter 1 §1.4; §12.3 intussusception → Chapter 6 §6.10; §12.4 appendiceal technique → Chapter 6 §6.9; §12.5 portal hypertension complex → Chapter 4 §4.5; §12.5 cavernous transformation → Chapter 4 §4.9; §12.5 heterotaxy → Chapter 15; §12.7 renal vein thrombosis → Chapter 7 §7.5; §12.8 duplex system and Weigert–Meyer → Chapter 7 §7.1; §12.9 tumour thrombus discrimination → Chapter 3 §3.5; §12.10 intracavitary contrast → Chapter 9 §9.3.

Word count: approximately 10,400 excluding image prompt blocks, learning objectives, registry questions, and these notes.

Chapter 13: The Neonatal Brain, Spine, and Hip

Learning Objectives

On completing this chapter you should be able to:

1. Select the appropriate cranial acoustic window and perform the standard coronal and sagittal plane series.
2. Identify normal neonatal cranial anatomy by plane, including the caudothalamic groove and the normal echogenicity hierarchy.
3. Recognise and grade germinal matrix and intraventricular haemorrhage, and describe its evolution.
4. Distinguish periventricular leukomalacia from normal peritrigonal echogenicity, and explain why scan timing determines what is seen.
5. Recognise the patterns of hypoxic-ischaemic injury in the term infant and interpret the resistive index correctly.
6. Measure ventricular size, distinguish hydrocephalus from atrophy, and perform the fontanelle compression test.
7. Identify the major congenital malformations and the sonographic markers of congenital infection.
8. Perform a neonatal spinal ultrasound, identify the conus level, and assess cord motion.
9. Recognise the features of spinal dysraphism and tethered cord.
10. Obtain a valid standard coronal plane of the infant hip, measure the alpha and beta angles, and perform dynamic assessment.

Three Examinations with One Thing in Common

The neonatal brain, spine, and hip share a single enabling fact: **they are accessible to ultrasound only because ossification is incomplete.** The anterior fontanelle is an open window into the skull; the unfused posterior vertebral elements let sound reach the cord; the unossified femoral head lets the acetabulum be seen.

All three windows close. The fontanelle narrows through the first year, the spinal window is reliable only for the first few months, and the femoral head ossifies at around four to six months and obscures the hip. **Each of these examinations therefore has an expiry date**, which is why they are performed early, why timing appears throughout this chapter, and why a delayed request may simply be unanswerable by this modality.

13.1 Cranial Acoustic Windows and Scanning Planes

The windows

Window	Access	Best for
Anterior fontanelle	The primary window; diamond-shaped, at the junction of coronal and sagittal sutures	Supratentorial anatomy — ventricles, germinal matrix, periventricular white matter, midline structures
Mastoid fontanelle	Behind and above the ear, between temporal, parietal and occipital bones	**Posterior fossa** — cerebellum, fourth ventricle, cisterna magna. Substantially better than the anterior view for the cerebellum, and consistently underused
Posterior fontanelle	At the junction of sagittal and lambdoid sutures	Occipital horns and peritrigonal region; useful for occipital clot and for posterior periventricular echogenicity
Squamosal (temporal)	Above the ear	Axial images for midline shift; transcranial Doppler of the circle of Willis
Foramen magnum	Below the occiput, neck flexed	Craniocervical junction, cerebellar tonsils

The anterior fontanelle window degrades as it closes. Image quality falls progressively through the first year, and by the time it is closed the examination is no longer possible — a hard limit that should be stated in the report when the window is small.

Equipment and technique

Transducer: a **small-footprint sector or microconvex probe** at the highest frequency that penetrates. Preterm infants tolerate — and benefit from — higher frequencies than term infants. A high-frequency linear probe is a valuable **addition** for the superficial cortex, extra-axial spaces, and the superior sagittal sinus, and is routinely omitted.

Settings: depth set to the far side of the skull, single focal zone at the region of interest, harmonics on.

Neonatal care is part of the examination (Chapter 12 §12.1): warm gel, minimal handling, scanning through the incubator port where the infant is unstable, and short exposure times consistent with ALARA (Chapter 1 §1.7). Hand hygiene and probe cleaning between infants are non-negotiable in a neonatal unit.

The standard plane series

Coronal planes — probe oriented transversely across the fontanelle, marker to the patient's right, swept from front to back. Six planes are conventionally recorded:

1. **Frontal lobes**, anterior to the frontal horns
2. **Frontal horns and caudate heads**, with the cavum septi pellucidi

3. **Foramina of Monro and third ventricle**, with the thalami
4. **Bodies of the lateral ventricles**, with choroid plexus, hippocampi, tentorium and cerebellum
5. **Trigones**, with the glomus of the choroid plexus
6. **Occipital lobes**, posterior to the trigones

Sagittal and parasagittal planes — probe rotated 90°, marker anterior, angled from midline out to each side:

1. **Midline sagittal** — corpus callosum, cavum septi pellucidi, third ventricle, brainstem, cerebellar vermis, fourth ventricle, cisterna magna
2. **Parasagittal through the caudothalamic groove** — the single most important plane in preterm imaging (§13.3)
3. **Parasagittal through the lateral ventricle body and atrium**
4. **Far lateral** — periventricular white matter, insula and Sylvian fissure

Mastoid views are added routinely in any preterm study and whenever posterior fossa pathology is a question — **cerebellar haemorrhage is missed from the anterior fontanelle alone.**

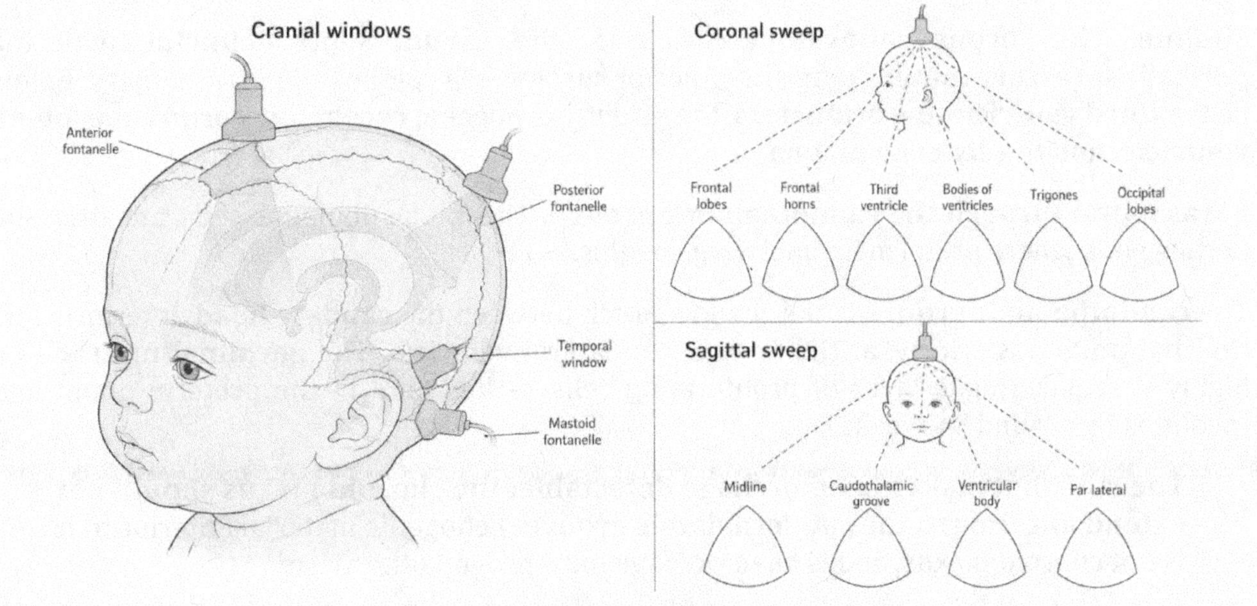

The cranial windows and the standard plane series.
Anterior, posterior and mastoid fontanelles, plus the temporal window. Coronal sweep: six planes from frontal to occipital regions. Sagittal sweep: midline to far lateral. Mastoid views assess the posterior fossa.

13.2 Normal Neonatal Cranial Anatomy by Plane

Coronal series, front to back

Plane 1 — frontal lobes. Symmetrical frontal lobes, the interhemispheric fissure in the midline, and the echogenic orbital roofs inferiorly. No ventricle yet.

Plane 2 — frontal horns. The frontal horns appear as thin slit-like anechoic spaces, separated by the **cavum septi pellucidi** — a normal midline fluid space in the neonate, particularly the preterm, which involutes over the first months. The **caudate heads** lie inferolateral to the frontal horns, and the **corpus callosum** forms the roof.

Plane 3 — foramina of Monro. The frontal horns communicate with the slit-like **third ventricle**; the **thalami** lie either side; the **Sylvian fissures** are seen laterally with pulsating **circle of Willis** vessels in the basal cisterns.

Plane 4 — ventricular bodies. The bodies of the lateral ventricles contain **echogenic choroid plexus**; the **hippocampi** lie inferomedially; the echogenic **tentorium** separates the cerebrum from the **cerebellum**, with the **fourth ventricle** between the cerebellar hemispheres.

Plane 5 — trigones. The **glomus of the choroid plexus** is large and brightly echogenic here **— a normal structure, and one of the commonest things mistaken for haemorrhage.** The periventricular white matter surrounds it.

Plane 6 — occipital lobes. Posterior periventricular white matter and occipital cortex.

Sagittal series

Midline. The **corpus callosum** arches over the **cavum septi pellucidi**, with the **pericallosal artery** running along its superior surface — a colour Doppler landmark. Below lie the **third ventricle**, the **brainstem**, the brightly echogenic **cerebellar vermis**, the **fourth ventricle**, and the **cisterna magna**.

Parasagittal through the caudothalamic groove. This plane demands separate attention because it is where preterm haemorrhage begins.

The **caudothalamic groove** is the shallow notch between the **caudate head** anteriorly and the **thalamus** posteriorly, at the floor of the lateral ventricle. The **germinal matrix** — a highly vascular, fragile layer of proliferating cells — lies here in the preterm infant and involutes by around 34 weeks.

> **The rule that makes haemorrhage detectable: the choroid plexus should not extend anterior to the caudothalamic groove.** Echogenic material anterior to it is not choroid plexus, and is haemorrhage until proven otherwise.

Parasagittal through the ventricular body and atrium, then **far lateral** through the periventricular white matter, insula and Sylvian fissure.

The echogenicity hierarchy

Normal relationships must be internalised, because almost all pathology in §13.3 and §13.4 is detected as a departure from them:

> **Choroid plexus and cerebellar vermis are the brightest normal structures. Periventricular white matter should be LESS echogenic than choroid plexus.**

Peritrigonal blush — a mild, **symmetrical**, ill-defined increase in echogenicity in the white matter behind and above the trigones — is a normal finding, is **less echogenic than choroid plexus**, exerts no mass effect, and fades on angling the probe. Distinguishing it from early periventricular leukomalacia is the subject of §13.4 and is one of the harder judgements in neonatal cranial ultrasound.

Ventricular size is assessed against gestational-age-referenced measurements (§13.5).

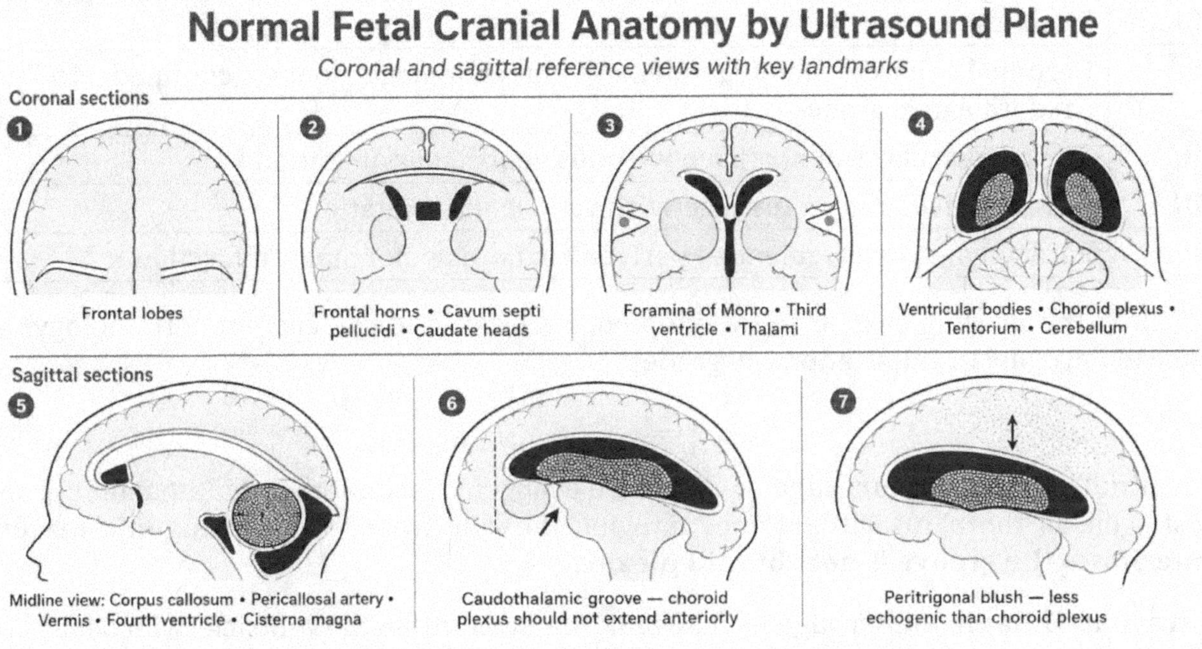

Normal anatomy by plane, and the two rules that make pathology detectable.

13.3 Germinal Matrix and Intraventricular Haemorrhage

Why it happens

The **germinal matrix** is a transient, highly cellular, richly vascularised structure at the caudothalamic groove, supplying neuronal and glial precursors. Its vessels are thin-walled and fragile, and it lies in a vascular watershed.

Preterm infants are at risk because the matrix is still present, cerebral autoregulation is immature, and the clinical course frequently involves fluctuating cerebral perfusion. Contributing factors include hypoxia, hypercapnia, hypotension and rapid volume expansion, patent ductus arteriosus, pneumothorax, and difficult resuscitation.

Timing: the majority of haemorrhages occur within the first few days of life, which is why screening protocols specify early scanning with defined repeat intervals. [VERIFY: current recommended screening schedule for cranial ultrasound in preterm infants, including gestational age thresholds and scan timing]

Grading

The long-established grading scheme divides haemorrhage into four grades. Grade IV is now understood not as simple extension of blood into the parenchyma but as **periventricular haemorrhagic infarction** — venous infarction of the periventricular white matter secondary to the germinal matrix haemorrhage obstructing the terminal veins — and many units now use that term.

Grade	Findings
I	Germinal matrix (subependymal) haemorrhage only, confined to the caudothalamic groove
II	Intraventricular haemorrhage **without** ventricular dilatation
III	Intraventricular haemorrhage **with** ventricular dilatation
IV	Parenchymal involvement — periventricular haemorrhagic infarction

[VERIFY: the grading system to be adopted, its exact criteria, current terminology, and reported prognostic implications by grade]

Findings

Germinal matrix haemorrhage — a rounded echogenic focus at the caudothalamic groove, best seen on the parasagittal plane, applying the rule from §13.2: **echogenic material anterior to the groove is not choroid plexus.**

Intraventricular haemorrhage — echogenic material within the ventricle, which may layer dependently, cast a clot within the ventricular lumen, or fill and distend the ventricle. Compare with the expected position and shape of choroid plexus; an irregular, bulky, or asymmetric "plexus" is clot.

Ventricular dilatation — assessed and measured as in §13.5, and compared with the previous study.

Periventricular haemorrhagic infarction — a **unilateral**, globular or fan-shaped echogenic region in the white matter adjacent to and contiguous with the dilated ventricle, typically on the side of the larger haemorrhage. Its distribution follows the terminal vein territory.

Cerebellar haemorrhage — increasingly recognised in very preterm infants and **missed from the anterior fontanelle**. It requires **mastoid views**, where it appears as a focal or diffuse echogenic area in the cerebellar hemisphere or vermis.

Evolution

Serial ultrasound is the standard of care, and knowing the expected evolution allows the age of a haemorrhage to be estimated:

1. **Acute** — echogenic, sometimes strikingly so

2. **Over one to two weeks** — the clot retracts and becomes progressively less echogenic, developing a hypoechoic centre
3. **Weeks to months** — liquefaction; a parenchymal infarct evolves into a **porencephalic cyst** communicating with the ventricle; intraventricular clot may leave **ventricular wall irregularity and intraventricular septations**

Complications to seek on follow-up: post-haemorrhagic ventricular dilatation (§13.5), porencephaly, and — where blood has provoked ependymal reaction — loculated ventricles that complicate later shunting.

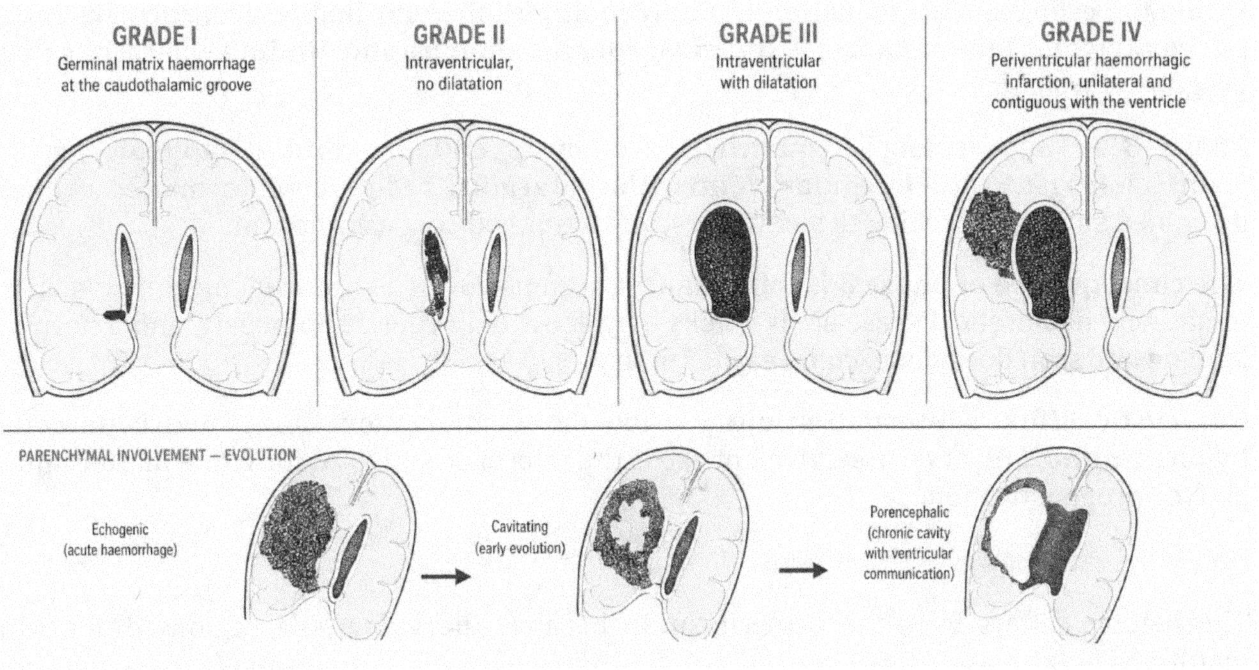

13.4 Periventricular Leukomalacia and Hypoxic-Ischaemic Injury

Periventricular leukomalacia

Ischaemic injury to the **periventricular white matter** — a vascular watershed in the preterm brain, and the site of the descending motor fibres to the lower limbs. This anatomical fact explains the characteristic clinical outcome: **spastic diplegia**.

The central teaching point of this section:

> **What you see depends entirely on when you scan relative to the insult.** A single study cannot exclude periventricular leukomalacia, and the timing of the scan must be interpreted against the timing of the clinical events.

The sequence:

Phase 1 — increased periventricular echogenicity (first days to first week or two). The white matter around the ventricles becomes echogenic.

To be significant rather than normal peritrigonal blush, the echogenicity should be:

- **Equal to or greater than the choroid plexus** in brightness — the comparison from §13.2
- **Globular, coarse, or asymmetric**, rather than smooth and symmetrical
- **Persistent** on repeat scanning beyond one to two weeks

Transient echogenicity that fades is common and usually of no consequence.

Phase 2 — cystic change (roughly two to six weeks after the insult). Small cysts appear within the echogenic white matter, typically multiple, bilateral, and periventricular. **Cystic periventricular leukomalacia is the most specific sonographic finding** and carries clear prognostic weight.

Phase 3 — late changes (months). The cysts collapse and disappear, leaving ventriculomegaly with **irregular ventricular margins**, reduced white matter volume, deepened sulci approaching the ventricles, and a thinned corpus callosum.

The consequence of phase 3 is important: a scan performed at term-equivalent age in an infant who had cystic disease at six weeks may show only ventriculomegaly, and a normal-looking late scan does not exclude earlier injury.

Non-cystic diffuse white matter injury is now the commoner form and is **poorly detected by ultrasound**. MRI at term-equivalent age is the reference standard for white matter injury and for prognostication.

Hypoxic-ischaemic injury in the term infant

The pattern differs from the preterm brain because the vulnerable regions differ with maturity.

Acute profound asphyxia injures the metabolically active deep structures: the **basal ganglia and thalami**, which become abnormally echogenic, and the perirolandic cortex.

Partial prolonged asphyxia injures the **parasagittal watershed** cortex and subcortical white matter.

Diffuse cerebral oedema produces a characteristic global appearance: **slit-like or effaced ventricles**, loss of sulcal and cisternal definition, blurring of grey–white differentiation, and diffusely increased parenchymal echogenicity — sometimes described as the "bright brain". It is a **subjective and difficult** assessment, best made by comparison with an earlier study in the same infant.

The resistive index in hypoxic-ischaemic encephalopathy

The Doppler behaviour is distinctive and prognostically useful, but only if the sequence is understood:

- **Early** — the resistive index may be **elevated**, reflecting raised cerebrovascular resistance and oedema

- **After roughly the first day** — as autoregulation fails and cerebral vasoparalysis develops, resistance falls and the resistive index becomes **abnormally low**. A markedly low resistive index in an encephalopathic term infant is an **adverse prognostic sign**

Therapeutic hypothermia alters this relationship, as do patent ductus arteriosus, sedative and inotropic drugs, hypercapnia, and heart rate — so the value must be interpreted in the full clinical context and never in isolation. [VERIFY: current resistive index thresholds and their prognostic performance in term hypoxic-ischaemic encephalopathy, including the effect of therapeutic hypothermia]

MRI remains the definitive modality for hypoxic-ischaemic injury, and the ultrasound report should direct there rather than attempting prognostication.

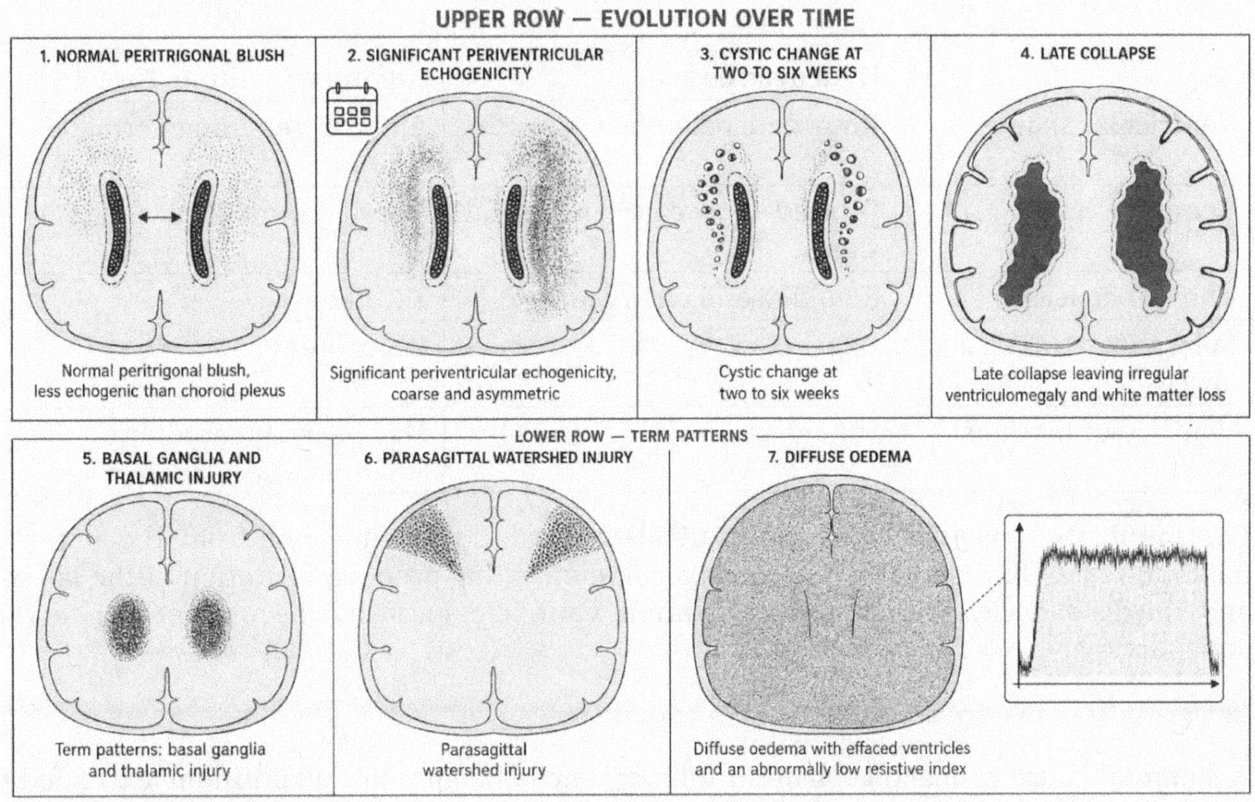

13.5 Ventriculomegaly, Hydrocephalus, and the Resistive Index

Measurement

Ventricular size is assessed reproducibly rather than impressionistically, and compared against **gestational-age-referenced charts** and against the infant's own previous studies.

The conventional measurements are taken on the **coronal plane at the level of the foramina of Monro**:

- **Ventricular index** — from the midline to the most lateral point of the anterior horn

- **Anterior horn width** — the diagonal width of the anterior horn
- **Thalamo-occipital distance** — on the parasagittal plane, from the thalamus to the occipital horn tip

[VERIFY: current reference ranges and intervention thresholds for ventricular index, anterior horn width, and thalamo-occipital distance, indexed to gestational age]

Reproduce the plane and the caliper convention exactly on serial studies (Chapter 1 §1.5). In post-haemorrhagic dilatation, the **rate of change** drives management decisions, and a measurement taken in a different plane is not a comparison.

Distinguishing hydrocephalus from atrophy

Both enlarge the ventricles, and the distinction is made on the surrounding structures rather than on ventricular size:

	Hydrocephalus	**Atrophy / volume loss**
Ventricular shape	**Rounded**, ballooned	Angular, retaining normal contour
Temporal horns	**Dilated** — an early and useful sign	Normal or mildly prominent
Third ventricle	Rounded and enlarged	Slit-like
Sulci and extra-axial spaces	**Effaced**	**Prominent**
Ventricular margins	Smooth	May be irregular after leukomalacia

Communicating versus non-communicating dilatation is inferred from the pattern: dilatation of all four ventricles suggests a communicating process; dilatation of the lateral and third ventricles with a **normal fourth ventricle** localises the obstruction to the aqueduct.

Benign enlargement of the subarachnoid spaces

A common cause of macrocephaly in infancy, and a benign one. **Prominent extra-axial cerebrospinal fluid** over the frontal convexities, with normal or only mildly prominent ventricles, in a well infant with a large head and normal development.

The discriminating sign is vascular: in benign enlargement, **cortical veins are seen traversing the widened space** to reach the dural sinuses. In a **subdural collection**, the veins are **displaced against the cortical surface** and the fluid lies outside them. Colour Doppler with a high-frequency linear probe over the anterior fontanelle demonstrates this directly and settles the question.

The resistive index and the fontanelle compression test

Measurement: interrogate the **anterior cerebral artery** on the midline sagittal plane as it courses around the corpus callosum, or a middle cerebral artery through the temporal window. Calculate the resistive index as in Chapter 7 §7.2, where angle correction is again unnecessary because the angle term cancels in the ratio.

Normal neonatal values are higher than adult values and fall with increasing age. [VERIFY: current normal resistive index ranges for term and preterm neonates by postnatal age]

Raised intracranial pressure elevates the resistive index by reducing diastolic flow.

The fontanelle compression test exploits this. Apply **gentle, graded pressure with the transducer over the fontanelle** while recording the waveform, and compare with the relaxed trace.

- **Normal compliance:** the resistive index changes little.
- **Reduced compliance / raised intracranial pressure:** the resistive index **rises significantly** with compression.

This is a genuinely useful bedside adjunct when deciding whether ventricular dilatation is under pressure — a question that measurement alone cannot answer. [VERIFY: the magnitude of resistive index change on fontanelle compression regarded as significant]

Confounders that must be excluded before interpreting any neonatal resistive index: a **patent ductus arteriosus** with diastolic steal (which raises the index independently of intracranial pressure), hypercapnia, sedative and vasoactive drugs, therapeutic hypothermia, heart rate, and hydration status.

Management context

Post-haemorrhagic ventricular dilatation is followed with serial head circumference and serial ultrasound. Intervention — ventricular access device, reservoir, external drainage, or ventriculoperitoneal shunt — is triggered by a combination of measurement trajectory, head circumference growth, and clinical signs.

Shunt complications that ultrasound can address include obstruction with re-expansion of the ventricles, and **over-drainage** producing slit-like ventricles and, occasionally, subdural collections.

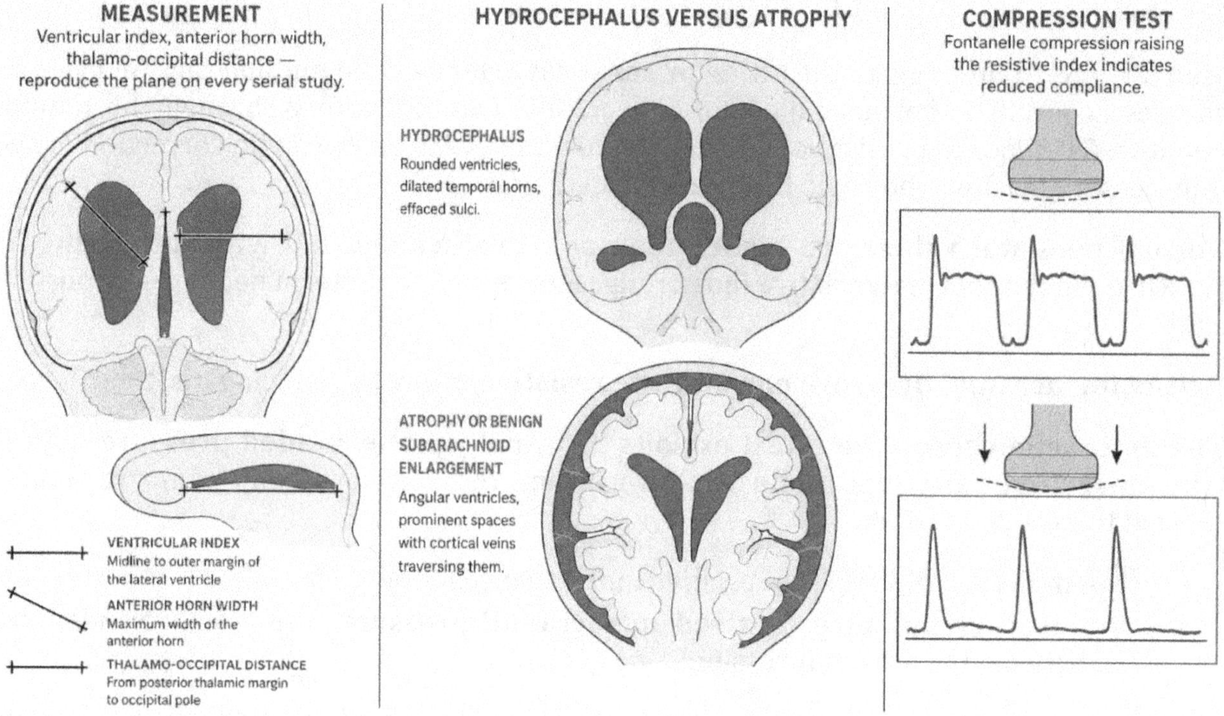

13.6 Congenital Malformations and Congenital Infection

Agenesis of the corpus callosum

A frequently encountered malformation with a recognisable constellation:

- **Absent cavum septi pellucidi** — often the first clue, and any absent cavum should prompt a careful midline assessment
- **Widely separated, parallel frontal horns** on coronal imaging, described as a steer-horn or Viking-helmet configuration
- **Colpocephaly** — disproportionate dilatation of the occipital horns and atria relative to the frontal horns
- **A high-riding third ventricle** extending upward between the separated lateral ventricles
- **On midline sagittal**, absence of the normal arching corpus callosum, with **medial hemispheric sulci radiating in a spoke-like pattern** toward the third ventricle
- **Colour Doppler** showing an abnormal course of the pericallosal artery, which no longer arches

Posterior fossa malformations

Chiari II malformation — almost always accompanying an open spinal dysraphism (§13.8). A **small posterior fossa** with **inferior displacement of the cerebellar vermis** through the foramen magnum, an **obliterated cisterna magna**, ventriculomegaly with colpocephaly, and a cerebellum wrapping anteriorly around the brainstem. **Mastoid views are essential** to assess it.

Dandy–Walker continuum — vermian hypoplasia or agenesis with **cystic dilatation of the fourth ventricle** communicating with an enlarged posterior fossa, and elevation of the tentorium and torcula.

The differential for a posterior fossa fluid collection must be worked through carefully, because the entities differ greatly in significance: **mega cisterna magna** (normal vermis, no mass effect), **Blake pouch cyst**, **arachnoid cyst** (mass effect, normal vermis), and true Dandy–Walker malformation (abnormal vermis). **Assessment of the vermis is the discriminator**, and it requires mastoid or midline sagittal views.

Other malformations

Holoprosencephaly — failure of forebrain cleavage, graded alobar, semilobar and lobar, with **absent midline structures, a monoventricle, and fused thalami** in the severe forms, and characteristic associated facial anomalies.

Vein of Galen malformation — a midline posterior anechoic or tubular structure that on greyscale resembles a cyst. **Colour Doppler is diagnostic: the "cyst" fills completely with turbulent high-velocity flow.** The neonate typically presents with **high-output cardiac failure**, and the associated dilated straight sinus and feeding vessels should be documented. **Any midline posterior fluid structure in a neonate must have colour Doppler applied before it is called a cyst.**

Schizencephaly, lissencephaly, grey matter heterotopia, arachnoid cysts, and **choroid plexus cysts** complete the list; ultrasound is limited for cortical malformations and MRI is required.

Congenital infection

Sonographic markers are non-specific individually but suggestive in combination, and the pattern of calcification helps:

Infection	Characteristic findings
Cytomegalovirus	**Periventricular calcification**, ventriculomegaly, germinolytic (subependymal) cysts, migrational anomalies, cerebellar hypoplasia, lenticulostriate vasculopathy
Toxoplasmosis	**Scattered parenchymal calcification** throughout the brain rather than periventricular, with hydrocephalus
Zika virus	**Microcephaly** with coarse calcification, often at the grey–white junction, ventriculomegaly, and cortical malformation
Herpes simplex	Diffuse oedema acutely, evolving to widespread cystic encephalomalacia

Lenticulostriate vasculopathy — fine, linear, branching echogenic lines within the basal ganglia and thalami, following the lenticulostriate vessels. It is **highly non-specific**, occurring in congenital infection, chromosomal abnormality, hypoxic injury, drug exposure, and in otherwise well infants. **Report it, and do not over-interpret it.**

Germinolytic and subependymal cysts along the caudothalamic groove are often incidental and benign, but may accompany congenital infection or metabolic disease, and warrant correlation.

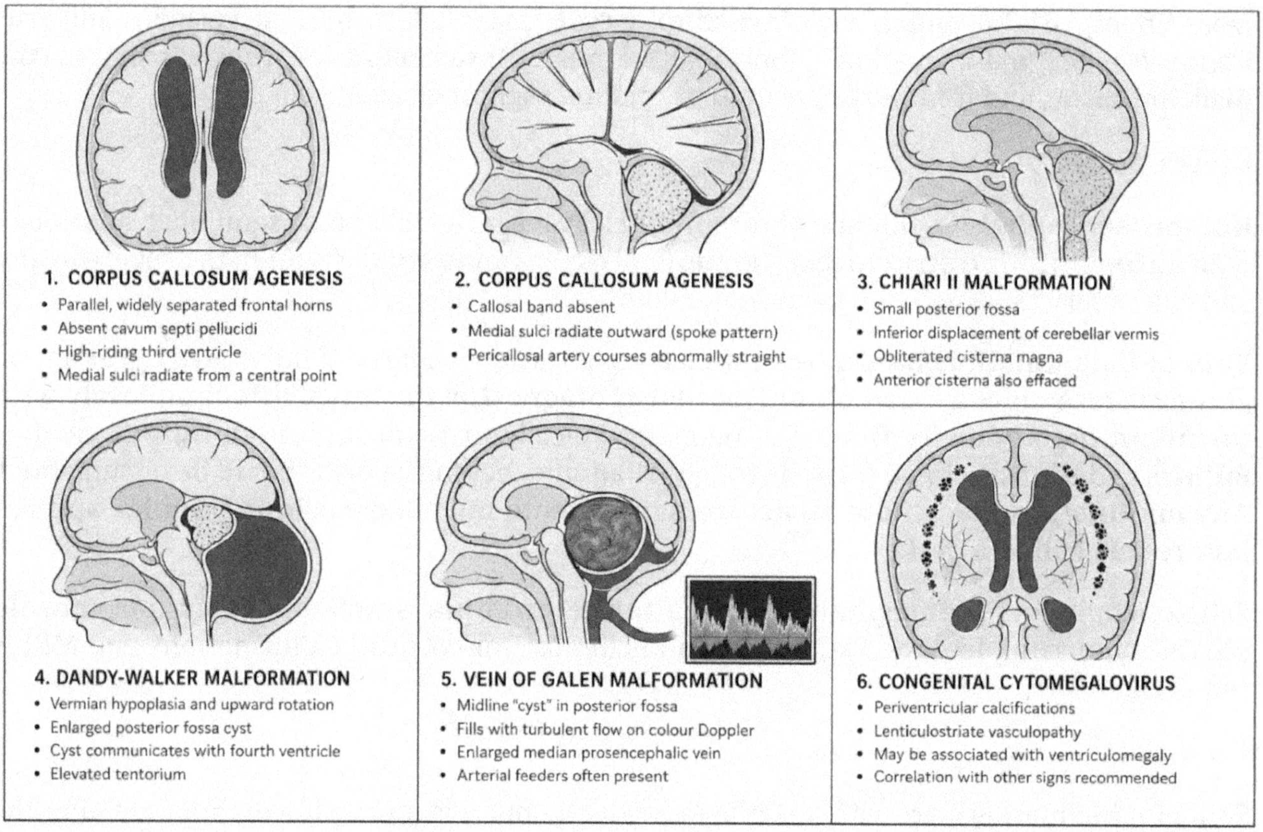

13.7 The Neonatal and Infant Spine: Technique and Normal Anatomy

Why and when

The window is time-limited. Ultrasound reaches the spinal canal through the **incompletely ossified posterior vertebral elements**, and that acoustic access closes progressively over the first months of life. The examination is most reliable in the early weeks and becomes unreliable thereafter. [VERIFY: current recommended upper age limit for diagnostic spinal ultrasound]

Indications:

- **Cutaneous stigmata over the spine** — the commonest referral. Atypical dimples, hair tufts, capillary malformations, subcutaneous lipomas, skin tags, and a deviated gluteal cleft

- **Anorectal and cloacal malformations**, and the **VACTERL** association
- **Sacral agenesis** and caudal regression, including infants of diabetic mothers
- **Postoperative assessment** after myelomeningocele repair
- **Neurological or urological signs** suggesting cord tethering

Technique

Position: prone, with a **roll beneath the abdomen** to flex the spine and open the interlaminar spaces. A settled, ideally feeding infant.

Transducer: high-frequency linear, the highest available.

Sweeps: continuous **longitudinal** midline sweep from the craniocervical junction to the coccyx, and **transverse** sweeps through the same range.

Counting levels is the part most often done poorly, and the report should state the method used. Options include counting **down from the last rib-bearing vertebra (T12)** and counting **up from the lumbosacral junction or the coccyx. Count in both directions and reconcile them**, because miscounting by one level changes the interpretation of the conus position.

Normal anatomy

The spinal cord appears as a hypoechoic tubular structure with a bright **central echo complex** — a linear echogenic line representing the interfaces around the central canal, not a lumen.

The cord terminates at the conus medullaris, tapering to the **filum terminale**, a thin echogenic strand descending to the coccyx. The **cauda equina** nerve roots surround it, and in normal circumstances are seen **floating freely and moving** in the cerebrospinal fluid.

Two normal findings must be assessed and reported:

1. Conus level. The conus should lie **at or above the L2–L3 level** in a term infant. A conus below this is abnormal and indicates tethering. [VERIFY: current normal conus level criteria by gestational and postnatal age]

2. Cord and nerve root motion. Observed in real time, the cord and nerve roots show **continuous pulsatile and oscillatory movement** with cardiac and respiratory cycles.

> **Absent or markedly reduced cord motion is a sign of tethering, and it is a dynamic finding that a still image cannot capture.** Record a cine clip.

Filum thickness is measured on the transverse or longitudinal image; a thickened filum is abnormal. [VERIFY: current upper limit of normal filum terminale thickness]

Normal variants

Ventriculus terminalis — a small ovoid cystic space within the conus, a normal remnant of the central canal, without mass effect and typically resolving.

Filar cyst — a small cyst within the filum terminale, generally benign.

A simple coccygeal pit lying within the gluteal cleft, low, small, and with no other cutaneous marker, is a low-risk finding — in contrast to the atypical dimples that warrant imaging (§13.8).

13.8 Spinal Dysraphism and Tethered Cord

The classification that matters

Open dysraphism — neural tissue exposed, with no skin covering. **Myelomeningocele** is the archetype, is usually diagnosed antenatally or clinically at birth, and goes to surgery. Ultrasound's role is **postoperative**: assessing the repair site, and — importantly — the associated **Chiari II malformation and hydrocephalus** (§13.6), which frequently determine the clinical course.

Closed dysraphism — skin-covered, and this is where ultrasound screening earns its place, because the lesion may be occult apart from a cutaneous marker.

Tethered cord

The unifying functional diagnosis, defined by three findings which should be sought together:

1. **Low conus** — below the L2–L3 level
2. **Thickened filum terminale**
3. **Reduced or absent cord motion** on real-time observation

Any one alone is suggestive; together they are convincing. **The motion assessment is the one most often omitted**, and it is the one that a still-image report cannot convey.

The lesions

Filum lipoma and lipomyelomeningocele — an **echogenic fatty mass** continuous with the subcutaneous fat, extending through a posterior bony defect, with the cord tethered into it. The echogenicity of fat makes these among the more conspicuous lesions.

Dermal sinus tract — a hypoechoic tract extending from a skin dimple toward or into the canal. **The significance is infective as much as neurological**: an open tract is a route for meningitis and for intraspinal dermoid formation, which is why atypical dimples are imaged.

Diastematomyelia (split cord malformation) — the cord divided into **two hemicords**, sometimes separated by a bony or fibrocartilaginous septum. **This is a transverse-plane diagnosis** — on longitudinal images the split can be missed entirely, which is the reason transverse sweeps are mandatory rather than supplementary.

Caudal regression and sacral agenesis — an abruptly terminating, blunt-ended cord with absent sacral segments. Strongly associated with maternal diabetes.

Meningocele and terminal myelocystocele — cystic posterior lesions, the latter with the cord central canal expanded into the sac.

Syringohydromyelia — dilatation of the central canal, appearing as an anechoic expansion within the cord.

Which dimples need imaging

A practical point that generates a large proportion of referrals. **Simple, small, midline coccygeal pits lying within the gluteal cleft and close to the anus carry a low risk** and generally do not require imaging. **Atypical markers do** — those that are high (above the gluteal cleft), large, off-midline, associated with a hair tuft, lipoma, vascular malformation, skin tag, or deviated gluteal cleft, or occurring in combination.

Local pathways differ and should be followed. [VERIFY: current criteria distinguishing low-risk simple coccygeal dimples from atypical cutaneous markers requiring imaging]

The modality relationship

MRI is the definitive study. Ultrasound is the **screening test**, with a high negative predictive value when performed within the age window, in a good acoustic setting, with the conus level and cord motion both assessed. A technically limited or late study should be reported as such and referred onward rather than treated as reassuring.

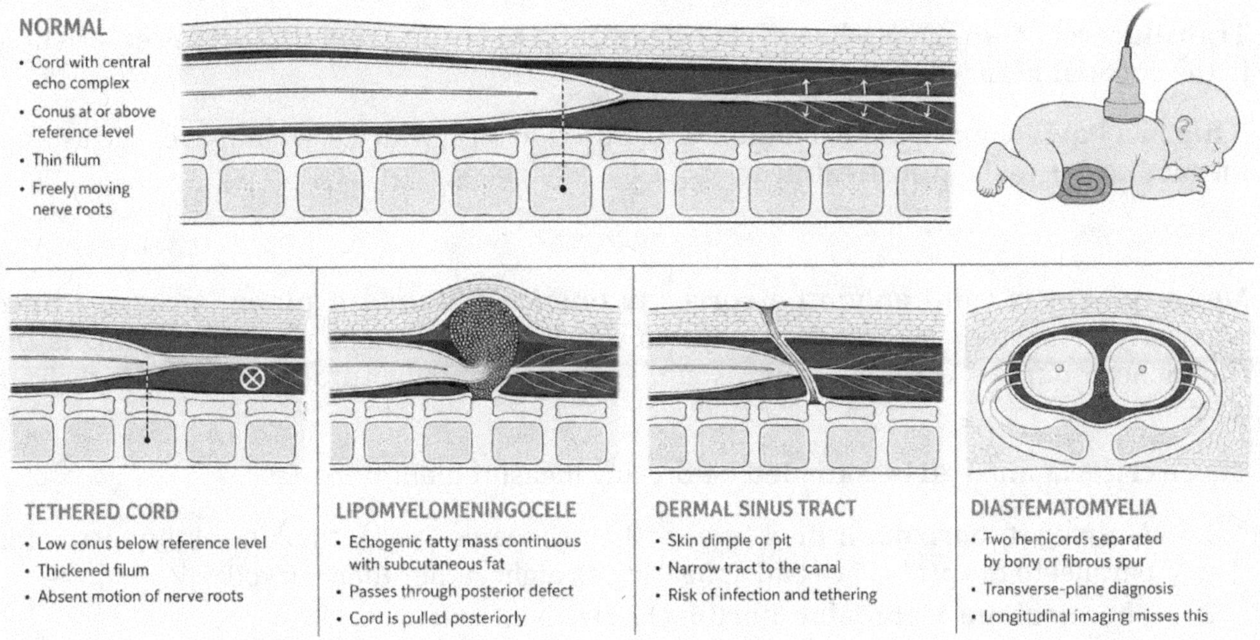

13.9 Developmental Dysplasia of the Hip: Scanning Technique

Who is scanned, and when

Risk factors prompting screening include **breech presentation**, a **family history** of developmental dysplasia, **female sex**, firstborn status, oligohydramnios, and swaddling practices that hold the hips in extension and adduction. Clinical instability on the Ortolani or Barlow manoeuvres prompts imaging regardless of risk factors.

Timing matters in both directions. Scanning **too early** — in the first weeks — produces false positives, because physiological laxity and incomplete ossification are normal at that stage. Scanning **too late** is limited by ossification of the femoral head. The conventional window opens at around six weeks. [VERIFY: current recommended timing for hip ultrasound screening and the criteria for earlier imaging]

The window closes as the **femoral head ossifies at around four to six months**, after which the ossific nucleus shadows the acetabulum and **radiography replaces ultrasound**.

Position and approach

Position: the infant in **lateral decubitus with the hip to be examined uppermost**, or supine, with the hip flexed to roughly 15 to 30 degrees and in neutral rotation. The infant should be calm — a crying, kicking infant cannot be assessed, and feeding or a pacifier is a legitimate part of the technique.

Transducer: high-frequency linear, placed **laterally over the greater trochanter**, oriented in the **coronal plane** of the body.

A hip in a Pavlik harness can usually be scanned in situ, which is what makes ultrasound the monitoring tool during treatment.

The standard coronal plane — and why it is non-negotiable

Measurement is valid only on a correctly obtained standard plane. An image tilted anteriorly or posteriorly produces a systematically different alpha angle, and this is the commonest source of error in hip ultrasound — a wrong number produced confidently from a wrong image.

Three criteria must all be satisfied before any measurement is made:

1. **A straight, horizontal iliac line** — the echogenic line of the lateral ilium running parallel to the probe face and appearing straight rather than curved
2. **The tip of the acetabular labrum** clearly visualised
3. **The transition of the ilium into the triradiate cartilage** at the deepest point of the acetabular fossa

If any is absent, adjust the probe and reacquire. **Do not measure an invalid image.**

Landmarks

Working from the top of the image downward and from lateral to medial:

- **Gluteal muscles** superficially
- **The iliac wing**, with its straight echogenic lateral cortex forming the baseline
- **The bony acetabular roof**, and its lateral edge — the **bony rim or promontory**
- **The cartilaginous acetabular roof**, hypoechoic, extending laterally from the bony rim
- **The labrum** — a small echogenic triangle at the lateral tip of the cartilaginous roof
- **The femoral head** — a rounded hypoechoic structure with fine internal stippled echoes
- **The triradiate cartilage**, at the floor of the acetabulum, marking the transition point
- **The greater trochanter** and the femoral metaphysis inferiorly

Both hips are examined and documented, whatever the clinical concern.

13.10 Hip Measurement, Classification, and Dynamic Assessment

The angles

Two angles are constructed from three lines on the valid standard coronal plane:

The baseline — drawn along the straight lateral cortex of the ilium.

The bony roof line — from the lower limb of the ilium at the acetabular floor, along the bony acetabular roof, to the bony rim.

The cartilaginous roof line — from the bony rim through the middle of the labrum.

Angle	Between	Measures	Direction of abnormality
Alpha (α)	Baseline and bony roof line	**Bony acetabular coverage**	**Lower is worse** — a shallow bony roof
Beta (β)	Baseline and cartilaginous roof line	**Cartilaginous coverage**	**Higher is worse** — the cartilaginous roof displaced upward

A mature hip has a high alpha and a low beta. As the head displaces laterally and superiorly, the bony roof becomes shallower (alpha falls) and the cartilaginous roof is pushed up and out (beta rises).

Femoral head coverage — the proportion of the femoral head lying medial to the iliac baseline — is used in some practices as an adjunct or alternative measurement.

Classification

The widely used morphological classification assigns each hip to a type based on the alpha angle, the beta angle, the appearance of the bony rim, and the position of the labrum, with age modifying the interpretation of borderline values:

- **Mature hips** — a well-formed bony roof with an angular rim and a covering cartilaginous roof
- **Physiologically immature and delayed-ossification hips** — a rounded bony rim with a still-covering cartilaginous roof, where **the infant's age determines whether the finding is normal for age or requires treatment**
- **Critical and decentring hips** — a deficient bony roof with the cartilaginous roof progressively displaced
- **Eccentric (subluxed) hips** — the head displaced with the cartilaginous roof pushed upward
- **Dislocated hips** — the head out of the acetabulum, with the labrum interposed or pressed downward

The exact angle ranges, type definitions, and the age thresholds that separate physiological immaturity from pathology are specified by the classification system and must be taken from it. [VERIFY: the hip classification system to be adopted, its precise alpha and beta ranges by type, the age thresholds applied, and the associated management recommendations]

As with the thyroid nodule and urinary tract dilatation systems elsewhere in this book, a department must adopt one system and apply it consistently, and the report should state which is in use.

Dynamic assessment

Morphology describes the shape of the joint; **dynamic assessment describes its stability**, and the two are complementary rather than alternatives.

The manoeuvre: with the hip flexed, apply a **posteriorly directed stress with adduction** — the sonographic equivalent of the Barlow manoeuvre — while imaging in the coronal or transverse plane, and observe whether the femoral head displaces from the acetabulum.

Categories:

- **Stable** — no displacement on stress
- **Subluxable** — partial displacement that reduces on release
- **Dislocatable** — the head displaces out of the acetabulum on stress
- **Dislocated** — the head lies out of the acetabulum at rest, and may or may not be reducible

Record a cine clip. A dynamic finding documented only as a still image is not documented.

Reporting

For each hip: the alpha angle, the beta angle, the assigned type, the stability on dynamic testing, and the infant's exact age — since age determines the significance of borderline findings. State the classification system used.

Pitfalls

Measuring from an invalid plane — the dominant error, and the reason the three plane criteria in §13.9 exist.

Excessive transducer pressure, which can reduce a subluxable hip and mask instability.

Scanning too early, over-calling physiological immaturity.

Over-reliance on angles without dynamic testing, missing an unstable hip with acceptable morphology.

Failing to examine both hips, missing bilateral disease — where the absence of asymmetry removes the clinical clue.

The older infant and child

Beyond the ossification window, ultrasound's hip role changes to **effusion detection**: an anterior approach along the femoral neck, measuring the **capsule-to-bone distance** and comparing with the contralateral side. It is the standard investigation in the irritable hip.

Ultrasound identifies an effusion; it cannot distinguish transient synovitis from septic arthritis. Where infection is suspected, the effusion must be **aspirated** for definitive diagnosis, and ultrasound guides that aspiration (Chapter 9 §9.5; Chapter 11 §11.10).

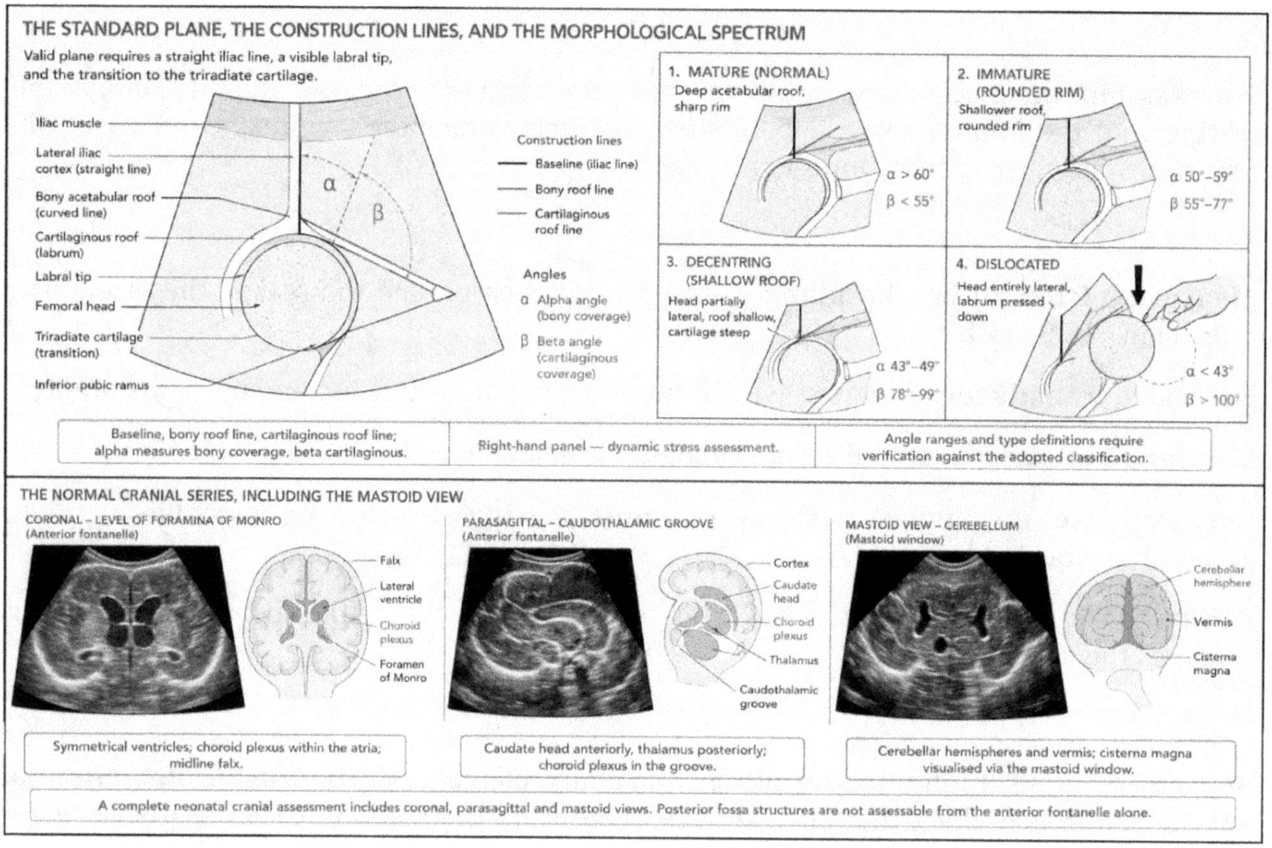

Key Points

1. All three examinations in this chapter depend on incomplete ossification, and all three windows close. Each has an expiry date, and a late request may be unanswerable.
2. The posterior fossa is not adequately assessed from the anterior fontanelle. Use mastoid views, and use them routinely in preterm infants — cerebellar haemorrhage is otherwise missed.
3. Choroid plexus should not extend anterior to the caudothalamic groove. Echogenic material there is haemorrhage until proven otherwise.
4. Periventricular white matter should be less echogenic than choroid plexus. That single comparison separates normal peritrigonal blush from significant echogenicity.
5. Grade IV haemorrhage is periventricular haemorrhagic infarction — a venous infarct — not simple extension of blood into brain.
6. In periventricular leukomalacia, what you see depends on when you scan. Cysts appear at two to six weeks and later collapse, so a normal late scan does not exclude earlier injury.
7. In term hypoxic-ischaemic encephalopathy the resistive index rises early and then falls; an abnormally low index after the first day is an adverse sign. Hypothermia and a patent ductus both confound it.
8. Hydrocephalus rounds the ventricles, dilates the temporal horns, and effaces the sulci. Atrophy leaves the ventricles angular and the spaces prominent.

9. In benign subarachnoid enlargement, cortical veins traverse the widened space. In a subdural collection they are displaced against the cortex. Colour Doppler settles it.
10. The fontanelle compression test answers a question that measurement cannot: whether dilated ventricles are under pressure.
11. An absent cavum septi pellucidi should prompt a deliberate search for corpus callosum agenesis.
12. Apply colour Doppler to any midline posterior fluid structure in a neonate before calling it a cyst — a vein of Galen malformation fills completely with turbulent flow.
13. Lenticulostriate vasculopathy is non-specific. Report it; do not over-interpret it.
14. On spinal ultrasound, assess both the conus level and cord motion, and record motion as a cine clip. Absent motion suggests tethering and cannot be shown on a still image.
15. Diastematomyelia is a transverse-plane diagnosis. Longitudinal sweeps alone will miss it.
16. Count spinal levels in both directions and state the method used. A one-level error changes the interpretation.
17. Never measure a hip from an invalid plane. The straight iliac line, labral tip, and triradiate transition must all be present first.
18. Alpha falls and beta rises as a hip decentres. Age determines whether a borderline value is physiological immaturity or pathology.
19. Morphology and stability are separate assessments. A hip with acceptable angles can still be unstable on stress.
20. Excessive transducer pressure can reduce a subluxable hip and conceal instability.
21. Ultrasound detects a hip effusion but cannot distinguish transient synovitis from sepsis. Aspiration makes that diagnosis.

Registry Check

1. On the parasagittal view of a preterm neonate, echogenic material is seen extending anterior to the caudothalamic groove. This most likely represents:

A. Normal choroid plexus **B.** Germinal matrix haemorrhage **C.** Periventricular leukomalacia **D.** Lenticulostriate vasculopathy

> **Answer: B.** Choroid plexus does not extend anterior to the caudothalamic groove, so echogenic material in that position is haemorrhage until proven otherwise. The germinal matrix lies at the groove in preterm infants and involutes by around 34 weeks.

2. Cerebellar haemorrhage in a preterm infant is most reliably detected using:

A. The anterior fontanelle in the coronal plane **B.** The anterior fontanelle in the sagittal plane **C.** The mastoid fontanelle **D.** The temporal window

> **Answer: C.** The posterior fossa is poorly assessed from the anterior fontanelle, and cerebellar haemorrhage is characteristically missed when mastoid views are

omitted. The mastoid window provides substantially better cerebellar and fourth ventricular detail.

3. Increased periventricular echogenicity is noted in a preterm infant. Which feature best distinguishes significant white matter injury from normal peritrigonal blush?

A. Bilateral distribution **B.** Echogenicity equal to or greater than choroid plexus, coarse and asymmetric, persisting beyond one to two weeks **C.** Any echogenicity in the periventricular region **D.** Associated ventricular dilatation

Answer: B. Normal peritrigonal blush is symmetrical, ill-defined, and less echogenic than choroid plexus, and it fades. Echogenicity that equals or exceeds choroid plexus, is coarse or asymmetric, and persists on repeat scanning is the pattern of significant injury.

4. A term infant with encephalopathy has an abnormally low anterior cerebral artery resistive index at 36 hours of age. This finding:

A. Excludes hypoxic-ischaemic injury **B.** Indicates raised intracranial pressure **C.** Suggests loss of cerebrovascular autoregulation and is an adverse prognostic sign **D.** Is a normal finding at this age

Answer: C. After the first day, failure of autoregulation with cerebral vasoparalysis reduces cerebrovascular resistance and lowers the index. It carries adverse prognostic weight, but must be interpreted alongside therapeutic hypothermia, patent ductus arteriosus, and medication effects.

5. An infant with macrocephaly has prominent frontal extra-axial fluid. Cortical veins are seen crossing the fluid space from the brain surface to the skull. This indicates:

A. Subdural haematoma **B.** Subdural effusion **C.** Benign enlargement of the subarachnoid spaces **D.** Communicating hydrocephalus

Answer: C. In benign subarachnoid enlargement, the fluid is within the subarachnoid space and cortical veins traverse it. In a subdural collection, the fluid lies superficial to the veins, which are displaced against the cortical surface. Colour Doppler demonstrates the distinction directly.

6. On neonatal spinal ultrasound, the conus lies below the L2–L3 level, the filum is thickened, and no cord or nerve root motion is seen. This indicates:

A. Normal variation **B.** Tethered cord **C.** Ventriculus terminalis **D.** Diastematomyelia

Answer: B. The triad of low conus, thickened filum, and reduced or absent cord motion defines tethering. Cord motion is a dynamic finding requiring real-time observation and cine recording, and is the element most often omitted.

7. Before measuring the alpha angle on an infant hip ultrasound, the operator must confirm:

A. The femoral head is fully ossified **B.** A straight iliac line, a visible labral tip, and the transition of the ilium to the triradiate cartilage **C.** The hip is in full extension **D.** Both hips appear symmetrical

> **Answer: B.** Measurement is valid only on a correctly obtained standard coronal plane, defined by those three criteria. Anterior or posterior tilting alters the alpha angle systematically, and measuring from an invalid image is the commonest error in hip sonography.

8. An infant hip has an alpha angle within the mature range, but on posteriorly directed stress with adduction the femoral head displaces from the acetabulum and reduces on release. The correct assessment is:

A. Normal hip **B.** Morphologically acceptable but subluxable — an unstable hip **C.** Dislocated hip **D.** Physiological immaturity

> **Answer: B.** Morphology and stability are separate assessments. A hip with acceptable angles may still be unstable, which is why dynamic stress testing is performed in addition to measurement and why the finding should be recorded as a cine clip.

Chapter Notes for the Editorial Pass

Verification queue. In priority order: **the hip classification system to be adopted**, with its precise alpha and beta ranges by type, the age thresholds separating physiological immaturity from pathology, and the management recommendations attached to each type (§13.10) — this is the chapter's most consequential decision and follows the same pattern as the thyroid nodule and urinary tract dilatation systems in Chapters 11 and 12; **the intraventricular haemorrhage grading system, its criteria, current terminology, and prognostic implications** (§13.3); **cranial ultrasound screening schedules for preterm infants** (§13.3); **ventricular measurement reference ranges and intervention thresholds indexed to gestational age** (§13.5); **normal neonatal resistive index ranges and the change on fontanelle compression regarded as significant** (§13.5); **resistive index thresholds in term hypoxic-ischaemic encephalopathy and the effect of therapeutic hypothermia** (§13.4); **normal conus level criteria and filum thickness** (§13.7); **the upper age limit for diagnostic spinal ultrasound** (§13.7); **criteria distinguishing low-risk coccygeal dimples from atypical markers requiring imaging** (§13.8); and **hip screening timing** (§13.9).

A pattern worth noting across the book. Three chapters now describe a formal classification system without committing to one — thyroid nodules (§11.3), urinary tract dilatation (§12.8), and infant hips (§13.10). In each case competing systems exist with materially different thresholds. **These three decisions should be made together before layout**, since a book that adopts one system in one chapter and hedges in another will read inconsistently, and readers will apply whichever they already know.

Figure count: 8 Lane A, 2 Lane B. Both Lane B slots would benefit substantially from **cine clips** rather than stills — the hip stress manoeuvre and, in the spine section, cord motion.

This is the first chapter where the static-image format is a real limitation on what can be taught, and it is worth deciding early whether the digital edition will support video.

Cross-reference targets to fix at layout: §13.1 neonatal handling and ALARA → Chapter 1 §1.7 and Chapter 12 §12.1; §13.5 resistive index calculation → Chapter 7 §7.2; §13.6 Chiari II → §13.8; §13.8 myelomeningocele → §13.6; §13.10 hip aspiration and effusion → Chapter 9 §9.5 and Chapter 11 §11.10.

Word count: approximately 10,400 excluding image prompt blocks, learning objectives, registry questions, and these notes.

Chapter 14: Cardiac Anatomy, Hemodynamics, and Echocardiographic Technique

Learning Objectives

On completing this chapter you should be able to:

1. Describe the position of the heart within the thorax and explain why the standard acoustic windows exist where they do.
2. Identify the cardiac chambers, valves and great vessels, and distinguish the morphological right ventricle from the left.
3. Relate the phases of the cardiac cycle to valve motion and to the ECG, and explain why an ECG trace is mandatory.
4. Apply the simplified Bernoulli and continuity equations, and calculate right ventricular systolic pressure.
5. Obtain the standard parasternal, apical, subcostal and suprasternal views, and recognise foreshortening.
6. Select appropriately between M-mode, two-dimensional imaging, colour, pulsed-wave, continuous-wave and tissue Doppler.
7. Perform chamber quantification using the recommended methods and conventions.
8. Assess left and right ventricular systolic function and grade diastolic function.
9. Recognise the artifacts and normal structures that are mistaken for pathology.

A Different Set of Rules

Echocardiography departs from general sonography in ways that catch out experienced abdominal and vascular sonographers, and it is worth naming them at the outset.

The orientation conventions differ. The transducer marker relationships and screen conventions established in Chapter 2 §2.6 do not carry over, and applying them produces mirrored images.

Angle correction is not used. In vascular work the angle cursor corrects a known insonation angle (Chapter 2 §2.5). In echocardiography the operator **moves the probe until the beam is parallel to flow** and accepts whatever velocity that alignment yields. Angle-correcting a cardiac Doppler trace is an error, not a refinement.

Temporal resolution frequently matters more than spatial resolution. The heart moves, and the whole diagnostic apparatus of M-mode, timing against the ECG, and frame-rate optimisation exists because of it.

Measurement is protocolised to an unusual degree, because the numbers feed directly into guideline thresholds for surgery, device implantation, and drug therapy. Reproducibility is not an aspiration here; it is the point.

14.1 Anatomic and Physiologic Relationships of the Thoracic Cavity

Position

The heart lies in the **middle mediastinum**, enclosed in the pericardium, with roughly two-thirds of its mass **to the left of the midline**.

Its orientation is oblique: the **base** is superior, posterior and to the right; the **apex** is inferior, anterior and to the left, normally lying in the **fifth intercostal space at the midclavicular line**. The cardiac long axis therefore runs from right-posterior-superior to left-anterior-inferior — which is why no standard body plane gives a useful cardiac image, and why echocardiographic planes are defined relative to the **heart** rather than to the body.

Surfaces and their contents matter for interpretation:

- **Sternocostal (anterior)** — predominantly **right ventricle**. This is the chamber nearest the transducer in parasternal views, and the reason the RV is the chamber most affected by near-field artifact
- **Diaphragmatic (inferior)** — left and right ventricles
- **Base (posterior)** — predominantly **left atrium**, which lies immediately anterior to the oesophagus. This relationship is the entire basis of transoesophageal echocardiography

The pericardium

A fibrous outer layer and a serous inner layer, the latter reflected as parietal and visceral (epicardial) layers with a **potential space** between them normally containing only a small volume of lubricating fluid.

The fibrous pericardium is relatively non-compliant acutely, which is why a **rapidly accumulating** effusion causes tamponade at a volume that a slowly accumulating one would not. Chronic effusions can become large without haemodynamic consequence.

Relations that create and destroy acoustic windows

The obstacles are ribs, sternum, and aerated lung. **The windows** exist where the heart abuts the chest wall without intervening lung, or where sound can travel around the lung:

Window	Why it works
Parasternal	The **cardiac notch** of the left lung leaves the heart in contact with the anterior chest wall
Apical	The apex lies against the chest wall inferolaterally
Subcostal	Sound passes beneath the ribs, using the **liver as an acoustic window**
Suprasternal	Above the manubrium, reaching the aortic arch

Respiration is a tool, not an inconvenience. Inspiration lowers the diaphragm and improves **subcostal** access; expiration brings the heart closer to the chest wall and generally improves **parasternal** views by moving lung aside. Instruct the patient deliberately.

Left lateral decubitus positioning rotates the heart anteriorly and laterally against the chest wall and displaces lung — it is the single most effective positional manoeuvre in echocardiography and is standard for parasternal and apical imaging.

Situs and cardiac position

Two independent questions that must not be conflated:

Situs — the arrangement of the viscera and atria. **Situs solitus** is normal; **situs inversus** is mirror-image; **situs ambiguus** (heterotaxy) has indeterminate arrangement, frequently with polysplenia or asplenia (Chapter 6 §6.5) and complex cardiac defects.

Cardiac position — where the heart sits and which way the apex points: **levocardia** (normal), **dextrocardia** (apex to the right), **mesocardia** (midline).

Determine situs from the abdomen first, in a subcostal transverse view: **the aorta lies to the left of the spine and the IVC to the right** in situs solitus, and the relationship reverses in situs inversus. This takes seconds and prevents the entire study being interpreted with reversed laterality.

Dextroposition — the heart displaced to the right by an extracardiac process such as a right lung hypoplasia or a large left effusion — is not dextrocardia, and the distinction is made by the direction of the apex.

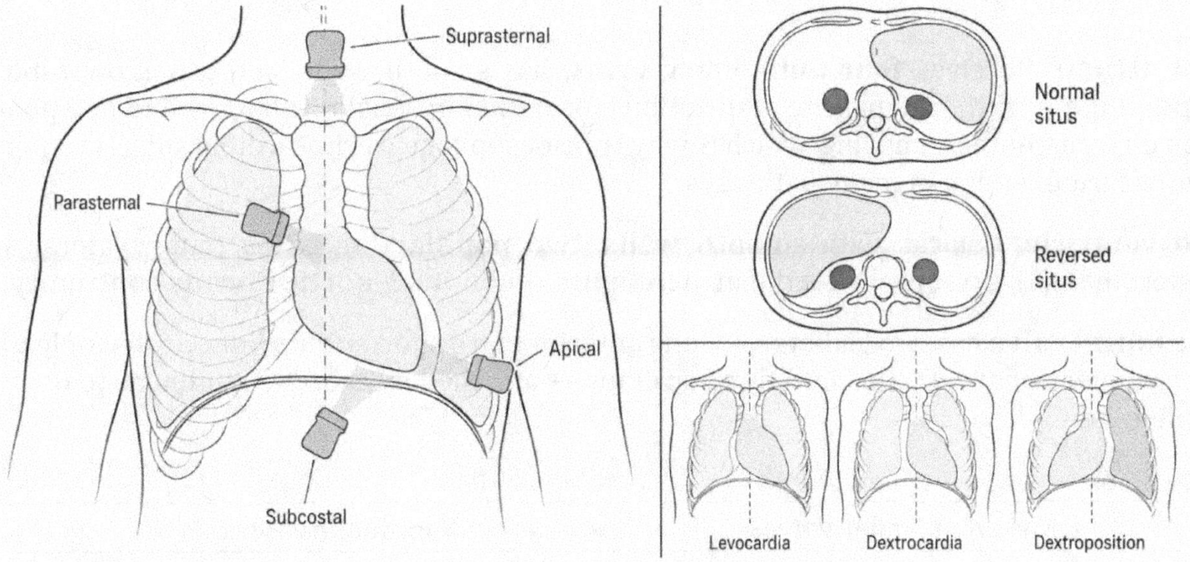

Why the windows exist where they do, and how to establish situs before anything else.
Cardiac notch of the left lung permitting the parasternal window; apical, subcostal and suprasternal approaches.
Abdominal situs is determined from the aorta and IVC relative to the spine.
Levocardia, dextrocardia and dextroposition are distinct patterns; dextroposition is displacement rather than malposition.

14.2 Cardiac Chambers, Valves, and Great Vessels

The right heart

Right atrium. Receives the **superior and inferior venae cavae** and the **coronary sinus**. Its internal features include the **crista terminalis, pectinate muscles**, the **fossa ovalis** in the interatrial septum, and two embryological remnants that are commonly mistaken for pathology (§14.9): the **Eustachian valve** at the IVC orifice and the filamentous **Chiari network.**

Right ventricle. Heavily **trabeculated**, crescentic in cross-section, wrapping around the left ventricle. Three features identify it morphologically:

- **The moderator band** — a prominent muscular band crossing from the interventricular septum to the anterior papillary muscle near the apex. **The single most reliable marker of the morphological right ventricle**
- **Coarse apical trabeculation**
- **Papillary muscle attachments to the septum**, which the left ventricle does not have

The tricuspid valve has three leaflets, and its **septal leaflet inserts more apically than the anterior mitral leaflet** — the **atrioventricular offset**. This offset is a defining normal relationship: its **absence** indicates an atrioventricular septal defect, and its **exaggeration** indicates Ebstein anomaly.

The **right ventricular outflow tract (infundibulum)** is a muscular conduit leading to the pulmonary valve — unlike the left, where mitral and aortic valves are in **fibrous continuity**.

The left heart

Left atrium. Receives **four pulmonary veins**, has smooth walls, and a narrow tubular **appendage** — the principal site of thrombus formation in atrial fibrillation, and one poorly seen on transthoracic imaging, which is why transoesophageal echocardiography is required before cardioversion in many pathways.

Left ventricle. Conical, with **smooth walls**, **two papillary muscles** (anterolateral and posteromedial), **no septal chordal attachments**, and **mitral–aortic fibrous continuity**.

The mitral valve has two leaflets — a long anterior and a shorter but wider posterior leaflet, each conventionally divided into three scallops — attached by chordae tendineae to the two papillary muscles.

The valves and the cardiac skeleton

	Atrioventricular valves	Semilunar valves
Which	Mitral, tricuspid	Aortic, pulmonary
Support	Chordae tendineae and papillary muscles	None — supported by the sinuses
Open in	Diastole	Systole

The **aortic valve** has three cusps — right coronary, left coronary and non-coronary — and a **bicuspid** configuration is a common congenital variant with important consequences for stenosis and aortopathy.

The valves are anchored in the **fibrous cardiac skeleton**, which also electrically insulates the atria from the ventricles.

The great vessels

The aortic root comprises the **annulus**, the **sinuses of Valsalva** (from which the coronary arteries arise), and the **sinotubular junction**, continuing as the **ascending aorta**, **arch** — giving off the brachiocephalic, left common carotid and left subclavian arteries — the **isthmus**, and the **descending aorta**.

The pulmonary trunk arises anterior and to the left of the aorta and bifurcates into right and left pulmonary arteries.

Coronary arteries: the **left main** divides into the **left anterior descending** and **circumflex**; the **right coronary artery** arises from the right sinus. Their territories map onto the wall segments used in regional function assessment (§14.8).

Septa and shunts

The **interatrial septum** contains the **fossa ovalis**; a **patent foramen ovale** persists in a substantial proportion of adults and is a potential route for paradoxical embolism.

The **interventricular septum** has a small **membranous** portion and a large **muscular** portion; ventricular septal defects are classified by which part they involve.

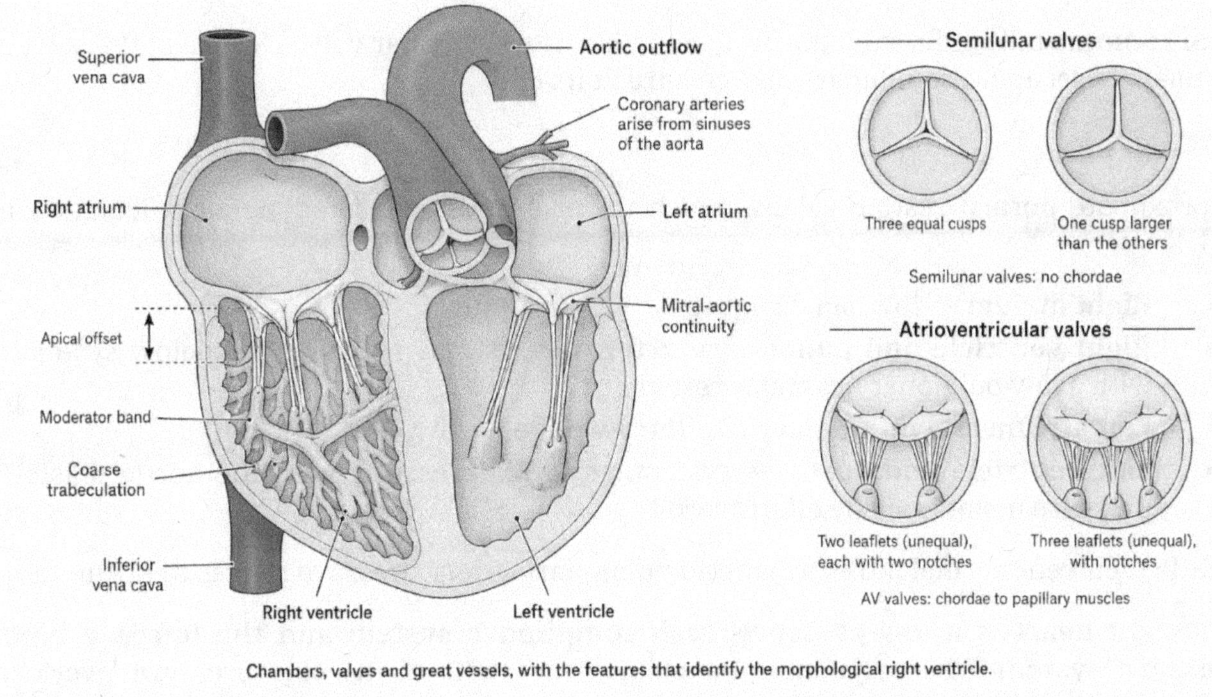

Chambers, valves and great vessels, with the features that identify the morphological right ventricle.

14.3 The Cardiac Cycle and Conduction System

The cycle, and the principle that governs it

Valves open and close because of pressure crossings, not because of active contraction. Every valve event in the cycle occurs at the instant the pressure on one side exceeds the pressure on the other. Hold that, and the sequence becomes derivable rather than memorised.

Phase	Pressure relationship	Valves
Atrial systole	Atrial pressure slightly exceeds ventricular; contributes the final portion of filling	AV open, semilunar closed
Isovolumic contraction	Ventricular pressure rises rapidly but is still below arterial	**All four closed**
Ejection	Ventricular exceeds arterial	Semilunar open, AV closed
Isovolumic relaxation	Ventricular pressure falls but is still above atrial	**All four closed**
Rapid filling	Atrial exceeds ventricular; the ventricle recoils and sucks	AV open, semilunar closed
Diastasis	Near equalisation; slow filling	AV open

Atrial contraction contributes a meaningful proportion of ventricular filling — a contribution that is lost in atrial fibrillation, which is one reason patients with stiff ventricles deteriorate when they lose sinus rhythm.

Heart sounds follow directly: the first sound is atrioventricular valve closure at the start of systole; the second is semilunar valve closure at its end.

Normal pressures

Approximate normal resting values, which underpin every haemodynamic calculation in §14.4:

- **Right atrium** — low, single figures
- **Right ventricle and pulmonary artery** — systolic pressures far below systemic, with a low pulmonary vascular resistance
- **Left atrium and pulmonary capillary wedge** — low
- **Left ventricle and aorta** — systemic systolic pressure, with the aortic diastolic pressure maintained by elastic recoil

[VERIFY: current normal intracardiac and pulmonary artery pressure ranges to be quoted]

The right heart is a low-pressure, high-compliance system and the left is a high-pressure system. That asymmetry explains why right ventricular pressure overload manifests as septal flattening, and why tricuspid regurgitation velocity is such a sensitive index of pulmonary pressure (§14.4).

Conduction

Impulses originate in the **sinoatrial node** in the right atrium near the superior vena cava, spread across the atria, and are delayed at the **atrioventricular node** — a delay that allows atrial contraction to complete before ventricular systole. Conduction then passes through the **bundle of His**, the **bundle branches**, and the **Purkinje network**.

Why the ECG is mandatory

Echocardiographic measurement is defined by cardiac timing, and the ECG is how timing is established.

- **End-diastole** is taken at the **onset of the QRS complex**, or at the frame with the largest ventricular cavity. All diastolic dimensions are measured here.
- **End-systole** is taken at the smallest cavity, near the end of the T wave.

A study performed without an ECG trace cannot reliably identify these frames, and the resulting measurements are not comparable with any other study.

Rhythm changes what you must do:

Atrial fibrillation abolishes the A wave, and stroke volume varies beat to beat. **Average measurements over several consecutive beats** — typically five or more — rather than measuring a single one.

Left bundle branch block produces abnormal septal motion (septal dyssynchrony) that must not be reported as ischaemic wall motion abnormality.

Ventricular pacing produces a similar septal appearance for the same reason.

Tachycardia fuses the E and A waves of mitral inflow and invalidates several diastolic measurements (§14.8).

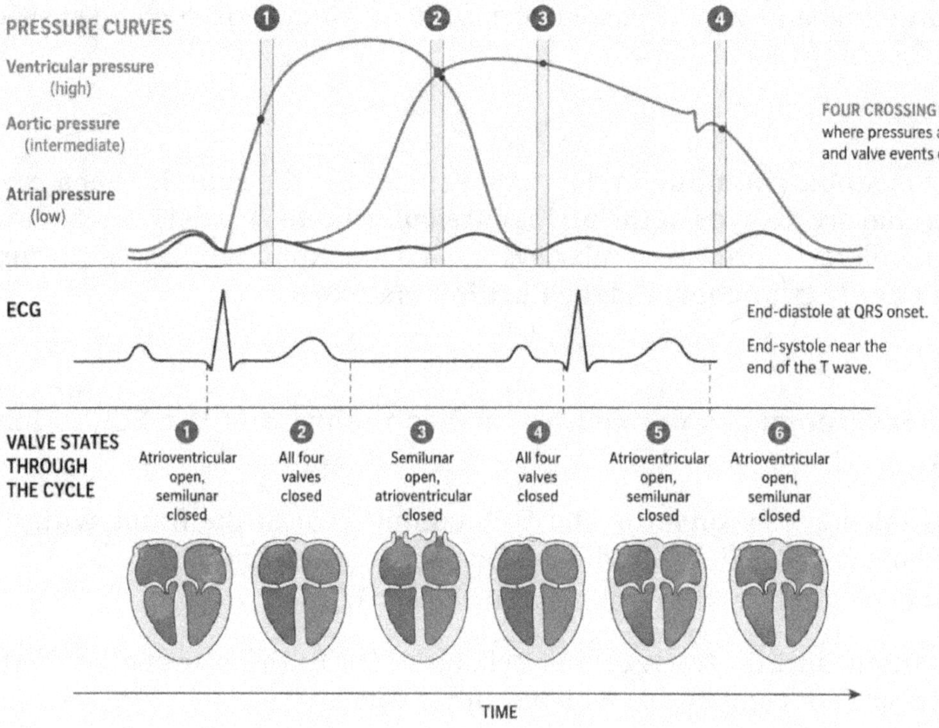

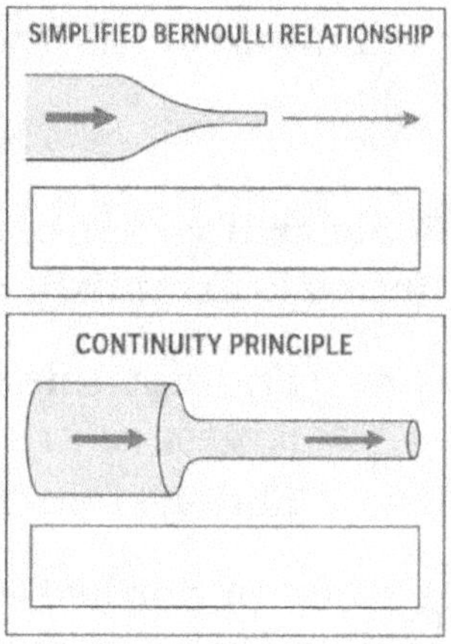

14.4 Hemodynamic Principles: Pressure, Flow, and Resistance

The simplified Bernoulli equation

Blood accelerating through a narrowing converts pressure energy into kinetic energy. The pressure drop across the narrowing can therefore be estimated from the velocity achieved:

$\mathbf{\Delta P = 4v^2}$, with pressure in mmHg and velocity in m/s

This single relationship converts a Doppler velocity into a pressure gradient, and it is the foundation of quantitative echocardiography.

Its assumption, which must be checked: the **proximal velocity is negligible**. Where the velocity approaching the narrowing is itself elevated — in a high-output state, in serial obstructions, or in a small outflow tract — the **expanded form** must be used:

$$\mathbf{\Delta P = 4(v_2^2 - v_1^2)}$$

Ignoring an elevated proximal velocity **overestimates the gradient**, and the error is not small.

The calculation used most

Right ventricular systolic pressure — and by extension pulmonary artery systolic pressure in the absence of outflow obstruction:

$$\mathbf{RVSP = 4(TR\ Vmax)^2 + right\ atrial\ pressure}$$

The **tricuspid regurgitation peak velocity** is obtained with continuous-wave Doppler, aligning the beam parallel to the regurgitant jet and interrogating from **several windows** to find the highest velocity — an underestimate here propagates directly into an underestimate of pulmonary pressure.

Right atrial pressure is estimated from the inferior vena cava — its diameter and its respiratory collapsibility (Chapter 3 §3.5) — with the same caveats about mechanical ventilation reversing the expected respiratory changes.

Two failure modes to state in the report: a **poor-quality or incomplete TR envelope** should not be measured, because a partially traced jet underestimates; and **trivial or absent TR** means the calculation cannot be performed at all, which should be reported as such rather than omitted silently.

The continuity equation

Flow is conserved along a conduit, so what passes one cross-section must pass the next:

$$A_1 \times V_1 = A_2 \times V_2$$

Its main application is **aortic valve area**:

$$\text{AVA} = (\text{LVOT area} \times \text{LVOT VTI}) / \text{Aortic valve VTI}$$

Why this matters clinically: the transvalvular gradient is **flow-dependent**, so a stenotic valve in a patient with a low cardiac output can produce a deceptively low gradient. **Valve area derived by continuity is far less flow-dependent** and is what identifies severe stenosis in the low-flow, low-gradient patient.

The dominant source of error is the **left ventricular outflow tract diameter**, because it is **squared** in computing the area. A one-millimetre measurement error produces a disproportionate error in the calculated area — so the LVOT is measured carefully, in the parasternal long axis, in mid-systole, inner edge to inner edge, immediately proximal to the valve.

Stroke volume and output

$$\text{Stroke volume} = \text{LVOT cross-sectional area} \times \text{LVOT velocity–time integral}$$
$$\text{Cardiac output} = \text{stroke volume} \times \text{heart rate}$$

The same LVOT diameter caveat applies. This calculation also underpins regurgitant volume estimation by comparing flow across two valves.

Other quantitative tools

Pressure half-time — the time for the peak gradient to fall by half. Used for **mitral valve area** in mitral stenosis and for grading **aortic regurgitation**, where a short half-time indicates rapid equalisation and therefore severe regurgitation.

Regurgitation quantification — **vena contracta width**, the **proximal isovelocity surface area (PISA)** method giving effective regurgitant orifice area and regurgitant volume, and regurgitant fraction. **Colour jet area alone is a crude measure** and is heavily influenced by machine settings (§14.9).

Alignment, not angle correction

In echocardiography, the operator achieves parallel alignment rather than correcting for a known angle. Cardiac jets are eccentric and their direction is not reliably known, so an angle-correction cursor introduces error rather than removing it.

The practical consequence: **interrogate from multiple windows** and take the **highest velocity** obtained, on the reasoning that the best alignment produces the highest recorded velocity. This is the opposite discipline to the vascular work of Chapter 2 §2.5 and Chapter 16, and confusing the two is a recurrent source of error in operators who move between the specialties.

14.5 Standard Echocardiographic Windows and Views

Preparation

Position: left lateral decubitus with the left arm raised for parasternal and apical imaging; **supine** for subcostal and suprasternal. A dedicated echocardiography bed with an apical cut-out improves the apical window materially.

ECG electrodes attached before starting (§14.3).

Transducer: phased array, low frequency in adults, higher in children and thin adults. Depth and sector width adjusted to maintain frame rate.

The windows and their views

Window	Views	Principally used for
Parasternal long axis	PLAX; RV inflow; RV outflow	LV linear dimensions, aortic root, mitral and aortic valves, LA size, pericardial effusion, and the descending aorta as a landmark
Parasternal short axis	Aortic valve level; mitral valve level; papillary muscle level; apical level	Aortic valve cusps, RVOT and pulmonary valve, tricuspid valve, mitral orifice, LV regional function and septal motion
Apical	4-chamber; 5-chamber; 2-chamber; 3-chamber (apical long axis)	Chamber volumes and ejection fraction, all four valves with Doppler, diastolic function, RV assessment
Subcostal	4-chamber; short axis; IVC long axis	The interatrial septum and shunts, pericardial effusion, IVC for right atrial pressure. **The rescue window** in obstructive lung disease and in ventilated patients
Suprasternal	Arch long axis; short axis	Aortic arch, coarctation, patent ductus, descending aorta flow

Window	Views	Principally used for
Right parasternal	With a non-imaging continuous-wave probe	Highest aortic velocity in aortic stenosis, where the jet is directed rightward

The subcostal window deserves particular emphasis for two reasons: it is often the only usable window in the patients who most need the study, and it is the best transthoracic view of the **interatrial septum**, making it the window for shunt assessment.

Foreshortening — the cardinal apical error

Apical views are the source of the volumes and ejection fraction that drive clinical decisions, and they are systematically degraded by a single, common technical fault.

What happens: the transducer is placed too **medially or too superiorly**, so the imaging plane cuts across the ventricle rather than through its true apex. The ventricle appears **shorter and more rounded** than it is.

The consequences:

- **Volumes are underestimated**
- **Ejection fraction is overestimated** — a foreshortened ventricle looks like it is contracting more than it is
- **Apical wall motion abnormalities and apical thrombus are missed**

The correction: move the transducer **laterally and inferiorly** to find the true apex — the point of maximal cardiac impulse, further round the chest than most operators expect. The correctly acquired apical four-chamber view shows the **longest** ventricle you can obtain, with the apex at the top of the sector and the ventricle not truncated.

A working test: if the ventricle looks round rather than elongated, it is foreshortened.

Other technical points

Off-axis parasternal long axis — cutting obliquely across the ventricle — underestimates linear dimensions. Align the plane through the true long axis, with the aortic and mitral valves and the LV cavity all in view.

Frame rate matters for rapidly moving structures: **narrow the sector** and **reduce depth** to raise it, particularly in tachycardic patients and in children.

Document every view, and state which windows were inadequate and why. In echocardiography, "poor acoustic windows" is a genuine and frequent limitation, and its specific consequences — which measurement could not be made — should be named (Chapter 1 §1.5).

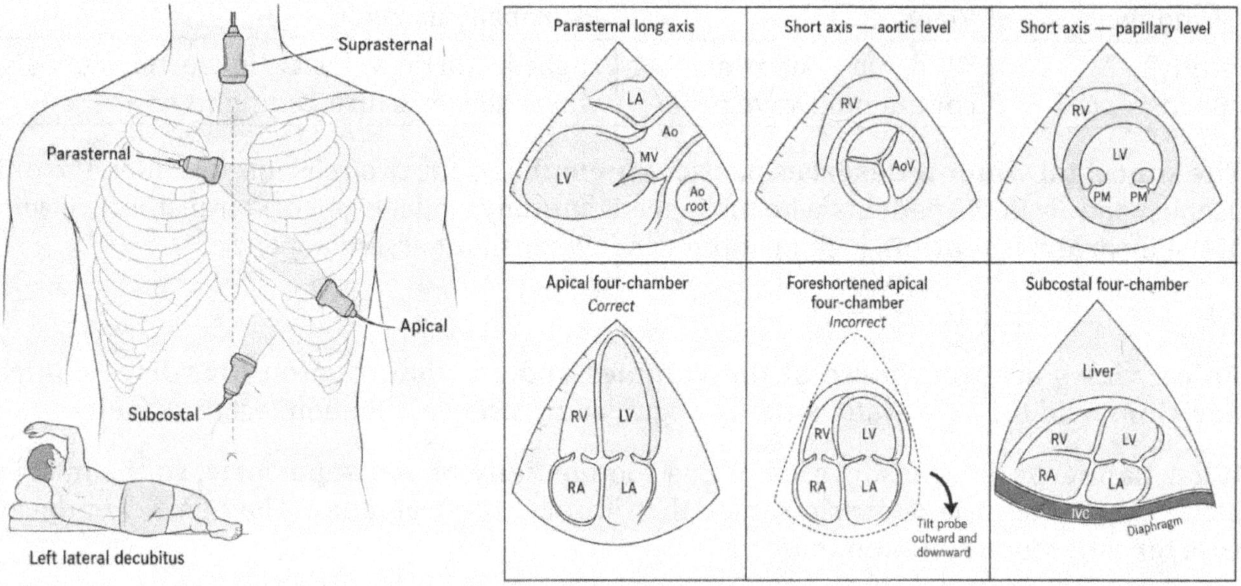

The standard transthoracic windows and the error that corrupts the most important measurements.
Foreshortening underestimates volumes, overestimates ejection fraction, and may hide apical pathology.

14.6 M-Mode, Two-Dimensional, and Doppler Technique

M-mode

A single scan line displayed against time, at a sampling rate far higher than two-dimensional imaging can achieve.

What it is for: temporal resolution. Rapid events — valve opening and closing, subtle wall motion timing, the systolic anterior motion of the mitral valve, fine mobile structures — are resolved by M-mode when they are blurred on 2D.

Standard applications: left ventricular linear dimensions; mitral valve leaflet motion; aortic root and left atrial dimensions; **TAPSE** through the lateral tricuspid annulus (§14.8); and inferior vena cava diameter and collapse.

Its limitation is alignment. The cursor samples a single line, and if that line is not **perpendicular to the structure**, dimensions are overestimated. **Anatomic (steerable) M-mode**, available on most systems, reconstructs a line at any angle from the 2D data and largely resolves this — at some cost in temporal resolution.

M-mode is a supplement, not a substitute. Chamber quantification guidelines have moved decisively toward volumetric methods (§14.7), and linear M-mode dimensions are no longer the basis for ejection fraction.

Two-dimensional imaging

The foundation of the study, and the basis of all volumetric measurement.

Frame rate is the parameter to protect. Cardiac motion is fast, and a low frame rate blurs systole and diastole together. **Narrow the sector**, **reduce depth**, and limit the number of focal zones. In children and in tachycardia this matters more than image beauty.

Harmonic imaging substantially improves endocardial border definition in difficult patients, at some cost in the appearance of thin structures.

Colour Doppler

Maps flow within a region of interest.

The setting that determines interpretation is the velocity scale (Nyquist limit). A low scale makes any regurgitant jet look large; a high scale makes it look small. **Regurgitation severity assessed from jet area is therefore highly settings-dependent**, which is why colour jet area is a crude tool and why the scale must be standardised and stated.

Keep the colour box as small as the question allows — a narrow box preserves frame rate.

Pulsed-wave Doppler

Samples a **defined location**. Used where the site matters and the velocity is modest: **mitral inflow** at the leaflet tips, **LVOT** velocity–time integral, pulmonary vein flow, and tissue Doppler.

Its limit is aliasing at the Nyquist limit (Chapter 2 §2.9), which is why it cannot record the high velocities of stenosis or regurgitation.

Continuous-wave Doppler

Transmits and receives continuously, recording **every velocity along the line** with **no aliasing limit** but **no depth localisation**.

Used for all high velocities: aortic stenosis, tricuspid regurgitation, mitral regurgitation, ventricular septal defect, and pulmonary gradients. A **dedicated non-imaging (Pedoff) probe** offers better sensitivity and is used from the right parasternal and suprasternal windows in aortic stenosis.

The practical discipline: interrogate from **multiple windows** and take the **highest velocity** (§14.4).

Tissue Doppler imaging

Reverses the usual filtering to record the **low-velocity, high-amplitude** motion of myocardium rather than blood.

Measured at the mitral annulus, septal and lateral, it yields:

- **s′** — peak systolic annular velocity, a longitudinal systolic function index
- **e′** — early diastolic annular velocity, a **relatively load-independent** marker of relaxation

- **a′** — late diastolic velocity with atrial contraction

e′ is the key measurement in diastolic assessment, because combining it with mitral inflow E velocity gives **E/e′**, a surrogate for left ventricular filling pressure (§14.8).

Advanced techniques

Speckle tracking and global longitudinal strain. Tracks myocardial deformation rather than motion, producing **GLS** — a more sensitive marker of early systolic dysfunction than ejection fraction, and now central to **cardio-oncology surveillance**, where it detects chemotherapy-related dysfunction before EF falls. **Values are vendor-dependent**, so serial studies must use the same vendor and preferably the same machine.

Three-dimensional echocardiography — more accurate chamber volumes and ejection fraction than 2D, and superior valve anatomy assessment.

Contrast echocardiography (Chapter 9) has two distinct cardiac uses:

1. **Left ventricular opacification** with a licensed contrast agent, to define the endocardial border in patients with poor windows and to detect **apical thrombus**. This converts a non-diagnostic study into a diagnostic one and is under-used.
2. **Agitated saline ("bubble study")** for shunt detection. Bubbles appearing in the left atrium **within a few beats** of right atrial opacification indicate an **intracardiac** shunt; **delayed** appearance suggests an **intrapulmonary** shunt such as a pulmonary arteriovenous malformation.

Stress echocardiography and **transoesophageal echocardiography** extend the examination where transthoracic imaging cannot answer the question — the latter particularly for the left atrial appendage, prosthetic valves, endocarditis, and the interatrial septum.

14.7 Chamber Quantification and Measurement Protocol

The governing principle

Measurements feed directly into guideline thresholds for intervention. A ventricular dimension, an atrial volume, or an ejection fraction determines whether a patient receives surgery, a device, or a drug. **Reproducibility therefore outranks convenience**, and the conventions below exist to make one operator's number comparable with another's.

All the reference values, measurement conventions, and indexing methods below are specified by a chamber quantification guideline that is periodically revised, and must be taken from its current edition rather than from memory. [VERIFY: current chamber quantification guideline, its reference ranges by sex, its measurement conventions, and its indexing requirements]

Timing

End-diastole — the frame at QRS onset, or the largest ventricular cavity. **End-systole** — the smallest ventricular cavity.

Left ventricular linear dimensions

Measured on the **parasternal long axis, perpendicular to the ventricular long axis**, at the level **immediately below the mitral leaflet tips**:

- **LVIDd** and **LVIDs** — internal diameter in diastole and systole
- **IVSd** — interventricular septal thickness
- **LVPWd** — posterior wall thickness

Take them from **2D-guided M-mode with correct perpendicular alignment**, or directly from the 2D image. **Oblique measurement overestimates**, and an off-axis parasternal view is the usual cause.

Left ventricular volumes and ejection fraction

The recommended method is the biplane method of discs (modified Simpson's rule), from the **apical four-chamber and apical two-chamber** views.

Technique:

1. Acquire both apical views **without foreshortening** (§14.5)
2. Trace the **endocardial border** at end-diastole and end-systole
3. **Include the papillary muscles and trabeculations within the cavity** — trace the compacted endocardial surface, not around the papillary muscles
4. Set the annular plane at the mitral hinge points, and the long axis to the apex

Linear methods (such as the Teichholz formula) are not recommended for ejection fraction, because they extrapolate a single dimension to a whole-ventricle volume, assuming a geometric shape that is invalid whenever regional wall motion abnormality is present — which is precisely the population in whom EF matters most.

Three-dimensional volumes are more accurate where image quality permits.

Left ventricular mass

Calculated from linear dimensions or from volumetric methods, and **indexed to body surface area**. Used to identify and grade hypertrophy and to define relative wall thickness and remodelling patterns.

Left atrial size

Left atrial volume, indexed to body surface area, is the measurement to report — anteroposterior linear dimension from the parasternal long axis is inadequate, because the atrium enlarges asymmetrically.

Method: biplane discs or area–length, from apical four- and two-chamber views, measured at **end-systole** when the atrium is largest, **excluding the appendage and the pulmonary vein confluences**.

Left atrial volume index is a powerful prognostic marker and is a core component of diastolic assessment (§14.8) — it reflects the cumulative effect of raised filling pressure over time, in the way that a single Doppler measurement cannot.

Right ventricle

The right ventricle is **not a simple geometric shape**, and 2D volume estimation is unreliable.

Measure: basal and mid-cavity diameters and longitudinal length from an **RV-focused apical four-chamber view** — acquired specifically for the purpose, rotating and angling to maximise the RV cavity rather than accepting the standard LV-centred view. **Right ventricular wall thickness** is measured from the subcostal view.

Three-dimensional echocardiography or cardiac MRI is preferred where RV volumes are required.

Aortic root

Measured at the **annulus, sinuses of Valsalva, sinotubular junction, and ascending aorta**.

Conventions differ — leading-edge to leading-edge versus inner-edge to inner-edge, and end-diastole versus mid-systole — and **the convention used must be stated**, because serial comparison across conventions is meaningless in a patient under surveillance for aneurysm. [VERIFY: the aortic measurement convention to be adopted and the timing within the cardiac cycle]

Indexing and serial comparison

Index to body surface area where the guideline requires it, and use **sex-specific reference ranges**.

For serial studies, **reproduce the plane, the caliper convention, and the timing** (Chapter 1 §1.5). In surveillance of aortic dimensions or ventricular size, the rate of change drives management, and a measurement taken differently is not a comparison.

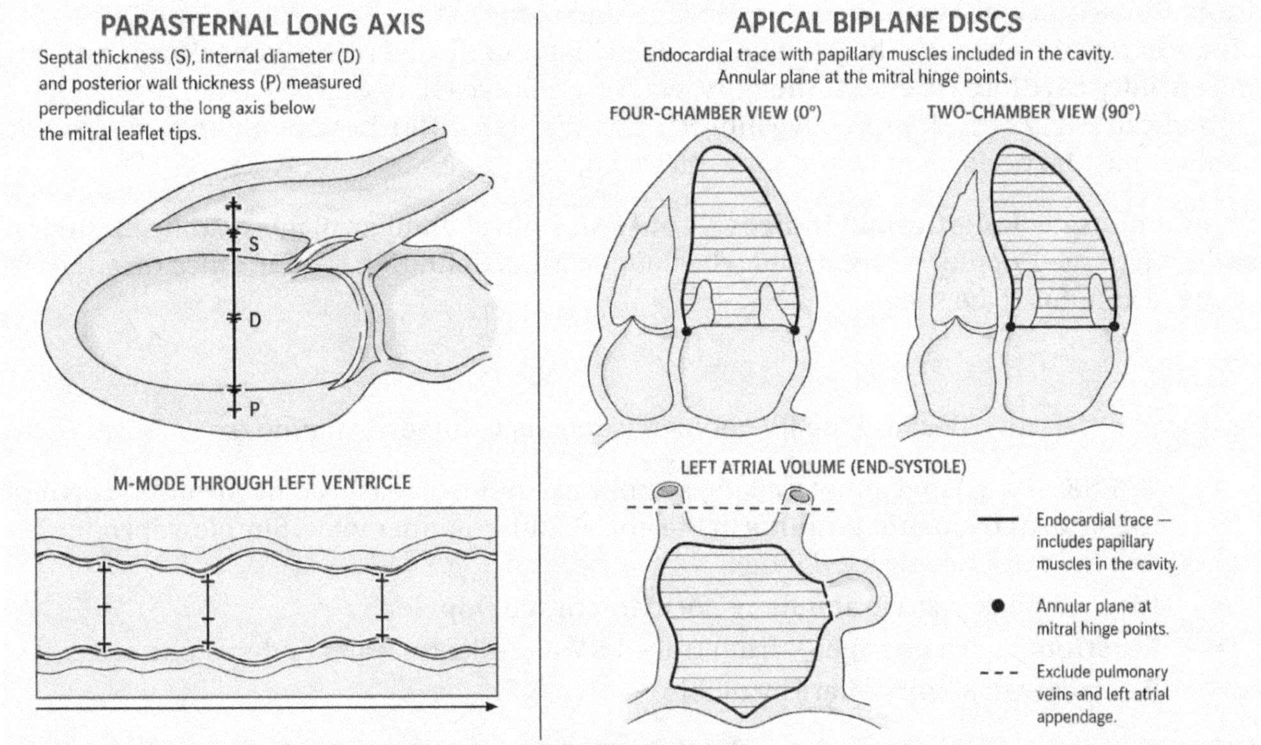

14.8 Systolic and Diastolic Function Assessment

Left ventricular systolic function

Ejection fraction is the primary index, calculated by biplane discs (§14.7) and reported against guideline categories. **It is not a measure of contractility** — it is load-dependent, and a patient with severe mitral regurgitation may maintain a normal-looking EF while the ventricle is failing, because the ventricle is ejecting into a low-pressure atrium.

Regional wall motion is assessed using a standardised segmental model, with each segment scored as normal, hypokinetic, akinetic, dyskinetic, or aneurysmal.

The segments map onto coronary territories, which is what makes regional assessment diagnostically useful:

Territory	Segments
Left anterior descending	Anterior and anteroseptal walls, and the apex
Right coronary	Inferior and inferoseptal walls
Circumflex	Lateral and posterolateral walls

A wall motion abnormality confined to a coronary territory suggests ischaemic disease; global hypokinesis suggests a non-ischaemic cardiomyopathy — a distinction with immediate management consequences.

Global longitudinal strain measures myocardial deformation and is **more sensitive than ejection fraction** to early dysfunction. Its principal established role is **surveillance during potentially cardiotoxic chemotherapy**, where a relative fall in GLS precedes any change in EF and can trigger cardioprotective intervention. **Values differ between vendors**, so serial studies must be performed on the same platform.

Supplementary longitudinal indices — MAPSE (mitral annular plane systolic excursion) and **s′** on tissue Doppler — are useful when endocardial definition is poor, since they require only the annulus to be seen.

Right ventricular systolic function

Assessed differently, because the RV geometry defeats volumetric methods:

- **TAPSE** — tricuspid annular plane systolic excursion, measured by **M-mode through the lateral tricuspid annulus** in the apical four-chamber view. Simple, reproducible, and the most widely used index
- **RV s′** — peak systolic annular velocity on tissue Doppler
- **Fractional area change** — from traced RV end-diastolic and end-systolic areas
- **RV free wall strain** where available

[VERIFY: current threshold values for TAPSE, RV s′, fractional area change, and RV strain]

Septal motion carries information about right heart pressure and volume: a **flattened interventricular septum** indicates RV overload — flattening predominantly in **diastole** suggests volume overload, and in **systole** suggests pressure overload, producing the D-shaped left ventricle in short axis.

Diastolic function

The question being answered is whether left ventricular filling pressure is raised — not simply whether relaxation is impaired. No single measurement answers it, so the assessment is deliberately multiparametric.

The four core parameters:

1. **Mitral inflow** by pulsed-wave Doppler at the **leaflet tips** — peak **E** and **A** velocities, the **E/A ratio**, and **deceleration time**
2. **Tissue Doppler e′** at the **septal and lateral mitral annulus**, and the derived **E/e′** ratio as a filling pressure surrogate
3. **Left atrial volume index** (§14.7)
4. **Peak tricuspid regurgitation velocity**, reflecting pulmonary pressure (§14.4)

The grading pattern:

Grade	Pattern	Physiology
Normal	Normal E/A, normal e′, normal LA volume	—

Grade	Pattern	Physiology
Grade I — impaired relaxation	**Reduced E/A**, prolonged deceleration time, reduced e′	Slowed relaxation, filling pressure not yet raised
Grade II — pseudonormal	**E/A appears normal**	Rising atrial pressure restores the E/A ratio — the trap
Grade III — restrictive	**High E/A**, short deceleration time	Markedly raised filling pressure, stiff ventricle

Pseudonormalisation is the central pitfall. As left atrial pressure rises, it pushes the E wave back up and the E/A ratio returns to an apparently normal value while the ventricle is in fact worse. **Mitral inflow alone therefore cannot grade diastolic function**, and this is precisely why e′, left atrial volume, and TR velocity are required — **e′ falls and does not pseudonormalise**.

The Valsalva manoeuvre reduces preload and unmasks a pseudonormal pattern, converting it back to the impaired relaxation appearance.

Confounders that invalidate or distort the assessment: age (e′ falls normally with age, so age-appropriate values must be used), **atrial fibrillation** (no A wave; average several beats), **tachycardia** (E and A fuse), significant **mitral valve disease or prosthesis**, heavy **mitral annular calcification**, and constrictive or restrictive physiology.

The diagnostic algorithms in this area have been substantially revised, and the current version must be applied rather than a remembered one. [VERIFY: current diastolic function assessment algorithm, its parameter thresholds, and the criteria for indeterminate results]

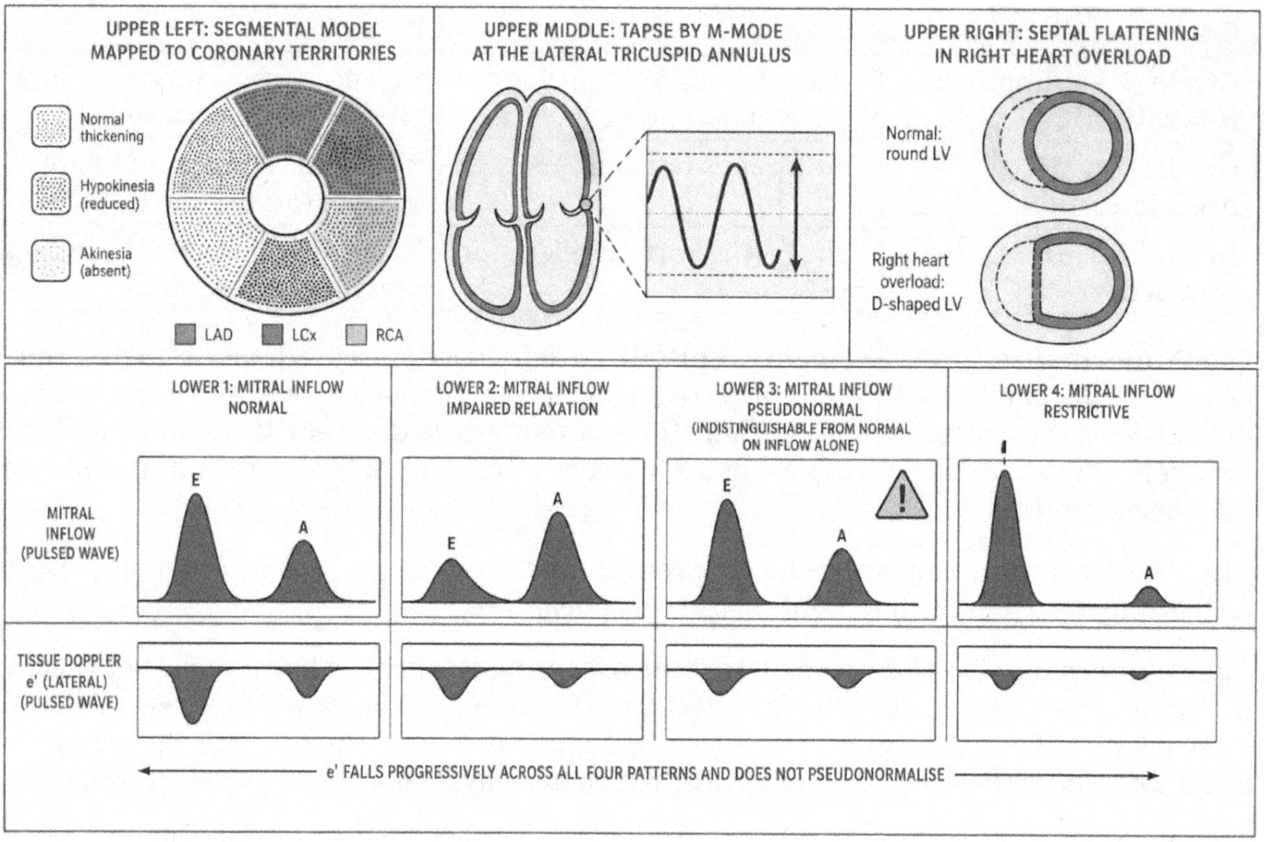

14.9 Echocardiographic Artifacts and Pitfalls

Artifacts, and where they cause trouble

The physics is Chapter 2; what follows is where each artifact does specific damage in the heart.

Reverberation and near-field clutter. Bright horizontal lines within the near field. In the heart these are mistaken for:

- **An intimal flap** in the ascending aorta — the commonest and most consequential false positive in aortic imaging
- **Apical thrombus**, in the near field of the apical view
- Layering within the left atrium

Resolve by changing the window and angle (Chapter 2 §2.8): a genuine flap persists and moves independently; a reverberation artifact disappears or shifts with a different approach. **A flap seen from only one window is not a flap.**

Side lobes. Curved arcs crossing chambers, producing false intracardiac structures, particularly in the atria. **They disappear on harmonic imaging** and on changing the angle.

Mirror imaging. Duplication of structures beyond a strong reflector — the descending aorta and the pericardium are the usual culprits. Doppler mirror artifact produces a symmetrical spectral trace above and below the baseline with unidirectional flow, usually from excessive gain or near-perpendicular insonation.

Acoustic shadowing. From **prosthetic valves**, annular and valvular **calcification**, ribs, and **pacemaker leads**. A mechanical mitral prosthesis shadows the entire left atrium behind it, which is why **transoesophageal echocardiography is required** to assess prosthetic mitral regurgitation — the transthoracic study is blind to exactly the region of interest. **Recognise the shadow and state its consequence in the report.**

Aliasing. In colour and pulsed-wave Doppler at the Nyquist limit. Distinguish it from true flow reversal by the colour transition: **aliasing passes through the pale tints of both colours, while true reversal passes through black** (Chapter 2 §2.9). Correct by raising the scale, shifting the baseline, or moving to continuous-wave.

Range ambiguity at high pulse repetition frequency, placing deep echoes at falsely shallow depths.

Settings that create disease

Colour gain and Nyquist setting determine apparent regurgitation severity. A high colour gain and a low velocity scale will make trivial regurgitation look moderate. **Standardise the scale**, set gain to just below the level at which random colour speckle appears in tissue, and never grade regurgitation from jet area alone.

Excessive 2D gain obscures fine structures and fills chambers with noise; insufficient gain drops out endocardium and exaggerates apparent wall motion abnormality.

Normal structures mistaken for pathology

This list accounts for a large share of unnecessary onward investigation:

Structure	Location	Distinguishing feature
Chiari network	Right atrium	Filamentous, highly mobile, attached near the IVC and coronary sinus
Eustachian valve	IVC orifice	A fixed ridge at a constant location
Crista terminalis	Right atrium, posterolateral	A smooth ridge continuous with the atrial wall
Moderator band	Right ventricular apex	Crosses from septum to free wall; a normal identifying feature
Lipomatous hypertrophy of the interatrial septum	Interatrial septum	Dumbbell-shaped, **sparing the fossa ovalis** — the sparing is the diagnostic feature
Left atrial ridge (between appendage and left upper pulmonary vein)	Left atrium	A smooth linear ridge with a bulbous tip; the classic pseudo-mass, resolved by recognising its constant location

Structure	Location	Distinguishing feature
False tendons	Left ventricular cavity	Thin linear structures crossing the cavity, of no significance
Pericardial fat pad	Anterior	**Echogenic** rather than anechoic, **anterior only**, and **moves with the heart**

Pericardial versus pleural fluid

A recurring and clinically important distinction, made on a single anatomical relationship in the parasternal long axis:

> **Pericardial fluid tracks anterior to the descending thoracic aorta. Pleural fluid lies posterior to it.**

The same principle appears in the trauma context in Chapter 8 §8.9, and it is worth being able to apply it instantly in both.

Technical limitations to report, not conceal

Poor acoustic windows are common in obstructive lung disease, obesity, chest wall deformity, and ventilated patients. The correct response is escalation of technique — reposition, use subcostal windows, use **contrast for left ventricular opacification** (§14.6) — and, where the study remains limited, an explicit statement of **which measurements could not be made** and what alternative is recommended.

"Technically difficult study" alone is not adequate; "endocardial border inadequately defined in the apical views; ejection fraction not quantifiable; consider contrast study or cardiac MRI" is (Chapter 1 §1.5).

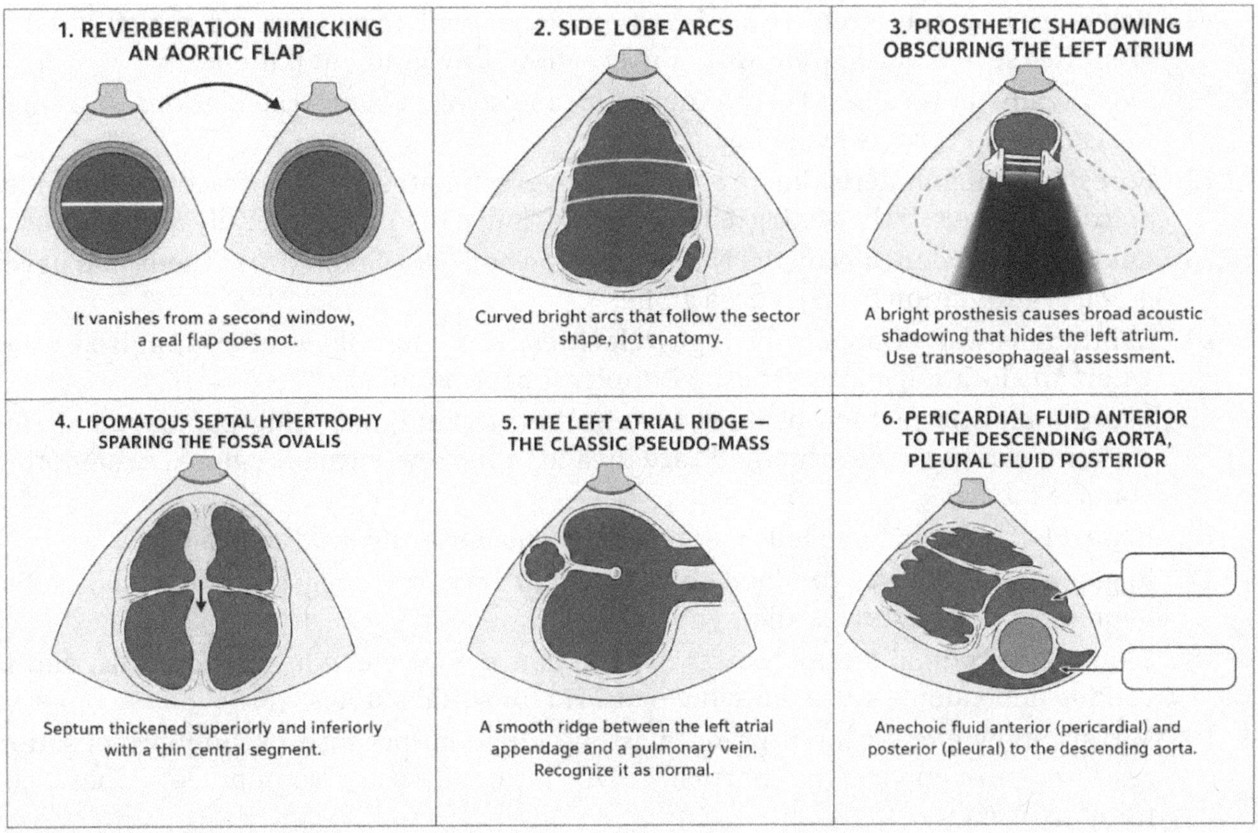

Key Points

1. Echocardiography does not follow the orientation conventions of general sonography, and it does not use angle correction — the operator aligns the beam with flow and takes the highest velocity obtained.
2. Establish abdominal situs before interpreting laterality: aorta left of the spine, IVC right, in situs solitus.
3. Left lateral decubitus positioning is the single most effective manoeuvre for parasternal and apical windows.
4. The moderator band, coarse trabeculation, and septal papillary attachments identify the morphological right ventricle. The atrioventricular offset is normal; its absence indicates an atrioventricular septal defect.
5. Valves open and close because of pressure crossings. That principle makes the whole cardiac cycle derivable.
6. An ECG trace is mandatory: end-diastole is at QRS onset, end-systole at the smallest cavity. Without it, measurements are not comparable.
7. In atrial fibrillation, average several consecutive beats. Do not measure one.
8. The simplified Bernoulli equation assumes a negligible proximal velocity. Where it is elevated, use the expanded form or the gradient will be overestimated.
9. RVSP is derived from the tricuspid regurgitation velocity plus estimated right atrial pressure. An incompletely traced envelope underestimates it, and trivial TR means the calculation cannot be made at all — say so.

10. Valve area by continuity is far less flow-dependent than gradient, which is what identifies severe aortic stenosis in the low-flow, low-gradient patient.
11. LVOT diameter is squared in the continuity and stroke volume calculations, so a small measurement error is magnified.
12. Foreshortening underestimates volumes, overestimates ejection fraction, and hides apical thrombus. If the ventricle looks round, move the probe laterally and inferiorly.
13. Colour jet area depends on the Nyquist setting and gain. Standardise them, and never grade regurgitation from jet area alone.
14. Continuous-wave Doppler for high velocities from multiple windows; pulsed-wave where the location matters; tissue Doppler for the annulus.
15. Use the biplane method of discs for ejection fraction, including papillary muscles within the cavity. Linear methods are invalid in the presence of regional wall motion abnormality.
16. Report left atrial volume index, not an anteroposterior linear dimension.
17. Regional wall motion confined to a coronary territory suggests ischaemia; global hypokinesis suggests a cardiomyopathy.
18. Global longitudinal strain detects dysfunction before ejection fraction falls, and is vendor-dependent — use the same platform for serial studies.
19. Mitral inflow alone cannot grade diastolic function, because pseudonormalisation restores an apparently normal E/A ratio. Tissue Doppler e′ does not pseudonormalise.
20. A reverberation flap disappears from a second window; a real dissection flap does not.
21. Pericardial fluid tracks anterior to the descending thoracic aorta; pleural fluid lies posterior to it.
22. A mechanical mitral prosthesis shadows the left atrium — the region you most need to see. State the limitation and refer for transoesophageal assessment.

Registry Check

1. Which finding most reliably identifies the morphological right ventricle?

A. Its anterior position **B.** The moderator band **C.** Two papillary muscles **D.** Fibrous continuity between the inflow and outflow valves

> **Answer: B.** The moderator band crossing from the interventricular septum to the anterior papillary muscle is the most reliable morphological marker of the right ventricle. Two papillary muscles and inflow-to-outflow fibrous continuity are features of the left ventricle, and chamber position is unreliable in congenital and malposition cases.

2. In estimating right ventricular systolic pressure from the tricuspid regurgitation jet, the value added to $4v^2$ is:

A. Pulmonary artery diastolic pressure **B.** Left atrial pressure **C.** Estimated right atrial pressure **D.** Mean arterial pressure

Answer: C. The modified Bernoulli calculation gives the pressure difference between right ventricle and right atrium during systole, so right atrial pressure must be added to obtain right ventricular systolic pressure. Right atrial pressure is estimated from inferior vena cava diameter and respiratory collapsibility.

3. An apical four-chamber view shows a left ventricle that appears short and rounded. The likely consequence for measurement is that ejection fraction will be:

A. Underestimated **B.** Overestimated **C.** Unaffected **D.** Unmeasurable

Answer: B. Foreshortening truncates the ventricle, reducing measured volumes and making the ventricle appear to contract more than it does, so ejection fraction is overestimated. It also conceals apical wall motion abnormality and apical thrombus. The correction is to move the transducer laterally and inferiorly to the true apex.

4. Aortic valve area calculated by the continuity equation is preferred over peak gradient in low-output states because:

A. It is easier to measure **B.** Gradient is flow-dependent and underestimates severity when cardiac output is low **C.** Continuity does not require the LVOT diameter **D.** Gradient cannot be measured in low-output states

Answer: B. The transvalvular gradient depends on flow, so a severely stenotic valve can generate a low gradient when stroke volume is reduced. Valve area by continuity is substantially less flow-dependent and identifies severe stenosis in the low-flow, low-gradient patient. The LVOT diameter is still required and remains the principal source of error, since it is squared.

5. Mitral inflow shows an E/A ratio within the normal range, but the tissue Doppler e′ is markedly reduced and the left atrial volume index is elevated. This pattern indicates:

A. Normal diastolic function **B.** Grade I diastolic dysfunction **C.** Pseudonormal filling — grade II diastolic dysfunction **D.** Constrictive pericarditis

Answer: C. Rising left atrial pressure restores an apparently normal E/A ratio while diastolic function is in fact worse — pseudonormalisation. Tissue Doppler e′ falls progressively and does not pseudonormalise, and left atrial volume reflects the cumulative effect of raised filling pressure, which is why both are required alongside mitral inflow.

6. A linear echo is seen crossing the lumen of the ascending aorta on a parasternal long-axis view. The most appropriate next step is:

A. Report an aortic dissection **B.** Increase the two-dimensional gain **C.** Re-image from a different window and angle to determine whether the line persists **D.** Apply colour Doppler alone

Answer: C. Reverberation artifact in the near field commonly mimics an intimal flap, and this is the most consequential false positive in aortic imaging. A genuine flap persists from multiple windows and moves independently through the cardiac cycle; an artifact disappears or shifts when the approach changes.

7. A thickened interatrial septum is noted with a dumbbell configuration and sparing of the fossa ovalis. This represents:

A. Atrial myxoma **B.** Lipomatous hypertrophy of the interatrial septum **C.** Thrombus **D.** An atrial septal aneurysm

Answer: B. Lipomatous hypertrophy thickens the septum superiorly and inferiorly while sparing the fossa ovalis, producing the characteristic dumbbell shape. The sparing of the fossa is the diagnostic feature, and the finding is benign.

8. In a parasternal long-axis view, an anechoic collection is seen tracking posterior to the descending thoracic aorta. This represents:

A. Pericardial effusion **B.** Pleural effusion **C.** Pericardial fat pad **D.** Dilated coronary sinus

Answer: B. The relationship to the descending thoracic aorta distinguishes the two: pericardial fluid tracks anterior to it, while pleural fluid lies posterior. The pericardial fat pad is echogenic rather than anechoic and lies anteriorly, moving with the heart.

Chapter Notes for the Editorial Pass

Verification queue. In priority order: **the chamber quantification guideline to be adopted**, with its reference ranges by sex, measurement conventions, and indexing requirements (§14.7) — every quantitative statement in Chapters 14 and 15 depends on it; **the diastolic function assessment algorithm**, its parameter thresholds, and the handling of indeterminate results (§14.8), which has been substantially revised and must not be reproduced from memory; **ejection fraction category boundaries** (§14.8); **right ventricular function thresholds** for TAPSE, s′, fractional area change and strain (§14.8); **normal intracardiac and pulmonary pressure ranges** (§14.3); **the aortic root measurement convention and cycle timing** (§14.7), which materially affects surveillance comparability; and **global longitudinal strain normal ranges and the relative-change threshold used in cardio-oncology** (§14.8).

Structural note. This chapter establishes the technique and quantification framework on which Chapter 15 entirely depends. The measurement conventions in §14.7 and the haemodynamic calculations in §14.4 should be finalised **before** Chapter 15 is edited, since valve severity grading, chamber remodelling criteria and pulmonary pressure estimation all inherit from them. Editing the two chapters in the opposite order will produce inconsistencies.

Figure count: 7 Lane A, 1 Lane B. Cardiac imaging is the most motion-dependent material in the book, and three of the teaching points here — foreshortening, pseudonormalisation unmasked by Valsalva, and the mobility of a genuine dissection flap — are demonstrated far better by cine than by still frames. This reinforces the recommendation made in the Chapter

13 notes: decide early whether the digital edition supports video, because Part V depends on it more than any preceding part.

Cross-reference targets to fix at layout: §14.1 heterotaxy and splenic anomalies → Chapter 6 §6.5 and Chapter 12 §12.5; §14.4 inferior vena cava assessment → Chapter 3 §3.5; §14.4 angle discipline contrasted with vascular practice → Chapter 2 §2.5 and Chapter 16; §14.6 contrast agents and bubble studies → Chapter 9 §9.1–9.3; §14.9 artifact mechanisms → Chapter 2 §2.7–2.9; §14.9 pericardial versus pleural fluid → Chapter 8 §8.9; §14.9 reporting of technical limitation → Chapter 1 §1.5.

Word count: approximately 10,400 excluding image prompt blocks, learning objectives, registry questions, and these notes.

Chapter 15: Clinical and Fetal Echocardiography

Learning Objectives

On completing this chapter you should be able to:

1. Assess mitral stenosis and regurgitation, and distinguish primary from secondary regurgitation.
2. Grade aortic stenosis, including the low-flow low-gradient patient, and assess aortic regurgitation.
3. Evaluate right-sided valves and recognise prosthetic valve dysfunction.
4. Identify pericardial effusion, apply the echocardiographic signs of tamponade, and distinguish constriction from restriction.
5. Recognise the principal cardiomyopathies and the features that identify cardiac amyloidosis.
6. Approach a cardiac mass systematically and distinguish thrombus, vegetation and tumour.
7. Perform the fetal cardiac screening sequence, including the outflow tracts and the three-vessel-and-trachea view.
8. Assess fetal rhythm using M-mode and interpret the fetal Doppler indices.
9. Recognise the septal and outflow tract defects, and explain the concept of duct dependence.
10. Describe the counselling pathway after a prenatal cardiac diagnosis and the sonographer's role within it.

Where This Chapter Sits

Everything here is built on Chapter 14. The windows, the measurement conventions, the Bernoulli and continuity calculations, and the artifact catalogue are assumed rather than repeated, and every severity assessment inherits from them.

Two organising ideas run through the whole chapter.

Severity is multiparametric. No single number grades a valve lesion. Guidelines specify a set of supportive and specific criteria, and the correct approach is to gather several and report where they agree and where they conflict. A lone measurement, quoted with confidence, is how patients get sent for the wrong operation.

The fetal sections are not a subspecialty appendix. Prenatal detection of duct-dependent lesions changes survival, because it allows delivery near a cardiac centre with prostaglandin available from birth. The screening sequence in §15.7 is the highest-yield material in this chapter.

15.1 Mitral Valve Disease

Mitral stenosis

Aetiology. Rheumatic disease remains the dominant cause worldwide, and its recognition matters most in populations where it is prevalent. Degenerative calcific disease with heavy mitral annular calcification is increasingly seen in older patients, and congenital, radiation-induced and drug-induced forms are uncommon.

The rheumatic morphology is characteristic:

- **Leaflet thickening, most marked at the tips**
- **Commissural fusion**
- **Chordal thickening and shortening**, restricting the subvalvular apparatus
- **Diastolic doming of the anterior leaflet** — the "hockey stick" appearance in the parasternal long axis, produced by a mobile leaflet body tethered at a fused tip
- A **fish-mouth orifice** on parasternal short axis

Assessment of severity uses several independent methods, and they should be compared rather than used singly:

Method	Technique	Caveats
Planimetry	Trace the orifice in parasternal short axis **at the leaflet tips** — the smallest orifice found on a careful sweep	The reference two-dimensional method; requires correct plane and adequate image quality
Pressure half-time	Mitral valve area derived from the deceleration of the diastolic gradient	**Invalidated by** significant aortic regurgitation, immediately after balloon valvuloplasty, by an atrial septal defect, by tachycardia, and by impaired left ventricular relaxation
Mean gradient	From the continuous-wave trace	**Heart-rate dependent** — report the heart rate alongside it
Continuity equation	As in Chapter 14 §14.4	Invalid in significant regurgitation of either valve

[VERIFY: current severity criteria for mitral stenosis, including valve area and mean gradient thresholds]

Also assess and report: left atrial size, **pulmonary artery systolic pressure** from the tricuspid regurgitation velocity, atrial fibrillation, spontaneous echo contrast, and the suitability of the valve for balloon valvuloplasty — for which a scoring system assessing leaflet mobility, thickening, calcification and subvalvular disease is used. [VERIFY: the valvuloplasty scoring system to be adopted and its thresholds]

Left atrial appendage thrombus must be excluded by transoesophageal echocardiography before valvuloplasty or cardioversion. The transthoracic study cannot do this (Chapter 14 §14.9).

Mitral regurgitation

The primary–secondary distinction determines everything that follows:

Primary (degenerative) regurgitation — the **valve itself is abnormal**. Myxomatous disease with prolapse, flail leaflet from ruptured chordae, rheumatic disease, endocarditis, or a cleft leaflet. **Treatment is directed at the valve.**

Secondary (functional) regurgitation — the **leaflets are structurally normal**, and regurgitation results from annular dilatation and leaflet tethering caused by left ventricular dilatation or regional dysfunction. **Treatment is directed at the ventricle**, and the severity thresholds differ from those used in primary disease.

Mitral valve prolapse is defined as displacement of a leaflet **beyond the annular plane by a defined margin**, and there is a technical trap: **the diagnosis must be made in the parasternal long axis or an apical long-axis view, not in the apical four-chamber**. The mitral annulus is **saddle-shaped**, and the four-chamber plane cuts through its lower saddle horn, making normal leaflets appear to prolapse. [VERIFY: current displacement threshold defining mitral valve prolapse]

Quantification — again multiparametric:

- **Vena contracta width** — the narrowest portion of the jet at the orifice
- **Proximal isovelocity surface area (PISA)** giving effective regurgitant orifice area and regurgitant volume
- **Regurgitant fraction**
- **Pulmonary venous flow — systolic blunting and, more specifically, systolic flow reversal** indicate severe regurgitation
- **Continuous-wave jet density and contour** — a dense, triangular, early-peaking envelope suggests severe regurgitation with rapid atrial pressure rise
- **Left ventricular and left atrial size** — chamber remodelling reflects chronic severity

The eccentric jet trap: an eccentric jet hugs the atrial wall and **appears far smaller than its true severity**, while a central jet of the same volume expands freely and looks larger. A wall-hugging jet should prompt escalation of quantification, not reassurance. This is a principal reason colour jet area alone is inadequate (Chapter 14 §14.9).

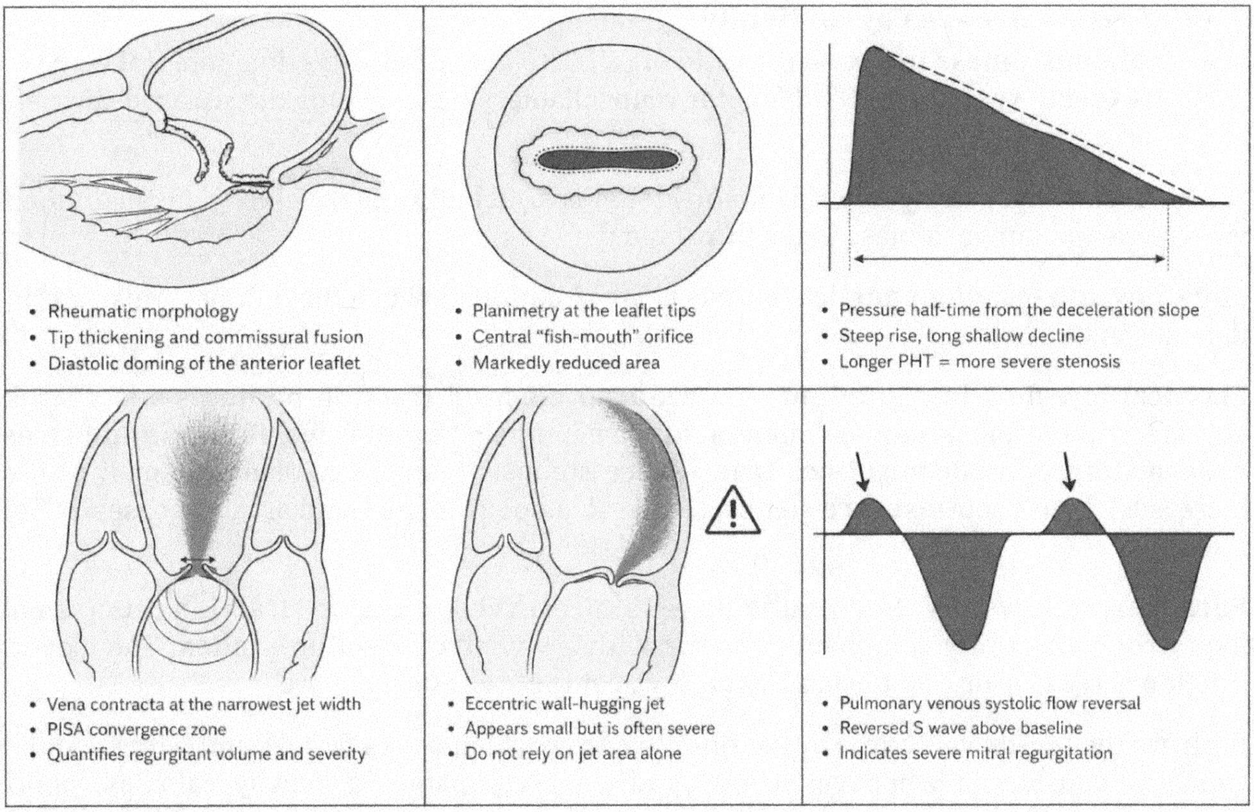

15.2 Aortic Valve Disease

Aortic stenosis

Aetiology. Calcific degenerative disease is much the commonest in older populations. **Bicuspid aortic valve** presents earlier, and **rheumatic disease** typically involves the mitral valve as well — a useful discriminator.

The bicuspid valve deserves separate emphasis because of what accompanies it:

- **Systolic doming** and an **eccentric closure line** on the long axis
- **Two cusps with a raphe** on the short axis in systole — the valve must be imaged in systole, since a raphe can make a bicuspid valve look trileaflet in diastole
- **Associated aortopathy — the ascending aorta must be measured in every bicuspid valve**, because dilatation and dissection risk are independent of the valve lesion and drive separate surgical thresholds
- **Association with coarctation** — assess the arch

Severity assessment:

- **Peak velocity** by continuous-wave Doppler, obtained from **multiple windows** including the **right parasternal position with a non-imaging probe**. Take the highest velocity — an underestimate here understates severity (Chapter 14 §14.4)
- **Mean gradient**

- **Aortic valve area by continuity**
- **Dimensionless index** — the ratio of LVOT to aortic velocity–time integral — which is useful when the LVOT diameter is unreliable, since it avoids the squared-diameter error

[VERIFY: current severity criteria for aortic stenosis, including peak velocity, mean gradient, valve area and dimensionless index thresholds]

Low-flow, low-gradient aortic stenosis is the situation in which the numbers mislead, and it comes in two forms:

Classical low-flow low-gradient — a **reduced ejection fraction** produces a low stroke volume, and therefore a low gradient across a genuinely severe valve. **Dobutamine stress echocardiography** distinguishes **true severe** stenosis (valve area remains small as flow increases) from **pseudosevere** stenosis (the valve opens further and area increases as flow rises).

Paradoxical low-flow low-gradient — a **preserved ejection fraction** in a small, hypertrophied, poorly compliant ventricle with a low **stroke volume index**. The ejection fraction is reassuring and the gradient is low, yet the stenosis is severe.

Both are the reason valve area by continuity matters (Chapter 14 §14.4), and both should be explicitly considered whenever a low gradient accompanies a heavily calcified, poorly mobile valve.

Subvalvular (discrete membrane or muscular) and **supravalvular** stenosis must be excluded when the gradient does not match the valve appearance.

Aortic regurgitation

Aetiology divides usefully into valve and root:

Valve — bicuspid, rheumatic, endocarditis, degenerative. **Root** — aortic dilatation of any cause, dissection, Marfan and related connective tissue disorders, and inflammatory aortitis.

This distinction changes the operation, so the root must be measured and described in every case of aortic regurgitation.

Severity assessment:

- **Vena contracta width**
- **Jet width relative to LVOT width** in the parasternal long axis
- **Pressure half-time** — a **short** half-time indicates rapid equalisation of aortic and ventricular pressures and therefore **severe** regurgitation
- **Holodiastolic flow reversal in the descending thoracic and abdominal aorta** — a relatively **specific** sign of severe regurgitation, and one obtainable from the suprasternal and subcostal windows
- **Regurgitant volume and fraction**
- **Left ventricular size and function**, which reflect chronicity and drive surgical timing

[VERIFY: current severity criteria for aortic regurgitation]

Acute severe aortic regurgitation presents differently and is a surgical emergency. Because the ventricle has not had time to dilate, the findings are: a **normal-sized left ventricle, tachycardia, premature closure of the mitral valve** as ventricular diastolic pressure rises above atrial pressure, and a **short pressure half-time**. The absence of ventricular dilatation is a sign of acuity, not of mildness — and this appearance in a patient with chest pain should prompt immediate consideration of **aortic dissection** and immediate escalation.

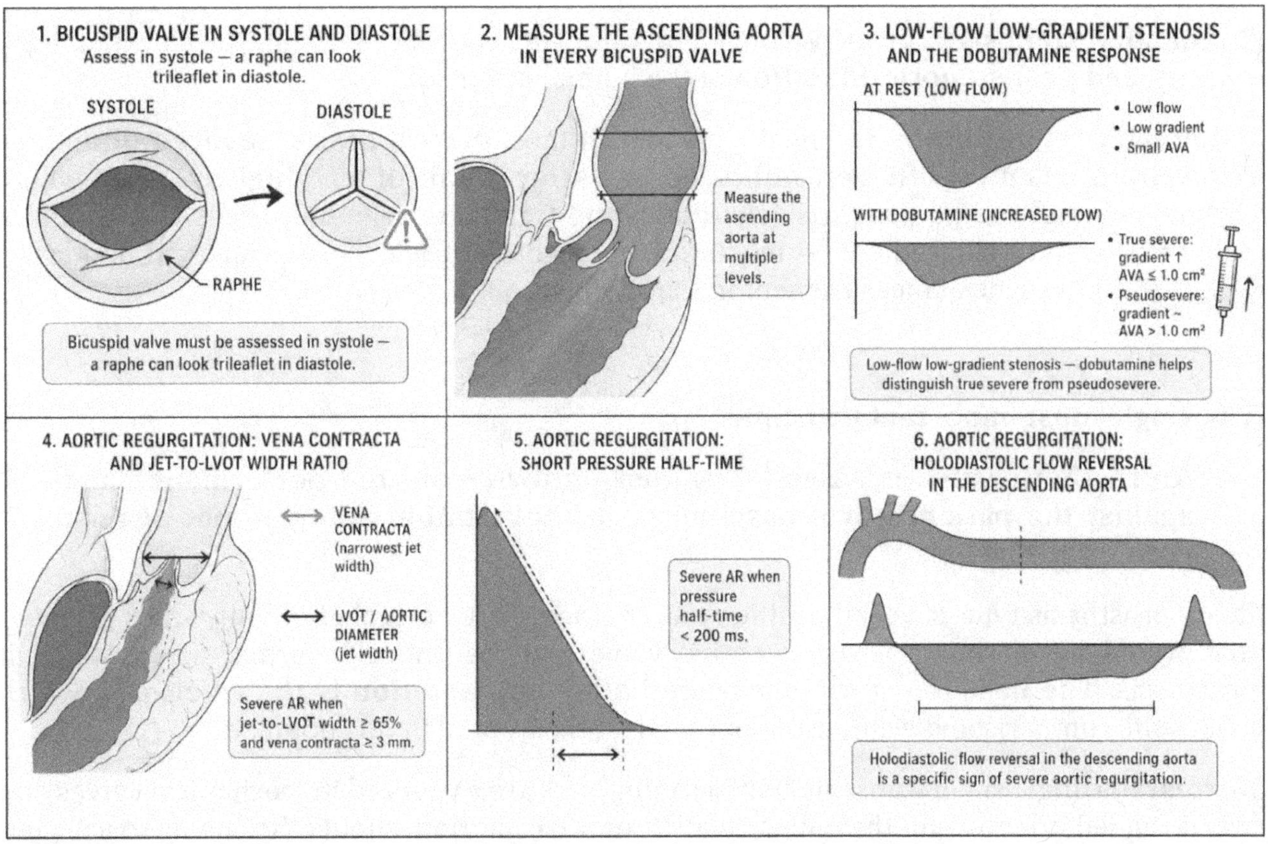

15.3 Right-Sided and Prosthetic Valve Assessment

Tricuspid regurgitation

Secondary regurgitation is far commoner than primary, arising from **annular dilatation** driven by right ventricular or right atrial enlargement — itself usually the consequence of left heart disease or pulmonary hypertension. The leaflets are normal.

Primary causes include **endocarditis** (particularly in people who inject drugs), **carcinoid** heart disease with thickened retracted leaflets, **Ebstein anomaly** (§15.10), **pacemaker or defibrillator lead** interference, rheumatic disease, and trauma.

Assessment: vena contracta, PISA-derived effective orifice area, jet area as a supportive measure only, right atrial and ventricular size, tricuspid annular diameter, and — a useful specific sign — **systolic flow reversal in the hepatic veins**, which indicates severe regurgitation and is readily obtained from the subcostal window (Chapter 3 §3.7).

The **tricuspid regurgitation velocity** remains the route to pulmonary pressure estimation (Chapter 14 §14.4), and severity of regurgitation and pressure estimation are separate assessments that must not be conflated.

Pulmonary and tricuspid stenosis

Tricuspid stenosis is uncommon, and is usually rheumatic or carcinoid.

Pulmonary stenosis is usually congenital, showing systolic doming, an elevated peak velocity, and **post-stenotic dilatation** of the pulmonary trunk.

Pulmonary regurgitation is trivially present in most normal hearts. **Severe pulmonary regurgitation is most often encountered late after repair of tetralogy of Fallot**, where chronic volume loading progressively dilates the right ventricle and drives the timing of pulmonary valve replacement — making serial right ventricular assessment (Chapter 14 §14.7–14.8) the central measurement in that population.

Prosthetic valves

The single most important principle:

> **A prosthetic valve is assessed against its own expected performance and against the patient's own baseline post-implantation study — not against native valve values.**

Every prosthesis type, size and position has characteristic normal gradients, and a gradient that would be alarming across a native valve may be entirely normal across a small prosthesis. **The baseline study performed after implantation is the reference**, which makes the comparison discipline of Chapter 1 §1.5 essential in this population.

Normal findings: small transvalvular "washing" jets are **expected** in mechanical valves and are designed to prevent thrombus; leaflet or disc motion should be symmetrical and unrestricted.

Dysfunction:

Problem	Findings
Obstruction	Raised gradient, **reduced dimensionless index**, prolonged acceleration time, reduced effective orifice area, restricted leaflet or disc motion
Transvalvular regurgitation	Jet arising **within** the sewing ring — pathological if more than the expected washing jets
Paravalvular regurgitation	Jet arising **outside** the sewing ring. The location is the diagnosis

Problem	Findings
Dehiscence	A **rocking** prosthesis, with abnormal motion of the whole valve — always significant
Thrombus versus pannus	Overlapping appearances; thrombus is usually more mobile and of lower echogenicity, pannus more fixed and echogenic. Distinguishing them determines thrombolysis versus surgery
Structural degeneration	In bioprostheses — leaflet thickening, calcification, and progressive stenosis or regurgitation over years

Patient–prosthesis mismatch — an effective orifice area that is adequate for the valve but too small for the patient's body size — produces high gradients with a normally functioning valve. It is identified by indexing effective orifice area to body surface area.

[VERIFY: expected normal gradients by prosthesis type, size and position, and the current criteria for prosthetic dysfunction]

The shadowing limitation is decisive. A mechanical mitral prosthesis shadows the left atrium behind it (Chapter 14 §14.9), which is exactly where paravalvular regurgitation and thrombus reside. **Transoesophageal echocardiography is required** for suspected mitral prosthetic dysfunction and for suspected prosthetic endocarditis, and the transthoracic report should say so rather than describing an inadequate assessment.

15.4 Pericardial Disease and Tamponade

Effusion

Detection is straightforward; the useful work is in characterisation.

Describe: **size** (by the end-diastolic separation of the pericardial layers), **distribution** (circumferential or loculated), **content** (anechoic, or complex with fibrin strands, debris, or thrombus suggesting exudate, haemorrhage or infection), and **haemodynamic effect**.

[VERIFY: current size categories for pericardial effusion by end-diastolic separation]

Distinguish from: pleural effusion by the relationship to the descending thoracic aorta (Chapter 14 §14.9), **pericardial fat** (echogenic, anterior, moving with the heart), and ascites on subcostal imaging.

Tamponade — physiology first

Pericardial pressure rises until it exceeds the pressure in a chamber during the phase when that chamber's pressure is lowest, and the chamber collapses. Everything else follows from that sentence.

- The **right atrium** has the lowest pressure in **systole** — so it collapses in systole
- The **right ventricle** has the lowest pressure in **early diastole** — so it collapses then
- The right-sided chambers are affected first because their pressures are lower

Because the pericardium is non-compliant, the total cardiac volume becomes fixed, so the ventricles compete for space — **interventricular dependence**. Inspiration increases right ventricular filling, which shifts the septum leftward and reduces left ventricular filling, producing exaggerated respiratory variation in flow.

The signs

Sign	Nature
Right atrial systolic collapse lasting more than about a third of systole	**Sensitive**, appears early
Right ventricular diastolic collapse	**Specific**
Dilated inferior vena cava with reduced inspiratory collapse	Reflects raised right atrial pressure; a normal collapsing IVC argues strongly against tamponade
Exaggerated respiratory variation in mitral and tricuspid inflow velocities	The echocardiographic correlate of pulsus paradoxus
Septal bounce with respirophasic shift	Interventricular dependence
Swinging heart in large effusions	Corresponds to electrical alternans

[VERIFY: current thresholds for respiratory variation in mitral and tricuspid inflow used to support tamponade]

The essential statement for the report:

> **Tamponade is a clinical diagnosis supported by echocardiography, not an echocardiographic diagnosis.** Report the effusion and the physiological signs present; the decision to drain is clinical.

Two important variants:

Low-pressure tamponade — in a hypovolaemic patient, tamponade physiology occurs at lower pericardial pressures and with less impressive-looking effusions.

Regional tamponade — most often after cardiac surgery, where a **loculated posterior collection or clot** compresses a single chamber, typically the left or right atrium. **The transthoracic study frequently misses it**, and a postoperative patient with unexplained haemodynamic deterioration and an apparently unremarkable transthoracic study needs transoesophageal assessment.

Pericardiocentesis follows the principles of Chapter 9 §9.4–9.6: a subcostal or apical approach chosen from where the fluid is deepest and closest, avoiding the internal mammary and intercostal vessels, with **agitated saline injection through the needle to confirm intrapericardial position** before dilating.

Constriction versus restriction

A classic and clinically important distinction, since one is surgically curable and the other is not.

	Constrictive pericarditis	Restrictive cardiomyopathy
Problem	A rigid pericardium constraining the heart	A stiff myocardium
Septal motion	**Septal bounce** with marked respirophasic shift	Normal septal motion
Respiratory variation in inflow	**Marked**	Minimal
Tissue Doppler e′	**Preserved or increased** — "annulus paradoxus"	**Reduced**
Medial versus lateral e′	**Medial ≥ lateral** — "annulus reversus"	Normal relationship preserved
Hepatic vein flow	**Expiratory diastolic flow reversal**	Inspiratory reversal
Pericardium	May be thickened — but ultrasound is insensitive to this	Normal

The tissue Doppler findings are the discriminators. In constriction the myocardium itself is normal, so longitudinal relaxation is preserved or even enhanced — a counterintuitive finding that separates it from restriction, where the myocardium is the problem and e′ falls.

Tamponade physiology and constriction–restriction discriminators

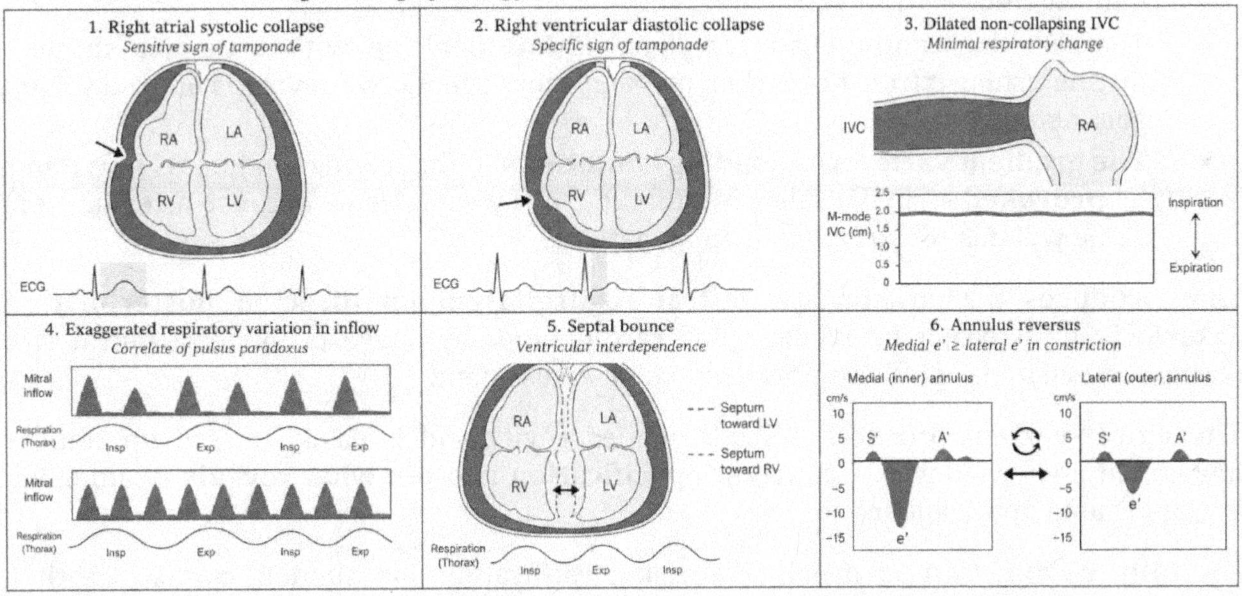

15.5 The Cardiomyopathies

Dilated cardiomyopathy

Findings: a dilated left ventricle with **globally reduced systolic function**, spherical remodelling with loss of the normal elliptical shape, **functional mitral regurgitation** from annular dilatation and leaflet tethering (§15.1), left atrial dilatation, and — in advanced disease — a **restrictive filling pattern** indicating high filling pressures.

Assess for apical thrombus, which is a real risk in a dilated akinetic ventricle and is a specific indication for **contrast opacification** (Chapter 14 §14.6).

The regional-versus-global distinction is the key interpretive step: regional wall motion abnormality confined to a coronary territory points to ischaemic cardiomyopathy, whereas **global hypokinesis** suggests a non-ischaemic cause — idiopathic, alcohol-related, anthracycline toxicity, myocarditis, peripartum, tachycardia-induced, or genetic.

Hypertrophic cardiomyopathy

The morphology: increased wall thickness not explained by loading conditions, most commonly **asymmetric septal hypertrophy**. Diagnostic thickness thresholds are lower where there is a family history. [VERIFY: current wall thickness diagnostic criteria for hypertrophic cardiomyopathy, including the family history modification]

Left ventricular outflow tract obstruction occurs in a substantial proportion and is **dynamic**:

- **Systolic anterior motion (SAM)** of the mitral valve drags the anterior leaflet into the outflow tract
- The resulting continuous-wave signal is **late-peaking with a dagger shape** — distinguishing it from the earlier-peaking, more symmetric envelope of fixed valvular aortic stenosis
- **The gradient varies with loading conditions.** If the resting gradient is low, it must be **provoked** — by Valsalva, by standing, or by exercise — because a resting study alone will miss obstruction in many patients

SAM produces a characteristic mitral regurgitation jet directed posteriorly. An **anteriorly** directed jet in hypertrophic cardiomyopathy suggests intrinsic mitral valve disease as well and should prompt closer valve assessment.

The apical variant produces a spade-shaped cavity and is easily missed on standard imaging in poor windows — **contrast opacification is often what reveals it**, along with any associated apical aneurysm.

Diastolic dysfunction is usual, and risk stratification for sudden cardiac death — incorporating wall thickness, apical aneurysm, outflow gradient and left atrial size — is a defined pathway that echocardiography feeds.

Athlete's heart is the principal differential: symmetric mild hypertrophy, a **larger** cavity rather than a small one, normal diastolic indices, and regression on detraining.

Restrictive cardiomyopathy and infiltration

Restrictive physiology: normal or small ventricular cavities with **normal wall thickness in the non-infiltrative forms, marked biatrial enlargement**, restrictive mitral filling, and reduced e′ (which is what separates it from constriction — §15.4).

Cardiac amyloidosis deserves separate treatment because it is increasingly recognised, treatable, and has a distinctive echocardiographic signature:

- **Increased wall thickness with low or normal ECG voltage** — the **voltage-thickness discordance** is a powerful clue, because true hypertrophy raises voltage
- **Biatrial enlargement**, thickened interatrial septum, thickened valves
- A **small pericardial effusion**
- A granular or sparkling myocardial texture — often described, but non-specific and dependent on machine settings
- **Apical sparing on longitudinal strain** — reduced strain in the basal and mid segments with **preserved apical strain**, producing a characteristic bullseye pattern. **This is the most specific echocardiographic finding**, and it is a direct clinical application of the strain imaging introduced in Chapter 14 §14.6

Other cardiomyopathies

Arrhythmogenic right ventricular cardiomyopathy — right ventricular dilatation, **regional right ventricular wall motion abnormality or aneurysm**, and reduced right ventricular function. Formal diagnostic criteria apply. [VERIFY: current diagnostic criteria for arrhythmogenic cardiomyopathy]

Left ventricular non-compaction — prominent trabeculation with deep intertrabecular recesses that fill with colour from the cavity, and a non-compacted to compacted myocardial ratio above a threshold. The criteria are debated and over-diagnosis is a recognised problem. [VERIFY: current criteria and their limitations]

Takotsubo syndrome — apical ballooning with basal hyperkinesis, typically following emotional or physical stress, with wall motion abnormality **extending beyond a single coronary territory** and characteristically **reversible** on follow-up imaging.

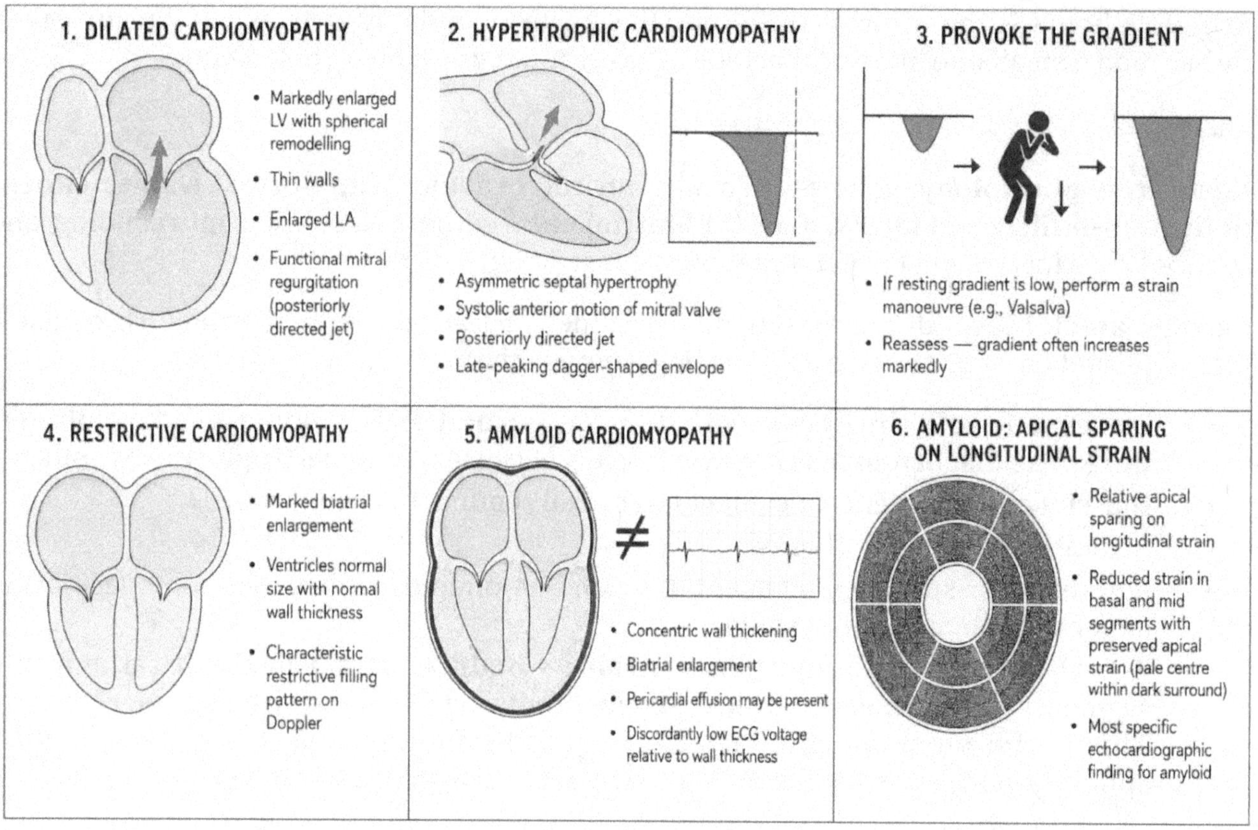

15.6 Cardiac Masses, Thrombi, and Vegetations

A systematic approach

Four questions, asked in order, resolve most cardiac masses:

1. **Where is it, and what is it attached to?** Location and attachment site are more discriminating than appearance.
2. **How does it move?** Independent oscillating motion suggests vegetation; a mass swinging on a stalk suggests myxoma; a mass moving with the wall suggests thrombus or intramural tumour.
3. **What is the clinical context?** Fever and bacteraemia, atrial fibrillation, recent infarction, known malignancy, or an indwelling line each reframe the differential entirely.
4. **Is it a normal structure or an artifact?** Work through the list in Chapter 14 §14.9 **before** anything else. The left atrial ridge, lipomatous septal hypertrophy, the Chiari network and the Eustachian valve account for a large share of referrals for "cardiac mass".

Thrombus

Left ventricular apical thrombus — in an **akinetic or aneurysmal apical segment**, most often after anterior myocardial infarction or in dilated cardiomyopathy. It is adherent, layered or protuberant, and lies adjacent to a wall motion abnormality.

Detection is substantially improved by contrast opacification, and the apex is exactly where foreshortening hides pathology (Chapter 14 §14.5) — so a suspected apical thrombus warrants a deliberately non-foreshortened apical view with contrast.

Left atrial appendage thrombus — associated with atrial fibrillation and mitral stenosis, frequently preceded by **spontaneous echo contrast** ("smoke"). **Transoesophageal echocardiography is required**; the transthoracic study cannot exclude it, and this determines anticoagulation and cardioversion decisions.

Right atrial thrombus — commonly associated with indwelling central catheters and pacing leads.

Vegetation

Appearance: an irregular, **oscillating** mass with **motion independent of the valve**, typically attached to the **upstream (low-pressure) side** of the valve — the atrial side of an atrioventricular valve, the ventricular side of a semilunar valve — with echogenicity similar to or lower than myocardium.

Complications to seek specifically, because they change management from medical to surgical: **perivalvular abscess** (particularly aortic root abscess), **leaflet perforation**, **fistula formation**, **prosthetic dehiscence**, and **mycotic aneurysm**.

Transthoracic sensitivity is limited, and **transoesophageal echocardiography is required** where the transthoracic study is negative but clinical suspicion is high, in all **prosthetic** valve endocarditis, and whenever a complication is suspected. Echocardiographic findings form part of formal diagnostic criteria alongside microbiological evidence.

Tumours

Myxoma — the commonest primary cardiac tumour. Characteristically in the **left atrium, attached to the interatrial septum at the fossa ovalis by a stalk**, mobile, and may **prolapse through the mitral valve** in diastole, causing intermittent obstruction. Multiple or atypically located myxomas raise the possibility of an associated syndrome.

Papillary fibroelastoma — small, mobile, frond-like, usually valve-associated, and clinically important because of **embolic risk** out of proportion to its size.

Rhabdomyoma — the **commonest cardiac tumour in fetal life and childhood**, typically multiple, strongly associated with **tuberous sclerosis**, and characteristically **regressing spontaneously** — which is why identification prompts genetic assessment rather than surgery in most cases.

Fibroma — usually solitary, intramural, in children, and may calcify.

Metastatic disease is far commoner than primary cardiac malignancy — melanoma, lung, breast, lymphoma, and renal cell carcinoma extending through the inferior vena cava (Chapter 7 §7.7). **A pericardial effusion is often the presenting finding.**

Angiosarcoma — the commonest primary malignancy, typically right atrial, aggressive and infiltrative.

15.7 Fetal Cardiac Anatomy and the Screening Sequence

Context and timing

Congenital heart disease is the commonest group of congenital anomalies, and a substantial proportion remains undetected before birth in many settings. **Detection rates depend heavily on whether the outflow tracts are examined**, which is why the sequence below matters more than any other content in this chapter.

Timing: the cardiac assessment forms part of the mid-trimester anomaly scan, with detailed fetal echocardiography offered earlier in high-risk pregnancies. [VERIFY: current recommended gestational age windows for routine cardiac screening and for specialist fetal echocardiography]

Indications for specialist fetal echocardiography include: a family history of congenital heart disease, **maternal diabetes**, maternal autoimmune disease with anti-Ro or anti-La antibodies, teratogen exposure, conception by assisted reproduction, **increased nuchal translucency**, an abnormality suspected on screening, an extracardiac anomaly, fetal arrhythmia, hydrops, and monochorionic twinning.

The screening sequence

Step 1 — Situs and cardiac position.

Establish fetal lie and laterality before anything else. Determine which side of the fetus is left, then confirm on a transverse abdominal section that the **stomach and descending aorta lie on the left** and the **inferior vena cava on the right**. Confirm the **cardiac apex points to the left**, and assess the **cardiothoracic ratio.**

Getting laterality wrong invalidates the entire subsequent examination — the same principle as adult situs assessment (Chapter 14 §14.1).

Step 2 — The four-chamber view.

Check, systematically:

- **Two atria and two ventricles of approximately equal size**
- **Two separate atrioventricular valves, both opening**
- **The offset of atrioventricular valve insertion** — the tricuspid valve inserting slightly more apically (Chapter 14 §14.2). **Loss of this offset is the marker of an atrioventricular septal defect**
- **An intact crux** — the central meeting point of the septa and valves
- **The moderator band** identifying the morphological right ventricle
- **The foramen ovale flap opening into the left atrium**
- **Pulmonary veins entering the left atrium**

- **An intact ventricular septum**
- **Normal rate and regular rhythm**

Step 3 — Left ventricular outflow tract. The **aorta arising from the left ventricle**, with **continuity between the anterior aortic wall and the interventricular septum.**

Step 4 — Right ventricular outflow tract. The **pulmonary artery arising from the right ventricle**, and — critically — **the great arteries crossing over one another** as they leave.

Normal great arteries cross. If they arise in parallel, suspect transposition.

This single observation is why four-chamber-only screening misses transposition of the great arteries entirely, since the four-chamber view in that condition is normal.

Step 5 — Three-vessel and trachea view. A transverse view of the upper mediastinum showing, from left to right, the **pulmonary artery, aorta and superior vena cava** in **decreasing calibre**, with the arch and duct forming a **V-shape to the left of the trachea**, and **forward flow in both.**

This view is highly informative for a small effort: vessel size discrepancy suggests outflow obstruction on one side, an abnormal V configuration or a vessel to the right of the trachea suggests arch anomaly, and reversed flow in either arm suggests a duct-dependent lesion.

Additional views — the aortic arch and ductal arch in long axis, and the systemic venous return — complete a detailed study.

Technique

Maternal habitus and fetal position dominate image quality. **Use harmonic imaging, a narrow sector with high frame rate, zoom on the heart rather than imaging the whole fetus, and record cine sweeps** — a sweep from the abdomen up through the four-chamber view to the three-vessel view captures the whole sequence and is reviewable.

Wait and re-approach. Fetal position changes, and a view that is impossible now may be straightforward in ten minutes.

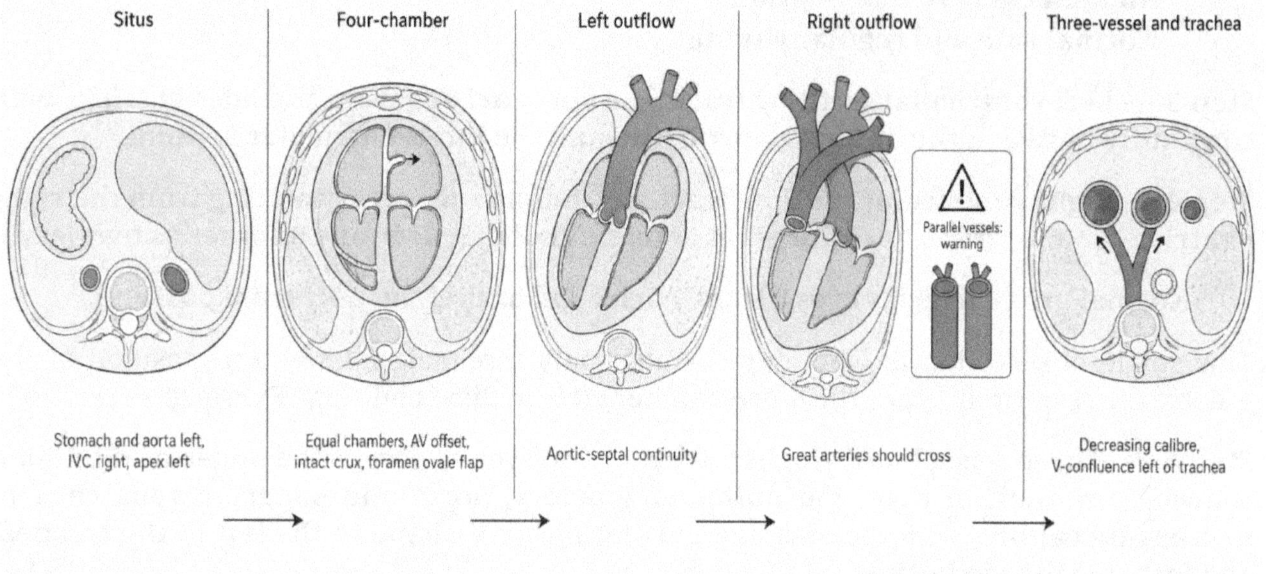

The normal fetal screening views as acquired.

15.8 Fetal Cardiac Function, Rhythm, and Doppler

Fetal circulatory physiology — and why it matters

The fetal circulation runs **in parallel** rather than in series, with three shunts diverting blood away from the non-functioning lungs:

- **Ductus venosus** — oxygenated umbilical venous blood bypassing the hepatic circulation
- **Foramen ovale** — right atrium to left atrium
- **Ductus arteriosus** — pulmonary artery to descending aorta

Pulmonary vascular resistance is high and systemic resistance is low, and the **right ventricle is dominant**, handling the larger share of combined cardiac output.

The consequence for congenital heart disease is fundamental:

> **Because the circulations are parallel and the duct is open, many severe lesions are haemodynamically silent in utero.** The fetus is well; the neonate collapses when the duct closes in the first days of life.

This is the physiological basis of **duct dependence** (§15.10), and the reason prenatal detection changes outcome.

Rhythm assessment

The technique: the fetal rhythm is characterised by demonstrating **the relationship between atrial and ventricular contraction**, which requires recording both simultaneously.

M-mode is the classic approach: place the cursor so that it passes through **an atrial wall and a ventricular wall simultaneously**, and read the timing of each contraction from the trace. **Simultaneous pulsed-wave Doppler** — sampling the left ventricular inflow and outflow together, or the superior vena cava and ascending aorta together — achieves the same and is often easier.

Normal fetal heart rate falls within a defined range that changes with gestation. [VERIFY: current normal fetal heart rate ranges by gestational age]

Rhythm	Findings	Significance
Ectopic beats	Usually atrial; an early atrial contraction, sometimes conducted, sometimes blocked	Common and usually benign; blocked ectopics cause an irregular slow rate that mimics bradycardia
Supraventricular tachycardia	Sustained rapid rate with **1:1 atrioventricular relationship**	Risk of hydrops; may require maternal antiarrhythmic therapy
Atrial flutter	Very rapid atrial rate with **variable block,** commonly 2:1	As above
Complete heart block	**Atrioventricular dissociation** — atria and ventricles beating independently	Associated with **maternal anti-Ro/anti-La antibodies**, and with structural disease including left atrial isomerism and atrioventricular septal defect. Requires specialist management

The association between complete heart block and structural disease means that a bradycardic fetus needs a full structural assessment, not just rhythm characterisation.

Fetal cardiac function

Assessment differs from postnatal practice because loading conditions and geometry differ:

- **Cardiothoracic area ratio** — a simple and reproducible marker of cardiomegaly
- **Ventricular shortening fraction**
- **Myocardial performance (Tei) index**, combining systolic and diastolic intervals
- **Atrioventricular valve regurgitation** — significant tricuspid regurgitation is an early sign of cardiac compromise
- **Signs of failure** — cardiomegaly, atrioventricular regurgitation, abnormal ductus venosus flow, and ultimately **hydrops** with effusions, ascites and skin oedema

Composite scoring systems combining these elements are used in specialist practice. [VERIFY: current fetal cardiovascular scoring systems and their thresholds]

The fetal Doppler indices

These are developed fully in Chapter 19 in the context of growth assessment; their cardiac relevance is summarised here:

Umbilical artery — reflects **placental resistance**. Progressive rise in resistance produces reduced, then **absent**, then **reversed end-diastolic flow**, each step marking deterioration.

Middle cerebral artery — falling pulsatility indicates **cerebral redistribution** ("brain sparing"). Separately, **peak systolic velocity** is the key measurement for **fetal anaemia**, where an elevated velocity reflects reduced blood viscosity and drives the decision to transfuse.

Ductus venosus — the **a-wave**, corresponding to atrial contraction. **Absent or reversed a-wave** indicates raised central venous pressure and is a late, high-risk sign.

Cerebroplacental ratio — combining the middle cerebral and umbilical indices, more sensitive than either alone.

15.9 Congenital Heart Disease: Septal and Outflow Tract Defects

Atrial septal defect

Types, defined by location, because location determines the surgical approach and the associated anomalies:

- **Secundum** — at the fossa ovalis; much the commonest, and often closable by device
- **Primum** — at the crux, part of the atrioventricular septal defect spectrum
- **Sinus venosus** — at the superior or inferior vena caval junction, **frequently associated with anomalous pulmonary venous drainage**, and poorly seen transthoracically
- **Coronary sinus** defect — rare

Findings: right atrial and right ventricular dilatation, **septal flattening with paradoxical motion** from right ventricular volume overload, and left-to-right colour flow across the defect. The shunt magnitude may be quantified as a pulmonary-to-systemic flow ratio.

A patent foramen ovale is not an atrial septal defect — it is a valve-like flap that can open under pressure, with no true tissue deficiency, and it does not cause volume overload.

Transoesophageal echocardiography and agitated saline contrast (Chapter 14 §14.6) are used for detection and characterisation, particularly for sinus venosus defects.

Ventricular septal defect

Types: perimembranous (commonest), **muscular**, **inlet** (part of the atrioventricular septal defect spectrum), and **outlet/subarterial**.

Assessment: size relative to the aortic annulus, and — importantly — whether the defect is **restrictive** (a small defect with a high-velocity jet and a large pressure gradient, protecting the pulmonary circulation) or **non-restrictive** (a large defect equalising ventricular pressures and exposing the lungs to systemic pressure).

Colour Doppler is essential — small muscular defects are frequently invisible on greyscale and are found only on a careful colour sweep.

Untreated large left-to-right shunts progress to pulmonary vascular disease and shunt reversal (Eisenmenger physiology), which is why shunt lesions are assessed and closed early.

Atrioventricular septal defect

A deficiency of the atrioventricular septum with a **common atrioventricular valve**, comprising a primum atrial defect, an inlet ventricular defect, and abnormal valve morphology in the complete form.

The prenatal marker is the loss of the normal atrioventricular valve offset (§15.7) — the valves insert at the same level rather than the tricuspid being more apical.

Strongly associated with trisomy 21, which makes its identification a trigger for genetic counselling.

Patent ductus arteriosus

In the preterm neonate this is a common and clinically significant problem rather than a congenital malformation. Assessment includes: **ductal diameter**, **continuous left-to-right flow** into the pulmonary artery, **left atrium to aortic root ratio** as a marker of volume loading, and — a useful systemic marker — **diastolic flow reversal in the descending aorta, and in the cerebral and mesenteric arteries**, indicating diastolic steal.

Tetralogy of Fallot

Four components arising from a single developmental abnormality: **a ventricular septal defect, an overriding aorta, right ventricular outflow tract obstruction, and right ventricular hypertrophy**.

The degree of outflow obstruction determines the clinical picture — from a minimally cyanotic infant to a duct-dependent pulmonary circulation in pulmonary atresia with ventricular septal defect, where pulmonary blood flow may depend on the duct or on major aortopulmonary collateral arteries.

Coarctation of the aorta

Postnatal findings: narrowing of the descending aorta, usually just distal to the left subclavian artery, with **a high-velocity jet showing a characteristic diastolic tail** (the sawtooth pattern of continuing forward flow into diastole), **arch hypoplasia**, and — a valuable and easily obtained sign — a **damped, delayed, low-amplitude waveform in the abdominal aorta** (Chapter 3 §3.7).

Associations: bicuspid aortic valve and **Turner syndrome**.

Prenatal diagnosis is genuinely difficult. The suggestive findings — **ventricular disproportion with the right larger than the left**, and a small aorta on the three-vessel view — are non-specific, and the **false positive rate is high**. Suspected fetal coarctation warrants specialist review rather than a definitive statement.

15.10 Complex Congenital Lesions and Counselling Pathways

Duct dependence — the organising concept

Some lesions produce a circulation that **cannot function once the arterial duct closes**:

Duct-dependent pulmonary circulation — pulmonary atresia, critical pulmonary stenosis, severe tetralogy. Pulmonary blood flow arrives through the duct.

Duct-dependent systemic circulation — hypoplastic left heart syndrome, critical aortic stenosis, interrupted aortic arch, severe coarctation. Systemic blood flow arrives through the duct.

Duct-dependent mixing — transposition of the great arteries, where the parallel circulations must communicate.

> **These neonates are well at birth and collapse in the first days of life as the duct closes.** Prenatal diagnosis allows delivery at or near a cardiac centre with **prostaglandin infusion available from birth**, and this is the single greatest contribution of fetal cardiac screening to survival.

The lesions

Transposition of the great arteries. The aorta arises from the right ventricle and the pulmonary artery from the left, producing two parallel circulations.

The four-chamber view is normal, which is precisely why outflow assessment is mandatory (§15.7). The findings are **parallel great arteries** rather than crossing ones, with the aorta anterior and to the right. Management is prostaglandin, balloon atrial septostomy to improve mixing, and arterial switch surgery.

Hypoplastic left heart syndrome. A small or absent left ventricle with mitral and aortic atresia or critical stenosis, and **retrograde flow in the aortic arch** supplied through the duct. **The four-chamber view is abnormal**, so this is detected by standard screening. It is duct-dependent, and follows a staged single-ventricle palliation pathway.

Ebstein anomaly. Apical displacement of the septal tricuspid leaflet — an exaggeration of the normal offset (Chapter 14 §14.2) — producing an atrialised right ventricle, a small functional right ventricle, severe tricuspid regurgitation, and marked right atrial enlargement with cardiomegaly.

Tricuspid atresia, double outlet right ventricle, truncus arteriosus, and interrupted aortic arch complete the common complex group.

Total anomalous pulmonary venous return. No pulmonary veins entering the left atrium, with a venous confluence draining elsewhere. **The obstructed form is a neonatal emergency** presenting with severe cyanosis and pulmonary oedema, and it is not improved by prostaglandin — a critical distinction from the duct-dependent lesions.

Single ventricle physiology — whatever the anatomy, a functionally univentricular heart follows a staged palliation pathway toward a Fontan circulation.

The counselling pathway

A prenatal cardiac diagnosis initiates a defined multidisciplinary process, and the sonographer's role within it is specific and bounded.

The team: fetal cardiologist, obstetrician, neonatologist, cardiac surgeon, specialist nurse, and clinical geneticist.

Genetic assessment is offered, because the associations are strong and specific — **trisomy 21 with atrioventricular septal defect**, and **22q11 deletion with conotruncal anomalies** including tetralogy, truncus, and interrupted arch. Karyotype and microarray are discussed.

The counselling covers: the diagnosis and its certainty, the expected natural history, the surgical pathway and its staging, survival and quality-of-life expectations, delivery planning — location, mode and timing — and the options available to the parents, including continuation with planned neonatal care, palliative care, and, where lawful, termination of pregnancy.

Written information, access to a second opinion, and psychological support are part of the pathway rather than optional additions.

The sonographer's role and boundary

Within scope: obtaining a technically complete study, recognising abnormality, escalating promptly and directly to the appropriate specialist, and documenting fully.

Outside scope: communicating a cardiac diagnosis or prognosis to the parents. This is the boundary set out in Chapter 1 §1.2, and it applies with particular force here, because the information is life-altering and the questions that follow — about surgery, survival and choices — require the specialist who can answer them.

What is required is the manner of the escalation, not silence. The approach set out in Chapter 1 §1.3 applies: explain that you need a colleague to review the images, that this is a normal part of the process, and that a specialist will speak with them — without confirming or denying a finding.

The ethical framework for obstetric imaging, including the handling of findings with implications for continuation of pregnancy, is developed in Chapter 18 §18.2.

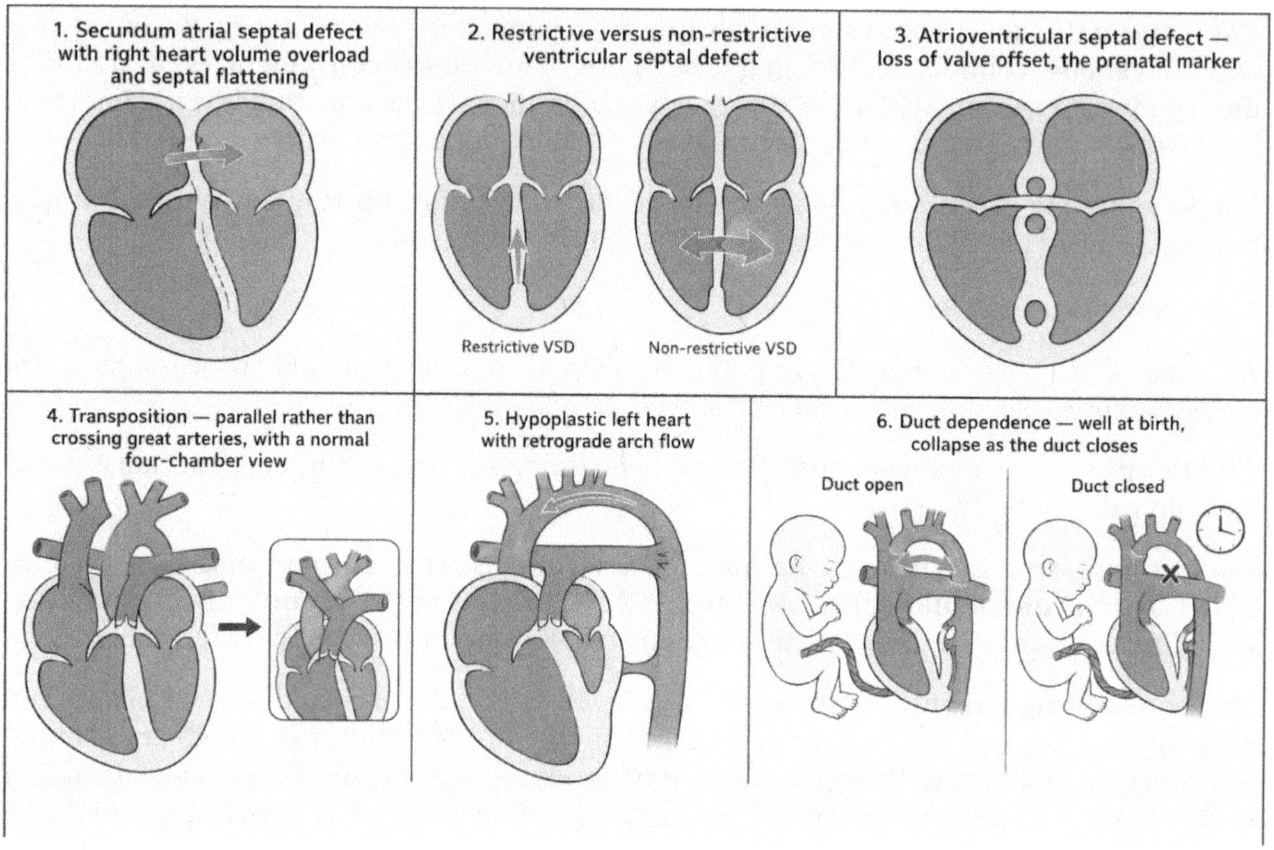

Key Points

1. Valve severity is multiparametric. Gather several criteria and report where they agree and where they conflict; a single confidently quoted number sends patients for the wrong operation.
2. Pressure half-time for mitral valve area is invalidated by significant aortic regurgitation, recent valvuloplasty, an atrial septal defect, tachycardia and impaired relaxation.
3. Diagnose mitral valve prolapse in the parasternal or apical long axis, never the four-chamber view — the saddle-shaped annulus produces false positives there.
4. An eccentric wall-hugging regurgitant jet looks smaller than it is. Treat it as a reason to escalate quantification, not to reassure.
5. Image a suspected bicuspid aortic valve in systole, and measure the ascending aorta in every case — the aortopathy carries its own surgical threshold.
6. In aortic stenosis, take the highest velocity from multiple windows including the right parasternal position. An underestimate here understates severity.
7. Low-flow low-gradient aortic stenosis occurs with both reduced and preserved ejection fraction. A low gradient across a heavily calcified immobile valve should prompt valve area assessment, not reassurance.
8. In acute severe aortic regurgitation the ventricle is normal-sized. That is a sign of acuity, not of mildness, and should prompt consideration of dissection.

9. Assess a prosthetic valve against its expected performance and the patient's own post-implantation baseline, never against native valve values.
10. A paravalvular jet arises outside the sewing ring; a rocking prosthesis indicates dehiscence. A mechanical mitral prosthesis shadows the left atrium, so transoesophageal assessment is required.
11. In tamponade each chamber collapses when its own pressure is lowest — right atrium in systole, right ventricle in diastole. A normally collapsing IVC argues strongly against it.
12. Tamponade is a clinical diagnosis supported by echocardiography. Report the effusion and the physiology; the decision to drain is clinical.
13. Preserved or increased e′, with medial exceeding lateral, distinguishes constriction from restriction — in constriction the myocardium itself is normal.
14. In hypertrophic cardiomyopathy the outflow gradient is dynamic. If the resting gradient is low, provoke it, or obstruction will be missed.
15. Increased wall thickness with discordantly low ECG voltage suggests infiltration, and apical sparing on strain is the most specific echocardiographic sign of cardiac amyloidosis.
16. Before reporting a cardiac mass, exclude the normal structures and artifacts of Chapter 14 §14.9 — they account for a large share of referrals.
17. Establish fetal situs before anything else. Getting laterality wrong invalidates the whole study.
18. Loss of the atrioventricular valve offset in the fetus indicates an atrioventricular septal defect.
19. Normal great arteries cross. Parallel great arteries suggest transposition — a lesion with a completely normal four-chamber view, which is why outflow views are mandatory.
20. Fetal complete heart block requires a full structural assessment, because of its association with left atrial isomerism and atrioventricular septal defect.
21. Because the fetal circulations are parallel and the duct is open, severe lesions are silent in utero and the neonate collapses when the duct closes. Prenatal detection allows delivery near a cardiac centre with prostaglandin from birth.
22. Obstructed total anomalous pulmonary venous return is a neonatal emergency that prostaglandin does not help — a critical distinction from the duct-dependent lesions.
23. The sonographer escalates a prenatal cardiac finding promptly and does not communicate the diagnosis or prognosis. Silence is not the alternative; explaining the process is.

Registry Check

1. Which finding is most specific for severe mitral regurgitation?

A. A large colour jet area **B.** Systolic flow reversal in the pulmonary veins **C.** Left atrial enlargement **D.** A dense continuous-wave Doppler envelope

Answer: B. Systolic flow reversal in the pulmonary veins indicates that regurgitant flow is sufficient to reverse the normal systolic pulmonary venous inflow, and it is a specific sign of severe regurgitation. Colour jet area is heavily influenced by machine settings and by jet eccentricity, and left atrial enlargement reflects chronicity rather than current severity.

2. Mitral valve prolapse should not be diagnosed from the apical four-chamber view because:

A. The frame rate is too low **B.** The mitral annulus is saddle-shaped, so this plane produces false positives **C.** The leaflets cannot be resolved **D.** Colour Doppler is unreliable in this view

Answer: B. The annulus is saddle-shaped, and the four-chamber plane passes through its lower horns, making normal leaflets appear displaced above the apparent annular line. The diagnosis is made in the parasternal long axis or an apical long-axis view.

3. A patient has a heavily calcified, poorly mobile aortic valve, a mean gradient below the severe threshold, and a reduced ejection fraction. The appropriate interpretation is:

A. Moderate aortic stenosis **B.** The gradient excludes severe stenosis **C.** Possible classical low-flow low-gradient severe stenosis, requiring valve area assessment and consideration of dobutamine stress echocardiography **D.** Aortic sclerosis without stenosis

Answer: C. Gradient is flow-dependent, so a reduced stroke volume lowers the gradient across a genuinely severe valve. Valve area by continuity is less flow-dependent, and dobutamine stress echocardiography distinguishes true severe stenosis, in which area remains small as flow rises, from pseudosevere stenosis, in which the valve opens further.

4. In cardiac tamponade, right ventricular collapse occurs in diastole because:

A. The right ventricle is the most anterior chamber **B.** Diastole is when right ventricular pressure is lowest and therefore most easily exceeded by pericardial pressure **C.** The right ventricle has the thinnest wall **D.** Venous return is greatest in diastole

Answer: B. Each chamber collapses during the phase in which its own pressure is lowest, so the right atrium collapses in systole and the right ventricle in early diastole. The right-sided chambers are affected first because their pressures are lower throughout the cycle.

5. Which finding distinguishes constrictive pericarditis from restrictive cardiomyopathy?

A. Biatrial enlargement **B.** Restrictive mitral inflow pattern **C.** Preserved or increased tissue Doppler e′ with medial exceeding lateral **D.** A dilated inferior vena cava

Answer: C. In constriction the myocardium itself is normal, so longitudinal relaxation is preserved or enhanced, and the medial annular velocity may exceed the lateral. In restriction the myocardium is the abnormality and e′ falls. Biatrial enlargement, restrictive filling and a dilated IVC occur in both.

6. An elderly patient has increased left ventricular wall thickness with low voltage on the ECG, biatrial enlargement, and a strain bullseye showing reduced basal and mid strain with preserved apical strain. This suggests:

A. Hypertensive heart disease **B.** Hypertrophic cardiomyopathy **C.** Cardiac amyloidosis **D.** Athlete's heart

> **Answer: C.** The discordance between increased wall thickness and low ECG voltage points to infiltration rather than true hypertrophy, and apical sparing on longitudinal strain is the most specific echocardiographic finding in cardiac amyloidosis. True hypertrophy raises voltage.

7. In the fetal outflow tract views, the great arteries are seen arising in parallel rather than crossing. This suggests:

A. Tetralogy of Fallot **B.** Transposition of the great arteries **C.** Atrioventricular septal defect **D.** Coarctation of the aorta

> **Answer: B.** Normally the great arteries cross as they leave the ventricles. Parallel origin is the hallmark of transposition, and because the four-chamber view is normal in this condition, it is missed entirely by four-chamber-only screening — which is why outflow views are mandatory.

8. A neonate with a duct-dependent systemic circulation is well at birth and deteriorates on day two. The explanation is:

A. Progressive pulmonary hypertension **B.** Closure of the arterial duct **C.** Development of pulmonary oedema **D.** Foramen ovale closure

> **Answer: B.** With the duct open, systemic perfusion is maintained despite the underlying lesion. Ductal closure in the first days of life removes that pathway and the neonate collapses. Prenatal diagnosis allows delivery near a cardiac centre with prostaglandin available from birth to maintain ductal patency.

Chapter Notes for the Editorial Pass

Verification queue. In priority order: **valve severity grading criteria for all four valves,** including the separate thresholds for primary and secondary mitral regurgitation and the low-flow low-gradient aortic stenosis definitions (§15.1–15.3) — these are the most consequential verifications in the book so far, since they determine surgical referral; **expected prosthetic valve gradients by type, size and position, and the criteria for dysfunction** (§15.3); **tamponade supporting thresholds for respiratory inflow variation and pericardial effusion size categories** (§15.4); **hypertrophic cardiomyopathy wall thickness criteria including the family history modification,** and the **arrhythmogenic cardiomyopathy and non-compaction criteria** (§15.5); **fetal cardiac screening gestational age windows and the indications for specialist fetal echocardiography** (§15.7); **normal fetal heart rate ranges by gestation and fetal cardiovascular scoring systems** (§15.8); and the **mitral valve prolapse displacement threshold** and **valvuloplasty scoring system** (§15.1).

Dependency note. Every quantitative statement in this chapter inherits from the measurement conventions and haemodynamic calculations established in Chapter 14 §14.4 and §14.7. Those must be settled first, as flagged in the Chapter 14 notes; editing this chapter against unresolved Chapter 14 conventions will produce internal inconsistency.

Overlap to resolve at layout. The fetal Doppler indices appear here in §15.8 in their cardiac context and again in Chapter 19 in the growth assessment context. This is deliberate rather than redundant, but the two treatments should be checked against each other, and §15.8 should refer forward rather than restating the thresholds.

Figure count: 7 Lane A, 1 Lane B. The video question raised in the Chapter 13 and 14 notes reaches its sharpest point here: **provoked outflow obstruction in hypertrophic cardiomyopathy, tamponade respiratory variation, the mobility of a vegetation, and the fetal screening sweep** are all dynamic phenomena that still frames represent poorly. If the digital edition supports video, the fetal sweep in `fig-15-6` is the single highest-value clip in the book.

Cross-reference targets to fix at layout: §15.1–15.3 haemodynamic calculations and measurement conventions → Chapter 14 §14.4, §14.7; §15.3 hepatic vein flow → Chapter 3 §3.7; §15.4 pericardial versus pleural fluid and prosthetic shadowing → Chapter 14 §14.9; §15.4 pericardiocentesis technique → Chapter 9 §9.4–9.6; §15.5 strain imaging → Chapter 14 §14.6; §15.6 contrast opacification and transoesophageal indications → Chapter 14 §14.6; §15.6 renal cell carcinoma with caval extension → Chapter 7 §7.7; §15.7 situs assessment → Chapter 14 §14.1; §15.8 fetal Doppler indices → Chapter 19; §15.10 obstetric clinical ethics and disclosure → Chapter 18 §18.2 and Chapter 1 §1.2–1.3.

Word count: approximately 10,400 excluding image prompt blocks, learning objectives, registry questions, and these notes.

Chapter 16: Cerebrovascular, Arterial, and Venous Evaluation

Learning Objectives

On completing this chapter you should be able to:

1. Perform a carotid and vertebral protocol and reliably distinguish the internal from the external carotid artery.
2. Apply velocity criteria for carotid stenosis, recognise the confounders that invalidate them, and characterise plaque.
3. Assess the postoperative and stented carotid, and explain why stent criteria differ from native criteria.
4. Identify the transcranial windows and the vessels accessible through each.
5. Describe the intracranial applications of transcranial Doppler, including vasospasm and sickle cell screening.
6. Perform a peripheral arterial duplex, calculate an ankle-brachial index, and recognise when it is falsely elevated.
7. Grade arterial stenosis by velocity ratio and recognise pseudoaneurysm and arteriovenous fistula.
8. Assess dialysis access and bypass grafts, including flow volume and the sites of stenosis.
9. Perform a venous compression protocol and interpret phasicity, augmentation and Valsalva response.
10. Distinguish acute from chronic thrombus and perform a reflux study in the correct position.

Returning to the Doppler Discipline

After two cardiac chapters, this one reverts to the rules of Chapter 2.

Angle correction returns. In echocardiography the operator aligns the beam with flow and takes the highest velocity (Chapter 14 §14.4). Here, the angle cursor is aligned to the vessel walls or to the visible jet, and **the insonation angle must be at or below 60°** for any velocity to be reportable. Above that, cosine changes so rapidly that small alignment errors produce large velocity errors — and in this chapter velocities are converted directly into stenosis grades that determine whether a patient has surgery.

Consistency across the examination matters as much as the individual value. A study performed at varying angles produces ratios that are not comparable, and most of the criteria below are ratios.

The archived image must show the angle cursor, correctly aligned (Chapter 1 §1.5). A velocity without a demonstrable angle is an uninterpretable number.

16.1 Extracranial Carotid and Vertebral Protocol

Anatomy

The **common carotid artery** arises from the brachiocephalic trunk on the right and directly from the aortic arch on the left — an asymmetry that matters when assessing the origins. It divides at a variable level, usually around the upper cervical spine, into the internal and external carotid arteries, with the **carotid bulb** at the origin of the internal carotid.

The **vertebral artery** arises from the subclavian artery and enters the transverse foramen at the sixth cervical vertebra, ascending in segments through the neck to the skull base.

Distinguishing internal from external carotid — the foundational skill

Getting this wrong invalidates the study, and it happens more often than is acknowledged. **Five discriminators**, used together:

	Internal carotid	**External carotid**
Branches in the neck	**None**	**Branches** — the superior thyroid artery is usually the first
Waveform	**Low resistance** — abundant continuous diastolic flow, supplying the brain	**High resistance** — sharp systolic peak with little or no diastolic flow
Calibre	Usually larger	Usually smaller
Position	Usually posterolateral	Usually anteromedial
Temporal tap	Little or no effect	**Oscillations transmitted** into the trace

The temporal tap — rhythmic tapping of the superficial temporal artery in front of the ear while recording the spectral trace — transmits a characteristic serrated oscillation into the external carotid and not into the internal. It is the confirmatory manoeuvre when the other features are ambiguous, and it takes seconds.

The branch rule is the most reliable single discriminator. The internal carotid has no cervical branches; if you can demonstrate a branch, you are on the external carotid.

Beware the exceptions: position is variable and cannot be relied upon alone; and a **severely stenosed internal carotid distal to a high-grade lesion may show a damped, high-resistance waveform** that resembles an external carotid — which is precisely when the branch rule and the temporal tap earn their place.

Technique

Position: supine, head slightly extended and rotated away from the side being examined, with the pillow removed or lowered.

Transducer: linear array. A small-footprint or curvilinear probe helps for high bifurcations, short necks, and the vessel origins.

Both planes: transverse for surveying plaque distribution and identifying the bifurcation level, and **longitudinal** for spectral sampling.

Sampling and documentation

Record spectral traces, with the angle cursor visible and correctly aligned, at:

- **Common carotid** — proximal, mid, and distal
- **Carotid bulb**
- **Internal carotid** — proximal, mid, and distal, and **through any stenosis and immediately distal to it**
- **External carotid**
- **Vertebral artery** — with **flow direction** explicitly documented
- **Subclavian arteries bilaterally**, for waveform comparison

Measure peak systolic and end-diastolic velocity at each site, and describe plaque wherever present.

Assess both sides, always. **Contralateral disease changes the interpretation of the side you are reporting** (§16.2), so a unilateral study is not an adequate carotid examination.

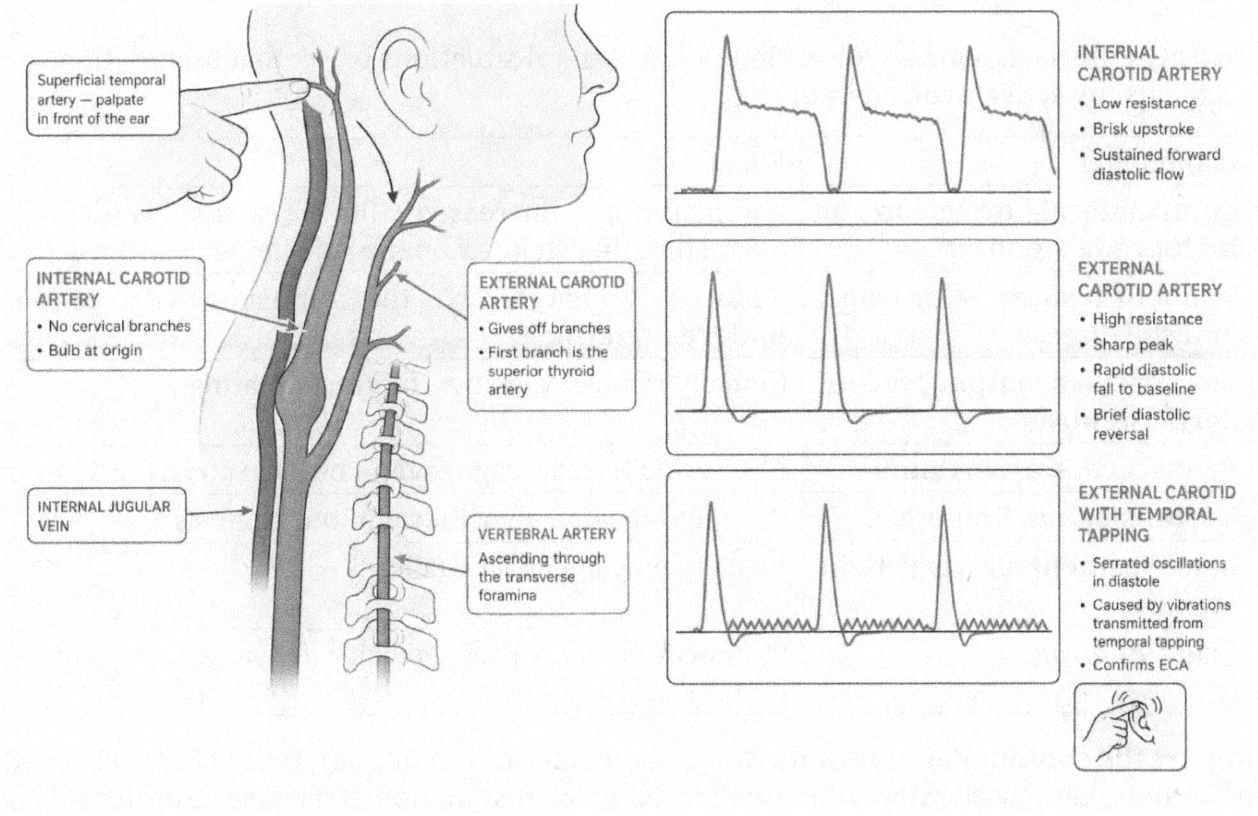

16.2 Carotid Stenosis Criteria and Plaque Characterisation

Velocity criteria

Stenosis grading rests on a small set of measurements combined into categories:

- **Internal carotid peak systolic velocity**
- **Internal carotid to common carotid peak systolic velocity ratio**
- **Internal carotid end-diastolic velocity**

These are combined into bands — typically below 50%, 50 to 69%, 70% or greater, near-occlusion, and occlusion — each with a defined management implication.

A department must adopt one published set of criteria and apply it consistently, stating in the report which set is in use. [VERIFY: the carotid velocity criteria to be adopted, the thresholds for each stenosis band, and the reference method (NASCET or ECST) against which they were validated]

The measurement method underlying the percentage matters, because published criteria were validated against a specific angiographic method, and the two historical methods yield different percentages for the same anatomical lesion. Quoting a percentage without knowing which convention it refers to is a real source of confusion between departments.

The confounders — when the numbers lie

Velocity criteria assume a typical circulation. Several situations break that assumption, and each must be actively considered:

Confounder	Effect
Contralateral occlusion or high-grade stenosis	Compensatory increased flow **raises velocities**, overestimating stenosis on the side being measured
Tandem lesions — proximal or distal disease	Reduce velocity at the interrogated lesion, **underestimating** it
Low cardiac output, severe aortic stenosis	Globally reduce velocities, underestimating
Bradycardia, arrhythmia	Alter velocities; average several beats in atrial fibrillation
Tortuosity and kinking	Produce elevated velocities without stenosis
Long-segment or very tight stenosis	Velocity may fall as flow falls
Prior stenting	Stiffened vessel raises velocity for a given stenosis (§16.3)

Report the confounder alongside the measurement. "ICA peak systolic velocity elevated; note contralateral occlusion, which may result in overestimation of the degree of stenosis" is a far more useful sentence than a bare number.

Near-occlusion and occlusion

Near-occlusion is the important trap. As the lesion becomes critical, flow falls, and **velocities may be normal or even low** — the opposite of what the grading logic expects. The distal internal carotid collapses, producing a **"string sign"** of a thread of flow.

The technique required: low pulse repetition frequency, **power Doppler**, careful slow interrogation of the distal vessel, and a **low wall filter**. Where doubt remains, **contrast-enhanced ultrasound** (Chapter 9 §9.3) or CT/MR angiography is required, because the distinction between near-occlusion and occlusion determines whether the patient is offered surgery.

Occlusion shows no detectable flow in the vessel despite optimised settings, sometimes with a **thump-like or staccato signal** in the proximal stump, **reversed flow in external carotid branches** supplying collateral pathways, and compensatory increased velocity in the contralateral vessel.

Plaque characterisation

Beyond the degree of stenosis, plaque morphology carries independent risk information:

Surface: smooth, irregular, or **ulcerated** — a defined crater with demonstrable flow within it.

Echogenicity:

- **Echolucent (hypoechoic)** — lipid-rich or containing haemorrhage; associated with **instability** and higher embolic risk. These plaques are also the hardest to see, so a lumen that looks unexpectedly narrow on colour with little visible plaque should raise suspicion
- **Heterogeneous** — mixed
- **Echogenic and calcified** — generally more stable, but **calcification shadows** and obscures the lumen behind it

Where calcified plaque shadows the lumen, work around it: change the angle of approach, use power Doppler, image from a different window, or use contrast.

Additional instability markers used in specialist practice include grey-scale median measurement, the juxtaluminal black area, and **plaque neovascularisation demonstrated on contrast-enhanced ultrasound** (Chapter 9 §9.3).

Vertebral and subclavian findings

Subclavian steal results from a stenosis or occlusion of the subclavian artery **proximal to the vertebral origin**, so that the arm is supplied by retrograde flow down the vertebral artery. It exists on a **spectrum**:

1. **Transient mid-systolic deceleration** — a notch in the systolic peak, sometimes called a bunny-ear waveform, indicating a pressure gradient without frank reversal

2. **Alternating (partial reversal)** flow
3. **Complete retrograde flow** throughout the cycle

Provocation: where the finding is equivocal, inflate a blood pressure cuff on the arm above systolic pressure for a period and then release, creating reactive hyperaemia that increases arm demand and unmasks or exaggerates the steal.

Always compare blood pressures in both arms — a significant difference supports the diagnosis and is free information.

Other carotid pathology

Dissection — an intimal flap with two lumina, a long tapered narrowing, or an eccentric **intramural haematoma**; the distal internal carotid waveform becomes high-resistance. Consider it in a young patient with neck pain, headache, Horner syndrome, or stroke.

Fibromuscular dysplasia — a **"string of beads"** appearance in the mid and distal internal carotid, characteristically sparing the bulb.

Carotid body tumour — a hypervascular mass at the bifurcation **splaying the internal and external carotid arteries apart**, a distinctive and near-specific sign.

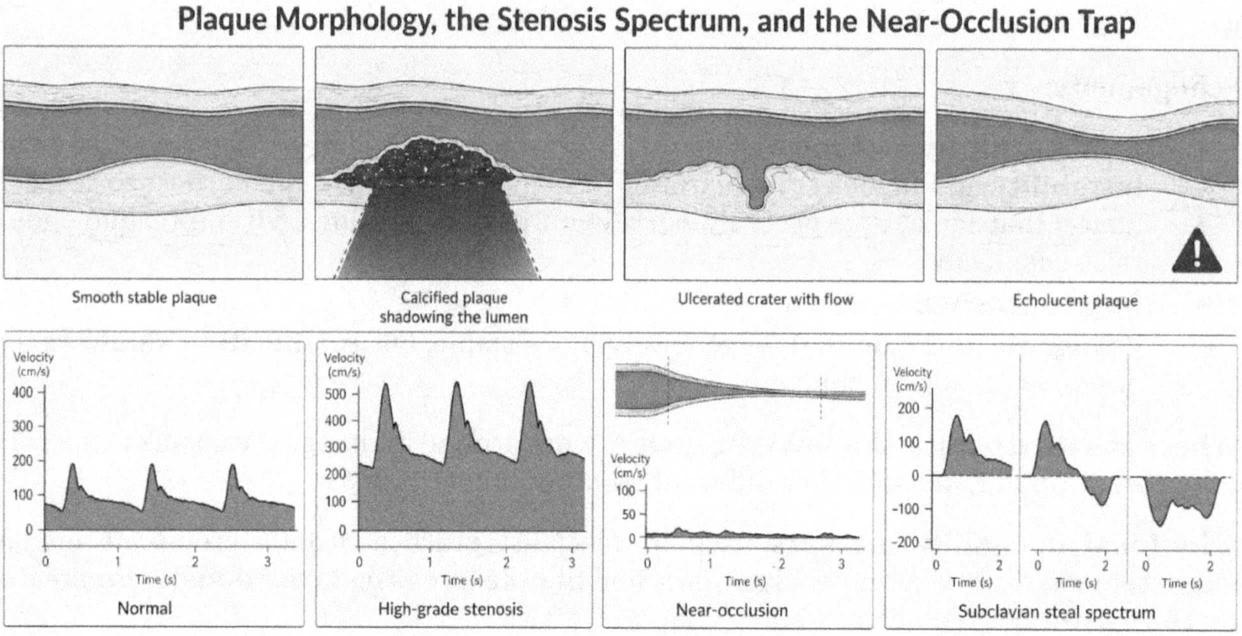

Carotid stenosis assessment with characteristic plaque appearances and spectral Doppler patterns.

16.3 Postoperative and Stent Surveillance

After endarterectomy

A baseline study is performed shortly after surgery, and everything subsequent is compared against it (Chapter 1 §1.5).

Assess for **residual stenosis** at the endarterectomy site, the appearance of any **patch**, and the distal end-point.

Two patterns of recurrent narrowing occur at different times and look different:

- **Myointimal hyperplasia** — within the first couple of years, appearing as **smooth, homogeneous, relatively hypoechoic** thickening
- **Recurrent atherosclerosis** — later, resembling the original disease with irregular, heterogeneous, often calcified plaque

After stenting

The essential technical point:

> **A stented artery is stiffer than a native artery, so velocities are higher for the same anatomical degree of stenosis. Applying native-vessel criteria to a stented carotid systematically overestimates stenosis.**

Stent-specific velocity criteria must be used, and the report should state which criteria are being applied. [VERIFY: current velocity criteria for in-stent carotid restenosis and their thresholds]

The post-procedure baseline study is more important here than anywhere else in the chapter, because the individual patient's post-stent velocities become their own reference, and a change from that baseline is more informative than an absolute value.

Assess: stent position and apposition to the wall, **in-stent restenosis** (which characteristically occurs at the stent ends), **stent deformity, kinking or fracture**, and velocities throughout the stent and at both ends.

Surveillance intervals are protocol-defined. [VERIFY: current surveillance intervals after carotid endarterectomy and stenting]

16.4 Transcranial Doppler: Windows and Technique

The two approaches

Non-imaging transcranial Doppler uses a low-frequency pulsed probe without an image, identifying vessels by **window, depth, flow direction, and response to compression manoeuvres**. It has better penetration and is the traditional tool for monitoring.

Transcranial colour-coded duplex adds a greyscale and colour image, allowing direct visualisation and angle correction, at some cost in penetration.

The windows

Window	Location	Vessels
Transtemporal	Above the zygomatic arch, anterior to the ear	Middle cerebral, anterior cerebral, posterior cerebral, terminal internal carotid

Window	Location	Vessels
Transorbital	Through the closed eyelid	Ophthalmic artery and carotid siphon
Suboccipital (transforaminal)	Below the occiput with the neck flexed	Vertebral arteries and basilar artery
Submandibular	Below the angle of the jaw	Distal extracranial internal carotid — used for the ratio in §16.5

The transorbital window requires specific safety discipline. The eye has low tolerance for acoustic energy, ophthalmic exposure limits are substantially lower than elsewhere, and **output power must be reduced to the minimum before insonating through the orbit** (Chapter 1 §1.7). This is one of the few examinations in the book where an ALARA failure could cause direct, immediate injury.

Vessel identification

Each vessel is identified by the combination of **window, sample depth, and flow direction relative to the transducer** — flow toward the probe in the middle cerebral artery, away in the anterior cerebral, and so on. **Compression of the ipsilateral common carotid** alters the signal in a predictable, vessel-specific way and confirms identification, though it is used cautiously in patients with carotid disease.

[VERIFY: current standard depth ranges and expected flow directions for each intracranial vessel by window]

Measurements and limitations

Mean flow velocity is the primary measurement in most applications, with peak systolic and end-diastolic velocities and the **pulsatility index** as adjuncts.

The principal limitation is the absent temporal window. A meaningful proportion of patients — more commonly older, female, and in some ethnic groups — have insufficient temporal bone thinning to permit insonation. **This is a hard technical limit, not a failure of technique**, and it must be reported as such rather than as a negative study. Contrast agents can sometimes rescue an inadequate window.

16.5 Intracranial Applications: Vasospasm, Sickle Cell Disease, Emboli

Vasospasm after subarachnoid haemorrhage

The principal indication for transcranial Doppler. Following aneurysmal subarachnoid haemorrhage, delayed cerebral vasospasm develops over days and causes ischaemic injury. Serial transcranial Doppler detects the **rising velocities** that accompany narrowing, allowing intervention before infarction.

The interpretive problem: velocity rises both when a vessel narrows (**vasospasm**) and when flow through it increases (**hyperaemia**), for example during induced hypertension or haemodilution therapy. Treating hyperaemia as vasospasm leads to harmful escalation.

The solution is a ratio:

> **Lindegaard ratio = middle cerebral artery mean velocity ÷ extracranial internal carotid mean velocity**

In vasospasm, the intracranial vessel is narrowed while the extracranial vessel is not, so the **ratio rises. In hyperaemia**, both rise together and the **ratio stays normal**. The submandibular window (§16.4) exists largely to provide the denominator.

An analogous ratio using the vertebral artery is applied to the basilar circulation.

[VERIFY: current mean velocity thresholds for vasospasm and current Lindegaard ratio thresholds]

Serial studies at defined intervals, with the same operator and technique where possible, are far more informative than a single value — the **trend** is the finding.

Sickle cell disease

One of the clearest examples in the whole of ultrasound of a screening test changing outcomes.

Children with sickle cell disease are at substantial risk of stroke. **Transcranial Doppler screening identifies elevated time-averaged mean velocities in the middle cerebral and distal internal carotid arteries**, and those children entered into a regular transfusion programme have a markedly reduced stroke rate.

This makes transcranial Doppler screening a standard of care in paediatric sickle cell disease, performed from early childhood at defined intervals, with velocity thresholds defining normal, conditional, and abnormal categories. [VERIFY: current screening ages, intervals, velocity thresholds and category definitions for transcranial Doppler in sickle cell disease]

Technique discipline matters here more than usual, because a management decision as consequential as lifelong transfusion follows from the number: insonate at the standard depths, record the time-averaged mean of the maximum velocity, and follow the protocol the thresholds were validated with.

Embolus detection

Circulating emboli produce **high-intensity transient signals** — brief, high-amplitude, unidirectional signals with a characteristic audible chirp — within the Doppler spectrum.

Applications: monitoring during carotid endarterectomy and stenting, and detecting an ongoing embolic source in patients with stroke of uncertain cause.

Right-to-left shunt detection

Agitated saline injected intravenously, with transcranial Doppler monitoring of the middle cerebral artery, detects microbubbles arriving in the cerebral circulation — indicating a right-to-left shunt, most often a patent foramen ovale.

The Valsalva manoeuvre is essential, since many shunts open only when right atrial pressure transiently exceeds left. **Timing distinguishes the level of the shunt**, as in the cardiac bubble study (Chapter 14 §14.6): early arrival suggests an intracardiac shunt, delayed arrival suggests an intrapulmonary one. The number of microbubbles is graded.

Other applications

Cerebral vasomotor reactivity — the response of velocity to a carbon dioxide challenge or breath-holding, assessing cerebrovascular reserve.

Cerebral circulatory arrest — in the context of suspected brain death, characteristic patterns of **oscillating (to-and-fro) flow and short systolic spikes** may be seen. **Transcranial Doppler is an ancillary test performed within a formal protocol**, never a primary determinant, and local law and policy govern entirely.

Monitoring during cardiac surgery and extracorporeal support.

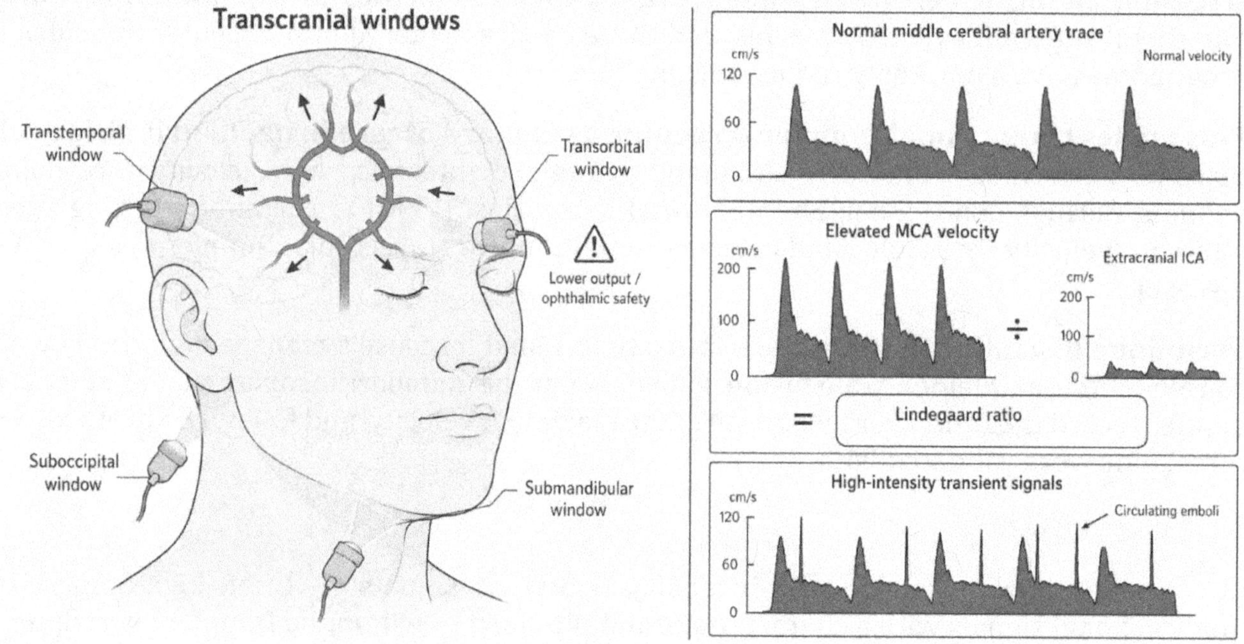

Transcranial windows and the ratio that separates vasospasm from hyperaemia.

16.6 Peripheral Arterial Protocol and Segmental Pressures

Anatomy

Lower limb: aorta → common iliac → external and internal iliac → **common femoral → superficial femoral** and **profunda femoris → popliteal → tibioperoneal trunk** and **anterior tibial → posterior tibial** and **peroneal → dorsalis pedis** and plantar arteries.

Upper limb: subclavian → axillary → brachial → **radial and ulnar** → palmar arches.

Duplex technique

Position: supine with the leg slightly externally rotated and the knee gently flexed; prone or lateral for the popliteal segment where access is difficult.

Transducer: linear for the femoral and distal vessels; **curvilinear for the iliacs and in larger patients**, where depth defeats the linear probe.

Sample systematically along the whole conduit — every few centimetres, and specifically **at every point where colour aliasing or a visible narrowing suggests a velocity change**. The lesion is found on colour and quantified on spectral.

Angle at or below 60°, cursor aligned to the vessel or to the visible jet, and — importantly — **use the same angle for the proximal reference and the stenosis**, since the criteria in §16.7 are ratios.

Waveforms — the fastest diagnostic information available

The waveform at a single site tells you about the whole conduit proximal to it, and the progression is the diagnosis (Chapter 3 §3.7):

Waveform	Interpretation
Triphasic — sharp systolic peak, early diastolic reversal, late diastolic forward flow	Normal compliant vessel with high peripheral resistance
Biphasic — loss of the reverse component	Reduced compliance or mild proximal disease
Monophasic, damped, delayed — slow upstroke, blunted rounded peak, continuous forward flow	**Significant proximal disease**

A damped monophasic waveform at the ankle establishes that there is significant disease somewhere proximal, before any velocity is measured. Working proximally to find where the waveform normalises localises the lesion.

Segmental pressures and the ankle-brachial index

The ankle-brachial index is calculated as:

> **the higher of the dorsalis pedis and posterior tibial pressures on that leg ÷ the higher of the two brachial pressures**

It is quick, quantitative, reproducible, and predictive of cardiovascular risk as well as limb outcome. [VERIFY: current ankle-brachial index interpretation categories and thresholds]

The critical pitfall:

> **Medial arterial calcification makes vessels incompressible, producing a falsely elevated or unobtainable index.** This occurs particularly in **diabetes and chronic kidney disease** — exactly the populations with the most severe peripheral arterial disease.

When the index is abnormally high or the vessels will not compress, use the toe-brachial index, since the digital arteries are usually spared from medial calcification. **Pulse volume recordings** and Doppler waveform analysis also remain valid when pressures are not.

Segmental pressures measured at the upper thigh, above the knee, below the knee and at the ankle **localise disease by level**: a significant pressure drop between adjacent cuffs indicates disease in the intervening segment. [VERIFY: current segmental pressure gradient thresholds indicating significant disease]

Exercise testing unmasks disease in patients with claudication and a normal resting index — the resting circulation is adequate, and the fall in index after exercise reveals the limitation.

Clinical context to record: claudication distance, rest pain, tissue loss, and — in the diabetic foot — the coexistence of neuropathy, which alters the presentation and the significance of the findings.

16.7 Stenosis, Occlusion, Aneurysm, and Pseudoaneurysm

Grading arterial stenosis

The peak systolic velocity ratio is the primary criterion:

> **PSV ratio = peak systolic velocity at the stenosis ÷ peak systolic velocity in a normal segment immediately proximal**

Ratio thresholds define stenosis bands, and are supported by **spectral broadening**, **post-stenotic turbulence**, and **distal waveform damping**. [VERIFY: current peak systolic velocity ratio thresholds for grading peripheral arterial stenosis]

Why a ratio rather than an absolute velocity: absolute velocities vary with vessel size, cardiac output and site along the limb, whereas the ratio normalises for the individual patient's flow state — the same logic that underlies the Lindegaard ratio in §16.5.

Occlusion

Findings: absent flow within the vessel despite optimised low-flow settings, often with echogenic material in the lumen, **collateral vessels** around the occluded segment, and **reconstitution** distally.

Identify and report the reconstitution point. The length of the occluded segment and where flow returns determine whether endovascular treatment or bypass is feasible, and where a distal anastomosis could be placed. This is the piece of information the vascular surgeon most needs from the study.

Aneurysm

Popliteal aneurysm is the commonest peripheral arterial aneurysm and carries two specific obligations:

1. **Examine the contralateral popliteal artery** — a substantial proportion are bilateral
2. **Examine the abdominal aorta** — the association with abdominal aortic aneurysm is strong

The risk is thromboembolic rather than ruptural — mural thrombus embolises distally and can cause acute limb ischaemia — so assess for thrombus and for distal runoff.

Measure outer wall to outer wall, perpendicular to the vessel axis, as in Chapter 3 §3.8.

Femoral aneurysms occur, often with popliteal disease.

Pseudoaneurysm

A contained arterial wall rupture, most commonly **following arterial puncture** for catheterisation, and increasingly common as endovascular procedures multiply.

The two diagnostic findings:

- **A "yin-yang" swirling pattern** within the sac on colour Doppler, as blood enters and leaves through a single neck
- **A "to-and-fro" spectral waveform in the neck** — forward flow into the sac in systole, reversed flow out in diastole. **This neck waveform is the diagnostic finding** and should be documented specifically

Measure and report: the sac dimensions, the **neck length and diameter**, the parent artery, and any surrounding haematoma.

Treatment is frequently ultrasound-guided — either compression of the neck under direct vision, or **ultrasound-guided thrombin injection** into the sac (Chapter 9 §9.5), which makes accurate delineation of the neck a procedural as well as a diagnostic requirement.

Arteriovenous fistula

Also usually post-puncture, and often coexisting with a pseudoaneurysm.

Findings:

- **High-velocity, low-resistance flow in the feeding artery** — the artery behaves as though supplying a low-resistance bed, because it is

- **Arterialised venous waveform** — pulsatile flow in the draining vein, which should not be pulsatile
- **Perivascular tissue vibration** producing a **mosaic of colour in the soft tissues around the communication** — a distinctive artifact and often the finding that first draws the eye

Other arterial pathology

Entrapment syndromes are **dynamic diagnoses**, and this is where ultrasound is uniquely capable:

- **Popliteal artery entrapment** — the artery compressed by an abnormal relationship with the gastrocnemius. **Assess with active plantarflexion and passive dorsiflexion**, looking for compression or occlusion that is absent at rest
- **Thoracic outlet syndrome** — subclavian artery or vein compression, assessed with the arm in provocative positions

Vasculitis:

- **Giant cell arteritis** — a **hypoechoic circumferential "halo"** around the lumen of the temporal artery representing wall oedema, and a **non-compressible artery** on gentle probe pressure (the compression sign). **Bilateral temporal and axillary artery assessment** is now an established diagnostic pathway and increasingly a first-line test, reducing reliance on biopsy. [VERIFY: current diagnostic criteria and protocol for temporal and axillary artery ultrasound in giant cell arteritis]
- **Takayasu arteritis** — long, smooth, concentric wall thickening of the great vessels

Dissection, **cystic adventitial disease**, and **arterial trauma** complete the differential.

16.8 Dialysis Access and Bypass Graft Surveillance

Preoperative mapping

Performed before access creation to select the site, and it examines both systems:

Arterial: patency, calibre, calcification, and waveform of the radial, ulnar and brachial arteries, with an assessment of the palmar arch to confirm that the hand will remain perfused if the radial artery is used.

Venous: calibre, patency, depth from the skin, and continuity through to the central veins, examining the cephalic and basilic systems along their length. **A vein that is too small, too deep, or has segmental narrowing from previous cannulation will not mature.**

Assessing maturation

A newly created fistula is assessed after a defined interval against criteria combining **flow volume, internal diameter, and depth from the skin** — a fistula must carry enough flow, be large enough to cannulate, and be superficial enough to reach. [VERIFY: current fistula maturation criteria — flow volume, diameter and depth thresholds — and the assessment interval]

Flow volume measurement:

Flow volume = cross-sectional area × time-averaged mean velocity

Measure in a **straight segment** of the feeding artery or the fistula body, avoiding turbulent regions near the anastomosis, using a **uniform insonation angle and a sample volume covering the whole lumen**. Take several measurements and average them — this is a noisy measurement and single values are unreliable.

Both extremes matter: low flow predicts thrombosis, while **very high flow** can cause distal steal and, over time, high-output cardiac failure.

Complications

Complication	Findings
Stenosis	**Juxta-anastomotic** in fistulae, **venous outflow** in grafts, and **central venous** in both. Diagnosed by elevated velocity with a raised velocity ratio, plus a fall in flow volume [VERIFY: current velocity ratio thresholds for access stenosis]
Thrombosis	Absent flow, echogenic material within the lumen
Aneurysm and pseudoaneurysm	From repeated cannulation at the same site; assess wall integrity and overlying skin
Steal syndrome	**Reversed flow in the artery distal to the anastomosis**, with symptoms of hand ischaemia. Assess with and without manual compression of the fistula — reversal that corrects on compression confirms the mechanism
Infection and perigraft collection	Complex fluid around a graft; a serious finding

Central venous stenosis deserves specific mention because it is easily missed: the stenosis itself is usually not directly visible, and the diagnosis rests on **indirect signs** in the accessible veins — **loss of respiratory phasicity and cardiac pulsatility** in the subclavian and axillary veins, elevated velocity where visible, and **collateral vessels** across the chest wall and shoulder. Arm swelling on the access side should prompt this specific assessment.

Bypass graft surveillance

Applies to lower limb vein and prosthetic grafts.

Scan the entire conduit — inflow artery, proximal anastomosis, the whole graft body, distal anastomosis, and outflow artery — because a lesion anywhere in that chain threatens the graft.

Criteria: an elevated **peak systolic velocity ratio** at a focal lesion, and — a separate and important marker — a **low uniform graft velocity**, which indicates poor overall flow and predicts imminent failure even without a demonstrable focal stenosis. [VERIFY: current velocity ratio thresholds and low-velocity criterion for bypass graft surveillance, and recommended surveillance intervals]

Vein grafts develop stenoses at valve sites and at anastomoses; prosthetic grafts fail predominantly at the **distal anastomosis** through myointimal hyperplasia.

The surveillance principle: a graft with a detected stenosis can be revised, whereas a thrombosed graft usually cannot be salvaged — which is the entire argument for programmatic surveillance, and the reason serial comparison against the immediate post-operative baseline matters (Chapter 1 §1.5).

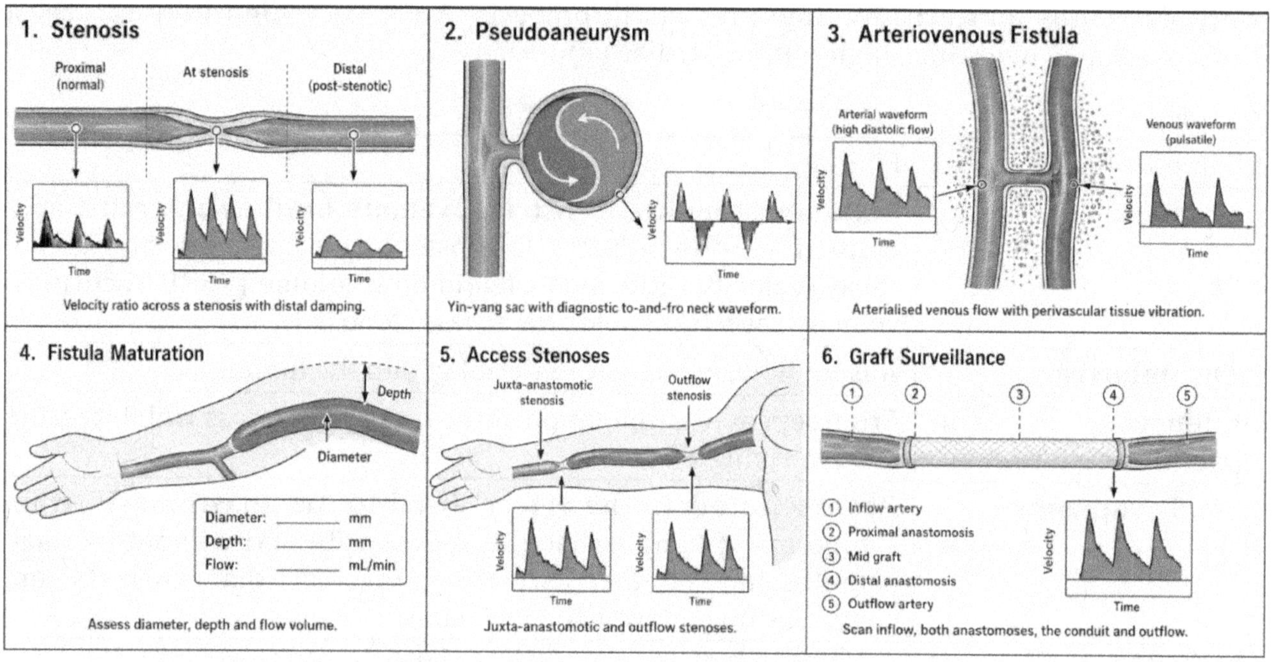

Arterial lesions, access complications, and where grafts fail.

16.9 Lower and Upper Extremity Venous Compression Protocol

Anatomy and a nomenclature warning

Deep system: common femoral vein, **femoral vein**, deep femoral (profunda) vein, popliteal vein, tibioperoneal trunk, and the paired posterior tibial, peroneal and anterior tibial veins, together with the soleal and gastrocnemius sinuses.

Superficial system: great saphenous vein, small saphenous vein, and accessory saphenous veins, connected to the deep system by **perforating veins**.

> **A nomenclature warning that has caused real clinical harm: the "superficial femoral vein" is a DEEP vein.** The historical term has led clinicians to withhold anticoagulation from patients with proximal deep vein thrombosis on the assumption that a "superficial" vein was involved. **Use "femoral vein"** and avoid the older term entirely.

Technique

Position: supine with **reverse Trendelenburg** tilt to distend the veins, the leg externally rotated and the knee slightly flexed. The popliteal segment is assessed prone, seated, or in lateral decubitus.

Transducer: linear for most of the limb; curvilinear for the iliac veins and in larger patients.

The compression manoeuvre — the core of the examination:

- **Compress in the TRANSVERSE plane**, not longitudinal. In longitudinal the probe slides off the vein and an incompressible-looking segment may simply be a vein you have moved past
- **Compress every 1 to 2 centimetres** along the course
- **The criterion for adequate compression:** the vein walls **coapt completely**, with sufficient pressure applied that the **adjacent artery is slightly deformed** — this confirms that enough force was used to have collapsed a normal vein
- Release and repeat along the vessel

Doppler assessment at the common femoral, femoral and popliteal veins: **spontaneous flow, respiratory phasicity, augmentation response, and Valsalva response.**

The stations

Work systematically from proximal to distal:

1. **Common femoral vein** at the inguinal ligament
2. **Saphenofemoral junction**
3. **Femoral vein** through its length, including the **adductor canal** — a segment that is deep, technically difficult, and consequently under-examined
4. **Popliteal vein**
5. **Tibioperoneal trunk**
6. **Paired calf veins** — posterior tibial, peroneal, and anterior tibial

Protocol extent — the genuine debate

Complete duplex examines the whole deep system including the calf. **Two-point compression** examines only the common femoral and popliteal veins. **Extended compression** covers the full length of the femoral and popliteal veins without formal calf assessment.

The trade-off is real and defensible in both directions. Complete studies detect isolated calf vein thrombosis, whose clinical significance and treatment remain debated, at the cost of time and of false positives. Limited studies are faster and reproducible but require a defined **repeat scan** protocol at a set interval to detect propagation.

What matters for the report is stating which protocol was performed, so that a negative study is understood for what it excludes and what it does not (Chapter 1 §1.5).

Phasicity — the most-missed finding

Normal lower limb venous flow is phasic with respiration, varying as intra-abdominal pressure changes.

> **Continuous, non-phasic flow in the common femoral vein means look proximal.** It indicates obstruction between the sampling site and the heart — iliac vein thrombosis, extrinsic compression by a pelvic mass, or a central lesion — none of which the compression protocol will find, because those veins are not compressible from the surface.

Compare the two sides. Asymmetry in phasicity is more informative than the appearance of either trace alone, and it is free.

Upper extremity

The same principles with anatomical adaptations:

Internal jugular, subclavian, axillary, brachial, basilic and cephalic veins. The **subclavian vein cannot be compressed** beneath the clavicle, so assessment there depends on **direct visualisation of thrombus, colour filling, phasicity, and the response to sniffing**.

Indirect signs of central obstruction — loss of cardiac pulsatility and respiratory phasicity, and chest wall collaterals — are the same as those used in dialysis access assessment (§16.8).

Consider Paget–Schroetter syndrome (effort thrombosis) in a young patient with arm swelling after exertion, and assess for thoracic outlet compression with provocative positioning.

16.10 Acute versus Chronic Thrombus and Venous Insufficiency

Distinguishing acute from chronic

Clinically consequential, because the question is usually whether this is a new event requiring anticoagulation or an old one requiring nothing:

	Acute	Chronic
Vein calibre	**Distended,** larger than the adjacent artery	**Contracted,** small, sometimes barely identifiable
Thrombus echogenicity	**Hypoechoic or anechoic** — frequently invisible on B-mode	**Echogenic**
Attachment	Loosely adherent; may have a **free-floating tail**	**Firmly adherent** to a thickened wall
Wall	Normal	**Thickened, irregular, rigid**
Recanalisation	Absent	**Channels** within the thrombus

	Acute	Chronic
Collaterals	Absent	**Present**
Compressibility	Non-compressible, "spongy"	Non-compressible, hard

The point that must be stated explicitly: acute thrombus is frequently **anechoic and therefore invisible on greyscale. The compression manoeuvre, not the appearance, makes the diagnosis** — which is why compression at close intervals is non-negotiable and why a study relying on B-mode appearance alone will miss thrombus.

Age-dating is imprecise. Report the features observed and their implication rather than asserting an age, and where a distinction between new and old is critical, **comparison with prior imaging** is far more reliable than morphology.

Also assess and report: the **proximal extent** of thrombus, whether it is **occlusive or non-occlusive**, and the presence of a **mobile free-floating component**.

Related conditions

Superficial vein thrombosis — the significant question is **proximity to the deep system**. Thrombus approaching the saphenofemoral or saphenopopliteal junction may warrant anticoagulation, so **measure and report the distance from the junction**.

May–Thurner syndrome — compression of the left common iliac vein by the overlying right common iliac artery, producing left-sided deep vein thrombosis characteristically in younger patients. Suspect it with isolated left iliofemoral thrombosis, and note that the compression itself is best demonstrated on cross-sectional imaging or venography.

Phlegmasia — massive thrombosis with limb-threatening venous outflow obstruction and compromised arterial inflow. A limb emergency.

Venous insufficiency and reflux

The single most important technical point in this section:

> **The reflux study is performed with the patient UPRIGHT — standing — or in steep reverse Trendelenburg. A supine reflux study underestimates or entirely misses reflux, and is not a valid examination.**

Gravity is the mechanism being tested; removing it removes the finding.

Technique:

1. **Patient standing**, weight borne on the contralateral leg, holding a support for balance, with the leg being examined relaxed and slightly externally rotated
2. Interrogate in **longitudinal** with the sample volume in the vessel
3. **Provoke** with distal augmentation — a manual calf squeeze or a rapid-inflation cuff — and **assess the flow on release**; or use **Valsalva** for the saphenofemoral junction and proximal deep veins
4. **Measure the duration of reversed flow** after release

Reflux is defined by duration thresholds, which differ for the superficial veins, the deep veins, and the perforators. [VERIFY: current reflux duration thresholds for superficial veins, deep veins and perforating veins]

Map the whole system for treatment planning: great saphenous vein from the junction to the point where reflux ceases, small saphenous vein and its junction, accessory and tributary veins, and **incompetent perforators** — which are located, measured and marked on the skin where intervention is planned.

Classify and report using the standard clinical classification for chronic venous disease, which combines clinical signs, aetiology, anatomy and pathophysiology. [VERIFY: current CEAP classification definitions]

Post-thrombotic syndrome — the late consequence of deep vein thrombosis, combining **deep venous reflux through damaged valves** and **residual obstruction**. Assess both components, because they carry different management implications.

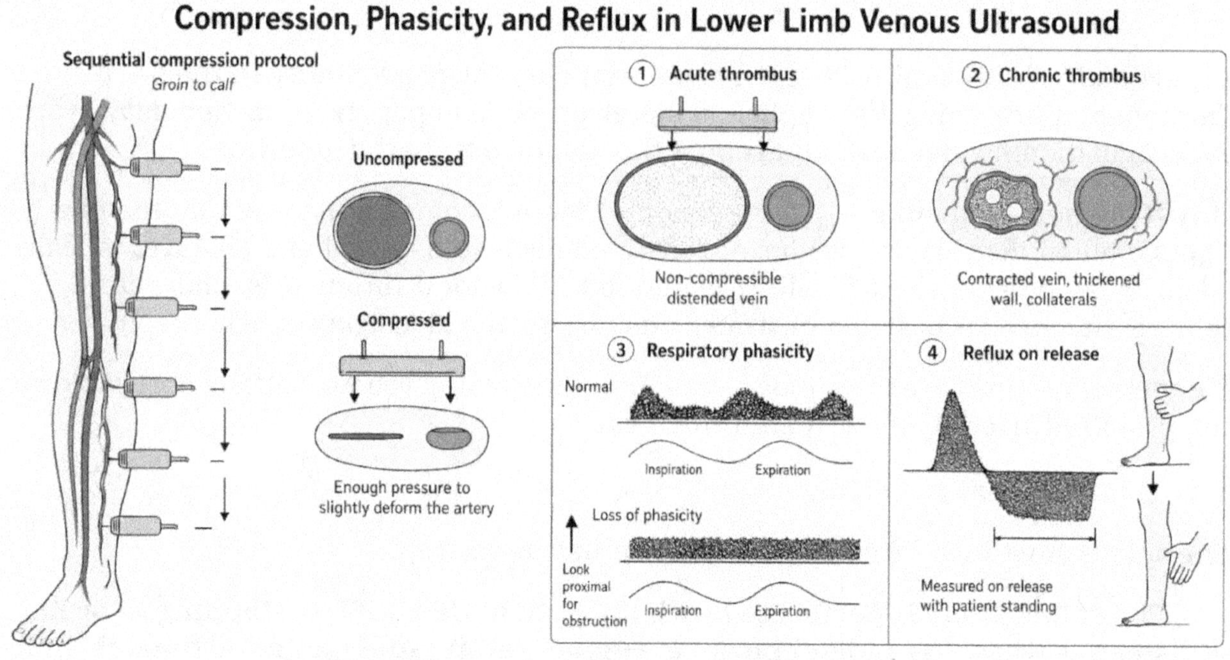

Compression protocol, dynamic venous findings, and machine-recorded Doppler patterns.

Key Points

1. Angle correction returns in this chapter. Keep the insonation angle at or below 60 degrees, use the same angle for a stenosis and its proximal reference, and archive the image with the cursor visible.
2. The internal carotid has no cervical branches and a low-resistance waveform; the external branches and is high-resistance. The temporal tap confirms it in seconds.
3. A high-grade internal carotid stenosis can produce a damped high-resistance distal waveform resembling an external carotid — which is when the branch rule matters most.

4. Contralateral occlusion raises velocities and overestimates stenosis. Report the confounder alongside the measurement.
5. Near-occlusion may show normal or low velocities. Use low PRF, power Doppler and, where needed, contrast — the distinction from occlusion decides whether surgery is offered.
6. Echolucent plaque is the least visible and the most unstable. An unexpectedly narrow colour lumen with little visible plaque should raise suspicion.
7. Stented arteries are stiffer, so velocities run higher for the same stenosis. Native criteria overestimate in-stent restenosis.
8. Reduce output before insonating through the orbit — ophthalmic exposure limits are substantially lower than elsewhere.
9. An absent temporal window is a hard technical limit, not a negative study, and should be reported as such.
10. The Lindegaard ratio separates vasospasm from hyperaemia, because hyperaemia raises the extracranial velocity too.
11. Transcranial Doppler screening in paediatric sickle cell disease reduces stroke — one of the clearest examples of screening changing outcome in this book.
12. A damped monophasic waveform at the ankle establishes significant proximal disease before any velocity is measured.
13. A falsely elevated ankle-brachial index means medial calcification, which is commonest in the patients with the worst disease. Use the toe-brachial index instead.
14. Grade peripheral stenosis by velocity ratio, not absolute velocity, because the ratio normalises for the individual's flow state.
15. In occlusion, find and report the reconstitution point — it is what the surgeon needs.
16. Popliteal aneurysm obliges you to examine the other popliteal artery and the abdominal aorta.
17. The to-and-fro neck waveform is the diagnostic finding in pseudoaneurysm, and delineating the neck is a procedural requirement as well as a diagnostic one.
18. Perivascular tissue vibration producing a colour mosaic in soft tissue is often what first reveals an arteriovenous fistula.
19. Access and graft stenoses occur at predictable sites: juxta-anastomotic in fistulae, venous outflow in grafts, distal anastomosis in prosthetic bypasses.
20. Central venous stenosis is diagnosed indirectly — loss of phasicity and pulsatility, and collaterals — because the lesion itself is usually not visible.
21. The "superficial femoral vein" is a deep vein. Use "femoral vein" and avoid a term that has caused patients to be denied anticoagulation.
22. Compress in the transverse plane, every one to two centimetres, with enough pressure to slightly deform the adjacent artery.
23. Acute thrombus is often anechoic. Compression, not appearance, makes the diagnosis.
24. Continuous non-phasic flow in the common femoral vein means look proximal — the compression protocol cannot reach the iliac veins.
25. Perform the reflux study standing. A supine reflux study is not a valid examination.

Registry Check

1. A cervical vessel shows a high-resistance waveform with minimal diastolic flow, and rhythmic tapping over the preauricular region produces serrated oscillations in the trace. This vessel is the:

A. Internal carotid artery **B.** External carotid artery **C.** Vertebral artery **D.** Common carotid artery

> **Answer: B.** A high-resistance waveform and transmission of the temporal tap identify the external carotid artery. The internal carotid supplies a low-resistance cerebral bed and shows abundant continuous diastolic flow, and the temporal tap is not transmitted into it.

2. Velocities in the right internal carotid artery are elevated. The left internal carotid is occluded. The correct interpretation is that the right-sided stenosis may be:

A. Underestimated **B.** Overestimated **C.** Accurately graded **D.** Impossible to assess

> **Answer: B.** Contralateral occlusion increases compensatory flow through the patent vessel, raising velocities independently of the local lesion and overestimating the degree of stenosis. The confounder should be reported alongside the measurement.

3. Applying native-vessel velocity criteria to a stented carotid artery will:

A. Underestimate the degree of restenosis **B.** Overestimate the degree of restenosis **C.** Have no systematic effect **D.** Be valid only beyond one year

> **Answer: B.** Stenting stiffens the arterial wall, raising velocities for any given anatomical narrowing. Stent-specific criteria must be used, and the patient's own post-procedure baseline study is the most useful reference.

4. In a patient with subarachnoid haemorrhage, the middle cerebral artery mean velocity is elevated. The Lindegaard ratio is normal. This suggests:

A. Vasospasm **B.** Hyperaemia **C.** Cerebral circulatory arrest **D.** Middle cerebral artery occlusion

> **Answer: B.** Vasospasm narrows the intracranial vessel while the extracranial internal carotid is unaffected, so the ratio rises. Hyperaemia raises velocities throughout, leaving the ratio normal. The distinction matters because treating hyperaemia as vasospasm leads to harmful escalation of therapy.

5. A diabetic patient with rest pain has an ankle-brachial index of 1.4. The appropriate interpretation is:

A. Normal arterial supply **B.** Mild arterial disease **C.** Falsely elevated due to medial calcification; obtain a toe-brachial index **D.** Measurement error requiring repetition

Answer: C. Medial arterial calcification renders the vessels incompressible, producing an abnormally high or unobtainable index, and it is most common in diabetes and chronic kidney disease — the populations with the most severe disease. The digital arteries are usually spared, making the toe-brachial index valid.

6. A pulsatile groin swelling after cardiac catheterisation shows a swirling colour pattern within a sac. The finding that confirms the diagnosis is:

A. The swirling colour pattern alone **B.** A to-and-fro waveform in the connecting neck **C.** Absence of flow in the sac **D.** Elevated velocity in the femoral artery

Answer: B. The to-and-fro spectral waveform in the neck — forward flow into the sac in systole and reversed flow out in diastole — is the diagnostic finding in pseudoaneurysm. The yin-yang appearance is suggestive but the neck waveform confirms it, and the neck must be delineated for thrombin injection or compression treatment.

7. Spectral Doppler in the common femoral vein shows continuous flow without respiratory variation, and the vein is fully compressible. The next step is to:

A. Report a normal study **B.** Assess for obstruction proximal to the sampling site **C.** Repeat the compression at closer intervals **D.** Perform a reflux study

Answer: B. Loss of respiratory phasicity indicates obstruction between the sampling site and the heart — iliac or central venous thrombosis or extrinsic compression — which the compression protocol cannot detect, since those veins are not compressible from the surface. Comparison with the contralateral side is informative.

8. A venous reflux study performed with the patient supine is likely to:

A. Overestimate reflux **B.** Underestimate or miss reflux **C.** Produce accurate results if Valsalva is used **D.** Be equivalent to a standing study

Answer: B. Gravity is the mechanism being tested, and removing it removes the finding. Reflux studies must be performed standing or in steep reverse Trendelenburg; a supine study is not a valid examination regardless of the provocation used.

Chapter Notes for the Editorial Pass

Verification queue. In priority order: **the carotid velocity criteria to be adopted**, with the thresholds for each stenosis band and the angiographic reference method against which they were validated (§16.2) — this determines surgical referral and is the chapter's most consequential decision; **in-stent restenosis criteria** (§16.3); **peripheral arterial velocity ratio thresholds** (§16.7); **dialysis access maturation criteria and stenosis velocity ratio thresholds** (§16.8); **bypass graft surveillance criteria including the low-velocity threshold and surveillance intervals** (§16.8); **ankle-brachial index categories and segmental pressure gradient thresholds** (§16.6); **venous reflux duration thresholds for**

superficial, deep and perforating veins, and the CEAP classification (§16.10); **transcranial vasospasm and Lindegaard thresholds** (§16.5); **sickle cell screening ages, intervals and velocity categories** (§16.5); **standard transcranial depths and flow directions** (§16.4); and the **temporal artery ultrasound protocol and criteria for giant cell arteritis** (§16.7).

A book-wide pattern, now at four. This chapter joins thyroid nodules (§11.3), urinary tract dilatation (§12.8) and infant hips (§13.10) in describing a classification framework without committing to a specific system — here, the carotid velocity criteria. As noted in the Chapter 13 editorial notes, **these decisions should be made together before layout.** The carotid criteria are arguably the most urgent of the four, since the resulting stenosis band determines whether a patient is offered an operation.

A deliberate contrast to preserve at layout. The opening of this chapter explicitly reverses the angle discipline established in Chapter 14 §14.4 — angle correction is used here and is not used in echocardiography. This is a genuine and important difference between the specialties, and the cross-references in both directions should be checked so that the contrast reads as intentional rather than as an inconsistency.

Figure count: 6 Lane A, 2 Lane B. The Lane B slots here are among the most straightforward acquisitions in the book — a compression pair and a phasicity pair are obtainable in any vascular laboratory in a single session — and they teach two findings that schematics convey only partially.

Cross-reference targets to fix at layout: §16.1 angle discipline → Chapter 2 §2.5, contrasted with Chapter 14 §14.4; §16.2 plaque neovascularisation and contrast → Chapter 9 §9.3; §16.4 ophthalmic exposure limits → Chapter 1 §1.7; §16.5 bubble study timing → Chapter 14 §14.6; §16.6 waveform progression → Chapter 3 §3.7; §16.7 aneurysm measurement → Chapter 3 §3.8; §16.7 thrombin injection → Chapter 9 §9.5; §16.8 and §16.9 central venous phasicity → each other; §16.10 Baker cyst as a DVT mimic → Chapter 11 §11.10.

Word count: approximately 10,400 excluding image prompt blocks, learning objectives, registry questions, and these notes.

Chapter 17: The Female Pelvis

Learning Objectives

On completing this chapter you should be able to:

1. Identify normal pelvic anatomy and locate the ovaries using their vascular landmarks.
2. Relate endometrial and ovarian appearances to the phase of the menstrual cycle, and time an examination accordingly.
3. Perform transabdominal and transvaginal examinations with appropriate consent, technique and infection control.
4. Apply Doppler to the pelvic vasculature and recognise its diagnostic limits.
5. Distinguish septate from bicornuate uterus and explain why the distinction matters.
6. Classify leiomyomas by location and recognise the features of adenomyosis.
7. Measure the endometrium correctly and assess it in postmenopausal bleeding.
8. Describe saline infusion sonohysterography and its indications.
9. Characterise ovarian lesions and apply the features associated with malignancy.
10. Recognise ectopic pregnancy, ovarian torsion, pelvic inflammatory disease and endometriosis.
11. Perform baseline and cycle-monitoring assessments in infertility.
12. Localise an intrauterine device and recognise malposition.

The Chapter's Two Recurring Themes

Timing determines what you see. More than any other region in this book, the normal appearance of the female pelvis changes week by week. An endometrium of a given thickness may be entirely normal or clearly abnormal depending on the cycle day, and an ovarian cyst may be a dominant follicle, a corpus luteum, or a lesion — the same image, three different reports. **Establish the cycle day and menopausal status before interpreting anything.**

Two emergencies run through the chapter. Ectopic pregnancy and ovarian torsion are both time-critical, both can look unremarkable at first glance, and both have a specific trap: in ectopic pregnancy the "ring of fire" is not specific, and in torsion **the presence of Doppler flow does not exclude the diagnosis**. These are dealt with in §17.10, but they should be in mind from the first image.

17.1 Normal Anatomy and Physiology of the Female Pelvis

The uterus

Divided into **fundus, body, isthmus** (the lower segment), and **cervix**, with three layers:

- **Endometrium** — the functional lining, echogenic, changing through the cycle (§17.2)
- **Myometrium** — three layers, of which the innermost, the **junctional zone**, appears as a thin hypoechoic band immediately deep to the endometrium. **The junctional zone is the key structure in adenomyosis** (§17.6)

- **Serosa** — a thin echogenic outer line

Orientation is described by two independent terms that are frequently confused:

- **Version** — the angle of the **cervix relative to the vagina**: anteverted or retroverted
- **Flexion** — the angle of the **body relative to the cervix**: anteflexed or retroflexed

A **retroverted uterus is harder to image transabdominally** — the fundus points away from the bladder window — and **easier transvaginally**, since it lies closer to the probe.

Size varies with parity and age. The prepubertal uterus is small with a **cervix longer than the body**, a ratio that reverses after puberty; the postmenopausal uterus atrophies. [VERIFY: current normal uterine dimensions by age and parity]

The ovaries — and how to find them

The ovaries lie in the **ovarian fossa** on the lateral pelvic sidewall. The landmark that finds them reliably:

> **The internal iliac vessels lie immediately posterior to the ovary, and the external iliac vessels anterosuperior.** When the ovary cannot be seen, find the internal iliac vessels transvaginally and the ovary is usually immediately anterior to them.

The ureter runs just posterior and is a useful additional landmark.

Ovarian volume is calculated by the ellipsoid formula and varies with age, falling markedly after menopause. **A postmenopausal ovary that cannot be identified is a common and usually normal finding**, and should be reported as not visualised rather than as absent. [VERIFY: current normal ovarian volume ranges by age]

The tubes, ligaments and spaces

The fallopian tubes — interstitial, isthmic, ampullary and infundibular segments with fimbriae — are **not normally visible** unless outlined by fluid. **A visible tube is usually an abnormal tube** (§17.10).

Supporting structures: broad, round, uterosacral and cardinal ligaments, the ovarian ligament, and the suspensory (infundibulopelvic) ligament carrying the ovarian vessels. **The uterosacral ligaments are a specific site of deep endometriosis** (§17.10).

The pouch of Douglas is the most dependent peritoneal space (Chapter 8 §8.1), and **a small volume of free fluid there is a normal finding** in reproductive-age women — particularly around ovulation.

Vascular anatomy

Uterine arteries arise from the internal iliac arteries and ascend alongside the uterus, branching into **arcuate** arteries in the outer myometrium, then **radial**, then **basal** and **spiral** arteries supplying the endometrium.

Ovarian arteries arise directly from the aorta. **Venous drainage is asymmetric** — the right ovarian vein to the inferior vena cava, the left to the left renal vein (Chapter 3 §3.5) — which is relevant to pelvic congestion (§17.4).

The two systems anastomose richly, and this **dual supply is the reason ovarian torsion can retain Doppler flow** (§17.10).

17.2 The Menstrual Cycle and Cyclic Sonographic Change

The endometrium through the cycle

Phase	Approximate days	Appearance
Menstrual	1–5	Thin, irregular, echogenic, often with a small amount of fluid or blood in the cavity
Early proliferative	6–9	Thin and uniformly echogenic, a single central line
Late proliferative / periovulatory	10–14	**Trilaminar ("triple line")** — a hypoechoic functional layer between echogenic basal layers, with a central echogenic line
Secretory	15–28	Thickest, **homogeneously echogenic**, with loss of the trilaminar pattern

The trilaminar appearance is the receptive pattern, and its presence and thickness are assessed in assisted reproduction cycles (§17.11).

The ovary through the cycle

Multiple small follicles are recruited in the early follicular phase. A **dominant follicle** emerges and enlarges by roughly a couple of millimetres a day, ovulating at a diameter in the high teens to low twenties of millimetres. [VERIFY: current normal dominant follicle diameter at ovulation and typical growth rate]

After ovulation the **corpus luteum** forms — a structure with a characteristically **thick, crenated (frilly) wall** and intense **peripheral vascularity**, the "ring of fire". It frequently contains internal haemorrhage, producing a lacy internal pattern.

> **The corpus luteum is the single most over-called structure in the female pelvis.** It is a normal cyclical finding, it has a ring of fire, and it can look alarming. Recognising it prevents both unnecessary follow-up and — importantly — mistaking it for an ectopic pregnancy (§17.10).

The practical consequence: when to scan

> **For endometrial assessment in a premenopausal woman, scan in the early proliferative phase — approximately days 4 to 6.**

At that point the endometrium is thinnest and most reproducible, focal lesions such as polyps stand out against a thin background, and the false positives generated by a thick secretory endometrium are avoided.

Scheduling the examination for the right cycle day is therefore part of the clinical service, not an administrative detail — and where a study was performed at the wrong point in the cycle, **the report should say so and state the limitation** (Chapter 1 §1.5).

Other states

Postmenopausal — a thin endometrium and small, often non-visualised ovaries.

Hormonal contraception — a thin, inactive endometrium.

Tamoxifen — subendometrial cystic change producing apparent thickening that is frequently not true endometrial pathology (§17.7).

Hormone replacement therapy — cyclical or continuous regimens alter appearance and the thresholds applied.

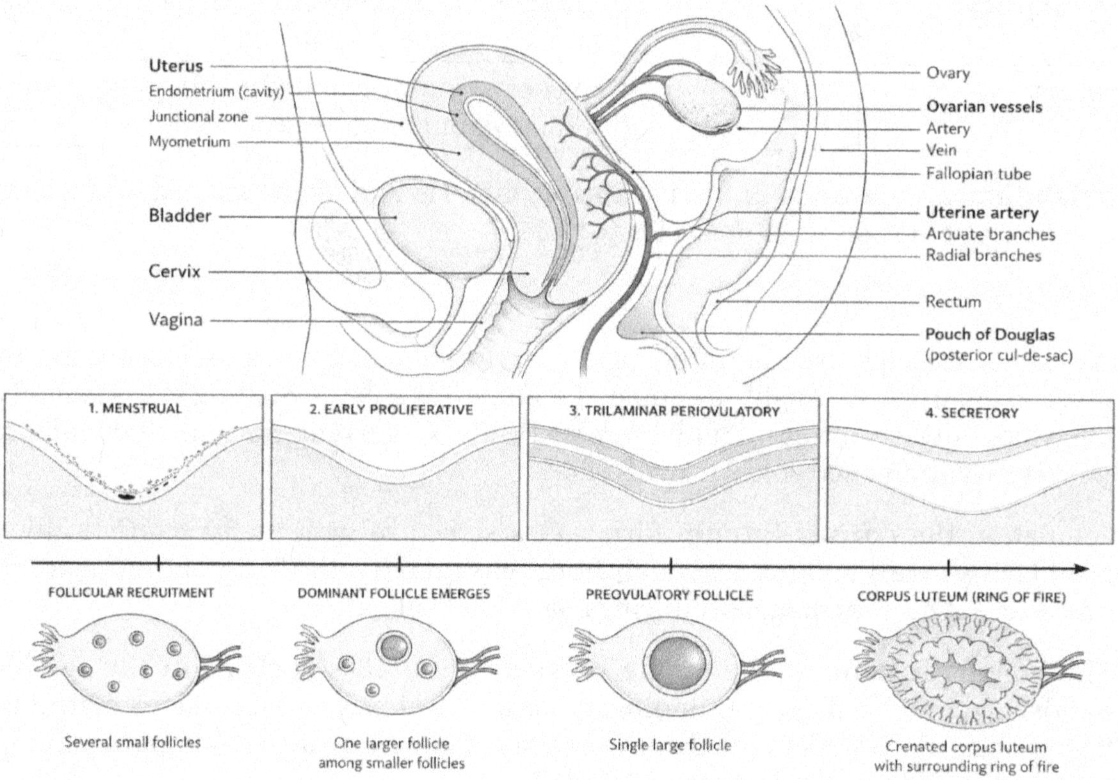

17.3 Transabdominal and Transvaginal Technique

Transabdominal

Requires a full bladder, which provides an acoustic window and displaces bowel from the pelvis. **An overfilled bladder distorts the anatomy** and compresses the uterus, so "as full as comfortable" is the instruction rather than "as full as possible".

Curvilinear transducer, sagittal and transverse sweeps covering the uterus, both adnexa, and the pelvic sidewalls.

Its role: an overview; **large masses that extend beyond the transvaginal field of view**; a high or enlarged uterus; and any situation where transvaginal imaging is not appropriate or is declined. A large fibroid uterus or a large ovarian mass **must** be assessed transabdominally, because the transvaginal probe cannot see its upper extent.

Transvaginal

Requires an empty bladder. Higher frequency and close proximity give far superior resolution, and this is the standard approach for detailed pelvic assessment.

Consent and dignity are not optional (Chapter 1 §1.3 and §1.5):

- **Explain what the examination involves before the patient undresses**
- Obtain **explicit verbal consent**, and state clearly that the examination can be stopped at any point
- **Offer the patient the option of inserting the probe herself**
- **Offer a chaperone and document the offer and the response**, including a decline
- Drape appropriately and expose only for as long as necessary

Infection control: a probe cover, appropriate gel, and — because the endocavitary probe is a **semicritical device — high-level disinfection between patients** (Chapter 1 §1.4). Sheath failure is assumed, and does not downgrade the requirement.

When transvaginal imaging is not appropriate — a patient who is not sexually active, a patient who declines, a child, or an imperforate hymen — the alternatives are a careful transabdominal study and, where needed, a **transperineal or translabial** approach.

Technique points

Rotate rather than sweep blindly. Obtain a sagittal image of the uterus, then rotate the probe through 90° for the coronal plane, and angle to each side for the adnexa.

Use gentle probe pressure deliberately as a diagnostic tool:

- **Sonographic tenderness** — localised pain reproduced under the probe, the pelvic equivalent of the sonographic Murphy sign (Chapter 5 §5.2)

- **Organ mobility and the sliding sign** — whether the uterus, ovaries and bowel glide freely against one another. **Loss of sliding indicates adhesions**, and is the basis of the pouch of Douglas assessment in deep endometriosis (§17.10)
- **The separation sign** — whether an adnexal mass moves independently of the ovary, distinguishing an ectopic from a corpus luteum (§17.10)

Three-dimensional imaging produces the **coronal plane of the uterus**, which cannot be obtained directly with a two-dimensional probe. It is the reference technique for **congenital anomalies** (§17.5) and for **intrauterine device localisation** (§17.12).

Documentation

Uterus in three dimensions with position and description; **endometrial thickness** with the cycle day recorded; both ovaries in three dimensions with volume and follicular appearance; the adnexa; the pouch of Douglas; and any lesion in **two planes with Doppler**.

17.4 Doppler Evaluation of the Pelvic Vasculature

Settings

Pelvic flow is slow. Use a **low velocity scale and a low wall filter**, and increase colour sensitivity. Abdominal Doppler settings will show no flow in structures that are normally perfused, and this is a common cause of a falsely "avascular" report.

The normal vessels

Uterine artery — sampled lateral to the cervix at the level of the internal os. In the non-pregnant state it is **high-resistance**, often with an early diastolic notch. Resistance falls somewhat in the luteal phase, and falls dramatically in pregnancy.

Ovarian arteries and intraovarian flow vary through the cycle, with **low-resistance flow in the dominant follicle and corpus luteum**.

Applications, and their limits

Ovarian torsion — reduced or absent flow supports the diagnosis, but **present flow does not exclude it**, because of the dual arterial supply (§17.1, §17.10). This is the single most important Doppler caveat in the chapter.

Adnexal mass characterisation — **vascularity within solid components, papillary projections or septations** raises concern for malignancy; flow confined to the periphery is more reassuring. Resistance indices alone are unreliable and have largely been superseded by morphological assessment (§17.9).

Ectopic pregnancy — the "ring of fire" of peripheral vascularity is **not specific**, since the corpus luteum shows the same pattern (§17.10).

Endometrial pathology — a **single dominant feeding vessel** entering a focal lesion, the "pedicle artery sign", supports a polyp; multiple irregular vessels within a thickened endometrium raise concern for malignancy (§17.7).

Leiomyoma — characteristically **peripheral rim vascularity**, in contrast to adenomyosis, where vessels **pass through** the affected myometrium (§17.6).

Retained products of conception and uterine arteriovenous malformation — high-velocity, low-resistance flow within the myometrium, an important finding because it identifies lesions at risk of catastrophic bleeding if instrumented.

Pelvic congestion — dilated, tortuous parauterine veins with **reflux on Valsalva**, often with ovarian vein incompetence, more common on the left for the anatomical reason given in §17.1. [VERIFY: current diameter and reflux criteria for pelvic venous congestion]

17.5 Congenital Uterine Anomalies

Embryology explains the classification

The uterus forms by **fusion of the paired Müllerian ducts** followed by **resorption of the intervening septum**. Anomalies arise from failure of either step:

- **Failure of formation** → agenesis or hypoplasia
- **Failure of one duct to develop** → unicornuate uterus, with or without a rudimentary horn
- **Failure of fusion** → didelphys or bicornuate uterus
- **Failure of septal resorption** → septate uterus

Formal classification systems exist and differ from one another, and a department should adopt one and state which it is using. [VERIFY: the Müllerian anomaly classification system to be adopted and its category definitions]

The distinction that matters clinically

> **Septate versus bicornuate is the key discrimination, because management differs entirely.** A septum is resected hysteroscopically; a bicornuate uterus is not, and requires abdominal surgery if anything.

The discriminator is the external fundal contour:

- **Septate uterus** — the **external contour is normal or only minimally indented**; the division is internal
- **Bicornuate uterus** — the external contour shows a **deep fundal cleft**, with two divergent horns

This requires seeing the fundal serosal contour and the cavity simultaneously, which a standard two-dimensional sagittal image cannot do.

> **Three-dimensional coronal reconstruction is the reference sonographic technique** for Müllerian anomalies, and a two-dimensional study should be reported as limited for this purpose.

The anomalies

Agenesis / hypoplasia — including Mayer–Rokitansky–Küster–Hauser syndrome, with an absent or rudimentary uterus and upper vagina, **normal ovaries** and normal secondary sexual characteristics, presenting with primary amenorrhoea.

Unicornuate uterus — a single banana-shaped cavity deviated to one side. **The rudimentary horn matters:** if it contains endometrium and does not communicate, it obstructs, causing **haematometra and cyclical pain**, and carries a **risk of ectopic implantation with rupture**.

Uterus didelphys — two separate uteri and two cervices, frequently with a longitudinal vaginal septum.

Bicornuate uterus — two horns sharing a single cervix, with the external fundal cleft.

Septate uterus — the commonest, and the one **most associated with recurrent pregnancy loss**; correctable hysteroscopically.

Arcuate uterus — a shallow smooth fundal indentation, generally regarded as a normal variant.

The mandatory additional examination

> **Assess the kidneys in every patient with a Müllerian anomaly.** Renal anomalies — agenesis, ectopia, duplication — accompany them frequently, because the Müllerian and mesonephric systems develop together.

The association is specific enough to have named syndromes, most notably **obstructed hemivagina with ipsilateral renal agenesis**, in which a young woman presents after menarche with cyclical pain and a pelvic mass from an obstructed hemivagina, and the absent kidney is the clue.

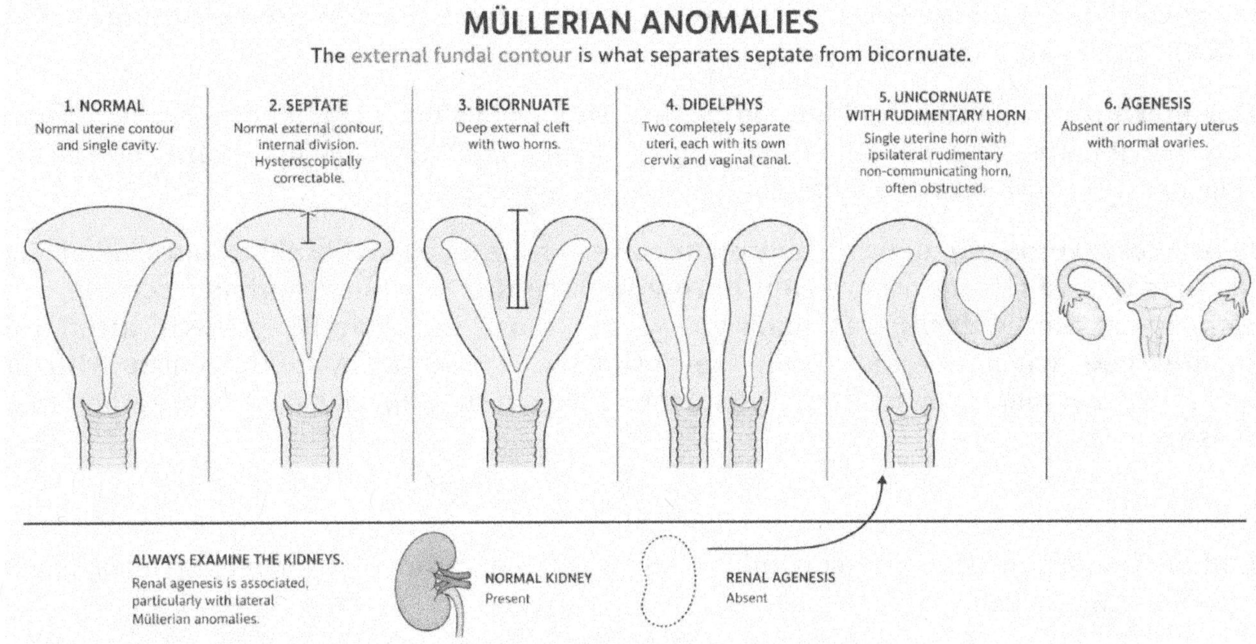

17.6 Myometrial Pathology: Leiomyoma and Adenomyosis

Leiomyoma

The commonest uterine tumour.

Appearance: a well-defined, usually **hypoechoic**, rounded mass with a **whorled internal texture**, characteristic **edge shadowing** and internal **fan-shaped or "venetian blind" shadowing**, and **peripheral rim vascularity**.

Location determines symptoms, and is what the report must specify. A standardised numerical classification is used, running from wholly intracavitary through submucosal, intramural and subserosal to pedunculated and cervical positions. [VERIFY: the leiomyoma location classification system to be adopted and its category definitions]

The clinical logic:

Location	Consequence
Submucosal / intracavitary	**Heavy bleeding and infertility** — distorts the cavity
Intramural	Bulk symptoms and bleeding, depending on size and cavity distortion
Subserosal / pedunculated	**Mass effect** on adjacent structures; may torse
Cervical	Obstructive symptoms, difficult surgery

Report: number, size of the largest and of any that are clinically relevant, **location by classification, relationship to the endometrial cavity**, and — for a submucosal fibroid being considered for hysteroscopic resection — the **distance from the outer edge of the fibroid to the serosa**.

Degeneration occurs as fibroids outgrow their supply: hyaline (commonest), cystic, myxoid, **red or carneous degeneration** (typically in pregnancy, causing acute pain), and calcific. Degenerating fibroids look heterogeneous and can be alarming.

Leiomyosarcoma cannot be reliably distinguished from a benign fibroid by ultrasound. The features that raise concern are **rapid growth, irregular margins, central necrosis, and rich irregular internal vascularity** — and, most importantly, **growth after the menopause**, when fibroids should be shrinking. A postmenopausal woman with an enlarging myometrial mass requires further imaging and specialist review rather than reassurance.

Adenomyosis

Endometrial glands and stroma within the myometrium, producing dysmenorrhoea, heavy bleeding, and infertility.

The features, several of which must be present:

- **Globular uterine enlargement** with **asymmetric myometrial thickening**, usually of the posterior wall
- **Myometrial cysts** — small anechoic spaces within the myometrium. **The most specific single feature**
- **Fan-shaped shadowing** — linear acoustic shadows radiating from the affected myometrium without a discrete mass to explain them
- **Heterogeneous myometrial echotexture**
- **Junctional zone thickening, irregularity or interruption**
- **Echogenic subendometrial lines and buds**
- **An indistinct endometrial–myometrial junction**
- **Translesional vascularity** — vessels running **through** the abnormal area

Standardised descriptive terminology exists and should be used so that reports are comparable. [VERIFY: the adenomyosis descriptive terminology and criteria to be adopted]

Distinguishing the two

This is a routine and important discrimination:

	Leiomyoma	**Adenomyosis**
Margins	**Well defined**, with a pseudocapsule	**Ill defined**, merging with normal myometrium
Shape	Rounded, mass-like	Diffuse or asymmetric thickening
Vascularity	**Peripheral rim**	**Translesional** — vessels pass through

	Leiomyoma	Adenomyosis
Shadowing	Edge shadows from a discrete mass	**Fan-shaped**, without a mass
Effect on cavity	Displaces or distorts	Ill-defined junction rather than displacement

The two frequently coexist.

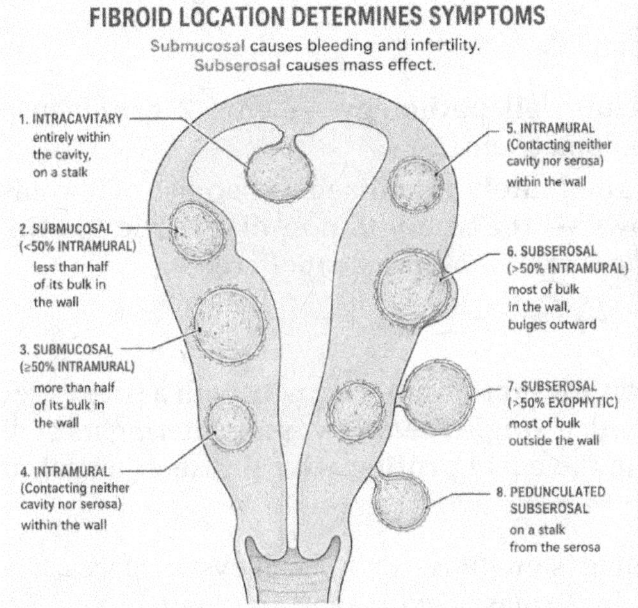

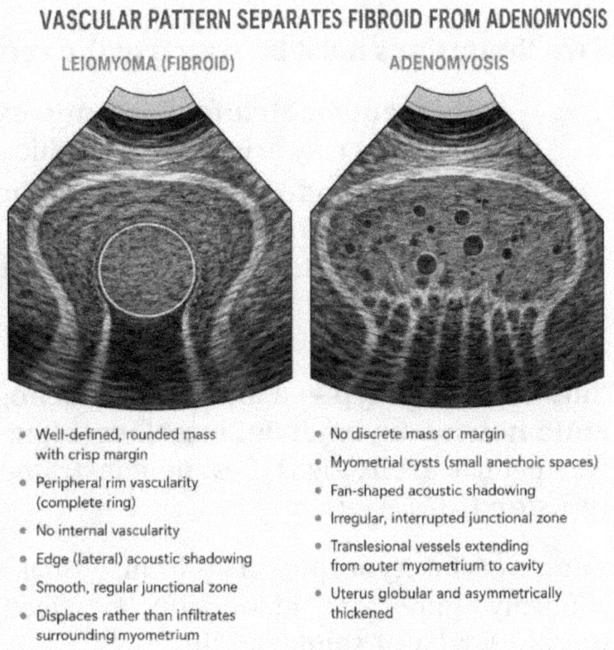

17.7 Endometrial Assessment and Pathology

Measurement technique

The convention:

1. **Midline sagittal plane**, transvaginally
2. Measure at the **thickest point**
3. **Anterior to posterior**, from one basal layer to the other, **perpendicular to the endometrial axis**
4. **Exclude any intracavitary fluid** — where fluid is present, measure the two layers **separately and add them**
5. **Exclude the hypoechoic junctional zone**, which is myometrium

Record the cycle day or menopausal status alongside the measurement. A number without that context cannot be interpreted (§17.2).

Postmenopausal bleeding

The dominant clinical scenario, and the one in which ultrasound has a defined triage role.

The logic is that endometrial carcinoma is very unlikely below a threshold endometrial thickness, so women below it may avoid invasive sampling, while those above it proceed to sampling or hysteroscopy.

The thresholds differ between guidelines and are modified by hormone replacement therapy use, and a different, lower-risk pathway applies to **incidental thickening in an asymptomatic postmenopausal woman**. [VERIFY: current endometrial thickness thresholds for investigation of postmenopausal bleeding, the modification for hormone replacement therapy, and the separate pathway for asymptomatic thickening]

Two limitations must be stated in the report:

- **A thin endometrium does not exclude all pathology** — type 2 endometrial carcinomas may arise in an atrophic endometrium
- **Where the endometrium cannot be adequately visualised** — because of fibroids, axial uterine position, or poor windows — **the study is non-diagnostic for this question**, and that must be stated rather than a measurement offered

Pathology

Endometrial polyp — a focal, usually **echogenic** lesion within the cavity with a **preserved endometrial–myometrial interface**, often with a **single feeding vessel** entering its stalk (the pedicle artery sign). Best demonstrated in the **early proliferative phase** or on **saline infusion** (§17.8).

Endometrial hyperplasia — diffuse thickening, sometimes with small cystic spaces. The clinically important distinction, between hyperplasia with and without atypia, is **histological, not sonographic**.

Endometrial carcinoma — a thickened, heterogeneous endometrium with an **irregular or indistinct endometrial–myometrial interface** suggesting myometrial invasion, **multiple irregular internal vessels**, and sometimes intracavitary fluid.

> **Ultrasound cannot exclude endometrial carcinoma.** In postmenopausal bleeding above the threshold, or where bleeding persists regardless of thickness, **tissue sampling is required**, and the report should direct to it.

Tamoxifen-associated change — **subendometrial cystic change** producing apparent endometrial thickening that frequently represents myometrial rather than endometrial pathology. **Transvaginal ultrasound performs poorly** in this group, and **hysteroscopy with sampling** is the preferred assessment in a symptomatic tamoxifen user.

Retained products of conception — echogenic intracavitary material with **demonstrable vascularity**, which distinguishes it from blood clot. The vascularity matters procedurally: markedly increased myometrial vascularity indicates a lesion at risk of heavy bleeding on instrumentation.

Intrauterine adhesions (Asherman syndrome) — bridging bands within the cavity, best demonstrated on saline infusion.

Endometritis, haematometra, pyometra, and endometrial fluid complete the differential; fluid in a postmenopausal cavity warrants assessment of the endometrium around it and consideration of cervical stenosis or obstruction.

Standardised descriptive terminology for the endometrium exists and improves reporting consistency. [VERIFY: the endometrial descriptive terminology to be adopted]

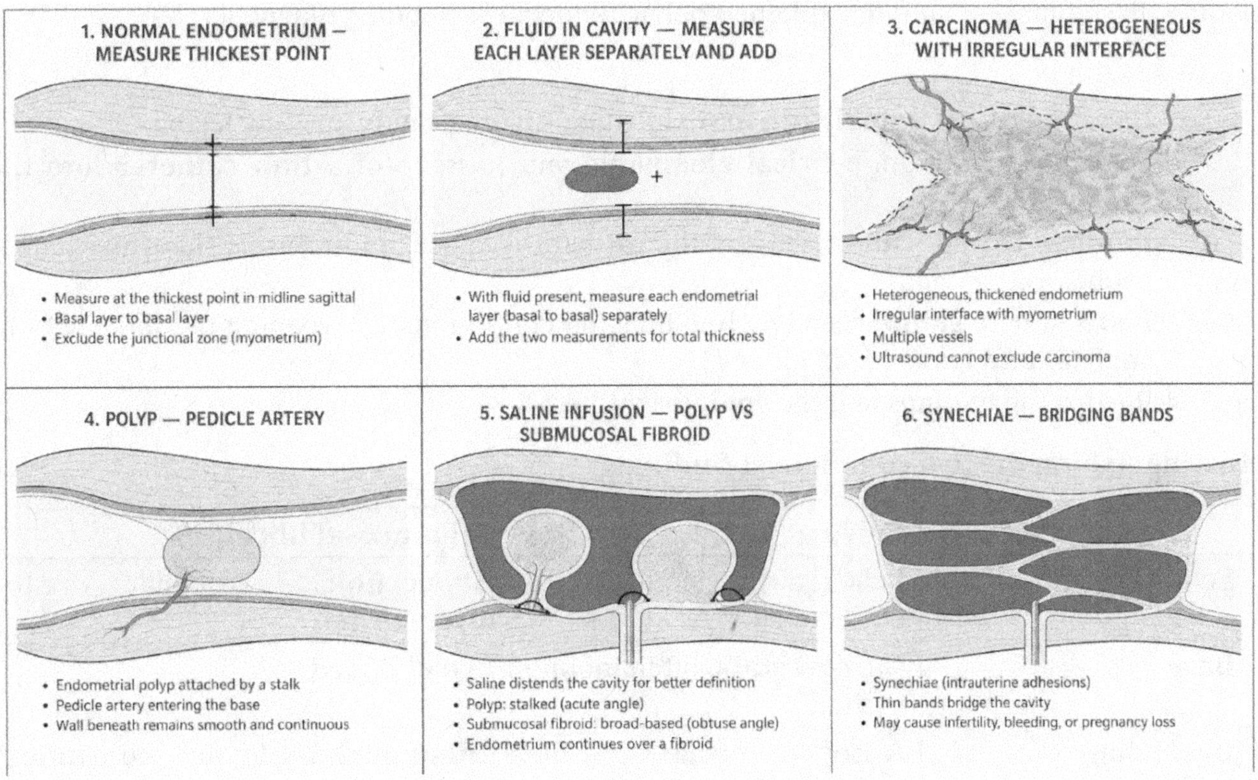

17.8 Sonohysterography and Saline Infusion Technique

Indications

Saline infusion sonohysterography distends the cavity, separating its walls so that focal lesions can be seen and characterised. It is indicated for:

- **Abnormal uterine bleeding** with a thickened or irregular endometrium
- **Distinguishing focal from diffuse** endometrial thickening
- **Polyp versus submucosal fibroid**, and defining the degree of intracavitary extension of a fibroid before hysteroscopic resection
- **Cavity assessment in infertility and recurrent pregnancy loss**
- **Suspected intrauterine adhesions**
- Cavity assessment after uterine surgery

Timing and contraindications

Perform in the early proliferative phase — after bleeding has stopped and before ovulation. The endometrium is thin, so lesions are conspicuous, and there is no risk of disturbing an early pregnancy.

Contraindications: pregnancy (exclude it), **active pelvic infection** — which the procedure would disseminate — and unexplained pelvic tenderness pending diagnosis.

Technique

1. **Baseline transvaginal scan** first, documenting the cavity and any lesion
2. Speculum insertion, **cervical cleansing**, and passage of a **thin catheter** into the cavity
3. **Remove the speculum**, leaving the catheter in place, and reinsert the transvaginal probe
4. **Instil sterile saline slowly** while imaging continuously, sweeping the full cavity in **sagittal and transverse** planes
5. Record the findings and the volume instilled

Distinguishing the two commonest findings:

	Polyp	**Submucosal fibroid**
Echogenicity	Echogenic, similar to endometrium	**Hypoechoic**, similar to myometrium
Base	**Narrow stalk**, often mobile in fluid	**Broad based**
Overlying endometrium	Arises from the endometrium	**Endometrial layer continues over its surface**
Angle with the wall	Acute	Obtuse

Tubal patency assessment

The same principle extended: **hysterosalpingo-contrast sonography**, using saline with an ultrasound contrast agent or a foam agent, allows **tubal patency** to be assessed by observing flow along the tube and spill into the peritoneal cavity.

It is an alternative to radiographic hysterosalpingography **without ionising radiation**, and it fits naturally into an infertility assessment already being performed by ultrasound (§17.11). [VERIFY: current recommendations, agents and technique for hysterosalpingo-contrast sonography]

Complications and aftercare

Cramping pain is usual and should be warned about in advance. **Vasovagal reactions**, minor bleeding, and — rarely — **infection** occur. **Failed cannulation** from cervical stenosis is the commonest technical failure, particularly in postmenopausal women.

Antibiotic prophylaxis follows local policy. Give clear post-procedure instructions covering expected symptoms and those that should prompt review.

17.9 Functional and Neoplastic Ovarian Lesions

Functional cysts — the majority

Follicular cyst — a simple anechoic cyst arising from a follicle that failed to ovulate. Thin-walled, unilocular, with posterior enhancement.

Corpus luteum cyst — the crenated thick-walled structure with a ring of fire described in §17.2. It **resolves**, and recognising it prevents unnecessary follow-up.

Haemorrhagic cyst — bleeding into a functional cyst, with a characteristic appearance:

- **Reticular, lacy or "fishnet" internal echoes** from fibrin strands
- A **retracting clot** with **concave or straight margins**, unlike the convex margin of a solid mural nodule
- **No internal vascularity**
- Posterior enhancement

It evolves and resolves over weeks, so **interval imaging after the next menstrual period** confirms the diagnosis without further intervention. The distinction from a solid nodule rests on the **absence of flow** and the **concave clot margin**.

Theca lutein cysts — bilateral, multiple, large, in states of **high human chorionic gonadotrophin**: molar pregnancy, multiple gestation, and ovarian stimulation.

Benign neoplasms

Mature cystic teratoma (dermoid) — highly recognisable when the signs are known:

- A **Rokitansky nodule** — an echogenic mural nodule, often shadowing
- **"Tip of the iceberg"** — dense shadowing obscuring the deep portion of the lesion, which can make it look smaller than it is or hide it entirely
- **Dermoid mesh** — fine echogenic dot-and-dash lines from hair
- **Fat–fluid levels** and floating echogenic spheres

It carries a torsion risk proportional to size, and bilateral in a minority.

Serous and mucinous cystadenoma — unilocular or multilocular; mucinous lesions tend to be larger, multilocular, and to contain low-level echoes.

Endometrioma — homogeneous low-level "ground glass" echoes with **no internal vascularity**, sometimes with punctate echogenic wall foci (§17.10).

Ovarian fibroma and thecoma — solid, hypoechoic, characteristically **shadowing**, and easily mistaken for a pedunculated fibroid. May be associated with ascites and pleural effusion.

Features associated with malignancy

Assessed morphologically rather than by resistance indices, which have proved unreliable alone:

- **Solid components or papillary projections** with **demonstrable internal vascularity** — the most important single feature
- **Thick, irregular septations**
- **Irregular internal wall**
- **Large size**
- **Ascites**
- **Peritoneal or omental deposits** (Chapter 8 §8.2)
- **Bilaterality**

Risk stratification systems combining these features into categories with defined management pathways are now standard, and they perform substantially better than unstructured impression. **A department should adopt one and apply it consistently, stating which is in use.** [VERIFY: the adnexal risk stratification system to be adopted, its descriptor definitions, category thresholds, and associated management recommendations]

Malignant types and the postmenopausal ovary

Epithelial tumours predominate, with serous carcinoma the commonest. **Germ cell tumours** occur in younger women. **Sex cord–stromal tumours** may be hormonally active. **Metastatic disease** — the Krukenberg tumour, characteristically **bilateral and solid**, from a gastrointestinal primary — must be considered when bilateral solid ovarian masses are found, and the abdomen assessed.

In a postmenopausal woman, any complexity carries greater weight, though **a simple unilocular cyst below a size threshold is common and generally managed by surveillance**. [VERIFY: current management thresholds for simple ovarian cysts in premenopausal and postmenopausal women]

Tumour markers support but do not replace imaging; CA-125 in particular has poor specificity in premenopausal women, where endometriosis, fibroids and pelvic inflammatory disease all elevate it.

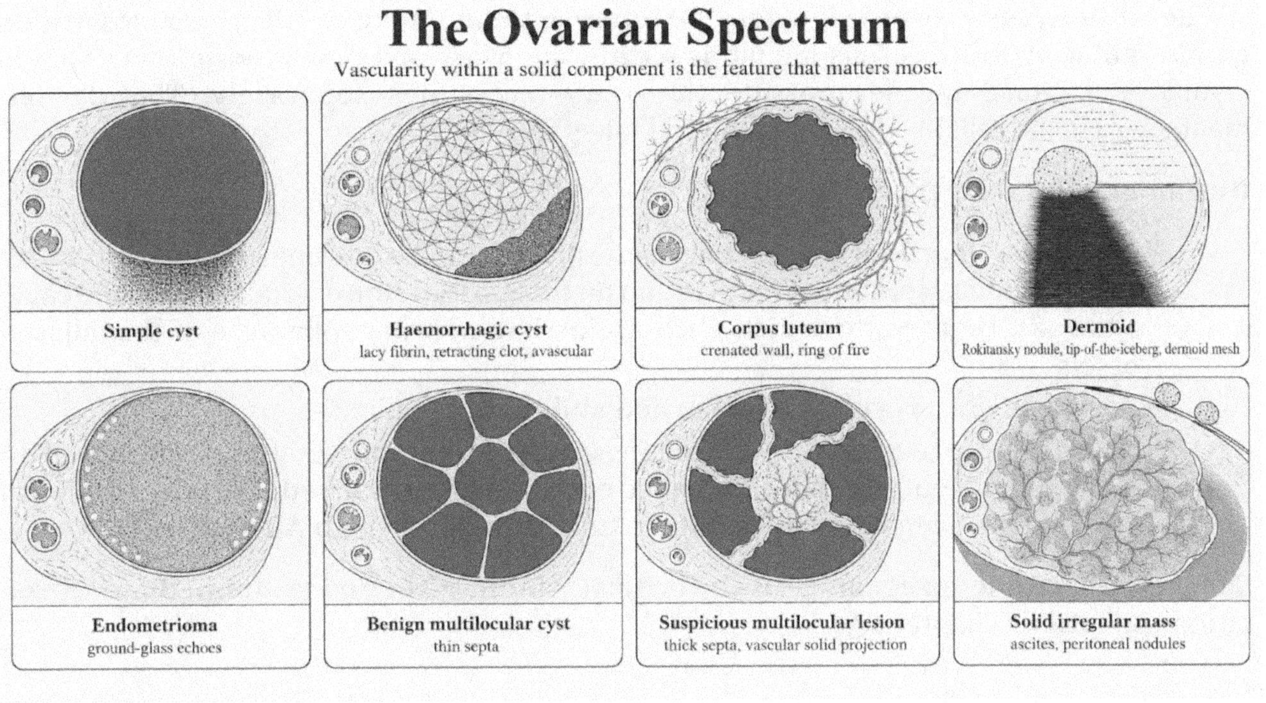

17.10 The Adnexa: Ectopic Pregnancy, Torsion, Inflammatory Disease, Endometriosis

Ectopic pregnancy

A positive pregnancy test with no intrauterine pregnancy is a pregnancy of unknown location until proven otherwise, and ectopic pregnancy must be actively excluded.

Findings, in ascending order of certainty:

- **An empty uterus** with a positive test
- A **decidual reaction** — a thickened endometrium without a gestational sac
- A **pseudogestational sac** — a central, ovoid fluid collection in the cavity **without** the eccentric position or double decidual sign of a true sac. It is decidual fluid, not a pregnancy, and mistaking it for one is a recognised cause of delayed diagnosis
- **An adnexal mass separate from the ovary**
- A **tubal ring** — an echogenic ring around a small sac in the adnexa
- **A yolk sac or embryo outside the uterus — definitive**
- **Free fluid**, particularly **echogenic** free fluid, indicating haemoperitoneum

Two discriminations that must be made deliberately:

1. The ring of fire is not specific. The corpus luteum has exactly the same peripheral vascularity, and the ectopic is usually on the same side as the corpus luteum. Doppler does not distinguish them.

2. The sliding (separation) sign does distinguish them. Apply **gentle pressure with the transvaginal probe**: a corpus luteum is **within** the ovary and moves **with** it, whereas an ectopic gestational sac lies **outside** the ovary and **slides separately**. This dynamic manoeuvre is the reliable discriminator and takes seconds.

Uncommon but dangerous sites:

- **Interstitial (cornual)** — eccentrically placed in the uterine cornu with a **thin surrounding myometrial mantle** and an **interstitial line** extending from the cavity to the sac. **High rupture risk with major haemorrhage**, because of the adjacent vessels
- **Caesarean scar**, **cervical**, **ovarian** and **abdominal** implantations
- **Heterotopic pregnancy** — coexisting intrauterine and ectopic pregnancy. Rare spontaneously but **substantially more common after assisted reproduction**, so **an intrauterine pregnancy does not exclude an ectopic in an ART patient**

Suspected ectopic pregnancy is a critical finding requiring immediate direct communication (Chapter 1 §1.5).

Ovarian torsion

A surgical emergency with a narrow window for ovarian salvage.

Findings:

- **An enlarged, oedematous ovary** — the most consistent finding, and often the only one
- **Peripherally displaced follicles** — the "string of pearls" appearance, as stromal oedema pushes follicles to the surface
- **Heterogeneous stroma**
- **Abnormal position** — the ovary displaced toward the midline or above the uterus
- **A whirlpool sign** in the twisted vascular pedicle — **specific** when present
- **Free fluid**
- **Marked tenderness** under the probe

> **The critical teaching point: Doppler flow may be entirely present in a torted ovary.** The ovary has a **dual arterial supply** — ovarian and uterine (§17.1) — and torsion is often intermittent and initially venous. **Absent flow supports the diagnosis; present flow does not exclude it.**

This is the direct analogue of testicular torsion (Chapter 11 §11.7), and the same error — reassurance based on preserved flow — occurs for the same reason.

A lead point — a dermoid, cyst or other mass — is present in most adult cases; in children the ovary is more often structurally normal.

Suspected torsion is a critical finding.

Pelvic inflammatory disease

The spectrum:

Endometritis — a thickened, heterogeneous endometrium, sometimes with fluid or gas, and tenderness.

Salpingitis and pyosalpinx — a **dilated, tortuous, tubular** adnexal structure with **incomplete septa** (a folded tube, not a septated cyst), containing debris. Two classic appearances: the **"cogwheel"** of thickened tubal folds in cross-section in acute disease, and **"beads on a string"** — flattened residual folds — in chronic disease.

Hydrosalpinx — the same tubular structure but anechoic, with a **"waist" sign** where the tube folds on itself.

Tubo-ovarian abscess — a **complex adnexal mass in which the tube and ovary can no longer be distinguished**, with debris, thick walls, marked hyperaemia, and severe tenderness.

Distinguishing a hydrosalpinx from a multilocular ovarian cyst is a common task: the hydrosalpinx is **tubular when swept through its length**, has **incomplete septa**, shows a **waist**, and — decisively — **a normal separate ipsilateral ovary can be identified**.

Endometriosis

Endometrioma — the ovarian form: **homogeneous ground-glass low-level echoes** with **no internal vascularity**, frequently bilateral. **A vascular mural nodule within an endometrioma raises the possibility of malignant transformation** and is a specific finding to look for.

Deep infiltrating endometriosis is assessed by a systematic protocol and produces findings that ultrasound is uniquely able to demonstrate:

- **Hypoechoic nodules** in the **uterosacral ligaments**, **rectovaginal septum**, **bladder**, and **rectosigmoid wall**
- **"Kissing ovaries"** — both ovaries adherent to one another behind the uterus, a strong marker of severe disease
- **The negative sliding sign — loss of the normal gliding of the uterus against the rectum and bowel on gentle probe pressure**, indicating obliteration of the pouch of Douglas

> **The sliding sign is a dynamic finding that only real-time ultrasound can provide**, and it is one of the clearest examples in this book of ultrasound outperforming cross-sectional imaging.

A structured consensus approach to reporting deep endometriosis exists and should be followed. [VERIFY: the deep infiltrating endometriosis assessment protocol and terminology to be adopted]

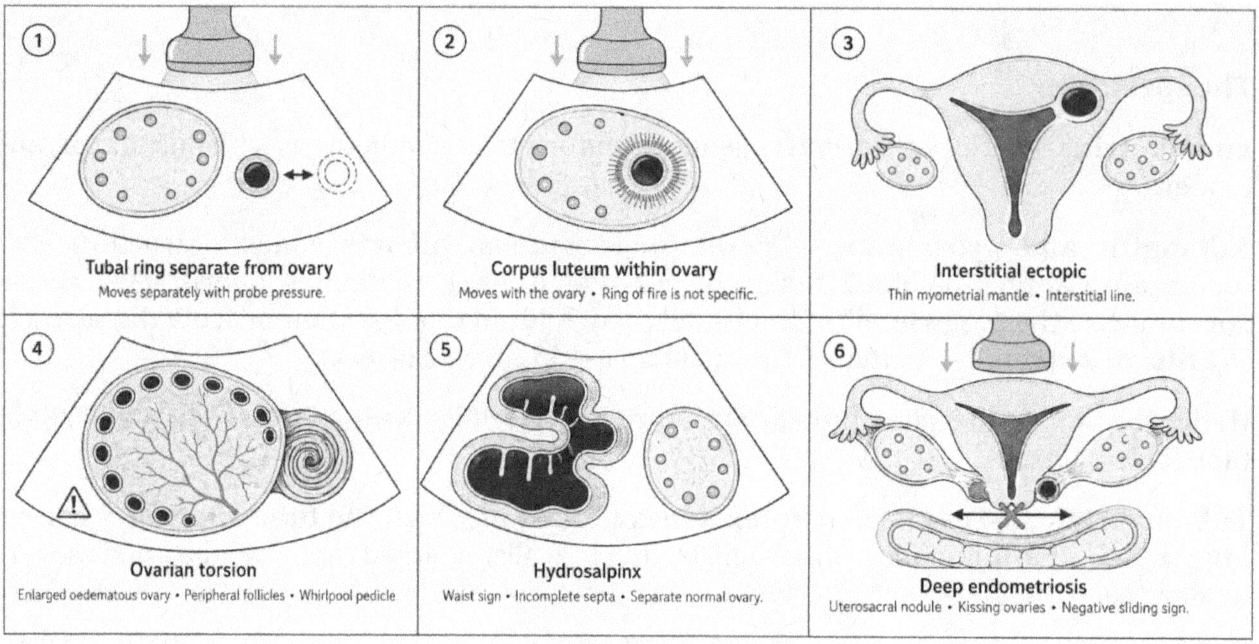

The adnexal emergencies, and the dynamic signs that resolve them.

17.11 Infertility Evaluation and Assisted Reproduction Monitoring

Baseline assessment

A structured baseline study addresses every element that could affect conception or implantation:

Uterus — **congenital anomaly** (§17.5, requiring three-dimensional assessment), **cavity-distorting fibroids** (§17.6), **polyps** (§17.7), **adenomyosis**, and **intrauterine adhesions**.

Endometrium — thickness and pattern, timed to the cycle.

Ovaries — volume, morphology, and **antral follicle count**.

Tubes — patency by contrast sonography where indicated (§17.8), and **hydrosalpinx**, which is important because it reduces implantation rates and is often treated before transfer.

Pelvis — endometriosis, adhesions, and the sliding sign (§17.10).

Antral follicle count

Technique: count all follicles measuring between approximately 2 and 10 mm in **both** ovaries, in the **early follicular phase**, using a systematic sweep through each ovary in a single plane so that follicles are neither missed nor counted twice.

It is a marker of **ovarian reserve** and predicts the response to stimulation, and it is used alongside anti-Müllerian hormone. **The count is technique-dependent**, which makes a systematic method and a stated cycle day essential. [VERIFY: current antral follicle count technique recommendations and the categories used to define low, normal and high reserve]

Polycystic ovarian morphology

Defined by follicle number per ovary above a threshold and/or increased ovarian volume. The threshold has been **revised upward as transducer resolution has improved** — modern high-frequency probes simply see more follicles than the equipment on which the original criteria were based, so an outdated threshold over-diagnoses. [VERIFY: current follicle number per ovary and ovarian volume thresholds for polycystic ovarian morphology, and their dependence on transducer frequency]

> **Polycystic ovarian morphology is not polycystic ovary syndrome.** The syndrome is a clinical and biochemical diagnosis requiring additional criteria, and the sonographic finding alone must not be reported as the syndrome.

Cycle monitoring

Follicular tracking — serial measurement of the **number and mean diameter of developing follicles** during stimulation, guiding gonadotrophin dosing and the timing of the trigger injection.

Endometrial assessment — thickness and pattern, since a thin or non-trilaminar endometrium at trigger affects the decision to proceed or to freeze all embryos.

Oocyte retrieval is performed under **transvaginal ultrasound guidance** with a needle guide (Chapter 9 §9.4–9.6), aspirating each follicle in turn.

Embryo transfer is commonly guided **transabdominally**, with a full bladder to straighten the uterocervical angle and visualise catheter placement.

Luteal phase and early pregnancy assessment follow, with the specific reminder that **heterotopic pregnancy is materially more likely after assisted reproduction** (§17.10).

Ovarian hyperstimulation syndrome

A complication of stimulation, ranging from mild to life-threatening: **enlarged ovaries containing multiple large follicles and cysts, ascites**, and in severe cases **pleural effusion** and haemoconcentration with thrombotic risk.

Ultrasound documents ovarian size, follicle number, and the volume of ascites, and is used to guide **paracentesis** where drainage is required (Chapter 8 §8.2 for site selection). **Avoid unnecessary transvaginal probe pressure on massively enlarged ovaries**, which are at risk of torsion and rupture.

17.12 Intrauterine Device Localisation

The devices

Copper devices are **strongly echogenic with dense posterior shadowing** and are easy to see.

Levonorgestrel-releasing devices are **less echogenic** — the hormone reservoir on the stem is poorly reflective, and the device may be much less conspicuous. **The transverse arms remain echogenic**, and **the shadow** is often what identifies the device when the device itself is faint. Knowing which type is present before scanning saves time.

Normal position

> **The device should lie entirely within the endometrial cavity, with the transverse arms at the fundus and the stem in the cavity — not extending into the cervical canal.**

Measure the distance from the top of the device to the **endometrial fundus**, and the distance from the device to the **serosa**, according to local convention. [VERIFY: current measurement conventions and thresholds defining acceptable intrauterine device position]

Why three-dimensional imaging matters here

A two-dimensional sagittal image shows the stem but cannot reliably show the arms. A device that is rotated, with one arm embedded in the myometrium, may look entirely normal in sagittal section.

> **The three-dimensional coronal reconstruction of the uterus displays the whole T-shape and the position of both arms in a single image, and it is the reference technique for device localisation.**

This is the same reason three-dimensional imaging is required for Müllerian anomalies (§17.5) — the coronal plane of the uterus cannot be obtained any other way.

Malposition and complications

Finding	Description
Low-lying / displaced	The device sits low in the cavity or extends into the **cervical canal**, reducing efficacy
Rotated	Arms not at the fundus, best appreciated in coronal reconstruction
Embedded	Part of the device — usually an arm — extends **into the myometrium**
Perforation	The device is partly or wholly **outside the uterus**. If not identified within the uterus and expulsion is not confirmed, it must be located
Expulsion	The device is absent from the uterus

"Lost threads" is the common presentation, and it has a defined logic:

1. **Scan for the device in the uterus.** If it is normally positioned, reassure and manage clinically
2. **If it is not in the uterus**, it has either been expelled or has perforated
3. **If expulsion was not witnessed, the device must be located** — an abdominal radiograph, or CT, will find an intraperitoneal device. **An unlocated device is not an acceptable endpoint**

Other complications: pain and bleeding, malposition-related failure, infection, and **pregnancy with a device in situ**. If a pregnancy occurs with a device present, **the proportion that are ectopic is increased**, so an intrauterine pregnancy must be confirmed and the device located relative to the sac.

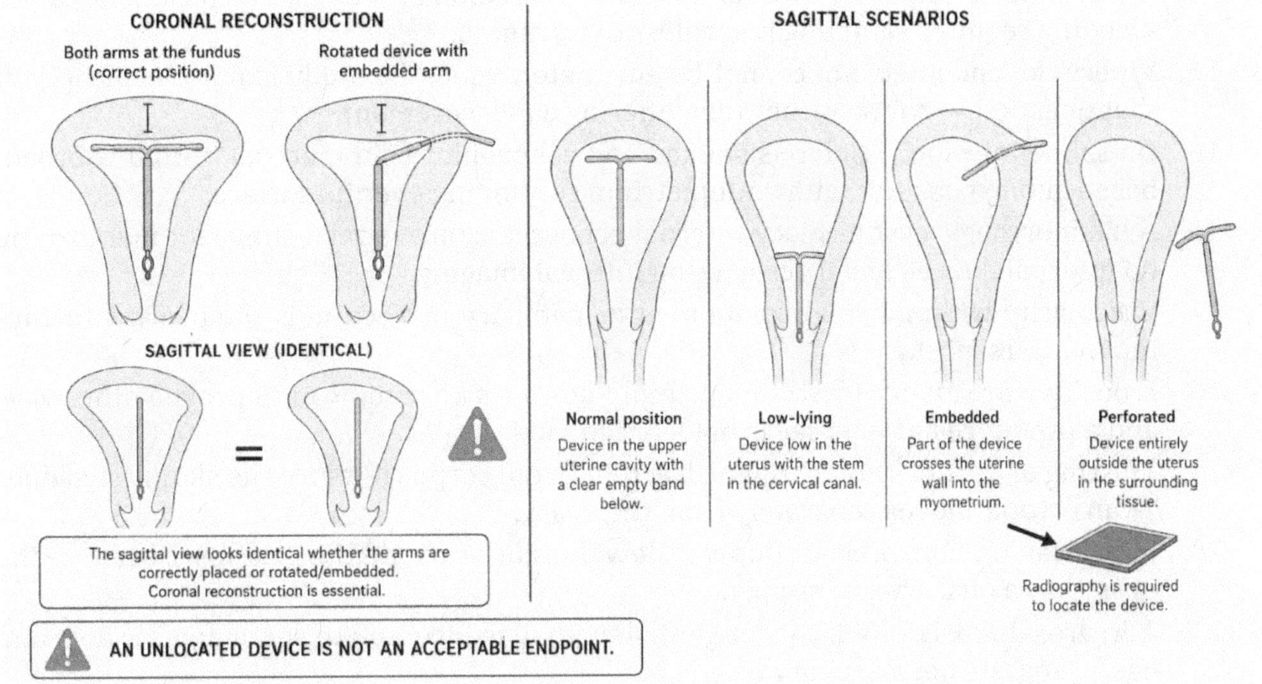

Key Points

1. Establish the cycle day and menopausal status before interpreting anything. The same image means different things on different days.
2. Find the ovary by finding the internal iliac vessels — it lies immediately anterior to them.
3. Scan the endometrium in the early proliferative phase, days 4 to 6. A study performed at the wrong point should say so.
4. The corpus luteum is the most over-called structure in the pelvis. It has a crenated wall, a ring of fire, and it resolves.
5. Transvaginal examination requires explicit consent, an offer of self-insertion, a documented chaperone offer, and high-level disinfection between patients.
6. Pelvic flow is slow. Abdominal Doppler settings will show no flow in normally perfused structures.
7. The external fundal contour separates septate from bicornuate uterus, and only three-dimensional coronal imaging shows contour and cavity together.
8. Examine the kidneys in every Müllerian anomaly.
9. Fibroid location determines symptoms — submucosal causes bleeding and infertility, subserosal causes mass effect. Report location by classification.
10. Fibroids have peripheral rim vascularity; adenomyosis has vessels passing through it. Myometrial cysts are the most specific sign of adenomyosis.

11. A myometrial mass that grows after the menopause is a red flag, because fibroids should be shrinking.
12. Measure the endometrium basal layer to basal layer at the thickest point, excluding fluid and excluding the junctional zone.
13. Ultrasound cannot exclude endometrial carcinoma. Persistent postmenopausal bleeding requires sampling regardless of thickness.
14. Where the endometrium cannot be adequately seen, the study is non-diagnostic for that question — say so rather than offering a measurement.
15. On saline infusion, a polyp is stalked and echogenic; a submucosal fibroid is broad-based and hypoechoic with endometrium continuing over its surface.
16. A haemorrhagic cyst has lacy internal echoes, a concave retracting clot margin, and no internal flow — and it resolves on interval imaging.
17. Vascularity within a solid component or papillary projection is the ovarian feature that matters most.
18. A positive pregnancy test with an empty uterus is an ectopic until proven otherwise, and a pseudogestational sac is not a pregnancy.
19. The ring of fire does not distinguish ectopic from corpus luteum. The sliding sign does — an ectopic moves separately from the ovary.
20. In ovarian torsion, present Doppler flow does not exclude the diagnosis, because the ovary has a dual arterial supply.
21. A hydrosalpinx is tubular through its length, has incomplete septa and a waist, and has a separate normal ovary beside it.
22. The negative sliding sign indicates an obliterated pouch of Douglas, and it is a dynamic finding only real-time ultrasound can provide.
23. Polycystic ovarian morphology is not polycystic ovary syndrome, and the follicle-number threshold has been revised upward as resolution improved.
24. Three-dimensional coronal reconstruction is the reference method for intrauterine device localisation — a sagittal image cannot show the arms.
25. A device that is not in the uterus and was not witnessed to be expelled must be located.

Registry Check

1. An endometrial thickness of 12 mm is measured in a 32-year-old woman on day 22 of a regular cycle. The appropriate interpretation is:

A. Endometrial hyperplasia **B.** A normal secretory endometrium for this cycle day **C.** Endometrial carcinoma **D.** Retained products of conception

> **Answer: B.** The secretory endometrium is thickest and homogeneously echogenic in the second half of the cycle, and this measurement is within normal limits for day 22. Endometrial assessment in premenopausal women should be performed in the early proliferative phase, when the endometrium is thin and most reproducible.

2. Which finding distinguishes a septate from a bicornuate uterus?

A. The length of the internal division **B.** The external fundal contour **C.** The presence of two cervices **D.** The number of endometrial cavities

> **Answer: B.** A septate uterus has a normal or minimally indented external contour with an internal division, whereas a bicornuate uterus has a deep external fundal cleft. The distinction determines management — a septum is resected hysteroscopically, a bicornuate uterus is not — and it requires three-dimensional coronal imaging to see contour and cavity together.

3. A myometrial abnormality shows ill-defined margins, myometrial cysts, fan-shaped shadowing, and vessels running through it. This represents:

A. Leiomyoma **B.** Adenomyosis **C.** Leiomyosarcoma **D.** Endometrial carcinoma with myometrial invasion

> **Answer: B.** Ill-defined margins, myometrial cysts, fan-shaped shadowing without a discrete mass, and translesional vascularity are the features of adenomyosis. A leiomyoma is well defined with edge shadowing and peripheral rim vascularity.

4. An adnexal cystic lesion contains lacy internal echoes and a wedge of material with a concave free margin, and shows no internal flow. This most likely represents:

A. Ovarian carcinoma **B.** Haemorrhagic cyst **C.** Endometrioma **D.** Tubo-ovarian abscess

> **Answer: B.** Reticular fibrin strands and a retracting clot with a concave margin, in the absence of internal vascularity, are characteristic of a haemorrhagic cyst. A solid mural nodule has a convex margin and demonstrable flow. Interval imaging after the next period confirms resolution.

5. A woman with a positive pregnancy test has an empty uterus and an adnexal ring-shaped structure with peripheral vascularity. The manoeuvre that distinguishes an ectopic pregnancy from a corpus luteum is:

A. Colour Doppler assessment of the ring **B.** Measuring the resistance index **C.** Gentle probe pressure to determine whether the structure moves separately from the ovary **D.** Measuring the endometrial thickness

> **Answer: C.** Both an ectopic and a corpus luteum show a ring of fire, so Doppler does not distinguish them. The sliding or separation sign does: a corpus luteum lies within the ovary and moves with it, whereas an ectopic lies outside the ovary and slides independently under gentle pressure.

6. An enlarged, oedematous ovary with peripherally displaced follicles is seen in a patient with acute pelvic pain. Colour Doppler demonstrates arterial and venous flow within the ovary. The correct interpretation is:

A. Torsion is excluded by the presence of flow **B.** Torsion remains possible, since the ovary has a dual arterial supply **C.** The findings indicate a haemorrhagic cyst **D.** The findings indicate pelvic inflammatory disease

Answer: B. The ovary is supplied by both the ovarian and uterine arteries, and torsion is frequently intermittent and initially venous, so flow may persist. Absent flow supports the diagnosis but present flow does not exclude it — the same trap as in testicular torsion.

7. A tubular adnexal structure shows a folded configuration with a waist, incomplete septa, and a separate normal ovary alongside it. This represents:

A. A multilocular ovarian cyst **B.** Hydrosalpinx **C.** Tubo-ovarian abscess **D.** Endometrioma

Answer: B. A dilated tube folds on itself, producing the waist sign and incomplete septa that project only part way across the lumen, and it is tubular when swept through its length. Identifying a separate normal ipsilateral ovary confirms that the structure is not ovarian.

8. An intrauterine device appears correctly positioned on a sagittal transvaginal image. Which additional assessment is required before the position can be confirmed as normal?

A. Transabdominal imaging with a full bladder **B.** Three-dimensional coronal reconstruction to assess the arms **C.** Colour Doppler over the device **D.** Measurement of endometrial thickness

Answer: B. The sagittal image demonstrates the stem but cannot reliably show the transverse arms, so a rotated device with an embedded arm can appear normal. The three-dimensional coronal plane displays the whole T-shape and both arm positions in a single image, and is the reference technique.

Chapter Notes for the Editorial Pass

Verification queue. In priority order: **the adnexal risk stratification system to be adopted**, with descriptor definitions, category thresholds and management pathways (§17.9) — this determines whether a woman is referred to gynaecological oncology and is the chapter's most consequential decision; **endometrial thickness thresholds for postmenopausal bleeding**, the hormone replacement modification, and the separate asymptomatic pathway (§17.7); **the Müllerian anomaly classification** (§17.5); **the leiomyoma location classification** (§17.6); **adenomyosis descriptive terminology** (§17.6); **endometrial descriptive terminology** (§17.7); **polycystic ovarian morphology thresholds**, noting explicitly their dependence on transducer resolution (§17.11); **antral follicle count technique and reserve categories** (§17.11); **simple ovarian cyst management thresholds** premenopausal and postmenopausal (§17.9); **the deep endometriosis assessment protocol** (§17.10); **intrauterine device position conventions** (§17.12); and **hysterosalpingo-contrast sonography recommendations** (§17.8).

A book-wide decision, now at five. This chapter's adnexal risk stratification system joins thyroid nodules (§11.3), urinary tract dilatation (§12.8), infant hips (§13.10) and carotid velocity criteria (§16.2) as frameworks described without commitment to a specific system. **These five decisions should be taken together in a single editorial session before**

layout. The adnexal and carotid systems are the two whose output most directly determines a referral or an operation.

Chapter size note. At twelve subchapters this is the largest chapter in the book, and several sections — particularly §17.3, §17.4, §17.8 and §17.12 — are treated more briefly than their clinical weight might warrant in order to hold the word budget. If the book expands in a second edition, splitting this chapter at the uterine/adnexal boundary is the most natural division, matching the split already suggested for musculoskeletal in the Chapter 11 notes.

Figure count: 8 Lane A, 1 Lane B. The Lane B slot deliberately requests a **paired image or clip demonstrating the ectopic separation sign**, because the discriminator described in §17.10 is dynamic and a single still cannot convey it — the same limitation flagged in Chapters 13 to 15.

Cross-reference targets to fix at layout: §17.1 gonadal vein asymmetry → Chapter 3 §3.5; §17.1 pouch of Douglas → Chapter 8 §8.1; §17.3 consent and chaperone → Chapter 1 §1.3 and §1.5; §17.3 endocavitary disinfection → Chapter 1 §1.4; §17.3 sonographic tenderness → Chapter 5 §5.2; §17.9 peritoneal deposits and omental caking → Chapter 8 §8.2; §17.10 dual supply and torsion → Chapter 11 §11.7; §17.10 right lower quadrant pain in women → Chapter 6 §6.9; §17.10 ectopic pregnancy → Chapter 18 §18.9; §17.11 guided oocyte retrieval → Chapter 9 §9.4–9.6; §17.11 paracentesis site selection → Chapter 8 §8.2.

Word count: approximately 10,400 excluding image prompt blocks, learning objectives, registry questions, and these notes.

Chapter 18: Principles and the First Trimester

Learning Objectives

On completing this chapter you should be able to:

1. State the purposes of obstetric sonography and the indications for first-trimester imaging.
2. Apply the ethical framework governing obstetric ultrasound, including consent, disclosure, and the handling of adverse findings.
3. Apply exposure discipline in early pregnancy, and state the rule governing spectral Doppler over the embryo.
4. Perform transvaginal and transabdominal first-trimester examinations systematically.
5. Recognise the normal developmental landmarks in sequence and relate them to gestational age.
6. Measure crown-rump length correctly and apply dating and redating rules.
7. Obtain a valid nuchal translucency measurement and describe first-trimester screening.
8. Distinguish findings that are diagnostic of early pregnancy failure from those that are only suspicious, and explain why the distinction exists.
9. Recognise ectopic pregnancy in its various sites, including caesarean scar implantation.
10. Identify gestational trophoblastic disease and subchorionic haemorrhage.
11. Determine chorionicity and amnionicity, and explain why the first trimester is the time to do it.

The Chapter With the Highest Stakes per Measurement

Two things make first-trimester sonography different from everything preceding it.

The consequences of error are asymmetric and severe. A misapplied viability criterion can end a wanted, viable pregnancy. A missed ectopic can kill a woman. A dating error propagates through every subsequent decision in the pregnancy, including the timing of delivery. This is why the viability criteria in §18.8 are deliberately conservative, why they are structured in two tiers, and why they must be taken from a current source rather than remembered.

The patient is rarely neutral about the examination. For the woman, a first-trimester scan is not a routine investigation. It is frequently the most emotionally significant appointment of her pregnancy, and the room in which she will learn whether it is continuing. The communication content of §18.2 is not adjacent to the clinical work; it is part of it.

18.1 The Role and Indications of Obstetric Sonography

What obstetric ultrasound is for

Across the pregnancy, the modality serves a defined set of purposes:

- **Confirm an intrauterine pregnancy** and its viability
- **Establish gestational age** — the foundation for everything that follows
- **Determine the number of fetuses and, in multiples, the chorionicity**
- **Screen for chromosomal abnormality**
- **Screen for structural anomaly** (Chapter 19 and Chapter 20)
- **Assess growth and fetal wellbeing** (Chapter 19)
- **Guide invasive procedures** — chorionic villus sampling, amniocentesis, fetal therapy
- **Investigate complications** — bleeding, pain, size–dates discrepancy

First-trimester indications

- **Pain or bleeding** in early pregnancy — the commonest urgent indication
- **Confirmation of location and viability**, particularly with previous ectopic pregnancy or after assisted reproduction
- **Dating**, where the menstrual date is uncertain
- **Nuchal translucency and combined screening** within its gestational window
- **Discrepancy between uterine size and dates**
- **Hyperemesis or markedly elevated human chorionic gonadotrophin**, raising the possibility of trophoblastic disease or multiples
- **Procedure guidance**

What it is not for

Non-medical or "keepsake" imaging has no clinical indication and therefore no justifiable exposure (§18.3, and Chapter 1 §1.7).

Fetal sex determination as a sole indication is restricted in some jurisdictions, and local policy governs (§18.2).

Screening programme structure — the number of scans, their timing, and what each includes — varies substantially between health systems. [VERIFY: the screening programme structure and scan timings for the intended jurisdiction]

18.2 Clinical Ethics, Consent, and Disclosure

The framework

Obstetric ultrasound involves an unusual ethical structure: findings concern a fetus, but **the patient is the pregnant woman**, and it is her autonomy that governs decisions.

The workable formulation is that the clinician has **beneficence-based obligations toward both the woman and the fetus**, but **autonomy-based obligations only to the woman**. She decides what screening she accepts, what information she receives, and what she does with it.

Consent to the examination

A scan is not automatically consented to by attendance. Before the examination the woman should understand:

- **What the scan is for**, and what it can and cannot detect
- **That screening components are optional** — nuchal translucency screening, in particular, is a choice, and declining it is a legitimate decision that must be recorded without pressure
- **That screening tests give risks, not diagnoses**, and that both false positives and false negatives occur
- **What might follow** a screen-positive result — further tests, some of which carry risk
- **That she may decline any part** of the examination

The consent conversation for **transvaginal** imaging — explicit verbal consent, the option of self-insertion, the offer of a chaperone, and the right to stop — is set out in Chapter 17 §17.3 and applies fully here.

Disclosure of findings

The scope boundary of Chapter 1 §1.2 applies: **the sonographer describes findings and does not deliver a diagnosis or a prognosis**. What differs in obstetrics is the intensity of the moment and the fact that the woman is watching the screen.

The rule for the ordinary scan is the one from Chapter 1 §1.3: explain at the start that you will be quiet while concentrating, that this means nothing about what you are finding, and who will give her the results.

Absent fetal cardiac activity is the situation to prepare for in advance, because improvising it goes badly.

- **The woman frequently already knows.** She is watching the screen and reading your face
- **Institutional policy varies** on whether the sonographer may confirm the finding. **Know your department's policy before it happens**
- **What is universally unacceptable is completing the examination in silence and leaving the room.** Stop the examination, tell her you need to ask a colleague to review the images, obtain the appropriate clinician promptly, and **stay with her**
- Where a second opinion is required before the finding is confirmed — as many protocols mandate — **say that a second opinion is routine practice**, which is true, rather than implying either reassurance or bad news

Specific ethical situations

Fetal sex. Policy varies, and in some jurisdictions disclosure is restricted because of the risk of sex-selective termination. **Know the local policy and apply it consistently**, rather than deciding case by case.

A companion in the room. The woman's consent to their presence is **not** consent to disclosure of every finding to them. Where a difficulty arises — and particularly where coercion is suspected — creating an opportunity to speak with her alone is appropriate.

Findings of uncertain significance, including minor markers, generate real anxiety. Report them proportionately and according to protocol rather than volunteering every equivocal observation.

Findings with implications for continuation of the pregnancy. Practitioners may hold conscientious objections to participation in termination, and provisions for this exist in most jurisdictions. **They do not extend to obstructing or delaying referral.** The obligation to escalate promptly and to ensure the woman reaches the clinician who can counsel her is unaffected.

Safeguarding. Pregnancy in a minor, indications of coercion, and disclosure of domestic abuse each trigger defined local pathways, and this obligation sits alongside the clinical one (Chapter 1 §1.3).

Images and confidentiality. The images are of the woman's pregnancy. Teaching and research use requires consent; sharing outside sanctioned pathways — including on personal devices or social media — is a breach (Chapter 1 §1.8).

18.3 Safety and Exposure Discipline in Early Pregnancy

Why the first trimester is different

The embryonic period is the period of **organogenesis**, and embryonic tissue is **poorly perfused** early — perfusion is what carries heat away (Chapter 1 §1.7). The combination makes this the point in the human lifespan at which exposure discipline matters most.

Ossification begins later in the first trimester, which changes which thermal index applies: **TIS** (soft tissue) is appropriate very early, and **TIB** (bone) becomes the relevant index once fetal bone is present in the beam.

The mode hierarchy, and the rule that follows

Acoustic output rises steeply across the modes (Chapter 1 §1.7):

B-mode < M-mode < colour Doppler < spectral (pulsed-wave) Doppler

Spectral Doppler holds a stationary sample volume and delivers a high pulse repetition frequency to one small location for as long as the trace runs. It is by a wide margin the highest-output mode.

Do not use spectral Doppler over the embryo to demonstrate cardiac activity. Document it with M-mode, or by direct B-mode observation.

This is a specific, widely endorsed recommendation, and it is the single most important safety rule in this chapter. There is no diagnostic information in a spectral trace of embryonic cardiac activity that M-mode does not provide. [VERIFY: current society statements on Doppler use in the first trimester]

Colour Doppler has legitimate first-trimester uses — locating an ectopic pregnancy, assessing a caesarean scar implantation, characterising retained products — and should be applied **briefly and purposefully** with a specific question in mind, not run continuously.

Practical discipline

1. **Use the correct obstetric preset**, which constrains output and displays the appropriate index
2. **Reach for receiver gain before transmit power**
3. **Keep the examination as short as is consistent with completeness** — dwell time is the operator-controlled variable
4. **Freeze the image before measuring.** Measurements are made on frozen frames at no additional exposure
5. **Watch the displayed indices**, and be able to justify continuing if they rise
6. **Do not scan without a clinical indication**

Talking to the woman about safety

An accurate answer, offered without either false absolutes or unnecessary alarm, is set out in Chapter 1 §1.7 and applies directly: ultrasound uses sound rather than radiation, has been used in pregnancy for decades without evidence of harm, does deposit a small amount of energy, and is therefore performed with the lowest settings and the shortest duration that answer the question.

18.4 Transvaginal and Transabdominal First-Trimester Technique

Which approach

Transvaginal imaging is the standard in early pregnancy. Proximity and higher frequency give the resolution required to identify a yolk sac, a small embryo, or a tubal ring — structures that transabdominal imaging will simply miss.

Transabdominal imaging remains necessary for: an overview of the whole uterus and adnexa; a **large or high uterus**, or one distorted by fibroids; a pregnancy beyond the early weeks; assessment of structures **beyond the transvaginal field of view**; and any situation where transvaginal imaging is declined or inappropriate (Chapter 17 §17.3).

In practice both are frequently required — a transabdominal overview followed by transvaginal detail. Where only one was performed and the study was limited by it, say so.

The systematic examination

Whatever the presentation, examine all of the following. **The commonest structural error in early pregnancy scanning is stopping once an intrauterine pregnancy is found.**

1. **The uterus** — position, myometrium, fibroids, and any **caesarean scar niche**
2. **The endometrial cavity** — the number, location and appearance of any gestational sac, and the relationship of a sac to the cavity and to any scar
3. **The sac contents** — yolk sac, embryo, cardiac activity, amnion
4. **Both adnexa** — the ovaries, the **corpus luteum**, and any separate mass
5. **The pouch of Douglas and paracolic gutters** — free fluid, and specifically whether it is **echogenic**
6. **The cervix**

Examine the adnexa and the pouch of Douglas even when a normal intrauterine pregnancy is seen. Heterotopic pregnancy, coincidental adnexal pathology, and unexplained free fluid all require it — and after assisted reproduction the heterotopic risk is materially raised (§18.9).

Measurement discipline

Magnify so that the structure being measured occupies a substantial proportion of the image — small structures measured on a small display carry proportionally large errors.

Measure on frozen images, take the required number of measurements, and follow the caliper conventions specified for each measurement (§18.6, §18.7).

Documentation

Sac location and mean diameter where relevant; yolk sac; embryo and crown-rump length; **cardiac activity documented by M-mode**; the number of sacs, embryos, yolk sacs and amnions; chorionicity where multiple; both ovaries; free fluid; and the cervix.

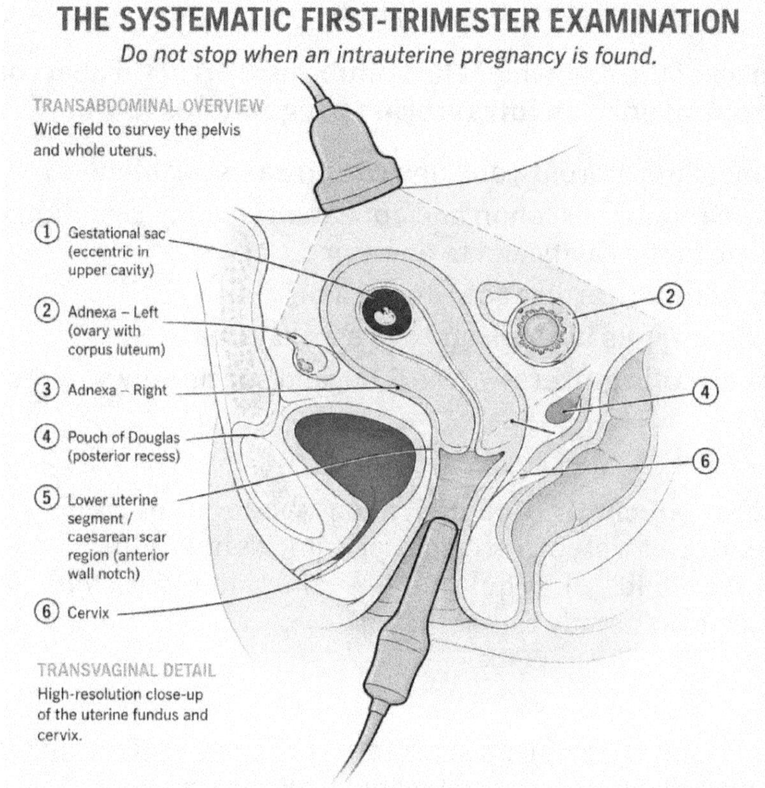

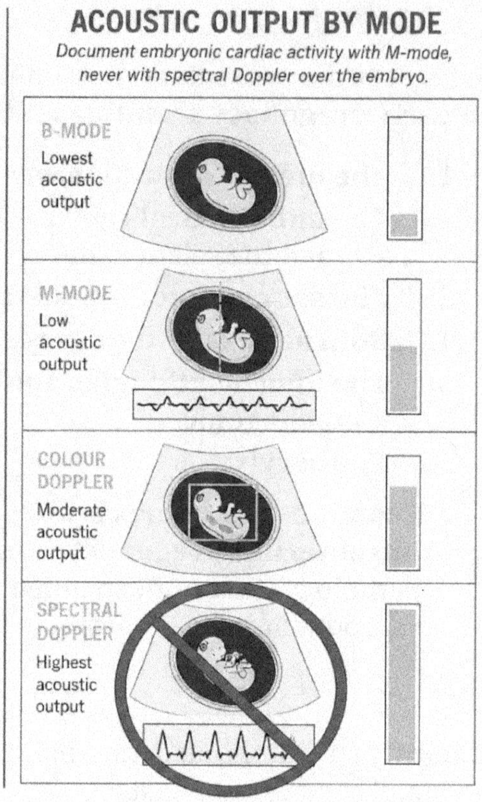

18.5 Normal Early Developmental Landmarks

The sequence

Early pregnancy has a highly predictable order of appearance, and knowing it allows a scan to be interpreted against expectation rather than in isolation.

Intradecidual sign — the earliest finding: a small fluid collection lying **eccentrically within the decidua**, adjacent to but not within the cavity line. Suggestive but not definitive.

Double decidual sac sign — two concentric echogenic rings around the sac, formed by the decidua parietalis and decidua capsularis. It supports an intrauterine pregnancy and helps distinguish a true sac from a **pseudogestational sac** (§18.9), but it is **not definitive** and is not always present.

Gestational sac — a rounded anechoic structure with an echogenic rim, **eccentrically placed** within the decidua. **Mean sac diameter** is the average of three orthogonal internal measurements.

Yolk sac — a round, echogenic-rimmed structure within the gestational sac. **This is the first finding that definitively confirms an intrauterine pregnancy**, because a pseudogestational sac cannot contain one.

Embryo with cardiac activity — the embryo first appears adjacent to the yolk sac, and cardiac activity is normally detectable from the point at which the embryo is measurable.

Amnion — a very thin membrane surrounding the embryo, closer to it than the chorion. It fuses with the chorion later in the first trimester, and an **"empty amnion"** — a visible amnion with no embryo within it — is an abnormal finding (§18.8).

Physiological midgut herniation — the midgut normally herniates into the base of the umbilical cord and returns to the abdomen during the early weeks.

> **Physiological midgut herniation must not be reported as an omphalocele before the gestation at which return is complete.** This is a specific and avoidable false positive. [VERIFY: the gestational age by which physiological midgut herniation should have resolved]

Cranial development — the **rhombencephalon** appears as a prominent cystic structure in the posterior head and is **normal**, not a posterior fossa cyst. The choroid plexuses and falx follow.

The thresholds at which each structure should be visible — by mean sac diameter and by crown-rump length — are defined and are the basis of the viability criteria in §18.8, and must be taken from the current source. [VERIFY: the mean sac diameter and crown-rump length thresholds at which yolk sac, embryo, and cardiac activity should be visible]

Human chorionic gonadotrophin and the discriminatory level

The "discriminatory level" is the serum hCG concentration above which an intrauterine pregnancy should be visible.

It must be used with considerable caution, and the modern position is materially more conservative than older teaching:

- **It varies with the assay, the operator, the equipment, and the patient**
- **It is unreliable in multiple pregnancy**, where a higher hCG accompanies each sac
- **A single value must never drive a decision to treat a presumed ectopic pregnancy**, because a viable intrauterine pregnancy can exist below the visualisation threshold at any given hCG

Current practice combines serial hCG measurement with serial ultrasound, and the pregnancy of unknown location pathway (§18.9) exists precisely because a single value cannot resolve the question. [VERIFY: current guidance on the use of hCG discriminatory levels in early pregnancy assessment]

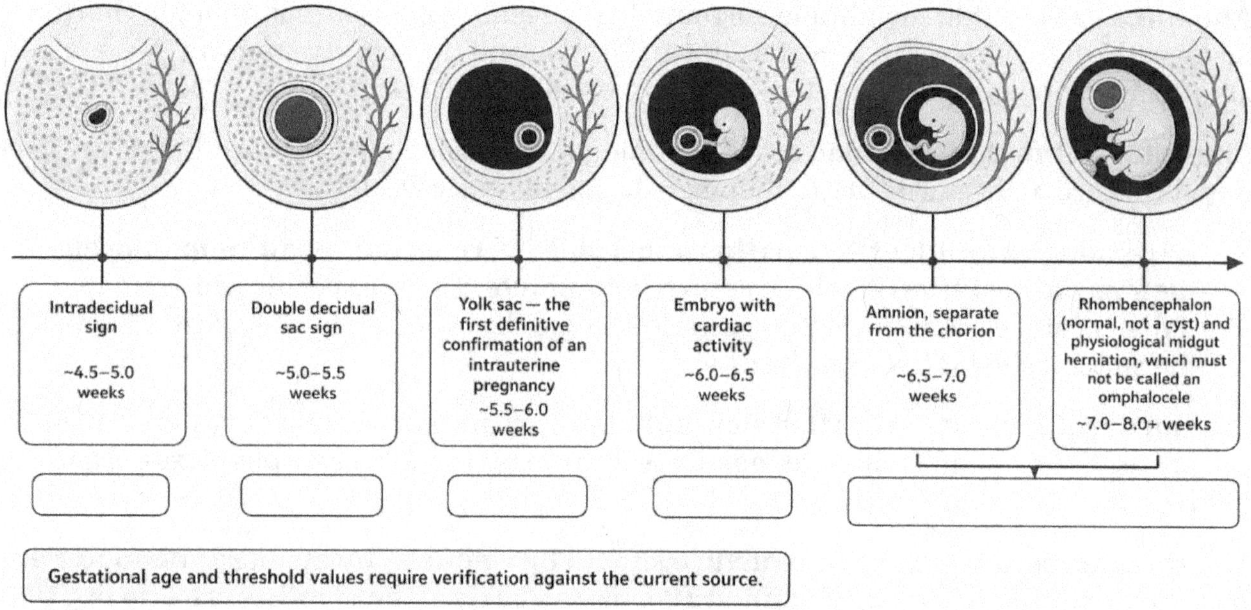

18.6 Crown-Rump Length and Establishing Dates

Why dating matters more than it appears to

Gestational age determines almost every subsequent decision in the pregnancy: the window for screening tests, the interpretation of growth measurements, the definition of preterm and post-term, and the timing of delivery. **A dating error propagates through the entire pregnancy** and cannot be corrected later without introducing inconsistency.

Crown-rump length is the most accurate method of dating available, and its accuracy is greatest early in the first trimester and declines as the fetus grows and begins to flex. [VERIFY: current stated accuracy of crown-rump length dating and the gestational range over which it is used]

Technique

The measurement is conventionally standardised, and the details matter:

1. **True midsagittal section** of the embryo
2. **Neutral position** — neither flexed nor hyperextended. A flexed embryo measures short; an extended one measures long
3. **Magnify** so the embryo fills a substantial part of the image
4. **Measure the maximum length**, from the outer margin of the **crown** to the outer margin of the **rump**
5. **Exclude the yolk sac and the limbs** — including the yolk sac is the classic error
6. **Take the required number of measurements and follow the local averaging convention**

[VERIFY: the current caliper convention and averaging protocol for crown-rump length]

Dating and redating rules

Where the crown-rump length differs from the menstrual dates by more than a defined margin, the pregnancy is redated by the scan. Below that margin, the menstrual dates are retained.

> **Once a pregnancy has been dated, it is not redated at subsequent scans.** A later scan showing a fetus smaller than expected is a growth finding, not a dating finding — and redating it would conceal exactly the problem the scan detected.

This is one of the most important procedural rules in obstetric ultrasound, and it is occasionally violated with serious consequence.

[VERIFY: the current discrepancy margin triggering redating, and the policy on redating at later gestations]

In pregnancies conceived by assisted reproduction, the date of fertilisation or transfer is known, and the pregnancy is dated from it. **These pregnancies are not redated by ultrasound.**

Beyond the first trimester

Crown-rump length becomes unreliable once the fetus flexes and grows beyond the range over which it was validated. **Head circumference, with or without biparietal diameter and femur length, replaces it** (Chapter 19).

Mean sac diameter dating is inferior to crown-rump length and should not be used once an embryo is measurable.

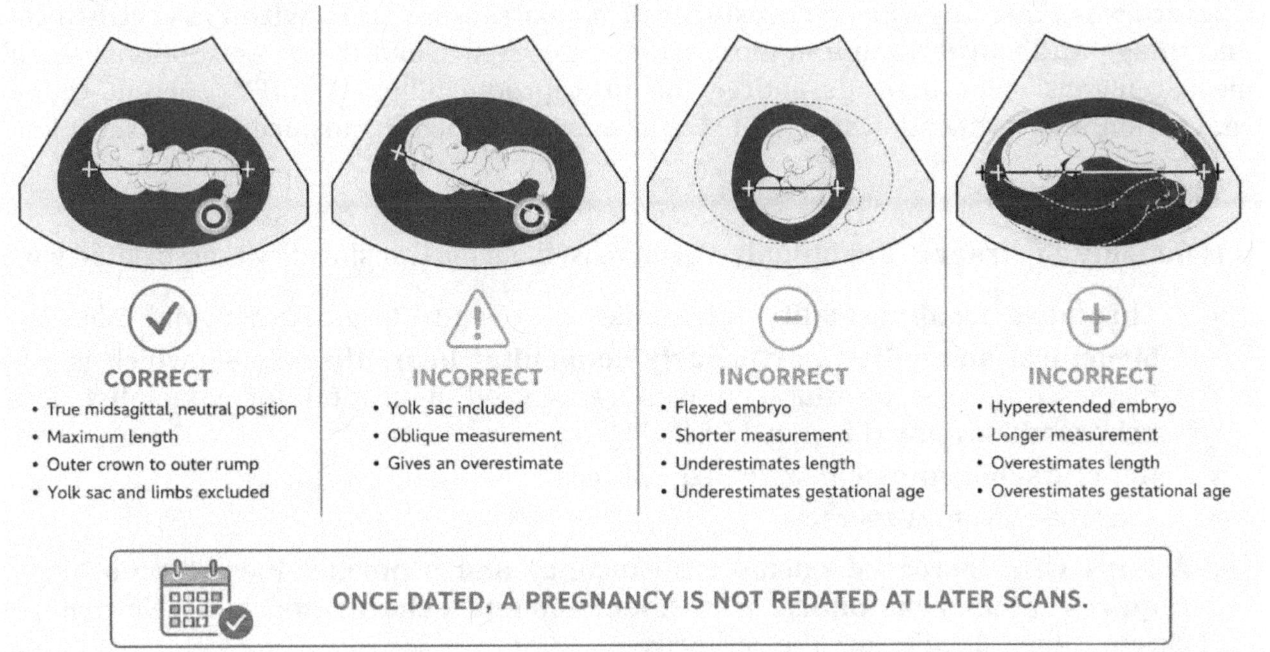

18.7 Nuchal Translucency and First-Trimester Screening

What is being measured

Nuchal translucency is the **subcutaneous fluid collection at the back of the fetal neck**, present in all fetuses, and measurable within a defined gestational window. **Increased thickness is associated with increased risk**, and the measurement is combined with maternal age and biochemistry to generate a risk figure.

The window is defined by crown-rump length, not by menstrual dates — and this is why accurate dating (§18.6) is a prerequisite for screening. [VERIFY: the current gestational and crown-rump length window for nuchal translucency measurement]

The criteria for a valid measurement

These are formally specified and audited, because measurement error translates directly into misclassified risk:

1. **True midsagittal plane** of the fetus
2. **Neutral fetal position** — neither flexed nor extended, since both alter the measurement
3. **Magnification** such that the fetal head and upper thorax fill most of the image
4. **The amnion must be visible and distinguished from the fetal skin** — measuring to the amnion instead of the skin is a specific and common error
5. **Calipers placed on the inner borders of the nuchal space**, perpendicular to the fetal body axis, at the **widest part**
6. **Several measurements taken**, with the largest valid measurement used

Operators performing nuchal translucency measurement work within a certification and image-audit programme in most screening systems, and this is not optional — the measurement's value depends entirely on its reproducibility. [VERIFY: current caliper convention, and certification and audit requirements for nuchal translucency measurement]

What an increased measurement means

It is not only a marker of aneuploidy. An increased nuchal translucency is associated with:

- **Chromosomal abnormality** — trisomies 21, 18 and 13, and Turner syndrome
- **Structural anomalies, particularly congenital heart disease** — which is why increased nuchal translucency is a recognised indication for **specialist fetal echocardiography** (Chapter 15 §15.7)
- **Genetic syndromes** and skeletal dysplasias
- Adverse outcome generally

A fetus with increased nuchal translucency and a normal karyotype still requires detailed anatomical assessment and fetal echocardiography. Normal chromosomes do not close the pathway.

Cystic hygroma is a distinct and more serious finding: a **large, septated** fluid collection extending along the fetal neck and back, with a substantially worse prognosis than isolated nuchal thickening.

The combined screening test and its alternatives

Combined first-trimester screening uses nuchal translucency, maternal age, and two serum markers — free beta-hCG and pregnancy-associated plasma protein A — to produce a risk estimate.

Additional first-trimester markers used in specialist settings include the **nasal bone**, the **ductus venosus a-wave**, and **tricuspid regurgitation**.

Cell-free DNA screening analyses placentally derived fetal DNA in maternal blood and offers high detection rates for the common trisomies.

> **Cell-free DNA is a screening test, not a diagnostic one.** A high-risk result requires confirmation by an invasive diagnostic test, and results can be affected by low fetal fraction, confined placental mosaicism, and vanishing twin. It also does not replace the ultrasound component, since nuchal translucency carries structural as well as chromosomal information.

[VERIFY: current detection rates and false positive rates for combined screening and cell-free DNA screening]

Diagnostic tests — chorionic villus sampling in the late first trimester and **amniocentesis** from the mid second trimester — provide a definitive karyotype and carry a small procedure-related loss risk, and are performed under ultrasound guidance (Chapter 9 §9.4–9.6). [VERIFY: current gestational windows and procedure-related loss rates]

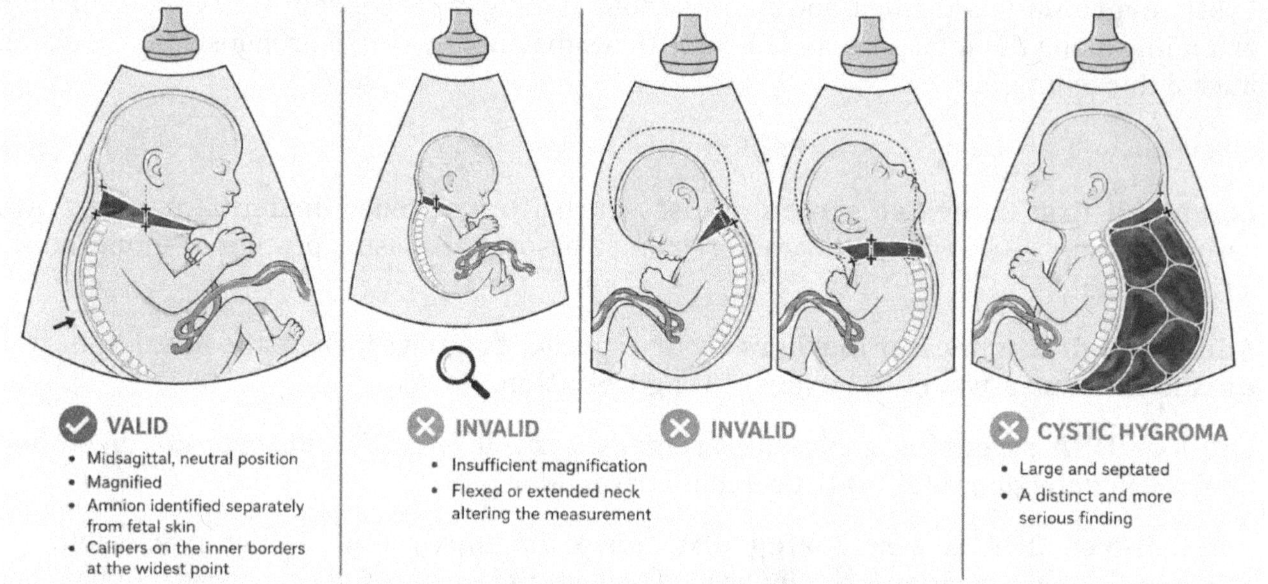

Increased translucency with a normal karyotype still requires detailed anatomy and fetal echocardiography.

18.8 Early Pregnancy Failure: Diagnostic versus Suspicious Criteria

Why this section is structured the way it is

This is the most medicolegally consequential material in the book.

The criteria for diagnosing early pregnancy failure were deliberately revised to be **more conservative** than those used historically, because the earlier thresholds carried a small but real risk of **misclassifying a viable pregnancy as failed** — and the consequence of that error is the termination of a wanted, viable pregnancy through medical or surgical management.

The resulting framework has **two tiers**, and understanding the distinction between them is more important than memorising any individual number:

Tier	Meaning	Action
Diagnostic of pregnancy failure	Findings that establish non-viability with essentially no false positives	Management of miscarriage may proceed
Suspicious for pregnancy failure	Findings that raise concern but are compatible, occasionally, with a viable pregnancy	**Interval follow-up scan — not intervention**

The governing rule: when a finding is suspicious but not diagnostic, the correct response is a follow-up scan at a defined interval, not intervention.

The categories of criteria

Diagnostic criteria are drawn from four types of observation:

1. **A crown-rump length at or above a threshold with no cardiac activity**
2. **A mean sac diameter at or above a threshold with no embryo**
3. **Absence of an embryo with cardiac activity a defined interval after a scan that showed a gestational sac without a yolk sac**
4. **Absence of an embryo with cardiac activity a defined interval after a scan that showed a gestational sac with a yolk sac**

Suspicious criteria include:

- A crown-rump length **below** the diagnostic threshold with no cardiac activity
- A mean sac diameter **below** the diagnostic threshold with no embryo
- **Absence of an embryo** at intervals **shorter** than the diagnostic ones
- An **enlarged yolk sac**
- A **small gestational sac relative to the embryo**
- **Expanded amnion sign** and the **empty amnion sign** — a visible amnion without an embryo within it
- A slow embryonic heart rate

> **The specific numerical thresholds and time intervals must be taken from the current multispecialty consensus criteria in force in the relevant jurisdiction, and must not be reproduced from memory or from an older text.** [VERIFY: the current diagnostic and suspicious criteria for early pregnancy failure, with all threshold values and time intervals, and the source and edition from which they are taken]

The hCG caveat, restated

> **A single serum hCG value must not be used to determine viability or to justify intervention.** The limitations set out in §18.5 apply directly, and a viable intrauterine pregnancy can exist at an hCG level above a nominal discriminatory threshold without yet being visible.

Related presentations

Pregnancy of unknown location — a positive pregnancy test with **no intrauterine or extrauterine pregnancy identified**. This is a **description of a state, not a diagnosis**, and it is managed with **serial hCG measurement and interval ultrasound** until the pregnancy is located or resolves. Every such patient is treated as a possible ectopic until proven otherwise (§18.9).

Incomplete miscarriage — echogenic material within the cavity with demonstrable vascularity, distinguishing retained products from blood clot. Marked vascularity indicates a lesion at risk of significant bleeding if instrumented (Chapter 17 §17.7).

Complete miscarriage — an empty uterus with a thin endometrium in a woman with a previously confirmed intrauterine pregnancy. **In a woman without a previously confirmed intrauterine pregnancy, an empty uterus is not a complete miscarriage — it is a pregnancy of unknown location.**

Communication

This is the scenario for which §18.2 exists. Know your department's policy on what the sonographer may say, obtain the clinician promptly, and **do not leave the woman alone with an unexplained silence**.

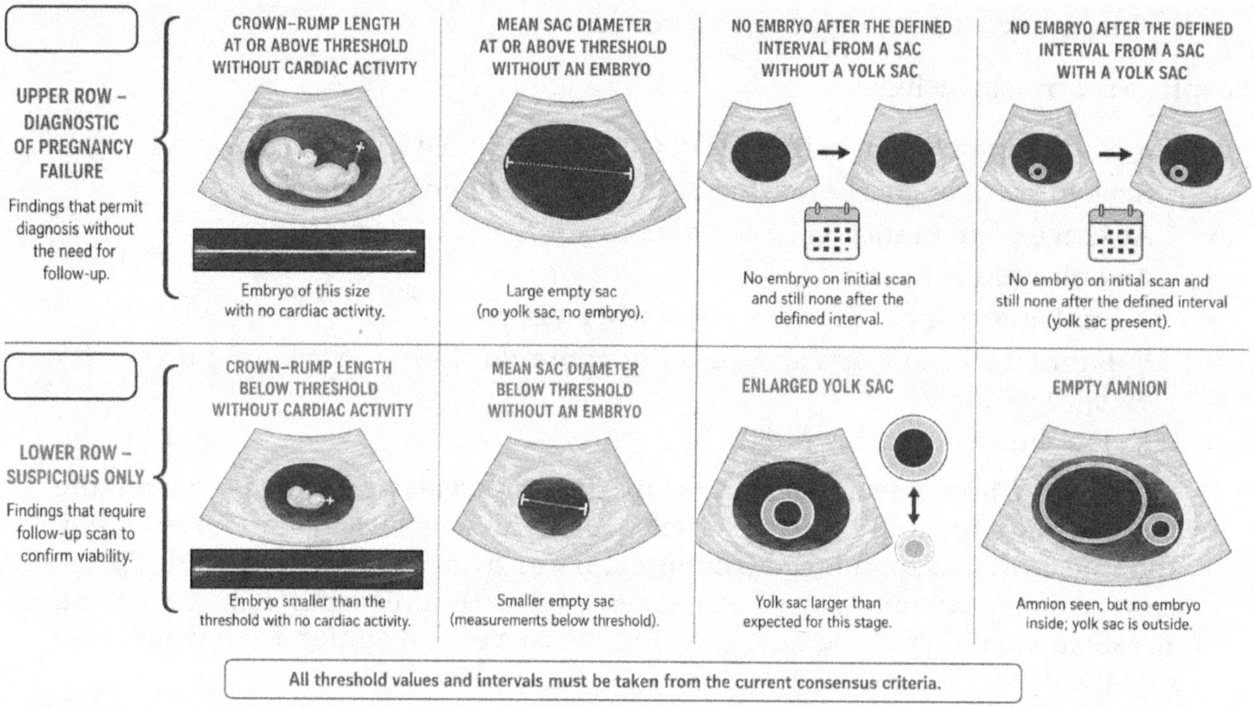

18.9 Ectopic and Heterotopic Pregnancy

The sonographic findings, the sliding sign, and the adnexal appearances are set out in **Chapter 17 §17.10** and are not repeated. What follows is the pregnancy-specific framing and the implantation sites that carry particular risk.

The governing statement

> **A positive pregnancy test with no visible intrauterine pregnancy is a pregnancy of unknown location, and ectopic pregnancy must be actively excluded before any other explanation is accepted.**

Ectopic pregnancy remains a leading cause of maternal death in early pregnancy, and the deaths are characteristically associated with delayed diagnosis rather than with an unusual presentation.

Findings, in ascending order of certainty

- An **empty uterus** with a positive test
- A **decidual reaction** without a sac
- A **pseudogestational sac** — a **centrally placed** collection lacking the eccentric position, the double decidual sign, and above all the **yolk sac** of a true intrauterine pregnancy

- An **adnexal mass separate from the ovary**, demonstrated by the **sliding sign**
- A **tubal ring**
- **A yolk sac or embryo outside the uterus — definitive**
- **Free fluid**, particularly **echogenic** fluid indicating haemoperitoneum

The corpus luteum trap from Chapter 17 §17.10 applies in full: the ring of fire does not distinguish an ectopic from a corpus luteum, and the ectopic is usually on the same side as it. **The sliding sign does distinguish them.**

The high-risk implantation sites

Interstitial (cornual) pregnancy — implanted in the intramural segment of the tube.

- **Eccentric sac position** high in the uterine cornu
- **A thin surrounding myometrial mantle**
- **The interstitial line sign** — an echogenic line running from the endometrial cavity outward to abut the sac

It ruptures late and catastrophically, because the myometrium allows it to grow before failing, and the adjacent uterine and ovarian vessels produce major haemorrhage.

Caesarean scar pregnancy — implantation within the niche of a previous caesarean scar. **Its incidence is rising with caesarean rates**, and it is easy to mistake for a low intrauterine pregnancy or a miscarriage in progress.

- Sac implanted **anteriorly in the lower uterine segment at the scar**
- **Thin or absent myometrium between the sac and the bladder** — the critical measurement
- **An empty endometrial cavity and an empty cervical canal**
- Prominent vascularity at the implantation site

It carries a high risk of catastrophic haemorrhage and uterine rupture, and it is the precursor lesion for **placenta accreta spectrum** if continued (Chapter 19). It requires prompt specialist referral, and blind uterine instrumentation is dangerous.

Cervical pregnancy — a sac implanted below the internal os, with an "hourglass" uterine configuration.

> **Distinguish it from a miscarriage in transit** using probe pressure: a **sac passing through the cervix slides**, while an **implanted cervical pregnancy does not**. This is the same sliding principle used in the adnexa, applied to a different question.

Ovarian and abdominal implantations are rare and difficult.

Heterotopic pregnancy

Coexisting intrauterine and ectopic pregnancy. **Rare in spontaneous conception, but substantially more common after assisted reproduction.**

In a woman who conceived by assisted reproduction, finding an intrauterine pregnancy does not exclude a concurrent ectopic. The adnexa must be examined and free fluid sought regardless — which is why §18.4 insists on completing the examination.

Escalation

Suspected ectopic pregnancy is a critical finding requiring immediate, direct communication (Chapter 1 §1.5). Where there is haemodynamic concern or substantial free fluid, the examination should be abbreviated rather than completed.

18.10 Gestational Trophoblastic Disease and Subchorionic Haemorrhage

Gestational trophoblastic disease

Complete hydatidiform mole:

- A **heterogeneous echogenic intrauterine mass** containing **multiple small cystic spaces**, classically described as a snowstorm or a cluster of grapes
- **No fetus and no amniotic sac**
- **Markedly elevated human chorionic gonadotrophin**, often far above that expected for gestation
- **Theca lutein cysts** — bilateral, large, multiseptate ovarian cysts driven by the high hCG (Chapter 17 §17.9)
- Clinically: bleeding, a uterus large for dates, **hyperemesis**, and occasionally **early pre-eclampsia** or thyrotoxicosis, both of which are unusual at that gestation and are clues

Partial mole:

- **A fetus or fetal parts are present**, frequently with structural abnormalities and growth restriction, reflecting triploidy
- **An enlarged, cystic placenta**
- hCG elevation is less marked

It is frequently mistaken for a missed miscarriage, which is why histological examination of products of conception matters.

Invasive mole and choriocarcinoma — myometrial invasion with **marked, low-resistance vascularity**, and in choriocarcinoma, metastatic disease (lung, liver, brain).

Management context worth knowing, because it explains the urgency of the diagnosis: patients are **registered with a trophoblastic disease service**, followed with **serial hCG until normalisation**, advised against pregnancy until cleared, and a proportion require chemotherapy.

The differential includes hydropic degeneration of a missed miscarriage, retained products of conception, and uterine arteriovenous malformation — the last distinguished by its high-velocity, low-resistance flow without trophoblastic tissue.

Subchorionic haemorrhage

A crescentic collection between the chorion and the uterine wall, elevating the chorionic membrane.

Appearance evolves with age: acutely it may be echogenic and easily overlooked against adjacent myometrium; it becomes progressively hypoechoic and then anechoic as it liquefies.

Report:

- **Its size relative to the gestational sac** — this is the parameter that correlates with outcome, and a proportion or an estimated volume is more useful than a linear measurement alone
- Its location, particularly whether it is **retroplacental**
- The gestational sac contents and viability

Most resolve, and the majority of pregnancies with a small subchorionic haemorrhage continue normally. **Larger collections are associated with an increased risk of loss**, and this should be conveyed by the clinician rather than the sonographer.

Distinguish it from:

- **A second gestational sac** — a subchorionic collection is **crescentic**, follows the uterine contour, and contains **no yolk sac or embryo**
- **Chorioamniotic separation** — a normal finding before fusion of the membranes
- **A retained sac from a vanishing twin**

18.11 Multiple Gestation: Chorionicity and Amnionicity

Why this is a first-trimester task

> **Chorionicity is the single most important determinant of risk in a multiple pregnancy, and it is most reliably determined in the first trimester.**

The membrane signs that establish it — the lambda and T signs — become progressively less reliable as the pregnancy advances and the membranes thin and the placentas grow. **A chorionicity determination made at the first-trimester scan and recorded clearly is one of the highest-value pieces of information generated in the whole pregnancy**, because it drives the entire surveillance schedule.

How to determine it

Count carefully and systematically:

- The **number of gestational sacs**
- The **number of yolk sacs** — which in the early weeks corresponds to the number of amnions
- The **number of embryos**

- The **number of amniotic cavities**

Then assess the membrane:

	Dichorionic diamniotic	Monochorionic diamniotic	Monochorionic monoamniotic
Dividing membrane	**Thick**	**Thin**	**Absent**
Membrane–placenta junction	**Lambda (twin peak) sign** — a triangular wedge of chorionic tissue extending into the base of the membrane	**T sign** — the membrane meets the placenta at a right angle, with no wedge	Not applicable
Placental masses	Two separate, **or one fused mass**	One	One
Risk profile	Lowest of the three	Higher — vascular anastomoses	**Highest** — cord entanglement

Two additional discriminators:

- **Different fetal sexes establish dichorionicity** — but this is a later-gestation observation and the same sex proves nothing
- **Two separate placental masses establish dichorionicity**, but **a single mass does not exclude it**, since adjacent dichorionic placentas fuse

Labelling

Label the fetuses consistently and describe the labelling clearly — by position (left/right, upper/lower) and by the relationship to the cervix — and **use the same labelling at every subsequent scan**. Inconsistent labelling between scans makes growth comparison impossible and has led to interventions on the wrong twin.

Complications by chorionicity

All multiples: preterm birth, growth restriction, pre-eclampsia, and the maternal complications of a multiple pregnancy.

Monochorionic pregnancies additionally, because they share a placental circulation with vascular anastomoses:

- **Twin-to-twin transfusion syndrome** — an imbalance in the shared circulation producing a discordant amniotic fluid volume, with a polyhydramnic recipient and an oligohydramnic, "stuck" donor
- **Twin anaemia–polycythaemia sequence**
- **Selective fetal growth restriction**
- **Twin reversed arterial perfusion (TRAP) sequence**

- **Following single fetal demise, a risk of neurological injury to the surviving co-twin** through acute transfusion at the time of death — which is why monochorionic pregnancies are managed and counselled differently after a loss

Monoamniotic pregnancies additionally: cord entanglement, which is essentially universal and drives an intensive surveillance and early delivery strategy.

Surveillance intervals differ substantially by chorionicity, with monochorionic pregnancies scanned far more frequently. [VERIFY: current surveillance intervals and protocols by chorionicity]

"Vanishing twin" — the early demise and resorption of one sac, seen in a proportion of multiple pregnancies detected in the first trimester, and worth documenting because it explains later biochemical and cell-free DNA anomalies.

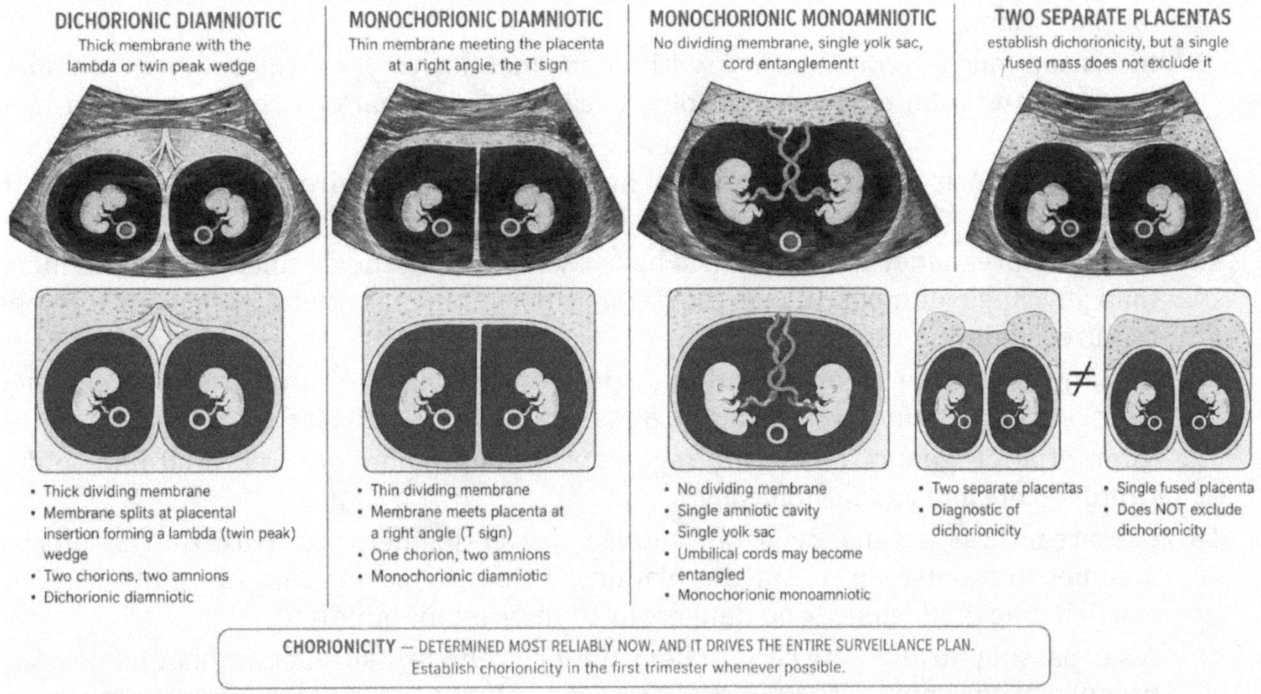

Key Points

1. The pregnant woman is the patient, and her autonomy governs. Screening is optional and declining it is a legitimate recorded decision.
2. Know your department's policy on disclosing absent fetal cardiac activity before you encounter it. Completing the scan in silence and leaving is never acceptable.
3. Do not use spectral Doppler over the embryo to document cardiac activity. Use M-mode or B-mode observation.
4. Freeze before measuring — measurements cost no additional exposure.
5. Do not stop the examination when an intrauterine pregnancy is found. Examine both adnexa and the pouch of Douglas every time.

6. The yolk sac is the first finding that definitively confirms an intrauterine pregnancy, because a pseudogestational sac cannot contain one.
7. Physiological midgut herniation is normal in the early weeks and must not be reported as an omphalocele.
8. The rhombencephalon is a normal cystic structure in the early fetal head, not a posterior fossa cyst.
9. A single hCG value must never determine viability or location, or justify intervention.
10. Crown-rump length is the most accurate dating method. Measure in true midsagittal, neutral position, crown to rump, excluding the yolk sac and limbs.
11. Once a pregnancy is dated, it is not redated at later scans. A small fetus later is a growth finding, not a dating finding.
12. Nuchal translucency requires the amnion to be identified separately from fetal skin, adequate magnification, and a neutral fetal position — and it is an audited measurement.
13. Increased nuchal translucency with a normal karyotype still requires detailed anatomy and fetal echocardiography, because it also marks structural and cardiac disease.
14. Cell-free DNA is a screening test. A high-risk result requires a diagnostic test to confirm it.
15. The early pregnancy failure criteria have two tiers, and the distinction matters more than any single number: diagnostic findings permit management, suspicious findings require a follow-up scan.
16. An empty uterus in a woman without a previously confirmed intrauterine pregnancy is a pregnancy of unknown location, not a complete miscarriage.
17. Interstitial pregnancy has a thin myometrial mantle and an interstitial line, and it ruptures late and catastrophically.
18. Caesarean scar pregnancy — an anterior lower-segment sac with thin or absent myometrium between it and the bladder, an empty cavity and an empty cervical canal. Rising in incidence and dangerous to instrument blindly.
19. A sac passing through the cervix slides under probe pressure; an implanted cervical pregnancy does not.
20. After assisted reproduction, an intrauterine pregnancy does not exclude a concurrent ectopic.
21. Hyperemesis, early pre-eclampsia, or an hCG far above that expected for gestation should prompt a deliberate look for trophoblastic disease.
22. Report a subchorionic haemorrhage by its size relative to the gestational sac, not by a linear measurement alone.
23. Determine chorionicity in the first trimester and record it clearly — the membrane signs degrade later, and it drives the whole surveillance plan.
24. Two separate placentas establish dichorionicity; a single fused mass does not exclude it.
25. Label multiples consistently and use the same labelling at every subsequent scan.

Registry Check

1. Which finding first definitively confirms an intrauterine pregnancy?

A. The intradecidual sign **B.** The double decidual sac sign **C.** A yolk sac within the gestational sac **D.** An eccentrically positioned anechoic sac

> **Answer: C.** A pseudogestational sac can mimic the appearance of an intrauterine sac and can produce a decidual reaction, but it cannot contain a yolk sac. The intradecidual and double decidual signs are supportive but not definitive.

2. Embryonic cardiac activity should be documented using:

A. Spectral pulsed-wave Doppler **B.** M-mode or direct B-mode observation **C.** Colour Doppler over the embryo **D.** Power Doppler

> **Answer: B.** Spectral Doppler carries the highest acoustic output of any routine mode and delivers it to a stationary sample volume. M-mode provides the same documentation of cardiac activity at far lower exposure, and its use in this situation is a specific and widely endorsed recommendation.

3. A crown-rump length measurement includes the yolk sac. The effect on the estimated gestational age is that it will be:

A. Unchanged **B.** Underestimated **C.** Overestimated **D.** Unmeasurable

> **Answer: C.** Including the yolk sac produces an oblique measurement longer than the true crown-rump length, giving a larger crown-rump length and therefore an overestimated gestational age. The yolk sac and the limbs are excluded, and the embryo must be in a neutral position.

4. A fetus dated at 12 weeks by crown-rump length is found at 32 weeks to measure small for the assigned dates. The correct response is to:

A. Redate the pregnancy using the current measurements **B.** Average the two estimates **C.** Retain the original dating and assess this as a growth finding **D.** Redate using femur length only

> **Answer: C.** Once a pregnancy has been dated, it is not redated at later scans. Redating at 32 weeks would conceal the very abnormality the scan has detected, since a growth-restricted fetus would simply be reassigned a younger gestational age.

5. During nuchal translucency measurement, the caliper is inadvertently placed on the amnion rather than the fetal skin. The measurement will be:

A. Falsely reduced **B.** Falsely increased **C.** Unaffected **D.** Invalid but unpredictable in direction

> **Answer: B.** The amnion lies outside the nuchal skin line, so measuring to it spans a greater distance and falsely increases the recorded translucency. Distinguishing

the amnion from fetal skin is a formal criterion for a valid measurement, and adequate magnification is what makes it possible.

6. A gestational sac with a mean sac diameter below the diagnostic threshold contains no embryo. The appropriate action is:

A. Diagnose early pregnancy failure and offer management **B.** Arrange a follow-up scan at a defined interval **C.** Measure serum hCG and manage on the basis of a single value **D.** Discharge with reassurance

> **Answer: B.** This finding is suspicious for, but not diagnostic of, pregnancy failure. The two-tier structure exists precisely to prevent intervention on findings that are occasionally compatible with a viable pregnancy, and the correct response to a suspicious finding is interval follow-up. A single hCG value cannot resolve the question.

7. A gestational sac is seen implanted anteriorly in the lower uterine segment, with minimal myometrium between it and the bladder, an empty endometrial cavity and an empty cervical canal. This represents:

A. A miscarriage in progress **B.** Cervical pregnancy **C.** Caesarean scar pregnancy **D.** A low intrauterine pregnancy

> **Answer: C.** Implantation within a caesarean scar niche produces an anterior lower-segment sac with deficient myometrium between it and the bladder, with both the cavity and the cervical canal empty. It carries a high risk of catastrophic haemorrhage and uterine rupture, and is the precursor of placenta accreta spectrum if the pregnancy continues.

8. In a twin pregnancy, the dividing membrane meets the placenta at a right angle with no wedge of chorionic tissue at its base. This indicates:

A. Dichorionic diamniotic twins **B.** Monochorionic diamniotic twins **C.** Monochorionic monoamniotic twins **D.** Chorionicity cannot be determined from this finding

> **Answer: B.** The T sign — a thin membrane meeting the placenta perpendicularly without an intervening wedge — indicates monochorionicity with two amnions. The lambda or twin peak sign, with a triangular wedge of chorionic tissue at the membrane base, indicates dichorionicity. Monoamniotic twins have no dividing membrane at all.

Chapter Notes for the Editorial Pass

Verification queue — and a specific instruction. The **early pregnancy failure criteria in §18.8 must be sourced directly from the current multispecialty consensus document in force in the intended jurisdiction, cited with its edition and date, and reproduced exactly.** They must not be paraphrased, rounded, or carried across from an earlier edition of any text. This is the single most consequential verification in the book: the criteria were revised specifically to reduce the risk of misclassifying viable pregnancies, and an outdated threshold printed in a handbook would be applied in practice.

Other verification items, in priority order: the **mean sac diameter and crown-rump length thresholds** at which each developmental landmark should be visible (§18.5); **hCG discriminatory level guidance**, which has moved substantially toward caution (§18.5); **crown-rump length caliper and averaging conventions, dating accuracy, and the redating margin** (§18.6); **the nuchal translucency window, caliper convention, and certification and audit requirements** (§18.7); **detection and false positive rates for combined and cell-free DNA screening**, and **procedure-related loss rates** for chorionic villus sampling and amniocentesis (§18.7); **the gestation by which physiological midgut herniation resolves** (§18.5); **surveillance intervals by chorionicity** (§18.11); and **the screening programme structure for the intended jurisdiction** (§18.1).

Jurisdictional dependence. This chapter is more jurisdiction-bound than any other in the book. Screening programme structure, fetal sex disclosure policy, conscientious objection provisions, termination law, and the applicable early pregnancy failure criteria all vary between health systems. §18.1, §18.2 and §18.8 should all be reviewed against the intended market before publication, and the text has been written to describe principles and to flag the decision points rather than to assert a single national practice.

Ethics cross-reference. §18.2 is the book's substantive obstetric ethics section, and Chapter 15 §15.10 refers forward to it for the counselling pathway after a prenatal cardiac diagnosis. Confirm at layout that the forward reference resolves and that the two sections read as complementary rather than overlapping.

Figure count: 6 Lane A, 1 Lane B. The Lane B request deliberately specifies **M-mode rather than spectral Doppler** for cardiac documentation, so that the acquired image demonstrates the §18.3 rule rather than contradicting it — a small point, but a published figure showing spectral Doppler over an embryo would undermine the chapter's most important safety statement.

Cross-reference targets to fix at layout: §18.2 scope and disclosure → Chapter 1 §1.2–1.3 and §1.8; §18.2 counselling after a cardiac diagnosis → Chapter 15 §15.10; §18.3 mode hierarchy and ALARA → Chapter 1 §1.7; §18.4 transvaginal consent and disinfection → Chapter 17 §17.3 and Chapter 1 §1.4; §18.6 second- and third-trimester dating → Chapter 19; §18.7 fetal echocardiography for increased nuchal translucency → Chapter 15 §15.7; §18.7 guided invasive procedures → Chapter 9 §9.4–9.6; §18.9 adnexal findings and the sliding sign → Chapter 17 §17.10; §18.9 caesarean scar pregnancy and accreta spectrum → Chapter 19; §18.10 theca lutein cysts → Chapter 17 §17.9; §18.10 retained products vascularity → Chapter 17 §17.7.

Word count: approximately 10,400 excluding image prompt blocks, learning objectives, registry questions, and these notes.

Chapter 19: The Second and Third Trimesters

Learning Objectives

On completing this chapter you should be able to:

1. Perform a systematic anatomic survey and report its limitations honestly.
2. Obtain the four standard biometric measurements in their correct planes.
3. Estimate fetal weight, state its error margin, and plot it appropriately.
4. Distinguish a constitutionally small fetus from fetal growth restriction, and recognise macrosomia.
5. Interpret umbilical, middle cerebral, ductus venosus and uterine artery Doppler, and describe the sequence of deterioration.
6. Perform and interpret a biophysical profile.
7. Recognise placental variants and pathology, including abruption.
8. Assess placental position and the accreta spectrum.
9. Evaluate the umbilical cord, including vessel number and insertion site, and recognise vasa previa.
10. Measure amniotic fluid and work through the causes of oligohydramnios and polyhydramnios.
11. Identify hydrops fetalis and structure its investigation.
12. Adapt surveillance to the principal high-risk maternal conditions.
13. Measure cervical length correctly and recognise funnelling.

Three Diagnoses That Prenatal Detection Transforms

Most of this chapter is surveillance. Three findings within it change outcomes decisively when found before delivery and are catastrophic when found during it:

- **Placenta accreta spectrum** (§19.8) — planned delivery in a specialist centre versus unanticipated massive haemorrhage
- **Vasa previa** (§19.9) — planned caesarean with excellent survival versus fetal exsanguination on membrane rupture
- **A short cervix** (§19.13) — an intervention that reduces preterm birth versus an unheralded delivery

Each is detectable with a deliberate look in a defined at-risk group, and each is missed by scanning past it. They are the reason this chapter's protocols specify what to look for rather than only what to measure.

19.1 The Standard Anatomic Survey Protocol

Purpose and timing

The mid-trimester survey screens for structural anomaly, confirms growth against the established dates, and assesses the placenta, amniotic fluid, cervix and, in multiples, each fetus. [VERIFY: the recommended gestational window for the anatomic survey in the intended jurisdiction]

It is a screening examination. Detection rates vary by anomaly, by gestation, by maternal habitus and by operator, and some anomalies are not detectable at this gestation at all. **The report should not imply that a normal survey excludes structural abnormality.**

The sequence

Work in a fixed order so that nothing is omitted under time pressure:

Orientation — fetal number, presentation, lie, situs (Chapter 14 §14.1), and cardiac activity.

Head and brain — skull shape and ossification; **cavum septi pellucidi**; lateral ventricles with **atrial diameter measured**; thalami; posterior fossa with **cerebellum and cisterna magna**; **nuchal fold**.

Face — orbits, upper lip, profile, nasal bone.

Chest — lungs, **diaphragm**, and the **cardiac sequence of Chapter 15 §15.7**: situs, four-chamber view, both outflow tracts, and the three-vessel and trachea view.

Abdomen — **stomach on the left**, bowel, **both kidneys and the bladder**, **cord insertion at the abdominal wall**, and the wall itself.

Spine — longitudinal and transverse, with overlying skin.

Limbs — all four, with femur and humerus, and the presence of hands and feet.

Adnexal structures — placenta and its cord insertion, amniotic fluid, cervix, and the maternal uterus and adnexa.

Reporting limitations

Maternal habitus, fetal position, advanced gestation, and oligohydramnios all degrade the survey.

Name what could not be seen, rather than issuing an unqualified normal report: *"Fetal heart outflow tracts and spine not adequately visualised due to fetal position; re-scan arranged."* An unremarked omission is read as a normal finding (Chapter 1 §1.5).

19.2 Obstetric Measurements and Gestational Age Assignment

The four standard measurements

Biparietal diameter and head circumference share a plane: a **transverse axial section** showing a symmetrical skull with the **midline falx**, the **cavum septi pellucidi** anteriorly, and the **thalami** — with the **cerebellum not visible**, since its presence indicates the plane is angled too far posteriorly.

- **BPD** is measured across the skull perpendicular to the falx, using the local caliper convention
- **HC** is an ellipse around the **outer skull perimeter**

Abdominal circumference — a **transverse section at the level of the stomach and the umbilical portion of the left portal vein**, where the vessel forms a short hook rather than extending to the anterior wall. The section should be **round rather than oval**, with symmetrical ribs, and **the kidneys should not be visible**. The ellipse follows the **outer skin surface**.

Femur length — the **full ossified diaphysis**, with the bone lying as close to perpendicular to the beam as possible, **excluding the unossified epiphyses** and any distal femoral point.

[VERIFY: the caliper conventions to be adopted for each biometric measurement]

The errors that matter

Error	Effect
Oblique or angled head plane	Distorts both BPD and HC
Cerebellum visible in the head plane	Plane too posterior — measurement invalid
Kidneys visible in the abdominal plane	Plane too low — AC underestimated
Oval rather than round abdominal section	Oblique plane — AC overestimated
Including subcutaneous oedema in AC	Overestimates, and matters in hydrops and diabetes
Foreshortened femur	Underestimates, and can falsely suggest skeletal dysplasia

Abdominal circumference is both the most influential measurement in weight estimation and the most error-prone — it deserves the most care.

Assigning and not reassigning gestational age

First-trimester crown-rump length remains the most accurate dating method (Chapter 18 §18.6). Beyond that window, **head circumference is the most robust single parameter**, used alone or in a composite.

> **A pregnancy dated in the first trimester is not redated in the second or third.** Restated here because the temptation is greatest when the fetus measures small — and redating at that point conceals growth restriction.

Dating accuracy declines with advancing gestation, because biological variation in size increases. [VERIFY: current stated dating accuracy by trimester]

Charts

Measurements are meaningless without a reference. **Population-based, customised, and international prescriptive standards** differ in what they consider normal, and therefore in how many fetuses they label small.

A service should adopt one chart system and use it consistently, stating which. [VERIFY: the biometric and growth chart standard to be adopted]

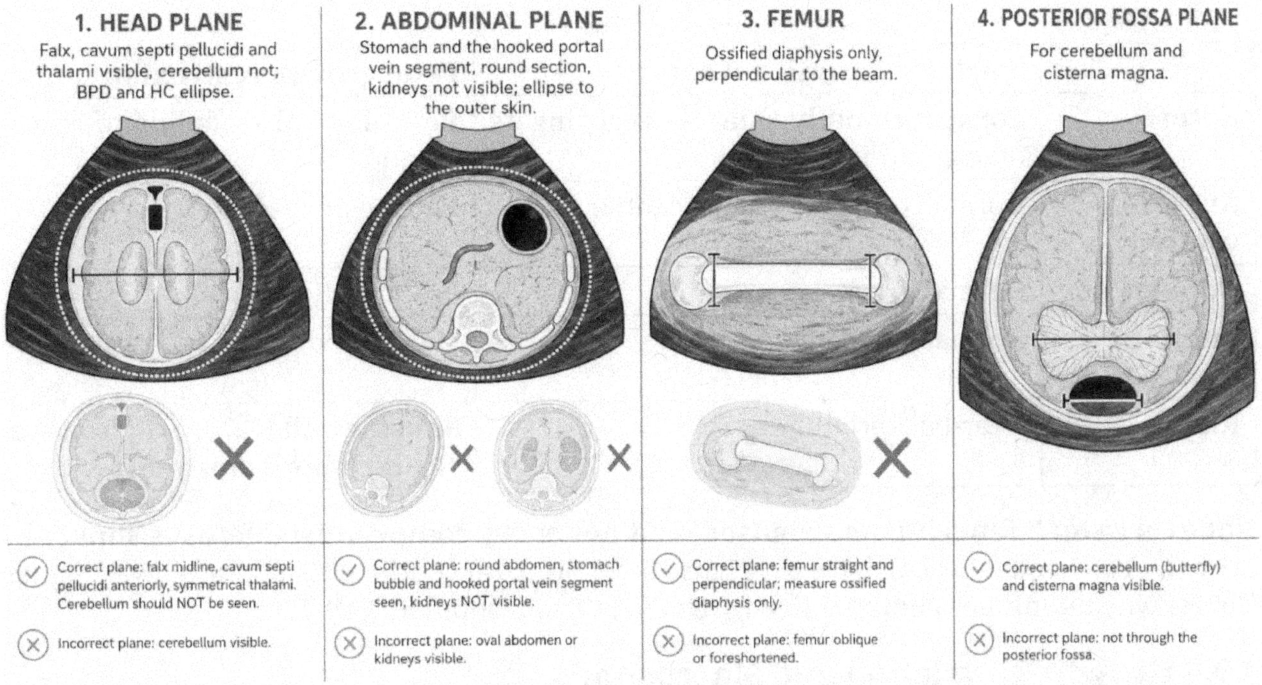

19.3 Fetal Growth Assessment and Estimated Fetal Weight

Estimating weight

Estimated fetal weight is calculated from combinations of the biometric measurements, with **abdominal circumference contributing most.**

> **Every estimated fetal weight carries a substantial error margin, and the report must state it.** Clinicians make delivery decisions on these numbers, and a weight quoted without its confidence interval invites false precision. **The error is proportionally greater at the extremes** — in the very small and the very large fetus, which are exactly the situations in which the estimate is being used. [VERIFY: current stated error margins for estimated fetal weight formulas, and any formula-specific differences]

Plotting and serial assessment

The percentile matters more than the absolute weight, and a single measurement plotted on a chart says less than a trajectory.

Serial measurements require an adequate interval. Repeating biometry too soon means the change measured is smaller than the measurement error, producing meaningless growth velocities and — worse — false reassurance or false alarm. [VERIFY: current minimum recommended interval between growth scans]

Growth velocity — the change in percentile or in absolute size over time — is more informative than a single point, and it is what distinguishes a small fetus growing normally from one that is falling away.

The distinction that organises everything after this

	Small for gestational age	**Fetal growth restriction**
Nature	**Constitutionally small** — reaching its own growth potential	**Pathological** — failing to reach its potential
Growth velocity	Normal, tracking along a centile	**Falling across centiles**
Doppler	Normal	Frequently abnormal
Amniotic fluid	Normal	May be reduced
Risk	Near-background	**Substantially increased stillbirth and morbidity**

Not every small fetus is compromised, and not every compromised fetus is small — a growth-restricted fetus can have a weight above the 10th centile if its potential was higher. This is why definitions combine size with velocity and Doppler (§19.4).

19.4 Growth Restriction and Macrosomia

Defining growth restriction

Contemporary definitions **combine several parameters rather than relying on a weight centile alone**: estimated fetal weight or abdominal circumference below a threshold centile, **growth velocity**, and **Doppler abnormality**, with different combinations applying at different gestations. [VERIFY: the consensus definition of fetal growth restriction to be adopted, with its parameter thresholds for early and late onset]

Early-onset and late-onset restriction behave differently

This distinction is more useful than the older symmetric/asymmetric framing:

Early-onset (before around 32 weeks)

- Usually reflects **significant placental disease**, frequently with **pre-eclampsia**
- **Umbilical artery Doppler is typically abnormal** and provides the surveillance signal
- Deterioration follows a **recognisable sequence** (§19.5), allowing timed intervention
- Higher perinatal mortality, but more predictable

Late-onset (from around 32 weeks)

- Milder placental disease
- **Umbilical artery Doppler is often normal**, which is the trap — a normal umbilical artery does not exclude late-onset restriction
- **Middle cerebral artery Doppler and the cerebroplacental ratio are more sensitive**
- Less predictable deterioration, and it accounts for a large share of the stillbirth burden precisely because it is harder to detect

The traditional symmetric versus asymmetric framing remains useful as a pointer: **asymmetric restriction with a disproportionately small abdominal circumference** suggests placental insufficiency with head sparing, while **symmetric smallness** raises the possibility of an early insult, aneuploidy, infection, or a constitutionally small fetus.

Assessment

Biometry with growth velocity; **Doppler** (§19.5); **amniotic fluid** (§19.10); **biophysical profile** where indicated (§19.6); a review of the **anatomy** for anomalies and markers of infection; and assessment of the **placenta**.

Macrosomia

Defined by an estimated weight above a centile threshold or above an absolute weight. [VERIFY: current definitions of macrosomia and large for gestational age]

Associations: maternal **diabetes** — pre-existing or gestational — obesity, excessive gestational weight gain, prior macrosomic infant, and post-term pregnancy.

Diabetic macrosomia has a characteristic pattern: disproportionate growth with an **increased abdominal circumference relative to head circumference**, **increased subcutaneous fat**, organomegaly, and **polyhydramnios**.

Risks: shoulder dystocia and birth injury, operative delivery, and neonatal hypoglycaemia.

> **The error in estimated fetal weight is greatest in the largest fetuses**, which is precisely where the number is used to decide mode of delivery. This limitation must be stated explicitly when reporting a macrosomic estimate.

19.5 Umbilical, Middle Cerebral, and Uterine Artery Doppler

Umbilical artery — placental resistance

Technique: sample a **free loop of cord**, in the absence of fetal breathing movements, with the angle as low as achievable. **Values differ between the free loop, the placental end and the fetal abdominal end**, so the sampling site must be consistent and stated.

The progression, in order of severity:

1. **Raised pulsatility index** — increased placental resistance

2. **Absent end-diastolic flow**
3. **Reversed end-diastolic flow** — the most severe, associated with a high risk of stillbirth and acidaemia

Absent or reversed end-diastolic flow is a major finding requiring prompt referral, and in the third trimester frequently prompts delivery.

Middle cerebral artery — redistribution and anaemia

Technique: sample in the **proximal third of the vessel near the circle of Willis**, with the beam as close to parallel with flow as possible.

> **Apply no undue transducer pressure on the fetal head.** Compression alters cerebral haemodynamics and falsifies the measurement — a specific technical trap in this measurement.

Two entirely separate applications:

Pulsatility index — cerebral redistribution. A **falling** middle cerebral artery pulsatility index indicates **brain sparing**: cerebral vasodilatation preserving perfusion at the expense of other territories. It is a sign of fetal adaptation to hypoxaemia.

Peak systolic velocity — fetal anaemia. An **elevated** peak systolic velocity, expressed in multiples of the median for gestation, indicates **fetal anaemia** — reduced viscosity increases velocity. This is the **key non-invasive test for fetal anaemia**, used in red cell alloimmunisation, parvovirus infection, and twin anaemia–polycythaemia sequence, and it has largely replaced invasive testing for surveillance. [VERIFY: current multiple-of-median thresholds for middle cerebral artery peak systolic velocity in fetal anaemia]

Cerebroplacental ratio — the middle cerebral artery pulsatility index divided by that of the umbilical artery. It falls when the brain is spared and placental resistance rises, and is **more sensitive than either vessel alone, particularly in late-onset growth restriction**.

Ductus venosus — cardiac decompensation

The **a-wave**, corresponding to atrial contraction, is the measurement of interest.

Absent or reversed a-wave indicates raised central venous pressure and **cardiac decompensation**. It is a **late and ominous sign**, and in early-onset growth restriction it is a principal trigger for delivery.

Uterine artery — the maternal side

Sampled in the first or second trimester, assessing the maternal uteroplacental circulation.

Raised pulsatility index and persistent early diastolic notching predict **pre-eclampsia and growth restriction**, and uterine artery Doppler is incorporated into first-trimester pre-eclampsia screening algorithms alongside maternal factors, blood pressure and biochemical markers. [VERIFY: current uterine artery Doppler thresholds and the composition of the screening algorithm to be described]

The sequence of deterioration

In **early-onset** growth restriction the changes typically progress in a recognisable order, which is what makes timed intervention possible:

> **Raised umbilical artery PI → absent end-diastolic flow → middle cerebral artery redistribution → reversed end-diastolic flow → abnormal ductus venosus a-wave → umbilical vein pulsations**

The sequence is typical, not invariable, and it does not apply to late-onset restriction, where deterioration is less orderly and the umbilical artery may remain normal throughout.

Safety: all of this is spectral Doppler, the highest-output mode. Use the obstetric preset, keep traces short, and observe the exposure discipline of Chapter 18 §18.3.

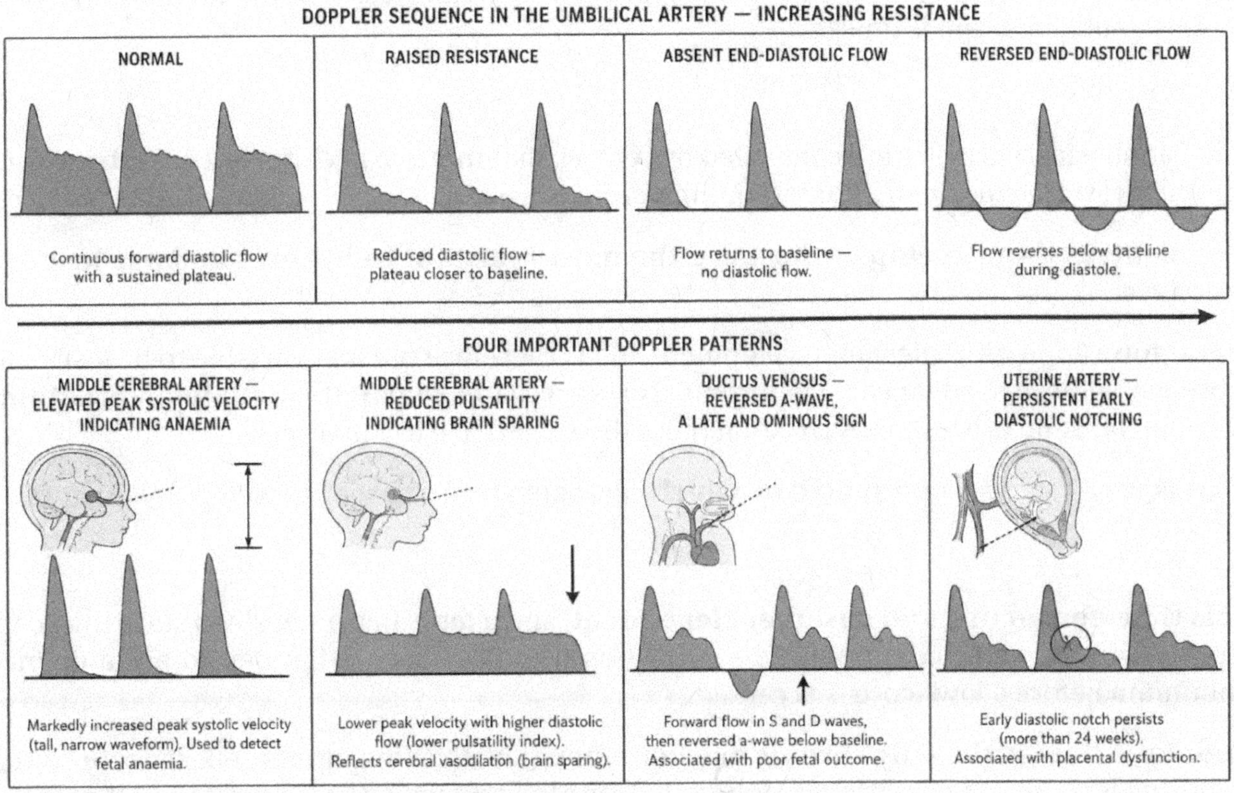

19.6 Biophysical Profile and Fetal Well-Being

The components

The biophysical profile scores five variables, each as present or absent, within a defined observation period:

Variable	Scored present when
Fetal breathing movements	Sustained rhythmic breathing episodes are observed

Variable	Scored present when
Gross body movements	A defined number of discrete body or limb movements occur
Fetal tone	An episode of active extension with return to flexion, or opening and closing of a hand
Amniotic fluid volume	An adequate pocket is present (§19.10)
Non-stress test (cardiotocography)	The trace is reactive

[VERIFY: current biophysical profile scoring criteria, observation period, score interpretation and associated management recommendations]

The modified biophysical profile combines the non-stress test with amniotic fluid assessment alone, and is quicker.

The physiological logic

The biophysical variables are controlled by centres that **mature at different gestations**, and they are lost to hypoxia in a corresponding order.

> **Centres that develop earliest are the most resistant to hypoxia and are lost last.**

Fetal tone appears earliest in development and is therefore the **last** variable to be lost — its absence indicates advanced compromise. **Heart rate reactivity and fetal breathing** develop late and are lost early, making them the sensitive early markers.

This is why a score is interpreted by **which** components are absent as well as by the total.

Limitations

It is time-consuming and observer-dependent, and a fetus in a quiet sleep state can score poorly without being compromised — which is why the observation period has a defined minimum before a low score is accepted.

Amniotic fluid is the only chronic marker among the five; the others reflect acute status. A profile is therefore interpreted **alongside Doppler and growth**, not instead of them.

Interpreting the score

The total score directs management, but two refinements matter more than the number alone:

Which components are absent. A score reduced only by an unreactive trace in an otherwise vigorous fetus is a different clinical situation from the same score produced by absent tone in a fetus with normal reactivity. **Absent tone indicates advanced compromise** and is not reassuring at any total.

Whether amniotic fluid is the deficient component. Because fluid is the chronic marker, **oligohydramnios with an otherwise normal profile indicates established placental insufficiency**, and it warrants escalation even when the acute variables are intact.

[VERIFY: current score bands and the management recommendation attached to each]

The relationship with other tests

Cardiotocography contributes the reactivity component and is the element most often performed independently. **Computerised analysis of short-term variation** is used in specialist units, particularly in preterm growth restriction, where visual interpretation of the trace is least reliable.

The contraction stress test — assessing the fetal heart rate response to induced uterine activity — is now rarely used, having been largely displaced by Doppler and the biophysical profile.

Doppler and the biophysical profile answer different questions. Doppler assesses the **placental circulation and fetal cardiovascular adaptation**, and it becomes abnormal comparatively early. The biophysical profile assesses **current central nervous system function**, and it deteriorates later.

> **In early-onset growth restriction, Doppler leads and the biophysical profile follows.** A normal profile does not override reversed umbilical artery end-diastolic flow, and a deteriorating profile in the presence of already abnormal Doppler indicates late compromise.

Practical limitations

Fetal sleep cycles produce transiently absent breathing and reduced movement, which is why the observation period has a defined minimum before a low score is accepted.

Maternal factors — sedative or opioid medication, smoking, hypoglycaemia, and corticosteroids given for fetal lung maturation — all transiently reduce biophysical activity, and **corticosteroid administration in particular is a recognised and temporary cause of a reduced score** that should not itself prompt delivery.

Gestation matters. Below the gestation at which heart rate reactivity normally develops, an unreactive trace is a maturational finding rather than a pathological one.

19.7 The Placenta: Anatomy, Variants, and Pathology

Normal appearance

A homogeneous, moderately echogenic structure with a smooth **chorionic plate** on the fetal side and a **retroplacental hypoechoic zone** between it and the myometrium — a normal interface whose **loss is a key sign in the accreta spectrum** (§19.8).

Placental thickness is assessed at the mid-portion, perpendicular to the myometrium. **A thick placenta** occurs in diabetes, hydrops, fetal anaemia, infection and triploidy; **a thin placenta** in pre-eclampsia and growth restriction.

Placental grading by calcification is of limited clinical value and is no longer widely used for management.

Variants

Succenturiate lobe — an accessory lobe separate from the main placental mass, connected by vessels. Two consequences: **retained lobe after delivery**, and **vasa previa** if the connecting vessels cross the internal os (§19.9). **Where a succenturiate lobe is found, examine the internal os with colour Doppler.**

Bilobed placenta — two roughly equal lobes.

Circumvallate placenta — the membranes insert inward from the placental edge, producing a rolled, raised margin. Associated with bleeding, abruption and preterm membrane rupture.

Placenta membranacea — a thin placenta covering most of the uterine surface; rare, associated with previa and accreta.

Pathology

Placental abruption — premature separation of the placenta.

> **The critical statement: a normal-appearing placenta does not exclude abruption.** Acute retroplacental haemorrhage is frequently **isoechoic with placental tissue and effectively invisible**; it becomes hypoechoic only as it evolves. Abruption is a **clinical diagnosis**, and ultrasound's role is to detect it when visible and to exclude other causes of bleeding — **not to rule it out**.

Where visible, a retroplacental collection elevates the placenta from the myometrium. Report its size and location, and specifically state that a normal study does not exclude the diagnosis.

Placental lakes — anechoic spaces with slow swirling flow, generally of no significance. **They must be distinguished from the lacunae of accreta spectrum** (§19.8), which are more numerous, irregular and turbulent.

Placental infarcts and **intervillous thrombi** — focal areas of altered echotexture, common and usually incidental unless extensive.

Chorioangioma — a well-defined, **hypervascular** placental mass. Large lesions act as arteriovenous shunts and can cause **polyhydramnios, fetal anaemia, cardiac failure and hydrops** (§19.11), so a placental mass warrants colour Doppler and fetal assessment.

19.8 Placenta Previa and the Accreta Spectrum

Terminology and measurement

The older four-grade classification has been abandoned in favour of two terms defined by the relationship of the placental edge to the internal os:

- **Placenta previa** — the placenta **covers** the internal os
- **Low-lying placenta** — the placental edge lies **within a defined distance of, but does not cover**, the internal os

[VERIFY: the current distance threshold defining a low-lying placenta, and the terminology to be adopted]

Measurement technique:

> **Transvaginal assessment is the standard and it is safe.** The probe is directed toward the cervix and does not need to be advanced against it, and the improved resolution resolves the question in almost every case.

Transabdominal assessment over-diagnoses previa for three reasons: an **overdistended bladder** apposes the anterior and posterior lower segment and falsely elevates the placental edge; a **myometrial contraction** mimics placental tissue; and the **fetal head shadows** the posterior lower segment. **A transabdominal impression of previa should always be confirmed transvaginally.**

Timing: assess at the anatomic survey, then **reassess in the third trimester**, because the lower segment lengthens and most low-lying placentas identified in the mid-trimester resolve. [VERIFY: current recommended timing of reassessment and the management thresholds]

Placenta accreta spectrum

Abnormally adherent or invasive placentation, ranging from adherence to the myometrium through invasion into it and beyond it. **It is a leading cause of massive obstetric haemorrhage and peripartum hysterectomy.**

The risk combination that must trigger a deliberate look:

> **An anterior placenta previa or low-lying placenta in a woman with a previous caesarean section.** The risk rises with the number of prior caesareans, and this combination should prompt targeted assessment in every case.

Other risk factors include prior uterine surgery or curettage, a prior caesarean scar pregnancy (Chapter 18 §18.9), advanced maternal age, and assisted reproduction.

The sonographic signs:

Sign	Description
Loss of the retroplacental clear zone	The normal hypoechoic interface between placenta and myometrium is absent
Myometrial thinning	Residual myometrium reduced to a very thin layer or not identifiable
Placental lacunae	Multiple irregular vascular spaces giving a "moth-eaten" or "Swiss cheese" appearance, with **turbulent flow** — distinguished from benign placental lakes by their number, irregularity and flow character
Bladder wall interruption	Loss of the smooth echogenic bladder–uterine interface, or bulging into the bladder
Placental bulge	Deviation of the uterine contour by placental tissue
Increased subplacental and bridging vascularity	Prominent vessels crossing the placental–myometrial interface and extending toward or into the bladder
Exophytic mass	Placental tissue extending beyond the serosa — percreta

Assessment technique: transabdominal **and** transvaginal, with a **partially filled bladder** to display the interface, using **colour Doppler at a low velocity scale** over the placental–myometrial and vesicouterine interfaces.

> **Prenatal diagnosis transforms outcome.** A planned delivery in a specialist centre, with an experienced multidisciplinary team, blood products available and a defined surgical plan, produces dramatically less morbidity than an unanticipated accreta encountered at caesarean. This is the same principle as prenatal detection of duct-dependent cardiac disease in Chapter 15 §15.10.

Where the diagnosis is suspected, **escalate to specialist assessment** rather than reporting the individual signs and leaving them to be assembled by someone else.

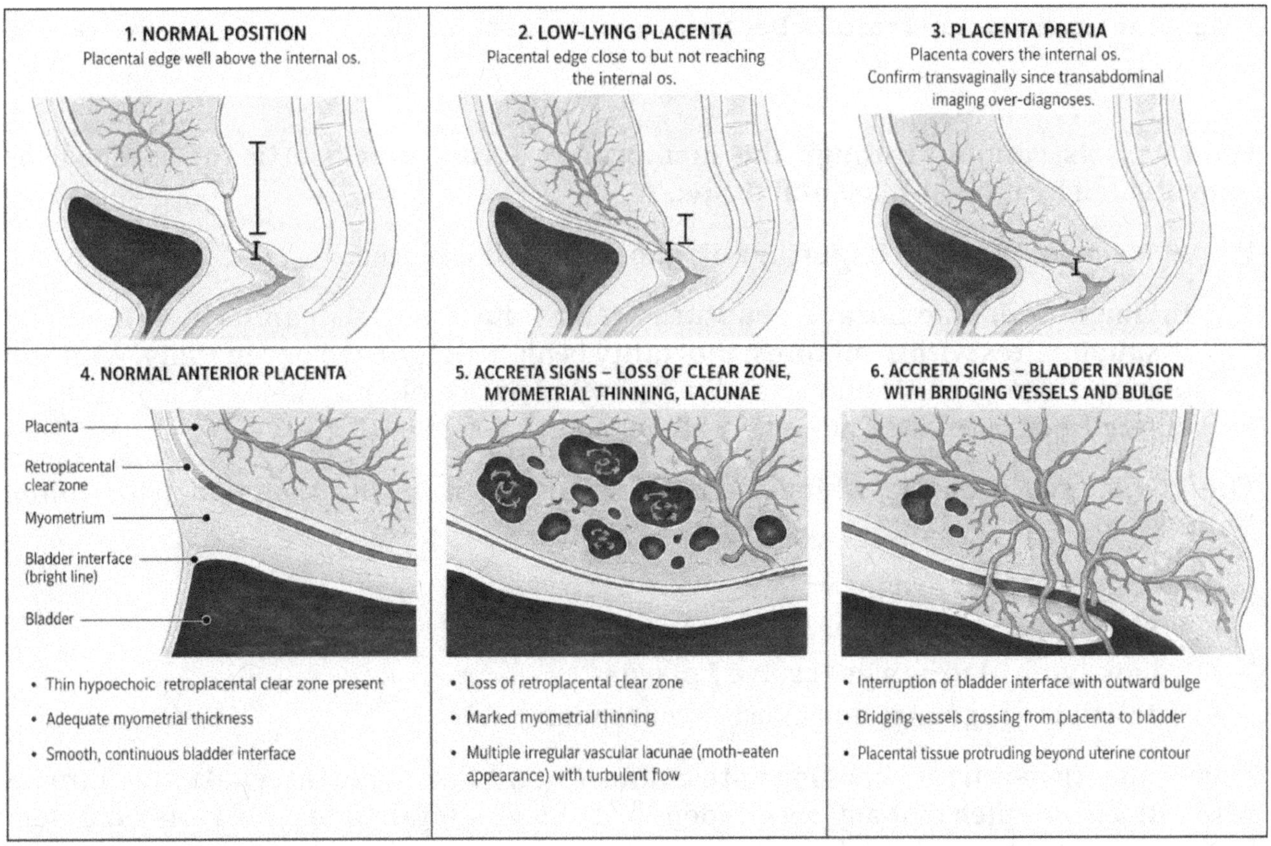

19.9 The Umbilical Cord

Vessel number

The normal cord contains **two arteries and one vein** within Wharton's jelly.

The standard technique for counting is not a transverse view of a free loop, which can mislead: **apply colour Doppler in a transverse view of the fetal pelvis and identify the two umbilical arteries coursing around either side of the bladder.** This is quick, reliable, and should be part of the routine survey.

Single umbilical artery is associated with an increased incidence of **other structural anomalies — particularly renal and cardiac — with aneuploidy, and with growth restriction.**

Where a single umbilical artery is found: perform a detailed anatomical review, and arrange **growth surveillance**, since even an isolated single umbilical artery carries a modestly increased risk of growth restriction. [VERIFY: current recommendations for surveillance following isolated single umbilical artery]

Insertion sites

Placental insertion is described as central, eccentric, **marginal (battledore)** — at the placental edge — or **velamentous**, in which the cord inserts into the membranes and the vessels run **unprotected by Wharton's jelly** before reaching the placenta.

Velamentous insertion matters because of what it can cause.

Vasa previa

Fetal vessels running through the membranes across or close to the internal os, unprotected by cord or placental tissue.

Why it is one of the most important diagnoses in this chapter:

> **Undiagnosed, membrane rupture tears the vessels and the fetus exsanguinates within minutes; mortality is high. Diagnosed antenatally, with planned caesarean before labour, survival is excellent.** Almost the entire difference in outcome is made by whether someone looked.

The at-risk situations in which the internal os must be interrogated with colour Doppler:

- **Velamentous cord insertion**
- **Succenturiate or bilobed placenta** (§19.7)
- **Low-lying placenta or resolved previa**
- **Multiple pregnancy** and assisted conception

Technique: transvaginal imaging with colour Doppler over the internal os, confirming with **pulsed Doppler** that any vessel identified shows a **fetal arterial waveform** at fetal heart rate — distinguishing it from a maternal vessel.

Other cord findings

Cord cysts — common early and usually resolving; persistent or multiple cysts warrant anatomical review.

True knots, **hypercoiling and hypocoiling**, and **nuchal cord** — the last is common and usually of no significance, and should be reported with proportion rather than alarm.

Abdominal wall insertion — assessed during the survey for abdominal wall defects (Chapter 20).

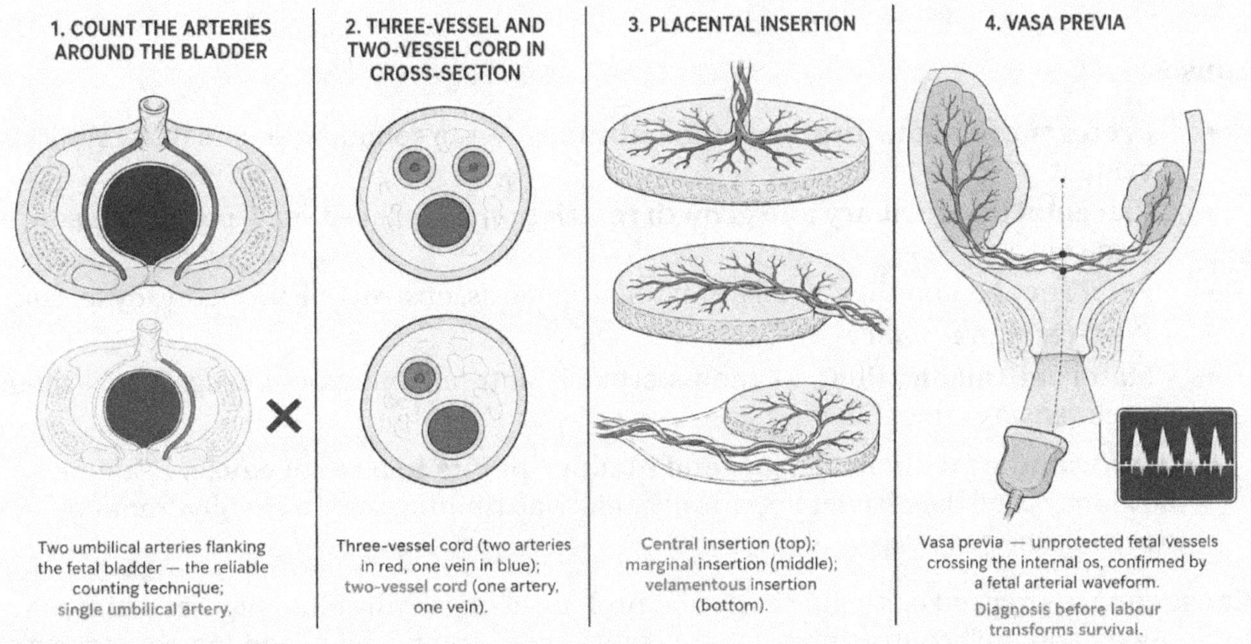

19.10 Amniotic Fluid Assessment

Physiology

After the first trimester, amniotic fluid is predominantly **fetal urine**, with a contribution from lung fluid, and it is removed by **fetal swallowing** and absorption.

This single fact organises the differential: reduced fluid points toward reduced production (renal or placental) or loss (membrane rupture); increased fluid points toward impaired swallowing or increased production.

Measurement

Amniotic fluid index — the sum of the deepest vertical pocket in each of four quadrants, with the transducer held **perpendicular to the floor** and aligned to the maternal sagittal axis.

Single deepest pocket — the deepest vertical pocket free of cord and fetal parts, meeting a minimum width requirement.

> **Current guidance favours the single deepest pocket**, because the amniotic fluid index **over-diagnoses oligohydramnios**, leading to more inductions and caesareans without demonstrable benefit to the fetus. [VERIFY: current preferred method, threshold values for oligohydramnios and polyhydramnios, and the evidence position]

Exclude cord loops from the measured pocket — colour Doppler confirms this and is a small step that prevents a systematic overestimate.

Oligohydramnios

Causes:

- **Preterm prelabour rupture of membranes** — the commonest, and often clinically evident
- **Placental insufficiency and growth restriction** — reduced renal perfusion reduces urine output
- **Fetal renal anomalies** — bilateral renal agenesis, obstructive uropathy, dysplasia
- **Post-term pregnancy**
- **Maternal medication** — non-steroidal anti-inflammatory drugs and renin-angiotensin system inhibitors

Anhydramnios with an absent fetal bladder points to a renal cause. Examine the kidneys and the bladder specifically before attributing severe oligohydramnios to membrane rupture.

Consequences depend on timing: early and prolonged oligohydramnios causes **pulmonary hypoplasia** and limb contractures; later, it causes cord compression and increases the risk of fetal distress.

Polyhydramnios

Causes:

- **Maternal diabetes**
- **Impaired swallowing** — oesophageal or duodenal atresia (the "double bubble"), other gastrointestinal obstruction, and neurological or neuromuscular conditions
- **Fetal anaemia and hydrops** (§19.11)
- **Twin-to-twin transfusion syndrome** in the recipient sac
- **Chorioangioma** (§19.7)
- **Idiopathic** — a substantial proportion

When polyhydramnios is found, look for a cause: review the swallowing pathway and the stomach, examine the heart, assess for hydrops, and measure the **middle cerebral artery peak systolic velocity** for anaemia (§19.5).

Consequences: preterm labour, malpresentation, cord prolapse at membrane rupture, and postpartum haemorrhage.

19.11 Fetal Membranes and Hydrops

Membranes

Chorioamniotic separation is normal before the membranes fuse in the early second trimester; **persisting or new separation later** is abnormal, and occurs after invasive procedures.

Amniotic band sequence — fibrous bands adherent to the fetus, producing **asymmetric, non-anatomical defects**: limb constriction rings or amputations, atypical facial clefts, and abdominal wall defects that do not conform to the usual patterns.

The discriminator from a benign band: a **uterine synechia** is a thick band with a free edge that the fetus moves freely around, causing no deformity, whereas an amniotic band is attached to the fetus and produces deformity.

Preterm prelabour rupture of membranes — ultrasound shows reduced fluid, but **the defect itself is not visible** and the diagnosis is clinical and biochemical.

Chorioamnionitis — intrauterine infection — is likewise a clinical and laboratory diagnosis. Ultrasound contributes supporting findings rather than confirmation: reduced fluid, **amniotic fluid sludge** near the internal os (§19.13), a short cervix, and — late — fetal tachycardia and reduced biophysical activity.

Uterine fibroids enlarge in pregnancy and may undergo **red degeneration**, presenting with acute pain (Chapter 17 §17.6). A fibroid in the lower segment is documented because of its implications for delivery.

Hydrops fetalis

Defined by abnormal fluid accumulation in two or more compartments:

- **Ascites**
- **Pleural effusion**
- **Pericardial effusion**
- **Skin oedema**

Frequently accompanied by placentomegaly and polyhydramnios, both of which should be documented.

The aetiological division:

Immune hydrops — red cell alloimmunisation causing fetal anaemia. Now less common where anti-D prophylaxis is available, but other antibodies persist.

Non-immune hydrops accounts for the large majority, and its causes group as:

Group	Examples
Cardiac	Structural disease, arrhythmia (Chapter 15 §15.8), cardiomyopathy
Chromosomal	Turner syndrome, trisomy 21 and others
Infection	**Parvovirus B19** (causing anaemia), cytomegalovirus, syphilis, toxoplasmosis
Thoracic	Congenital lung malformation, diaphragmatic hernia, effusions
Anaemia	Alpha thalassaemia — a major cause in populations where it is prevalent — and fetomaternal haemorrhage

Group	Examples
Twin-related	Twin-to-twin transfusion, twin anaemia–polycythaemia sequence
Tumours and vascular	Sacrococcygeal teratoma, chorioangioma, vascular malformations
Metabolic	Lysosomal storage disorders

The investigation is structured, and ultrasound leads it:

1. **Middle cerebral artery peak systolic velocity** — because **anaemia is the treatable cause** and intrauterine transfusion can reverse the hydrops
2. **Detailed anatomical survey and fetal echocardiography** including rhythm assessment
3. **Maternal antibody screen, infection serology, and testing for fetomaternal haemorrhage**
4. **Karyotype and microarray**

Identifying anaemia is the priority, because it converts an often-fatal condition into a treatable one. Measure the middle cerebral artery peak systolic velocity in every case of hydrops.

The treatable causes

Structuring the investigation around treatability is what makes it useful, because several causes have specific and effective interventions:

Cause	Intervention
Fetal anaemia — alloimmunisation, parvovirus, fetomaternal haemorrhage	**Intrauterine transfusion**, which can reverse hydrops completely
Fetal tachyarrhythmia	**Maternal antiarrhythmic therapy** (Chapter 15 §15.8)
Twin-to-twin transfusion syndrome	**Fetoscopic laser ablation** of the placental anastomoses
Large pleural effusion or lung lesion	**Thoracoamniotic shunting** or drainage
Chorioangioma	Interventional ablation in selected cases

Prognosis in non-immune hydrops is poor overall and depends heavily on the cause and the gestation at onset, which is why establishing an aetiology promptly matters more than characterising the fluid distribution in detail.

Reporting hydrops

Document **which compartments are involved and the severity of each**, the **placental thickness**, the **amniotic fluid volume**, the **middle cerebral artery peak systolic velocity**, the **cardiac assessment including rhythm**, and any structural abnormality identified.

Serial assessment tracks response to treatment, and the same measurements must be reproduced each time (Chapter 1 §1.5).

19.12 High-Risk Pregnancy: Maternal Conditions and Surveillance

Diabetes

Pre-existing diabetes carries an increased risk of **structural anomaly** — cardiac defects, neural tube defects, and caudal regression — making a **detailed anatomical survey and fetal echocardiography** standard.

Later in pregnancy, both pre-existing and gestational diabetes are associated with **macrosomia with a disproportionate abdominal circumference** (§19.4), **polyhydramnios**, and an increased **late stillbirth** risk, driving serial growth and surveillance.

Hypertensive disease

Pre-eclampsia and chronic hypertension produce **placental insufficiency**: growth restriction, oligohydramnios, abnormal umbilical artery Doppler, and an increased risk of **abruption**.

Uterine artery Doppler (§19.5) contributes to first-trimester risk prediction, and identified high-risk women enter serial growth and Doppler surveillance.

Maternal obesity

A technical rather than a pathological problem, and an under-acknowledged one. Anomaly detection rates fall substantially with increasing maternal body mass index.

The correct response is technique escalation and honest reporting: lower frequency, harmonic imaging, alternative windows including the umbilicus and suprapubic region, repositioning, and — where the survey remains incomplete — **a stated limitation and an arranged re-scan** rather than an unqualified normal report.

Autoimmune disease

Anti-Ro and anti-La antibodies carry a risk of **fetal complete heart block** (Chapter 15 §15.8), requiring rhythm surveillance during the vulnerable gestational window.

Antiphospholipid syndrome and lupus are associated with growth restriction, pre-eclampsia and loss, driving serial growth and Doppler assessment.

Previous caesarean section

Three specific assessments: **placental location and, if anterior and low, the accreta signs** (§19.8); **the caesarean scar**; and, in early pregnancy, **scar implantation** (Chapter 18 §18.9).

Multiple pregnancy

Surveillance is **determined by chorionicity** (Chapter 18 §18.11), with monochorionic pregnancies scanned substantially more frequently to detect **twin-to-twin transfusion syndrome** — staged by amniotic fluid discordance, bladder visibility, Doppler abnormality, hydrops and demise — and **twin anaemia–polycythaemia sequence**, detected by **discordant middle cerebral artery peak systolic velocities**. [VERIFY: current twin-to-twin transfusion staging system and surveillance intervals by chorionicity]

Infection and alloimmunisation

Congenital infection — cytomegalovirus, toxoplasmosis, parvovirus, Zika and syphilis — produces findings including growth restriction, intracranial calcification and ventriculomegaly (Chapter 13 §13.6), hepatosplenomegaly, and hydrops.

Red cell alloimmunisation is surveilled with **serial middle cerebral artery peak systolic velocity**, which has replaced invasive testing and directs the timing of intrauterine transfusion.

Other maternal conditions

Thyroid disease. Maternal Graves disease with transplacental passage of stimulating antibodies can produce **fetal thyrotoxicosis** — tachycardia, goitre, growth restriction and cardiac failure — while antithyroid medication can cause **fetal hypothyroidism with goitre**. A fetal goitre is visible as a symmetrical anterior neck mass, and its vascularity helps distinguish the hyperthyroid from the hypothyroid state.

Renal disease and chronic hypertension carry a substantially increased risk of growth restriction and pre-eclampsia, driving serial growth and Doppler surveillance from the mid-trimester.

Thrombophilia and antiphospholipid syndrome are associated with placental insufficiency, growth restriction and loss.

Intrahepatic cholestasis of pregnancy is a biochemical diagnosis, and ultrasound has no role in confirming it — but the associated stillbirth risk means these pregnancies enter surveillance pathways in which growth and fluid are monitored.

Epilepsy and antiepileptic medication — several agents are teratogenic, with **neural tube defects, cardiac and facial clefting** the principal associations, making a detailed anatomical survey and fetal echocardiography standard.

Substance use — alcohol, tobacco, opioids and stimulants — is associated with growth restriction, abruption and specific anomalies, and warrants growth surveillance.

A previous stillbirth is among the strongest predictors of recurrence, and these pregnancies typically enter intensive surveillance with serial growth, Doppler and fetal movement monitoring.

The principle underlying all of it

High-risk surveillance is not a longer scan; it is a differently targeted one. Each condition predicts a specific set of complications, and the examination is weighted toward them:

- **Anomaly risk** — a detailed anatomical survey and fetal echocardiography, performed early
- **Placental insufficiency risk** — serial growth, Doppler and amniotic fluid
- **Preterm birth risk** — cervical length surveillance (§19.13)
- **Bleeding and abnormal placentation risk** — placental site and accreta assessment (§19.8)

Knowing which of these applies before the patient arrives is what makes the appointment useful, and it is why the referral information matters as much as the images (Chapter 1 §1.3).

19.13 Cervical Length and Preterm Birth Risk

Why it is measured

A short mid-trimester cervix is one of the strongest predictors of spontaneous preterm birth, and — critically — **it identifies a group in whom intervention works**: progesterone, cervical cerclage, or a pessary, depending on the clinical picture and local protocol.

This is a screening measurement that leads to an effective intervention, which is what distinguishes it from measurement for its own sake.

Technique — an audited measurement

> **Transvaginal measurement is the reference standard.** Transabdominal measurement is unreliable — a full bladder artificially lengthens the cervix and apposes its walls — and translabial imaging is a fallback, not an equivalent.

The steps, and the reason for each:

1. **Empty the bladder.** A full bladder lengthens the cervix and can conceal funnelling
2. **Insert the transvaginal probe**, then **withdraw it until the image just blurs, and reapply only enough pressure to restore it**

   Excessive probe pressure is the dominant error. It compresses the cervix and artificially lengthens it, converting a short cervix into a normal-looking one.

3. **Obtain a sagittal view with the whole cervical canal visible**, both the internal and external os identified
4. **Magnify** so the cervix occupies most of the image
5. **Check that the anterior and posterior cervical widths are approximately equal** — marked asymmetry indicates an oblique plane
6. **Measure from the internal os to the external os along the canal.** Where the canal is curved, follow the local convention — either two straight segments or a traced line

7. **Take three measurements over several minutes and report the shortest**, because the cervix changes dynamically during the examination
8. **Apply provocation** — transfundal pressure, a cough, or standing — where a short cervix or funnelling is suspected but not seen at rest

[VERIFY: the current caliper and averaging convention, measurement duration, and the cervical length thresholds triggering intervention]

Funnelling

Dilatation of the internal os with the membranes protruding into the upper canal, progressing through recognised configurations as the process advances from a closed T-shape through Y and V to a U-shape.

> **Report the residual closed cervical length**, not the total length including the funnel. The closed portion is what carries the mechanical function and the predictive value.

Other findings

Amniotic fluid "sludge" — echogenic particulate material near the internal os — is associated with **intra-amniotic infection or inflammation** and with preterm birth, and should be reported when present.

Cerclage — where a suture is in place, document its position and the cervical length above and below it.

Serial surveillance is used in women with a history of spontaneous preterm birth or mid-trimester loss.

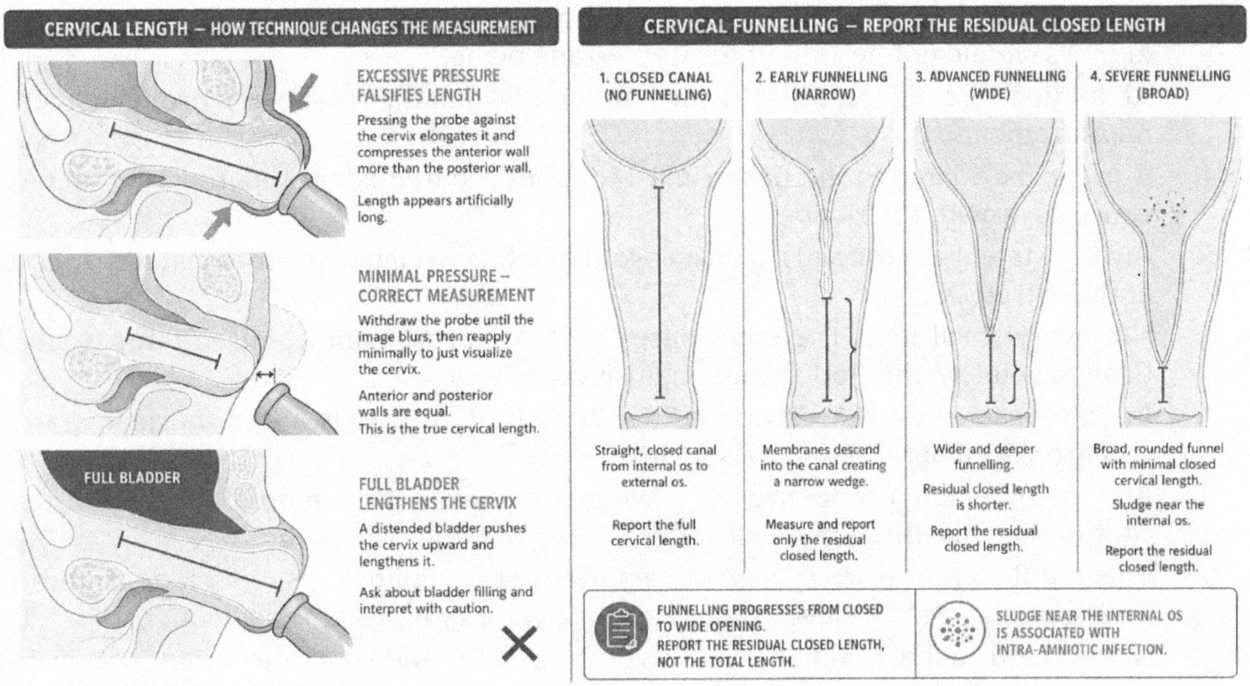

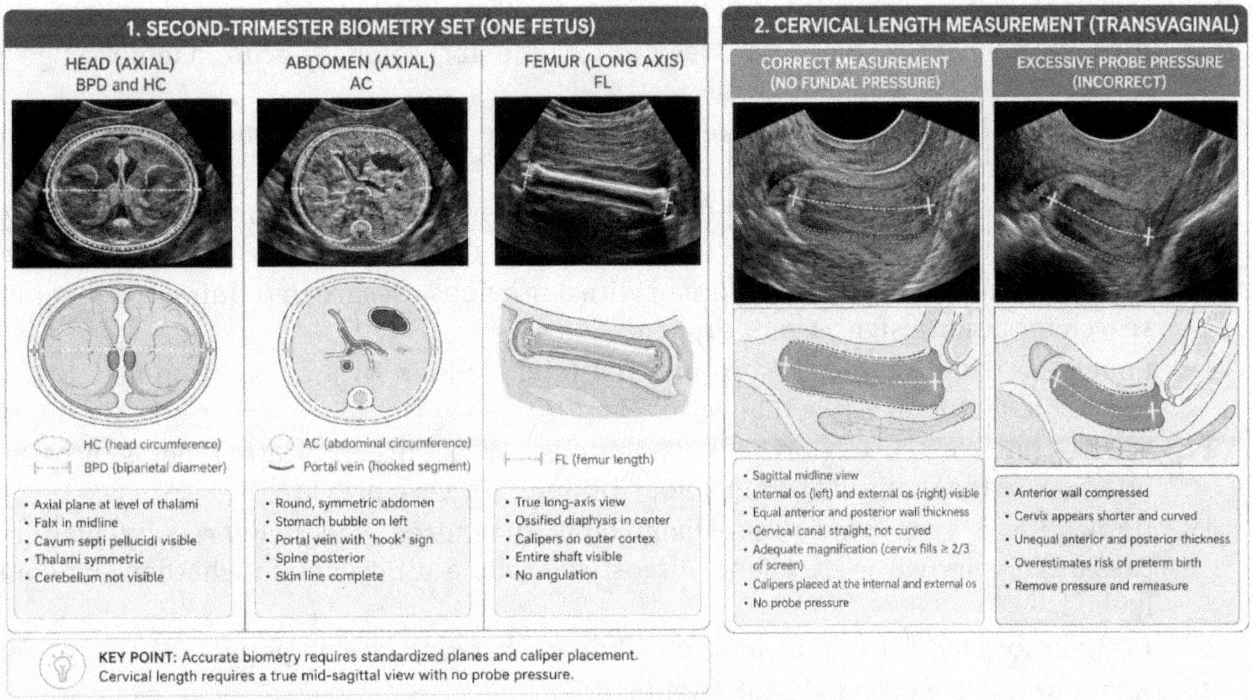

Key Points

1. The anatomic survey is a screening test. Name what could not be seen rather than issuing an unqualified normal report.

2. In the head plane, the cerebellum should not be visible; in the abdominal plane, the kidneys should not be. Both indicate a wrong plane.
3. Abdominal circumference is the most influential and the most error-prone biometric measurement.
4. A pregnancy dated in the first trimester is not redated later. Redating a small fetus conceals growth restriction.
5. Always state the error margin on an estimated fetal weight, and note that it is greatest at the extremes.
6. Not every small fetus is compromised, and not every compromised fetus is small. Growth velocity and Doppler distinguish them.
7. In late-onset growth restriction the umbilical artery is often normal — the cerebroplacental ratio is more sensitive.
8. Apply no undue probe pressure when measuring the middle cerebral artery; compression falsifies the result.
9. The middle cerebral artery has two separate uses: a falling pulsatility index indicates brain sparing, and an elevated peak systolic velocity indicates anaemia.
10. A reversed ductus venosus a-wave is a late and ominous sign of cardiac decompensation.
11. In the biophysical profile, the earliest-developing centres are the most hypoxia-resistant, so tone is lost last and heart rate reactivity and breathing are lost first.
12. A normal-appearing placenta does not exclude abruption — acute haemorrhage is frequently isoechoic and invisible.
13. Distinguish benign placental lakes from the numerous, irregular, turbulent lacunae of accreta spectrum.
14. Transabdominal imaging over-diagnoses placenta previa. Confirm transvaginally, which is safe.
15. An anterior low placenta in a woman with a previous caesarean requires a deliberate search for accreta signs, every time.
16. Count the umbilical arteries around the fetal bladder with colour Doppler — it is quicker and more reliable than a free loop.
17. Where the cord insertion is velamentous, or a succenturiate lobe is present, interrogate the internal os with colour Doppler for vasa previa.
18. Undiagnosed vasa previa is usually fatal; diagnosed and delivered by planned caesarean, survival is excellent. Almost the whole difference is whether someone looked.
19. Exclude cord loops from the amniotic fluid pocket with colour Doppler.
20. Anhydramnios with an absent fetal bladder points to a renal cause — examine the kidneys before blaming membrane rupture.
21. When polyhydramnios is found, look for a cause: the swallowing pathway, the heart, hydrops, and anaemia.
22. An amniotic band is attached to the fetus and causes deformity; a uterine synechia has a free edge and the fetus moves around it.

23. Measure the middle cerebral artery peak systolic velocity in every case of hydrops, because anaemia is the treatable cause.
24. In maternal obesity, escalate technique and report the limitation. Detection rates fall and an unqualified normal report is misleading.
25. Excessive transvaginal probe pressure artificially lengthens the cervix and is the dominant error in cervical length measurement. Take three measurements and report the shortest.
26. Report the residual closed cervical length, not the total length including a funnel.
27. In the biophysical profile, which components are absent matters as much as the total — absent tone indicates advanced compromise at any score.
28. Corticosteroids given for lung maturation transiently reduce biophysical activity, and that reduction should not itself prompt delivery.
29. Doppler and the biophysical profile answer different questions. In early-onset restriction Doppler leads and the profile follows; a normal profile does not override reversed end-diastolic flow.
30. Structure the hydrops investigation around the treatable causes — anaemia, tachyarrhythmia, twin-to-twin transfusion and effusions all have specific interventions.
31. High-risk surveillance is a differently targeted scan, not a longer one. Know which complications the condition predicts before the patient arrives.

Registry Check

1. A head circumference is measured in a plane in which the cerebellum is visible. The plane is:

A. Correct **B.** Angled too far posteriorly, and the measurement is invalid **C.** Angled too far anteriorly **D.** Correct if the falx is also seen

> **Answer: B.** The correct plane for biparietal diameter and head circumference contains the falx, cavum septi pellucidi and thalami, and specifically excludes the cerebellum. Visualisation of the cerebellum indicates a posteriorly angled plane, which distorts both measurements.

2. A fetus dated by first-trimester crown-rump length measures below the 10th centile at 30 weeks. The correct action is to:

A. Redate the pregnancy using current biometry **B.** Retain the original dating and assess growth velocity and Doppler **C.** Repeat the biometry the following day **D.** Report the fetus as appropriately grown for revised dates

> **Answer: B.** A pregnancy dated in the first trimester is never redated. Reassigning dates at 30 weeks would relabel a potentially growth-restricted fetus as normally grown for younger dates, concealing the finding the scan detected. Growth velocity over an adequate interval and Doppler assessment distinguish restriction from constitutional smallness.

3. In late-onset fetal growth restriction, which finding is most sensitive?

A. Reversed umbilical artery end-diastolic flow **B.** Absent ductus venosus a-wave **C.** A reduced cerebroplacental ratio **D.** Umbilical artery pulsatility index above the 95th centile

> **Answer: C.** Umbilical artery Doppler is frequently normal in late-onset restriction, which is the trap. The cerebroplacental ratio, combining middle cerebral artery and umbilical artery indices, detects cerebral redistribution and is more sensitive in this group. Reversed end-diastolic flow and an abnormal ductus venosus are late findings typical of early-onset disease.

4. An elevated middle cerebral artery peak systolic velocity in multiples of the median indicates:

A. Cerebral redistribution **B.** Fetal anaemia **C.** Raised intracranial pressure **D.** Cardiac decompensation

> **Answer: B.** Reduced blood viscosity in anaemia increases flow velocity, and the middle cerebral artery peak systolic velocity is the key non-invasive test for fetal anaemia. Cerebral redistribution is indicated by a fall in the pulsatility index, which is a separate measurement from the same vessel.

5. A woman with two previous caesarean sections has an anterior placenta covering the internal os. Which additional assessment is mandatory?

A. Measurement of cervical length **B.** A deliberate search for signs of placenta accreta spectrum **C.** Umbilical artery Doppler **D.** Amniotic fluid index

> **Answer: B.** Anterior placenta previa with a previous caesarean is the principal risk combination for accreta spectrum, and the risk rises with the number of prior caesareans. Loss of the retroplacental clear zone, myometrial thinning, irregular lacunae with turbulent flow, and bladder wall interruption must be sought specifically, because prenatal diagnosis transforms outcome.

6. A velamentous cord insertion is identified. The additional assessment required is:

A. Serial growth scans only **B.** Colour Doppler interrogation of the internal os for vasa previa **C.** Fetal echocardiography **D.** Amniotic fluid measurement

> **Answer: B.** Velamentous insertion is a principal risk factor for vasa previa, in which unprotected fetal vessels cross the internal os. Undiagnosed, membrane rupture causes fetal exsanguination; diagnosed antenatally with planned caesarean, survival is excellent. Colour Doppler over the internal os, confirmed with a fetal arterial waveform, makes the diagnosis.

7. Severe oligohydramnios is found with no visible fetal bladder on repeated observation. This suggests:

A. Preterm prelabour rupture of membranes **B.** A fetal renal cause **C.** Post-term pregnancy **D.** Maternal dehydration

Answer: B. After the first trimester amniotic fluid is predominantly fetal urine, so anhydramnios with a persistently absent bladder points to a renal cause — bilateral renal agenesis, obstruction, or dysplasia. The kidneys and bladder should be examined specifically before attributing severe oligohydramnios to membrane rupture.

8. During transvaginal cervical length measurement, excessive probe pressure will:

A. Shorten the measured cervix **B.** Lengthen the measured cervix **C.** Have no effect if the plane is sagittal **D.** Produce funnelling artefactually

Answer: B. Compression elongates the cervix and can make a short cervix appear normal, which is the dominant error in this measurement. The probe should be withdrawn until the image blurs and then reapplied with minimal pressure, with three measurements taken over several minutes and the shortest reported.

9. A biophysical profile is performed 12 hours after maternal corticosteroid administration and returns a reduced score, with absent fetal breathing and an unreactive trace. Fetal tone and movement are normal and Doppler is unchanged. The most appropriate interpretation is:

A. Fetal compromise requiring immediate delivery **B.** A recognised transient corticosteroid effect, to be reassessed rather than acted upon in isolation **C.** An invalid study requiring repetition immediately **D.** Evidence of chorioamnionitis

Answer: B. Corticosteroids given for fetal lung maturation transiently reduce biophysical activity, particularly breathing and heart rate reactivity, and this is a recognised and temporary effect. Preserved tone and movement, with unchanged Doppler, argue against acute compromise. The components affected, and the clinical context, matter as much as the total score.

Chapter Notes for the Editorial Pass

Verification queue. In priority order: the **fetal growth restriction consensus definition** with its early and late-onset criteria (§19.4); the **biometric and growth chart standard to be adopted** (§19.2) and the **estimated fetal weight error margins** (§19.3), since together these determine which fetuses are labelled abnormal; the **placenta previa terminology and distance threshold**, and the **timing of reassessment** (§19.8); **middle cerebral artery peak systolic velocity thresholds for anaemia** (§19.5); **amniotic fluid method and thresholds**, including the evidence position favouring single deepest pocket (§19.10); **cervical length thresholds and measurement convention** (§19.13); **biophysical profile scoring and management** (§19.6); **caliper conventions for each biometric measurement** (§19.2); **surveillance recommendations after isolated single umbilical artery** (§19.9); **twin-to-twin transfusion staging and chorionicity-based surveillance intervals** (§19.12); **uterine artery Doppler thresholds and the pre-eclampsia screening algorithm** (§19.5); and **macrosomia definitions** (§19.4).

Chapter size. At thirteen subchapters this is the longest chapter in the book, and §19.6, §19.11 and §19.12 in particular are compressed relative to their clinical weight. If a second edition expands, the natural division is between the fetal assessment material (§19.1–19.6) and the adnexal and maternal material (§19.7–19.13) — the third such split flagged, alongside musculoskeletal in Chapter 11 and the female pelvis in Chapter 17.

Three diagnoses to protect in editing. The chapter's opening frames accreta spectrum, vasa previa and short cervix as the findings where prenatal detection changes outcome most decisively. If space must be recovered during editing, it should not come from §19.8, §19.9 or §19.13.

Figure count: 5 Lane A, 1 Lane B. Lower than the chapter's breadth would suggest, because much of the material — growth definitions, biophysical scoring, maternal conditions — is tabular rather than visual. The Lane B request pairs a full biometry set with a cervical length measurement, and asks additionally for a deliberately over-compressed cervix, which teaches §19.13 better than a schematic can.

Cross-reference targets to fix at layout: §19.1 cardiac sequence → Chapter 15 §15.7; §19.2 first-trimester dating → Chapter 18 §18.6; §19.5 Doppler safety → Chapter 18 §18.3; §19.5 fetal Doppler in the cardiac context → Chapter 15 §15.8; §19.8 caesarean scar pregnancy as precursor → Chapter 18 §18.9; §19.8 prenatal detection principle → Chapter 15 §15.10; §19.11 fetal arrhythmia → Chapter 15 §15.8; §19.11 congenital infection CNS findings → Chapter 13 §13.6; §19.12 chorionicity-based surveillance → Chapter 18 §18.11; §19.13 cervical assessment technique → Chapter 17 §17.3.

Word count: approximately 10,400 excluding image prompt blocks, learning objectives, registry questions, and these notes.

Chapter 20: Fetal Anatomy and Congenital Anomalies

Learning Objectives

On completing this chapter you should be able to:

1. Distinguish screening from diagnosis, and explain why an anomaly must be classified as isolated or non-isolated.
2. Assess the fetal brain in the standard planes and recognise the major malformations.
3. Examine the fetal spine and use the cranial signs that detect open dysraphism.
4. Evaluate the fetal face and neck, and recognise the findings that require airway planning.
5. Recognise diaphragmatic hernia and the principal thoracic lesions, and state what determines prognosis.
6. Distinguish gastroschisis from omphalocele and explain why the distinction matters.
7. Recognise gastrointestinal obstruction and interpret echogenic bowel.
8. Assess the fetal urinary tract and recognise lower urinary tract obstruction.
9. Approach short long bones systematically and identify the measurement that predicts lethality.
10. Interpret soft markers appropriately in the era of cell-free DNA screening.
11. Describe the counselling pathway and the established fetal interventions.

The Last Chapter, and What It Assumes

This chapter completes the book, and it assumes almost all of it. The physics of Chapter 2 determines what can be resolved; the safety discipline of Chapter 1 §1.7 and Chapter 18 §18.3 governs how long you may look; the cardiac sequence of Chapter 15 §15.7 is part of every survey described here; and the ethical framework of Chapter 18 §18.2 governs everything that happens after a finding.

One principle organises the whole chapter:

> **Finding an anomaly is the beginning of the examination, not the end of it.** The prognosis, the aneuploidy risk, the genetic testing offered, and the counselling all depend on whether the finding is **isolated** — and that can only be established by a deliberate, complete search of every other system.

20.1 Principles of Prenatal Diagnosis and Genetic Correlation

Screening and diagnosis are different activities

The anatomic survey is a screening test. Detection rates vary widely by organ system, by anomaly, by gestation, by maternal habitus and by operator, and **some anomalies are simply not detectable at the time the survey is performed**.

Late-manifesting conditions are a specific category worth naming, because a normal mid-trimester survey does not exclude them: **achondroplasia**, some forms of **ventriculomegaly and microcephaly**, **bowel obstruction**, several **cardiac lesions** including coarctation, and progressive renal disease all develop or become apparent after the survey.

The report must not imply that a normal survey excludes structural abnormality, and the counselling that follows a normal scan should reflect that.

Isolated versus non-isolated — the classification that drives everything

When an anomaly is found, the immediate task is to determine whether it stands alone.

	Isolated anomaly	**Non-isolated anomaly**
Aneuploidy risk	Generally lower	**Substantially higher**
Prognosis	Often determined by the lesion itself	Often determined by the associated findings
Genetic testing	Offered according to the specific lesion	**Strongly indicated**
Counselling	Lesion-specific	Syndromic possibilities must be considered

This requires a complete re-survey after any anomaly is identified, including a detailed cardiac assessment, because the heart is the most commonly associated system and cardiac lesions carry the strongest aneuploidy associations.

Genetic correlation

Karyotype identifies aneuploidy and large structural rearrangements.

Chromosomal microarray detects submicroscopic copy number variants and has a **meaningfully higher diagnostic yield than karyotype in structurally abnormal fetuses**, which is why it is now standard in that setting.

Exome sequencing is increasingly offered where a structural anomaly is present and microarray is normal, particularly for skeletal dysplasias and multisystem patterns.

Cell-free DNA screening (Chapter 18 §18.7) is a **screening test for a limited set of conditions**, and it does not exclude the wide range of genetic causes underlying structural anomaly. **A normal cell-free DNA result must not be used to reassure in the presence of a structural abnormality.**

[VERIFY: current recommendations on genetic testing modality by indication, and reported diagnostic yields]

Recurring associations

Certain combinations recur and should prompt a specific search:

Anomaly	Associated aneuploidy
Atrioventricular septal defect, duodenal atresia	Trisomy 21
Clenched hands, choroid plexus cysts, diaphragmatic hernia, omphalocele	Trisomy 18
Holoprosencephaly, midline facial cleft, polydactyly	Trisomy 13
Cystic hygroma, coarctation, hydrops	Turner syndrome
Conotruncal cardiac lesions, thymic hypoplasia	22q11 deletion

Reporting discipline

Describe what you see; do not assign a syndrome. A named syndrome in an ultrasound report becomes the working diagnosis regardless of subsequent testing, and the diagnosis frequently changes. Report the individual findings, note the associations they raise, and escalate to fetal medicine.

Fetal MRI is a valuable adjunct, particularly for the **brain and the posterior fossa**, for thoracic lesions where lung volume matters, and where ultrasound is technically limited.

20.2 The Fetal Neural Axis: Brain

The standard planes and measurements

Three axial planes form the basis of screening:

- **Transventricular** — lateral ventricles, cavum septi pellucidi, choroid plexuses
- **Transthalamic** — the biometry plane (Chapter 19 §19.2)
- **Transcerebellar** — cerebellum, cisterna magna, and the nuchal fold

Measurements: atrial diameter of the lateral ventricle, **transcerebellar diameter**, **cisterna magna** depth, and **nuchal fold** thickness within its gestational window. [VERIFY: current normal ranges for atrial diameter, cisterna magna, transcerebellar diameter and nuchal fold]

Sagittal and coronal planes — obtainable transvaginally when the fetus is cephalic — are required for the corpus callosum and the cerebellar vermis, and a midline sagittal view should be sought whenever a midline abnormality is suspected.

Ventriculomegaly

Defined by the **atrial diameter**, and graded into mild, moderate and severe bands. [VERIFY: current threshold values and grading bands]

It is a finding, not a diagnosis, and the task is to find the cause:

- **Obstructive** — aqueduct stenosis

- **Associated with a malformation** — agenesis of the corpus callosum, open spina bifida with Chiari II, holoprosencephaly
- **Destructive** — haemorrhage, ischaemia, or infection with parenchymal loss
- **Chromosomal**
- **Infective** — cytomegalovirus and toxoplasmosis in particular

Isolated mild ventriculomegaly carries a broad range of outcomes and requires: **detailed anatomical review**, **infection screening**, **genetic testing**, **fetal MRI**, and **serial follow-up** to determine whether it is progressive — progression being the finding that most alters prognosis.

The major malformations

Agenesis of the corpus callosum — the features are set out in Chapter 13 §13.6 and apply prenatally: **absent cavum septi pellucidi**, **colpocephaly** with teardrop-shaped ventricles, a **high-riding third ventricle**, radiating medial sulci, and an abnormal pericallosal artery course.

> **An absent cavum septi pellucidi is the alerting sign**, and it should prompt a deliberate midline sagittal assessment rather than being noted in passing.

Holoprosencephaly — failure of forebrain cleavage, graded alobar, semilobar and lobar, with a **monoventricle and fused thalami** in the severe forms.

> **The face predicts the brain.** Holoprosencephaly is accompanied by a spectrum of midline facial anomalies — **hypotelorism, a single nostril or proboscis, and median cleft** — and finding either the facial or the cerebral abnormality obliges a careful look for the other. Strong association with trisomy 13.

Dandy–Walker continuum — vermian hypoplasia or agenesis with an enlarged posterior fossa communicating with the fourth ventricle, and an elevated tentorium. **The differential — mega cisterna magna, Blake pouch cyst, and arachnoid cyst — is resolved by assessing the vermis**, which requires a midsagittal view.

Chiari II malformation — accompanying open spina bifida, and detected through the cranial signs described in §20.3.

Encephalocele — herniation of meninges and brain through a skull defect, most often occipital. **Look for polydactyly and enlarged echogenic kidneys**, since the combination suggests Meckel–Gruber syndrome.

Acrania and anencephaly — absence of the cranial vault above the orbits, part of a sequence that is **detectable in the first trimester** and is one of the earliest anomalies diagnosable.

Microcephaly — a head circumference below a defined threshold with a sloping forehead. It is frequently **late-manifesting**, and it is a cardinal feature of congenital Zika infection.

Intracranial haemorrhage, porencephaly and schizencephaly — destructive lesions, often with a preceding vascular or infective insult.

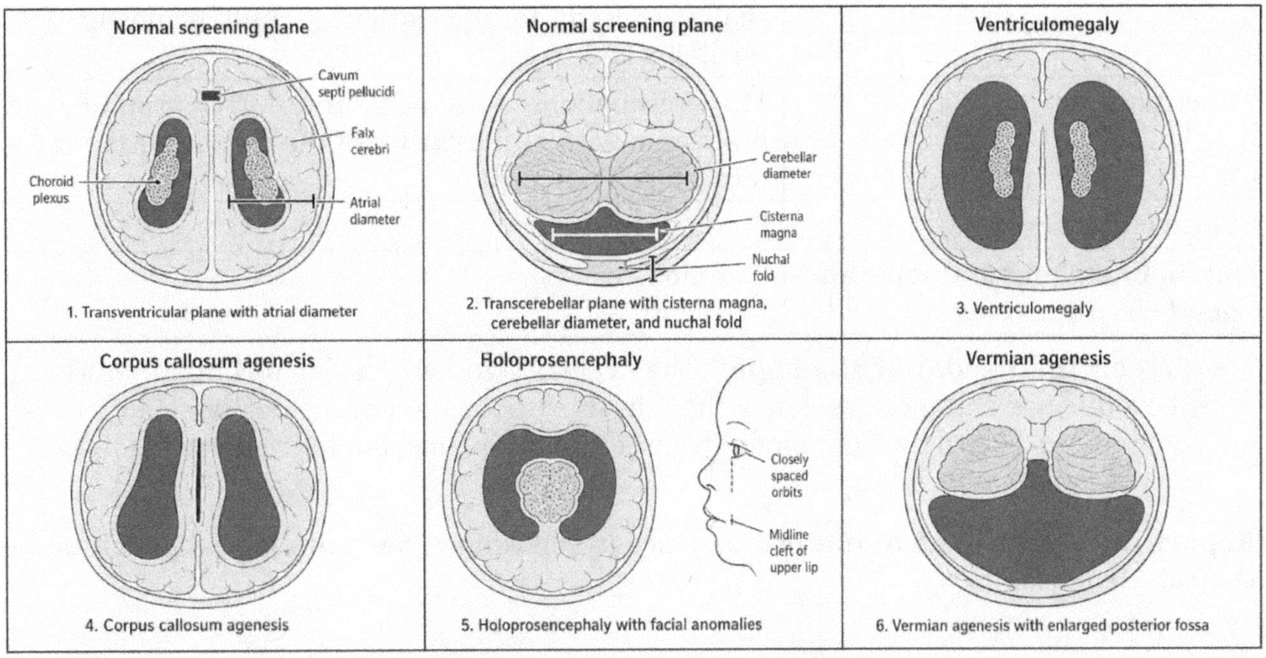

The screening planes and the malformations they detect.

20.3 The Fetal Neural Axis: Spine

Technique

Examine the spine in **three planes**, and do not accept one:

- **Sagittal** — alignment, curvature, and the **continuity of the overlying skin**
- **Coronal** — the parallel lines of the ossification centres, converging normally at the sacrum
- **Transverse** — the **three ossification centres** forming a closed triangle, with intact overlying soft tissue

Sweep the whole spine from the cervical region to the sacrum, and confirm the skin covering along its length.

Open spina bifida

The direct spinal signs:

- **Splaying of the posterior ossification centres** on transverse imaging — the U or V configuration replacing the closed triangle
- **Absence of the overlying skin**
- **A meningeal or meningomyelocele sac**, or a flat lesion with no sac

But the cranial signs are more sensitive, and they are what makes screening work:

Sign	Finding
Lemon sign	Scalloping of the frontal bones, giving the skull a lemon shape. Present in the earlier second trimester and resolving later
Banana sign	The cerebellum wrapped anteriorly around the brainstem with **obliteration of the cisterna magna** — the Chiari II deformity
Ventriculomegaly	Frequently present
Small biparietal diameter and head circumference	Common

> **Screen the head, not the spine.** The cranial signs are easier to obtain, more reproducible, and more sensitive than direct visualisation of the defect — and an obliterated cisterna magna on the transcerebellar plane should trigger a detailed spinal examination every time.

Report the upper level of the lesion, since it determines the neurological deficit and is central to counselling.

Closed dysraphism and other lesions

Closed (skin-covered) dysraphism — lipomyelomeningocele and tethering — is **substantially harder to detect** and is **not accompanied by the Chiari II cranial signs**, so the reassurance provided by a normal posterior fossa does not extend to it.

Sacrococcygeal teratoma — a mass arising from the sacrum, solid, cystic or mixed, classified by the proportion internal versus external. **Highly vascular lesions act as arteriovenous shunts and can cause high-output cardiac failure and hydrops**, so colour Doppler assessment and fetal cardiac surveillance are required. [VERIFY: current classification and prognostic criteria for sacrococcygeal teratoma]

Vertebral anomalies — hemivertebrae, segmentation defects and scoliosis — should prompt a search for the **VACTERL** associations: vertebral, anorectal, cardiac, tracheo-oesophageal, renal and limb.

Caudal regression sequence — absent sacral segments with an abruptly terminating cord, strongly associated with maternal diabetes.

Why prenatal diagnosis matters here

Prenatal repair of open spina bifida improves motor outcome and reduces the need for shunting, compared with postnatal repair, in appropriately selected cases. This makes accurate prenatal detection and prompt referral to a fetal surgical centre directly consequential (§20.11).

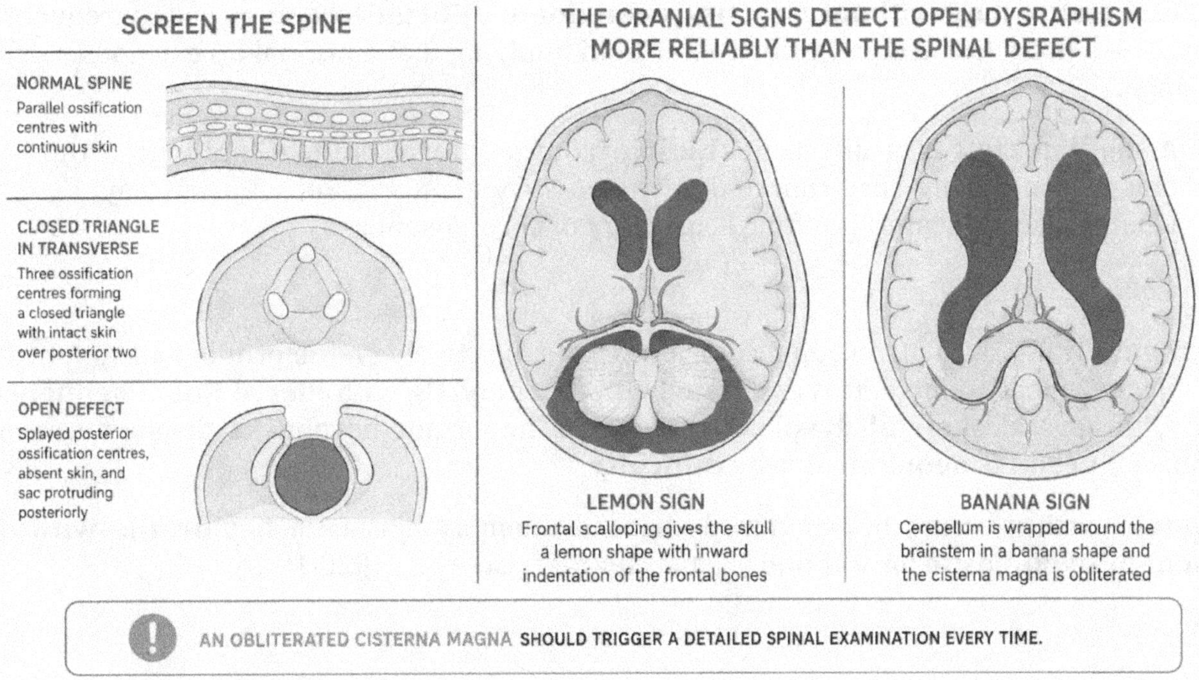

20.4 The Fetal Face and Neck

The planes

Axial — the **orbits**, assessing presence, symmetry, size and separation.

Coronal — the **retronasal triangle** and the upper lip, the plane in which cleft lip is detected.

Midsagittal — the **profile**: forehead, nasal bone, the shape of the jaw, and the relationship of the chin to the lip.

Three-dimensional imaging adds substantially to facial assessment, particularly for clefting and for demonstrating a finding to a parent or a surgical team.

Orbits

Hypotelorism — closely spaced orbits, a cardinal association of **holoprosencephaly** (§20.2).

Hypertelorism, **microphthalmia** and **anophthalmia** occur within syndromic patterns, and a cataract appears as an echogenic lens.

Clefting

Cleft lip with or without cleft palate is detected in the coronal view of the upper lip and confirmed in axial and three-dimensional views. Describe **laterality and extent**, and whether the alveolus is involved.

Isolated cleft palate without cleft lip is genuinely difficult to detect and is frequently missed — a limitation worth stating rather than implying that a normal lip excludes palatal clefting.

> **A median cleft is a different finding from a lateral cleft.** It sits within the holoprosencephaly spectrum and carries a strong association with trisomy 13, whereas isolated lateral clefting is usually not chromosomal.

The profile

Micrognathia — a small, receding chin, assessed subjectively on the profile and supported by objective measurement. It is associated with **trisomy 18**, with **Pierre Robin sequence**, and with several **skeletal dysplasias**, and it is important beyond its diagnostic value because it **predicts neonatal airway difficulty**.

Frontal bossing occurs in achondroplasia and other dysplasias; a **flat profile with an absent or hypoplastic nasal bone** is a marker for trisomy 21 (§20.10).

Neck masses

The differential is short and the management implications differ sharply:

Mass	Features
Cystic hygroma	**Posterior, septated**, often extending down the back; associated with **Turner syndrome**, other aneuploidy, and hydrops
Goitre	**Symmetrical, anterior, bilobed**, in the context of maternal thyroid disease or antithyroid medication (Chapter 19 §19.12). May cause hyperextension of the neck and polyhydramnios
Teratoma	Heterogeneous, often with **calcification** and cystic areas, usually anterior or lateral
Lymphatic malformation	Multiloculated, transspatial

> **Any large neck mass raises the question of neonatal airway obstruction**, and this changes delivery planning fundamentally. Where the airway is likely to be compromised, delivery is planned in a centre able to perform an **ex utero intrapartum treatment (EXIT) procedure** — securing the airway while placental circulation is maintained (§20.11).

Assess and report the **mass dimensions, its relationship to the airway, the position of the trachea, whether the neck is hyperextended, and the amniotic fluid volume**, since polyhydramnios suggests impaired swallowing.

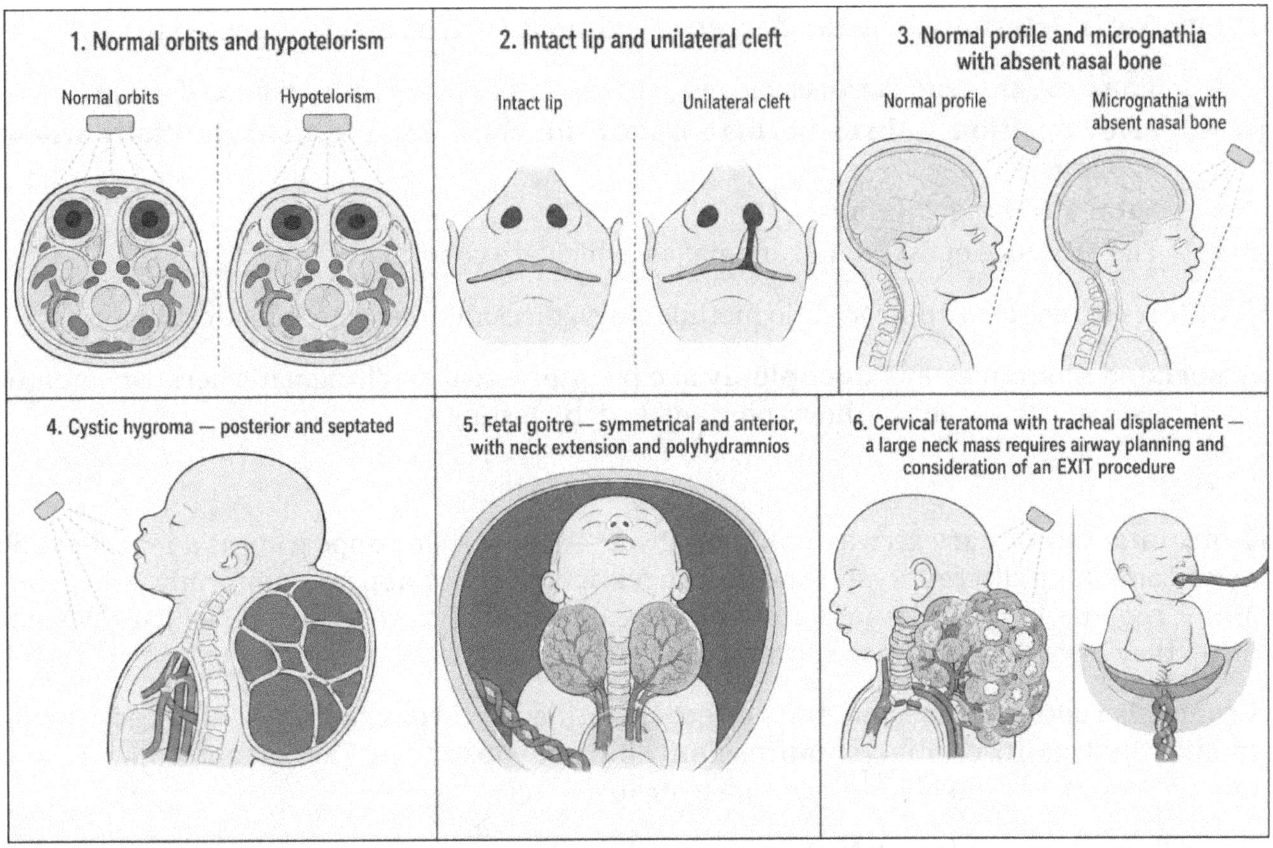

20.5 The Fetal Thorax and Diaphragm

Normal appearances

The lungs are **homogeneous and slightly more echogenic than the liver**, filling the thorax around a heart that occupies roughly a third of the chest area. **The diaphragm** appears as a smooth hypoechoic curved line separating thorax from abdomen, best seen in a sagittal or coronal plane.

Congenital diaphragmatic hernia

The key observation:

> **Abdominal contents visible at the same axial level as the heart.** In the four-chamber view, the presence of stomach or bowel alongside the heart is the finding that makes the diagnosis, and it is why the cardiac plane detects diaphragmatic hernia.

Supporting findings: mediastinal shift away from the lesion, **absence of the stomach bubble in its normal abdominal position**, loss of the smooth diaphragmatic line, and peristalsis within the thorax.

Left-sided hernias are commoner; right-sided hernias are harder to detect because herniated liver is close in echogenicity to lung.

Prognosis is determined by the degree of pulmonary hypoplasia, assessed by:

- **The lung-to-head ratio**, usually expressed as an observed-to-expected value
- **Liver position — liver herniated into the chest carries a substantially worse prognosis**
- **Fetal MRI lung volume**
- The presence of associated anomalies, which are common

[VERIFY: current lung-to-head ratio methodology, thresholds and prognostic categories]

Associated anomalies and aneuploidy are frequent, so a diaphragmatic hernia mandates a full re-survey, fetal echocardiography, and genetic testing.

Lung lesions

Congenital pulmonary airway malformation — a lung lesion appearing as a **macrocystic** mass containing discrete cysts, or a **microcystic** mass that appears uniformly echogenic. **Many regress or become less conspicuous** during the third trimester, which does not mean they have resolved anatomically.

Prognosis relates to size and mass effect, quantified by a volume ratio, with the risk being **mediastinal shift, cardiac compression and hydrops**. [VERIFY: current volume ratio methodology and thresholds predicting hydrops]

Bronchopulmonary sequestration — an echogenic lung mass which can look identical to a microcystic malformation on greyscale.

> **The discriminator is vascular: a sequestration has a systemic arterial supply arising from the aorta.** Colour Doppler demonstrating a feeding vessel from the descending aorta makes the diagnosis, and it should be sought in every echogenic lung lesion.

Congenital high airway obstruction sequence — laryngeal or tracheal atresia producing **bilaterally enlarged, uniformly echogenic lungs**, **flattened or everted diaphragms**, dilated airways below the obstruction, and hydrops. It requires **EXIT delivery planning**.

Pleural effusion — unilateral or bilateral, primary (chylothorax) or secondary to hydrops (Chapter 19 §19.11). Large effusions cause mediastinal shift and lung compression and may be treated by **thoracoamniotic shunting** (§20.11).

Pulmonary hypoplasia is the final common pathway of several conditions — prolonged oligohydramnios, skeletal dysplasia with a narrow thorax (§20.9), and diaphragmatic hernia — and it is the determinant of survival in each.

20.6 The Fetal Anterior Abdominal Wall

The baseline

Physiological midgut herniation resolves in the early first trimester (Chapter 18 §18.5), and an abdominal wall defect should not be diagnosed before it has done so.

The routine assessment is a **transverse view of the abdomen at the cord insertion**, confirming an intact wall with the cord inserting normally.

Gastroschisis versus omphalocele

This is the most consequential distinction in this section, because the two lesions differ in their genetic risk, their associations, and their management.

	Gastroschisis	**Omphalocele (exomphalos)**
Position	**Paraumbilical**, almost always to the **right** of the cord	**Central**, at the cord insertion
Covering membrane	**None** — bowel floats freely in amniotic fluid	**Present** — contents covered by a membrane
Cord insertion	**Normal**, separate from the defect	**Into the apex of the sac**
Contents	Bowel, occasionally other viscera	Bowel, and frequently **liver**
Aneuploidy risk	**Low**	**High** — and **higher still when the liver is NOT herniated**, that is, in bowel-only omphalocele
Associated anomalies	Usually isolated; bowel complications are the issue	**Frequent**, particularly **cardiac**
Maternal factors	Younger maternal age	—
Syndromic association	—	**Beckwith–Wiedemann syndrome**

> **The counterintuitive point worth remembering: a smaller, bowel-only omphalocele carries a higher aneuploidy risk than a large one containing liver.**

Management differs accordingly:

Gastroschisis — genetic risk is low, so the surveillance is directed at the bowel and growth: **fetal growth restriction is common**, and **progressive bowel dilatation and wall thickening** may indicate atresia, ischaemia or obstruction. Serial scanning and delivery planning at a surgical centre follow.

Omphalocele — the priority is **genetic testing and fetal echocardiography**, because the associated anomalies determine the outcome more often than the defect itself.

Other wall defects

Body stalk anomaly (limb–body wall complex) — a large defect with **evisceration, a short or absent umbilical cord, severe scoliosis, and the fetus adherent to the placenta**. It is lethal, and recognising the pattern prevents an inappropriate management pathway.

Bladder exstrophy — an **absent bladder despite normal amniotic fluid**, with a low anterior wall mass. The combination of a persistently non-visualised bladder and normal fluid is the alerting sign.

Cloacal exstrophy (OEIS complex) — omphalocele, exstrophy, imperforate anus and spinal defects.

Pentalogy of Cantrell — a high midline defect with **ectopia cordis**, in which the heart lies partly or wholly outside the thorax.

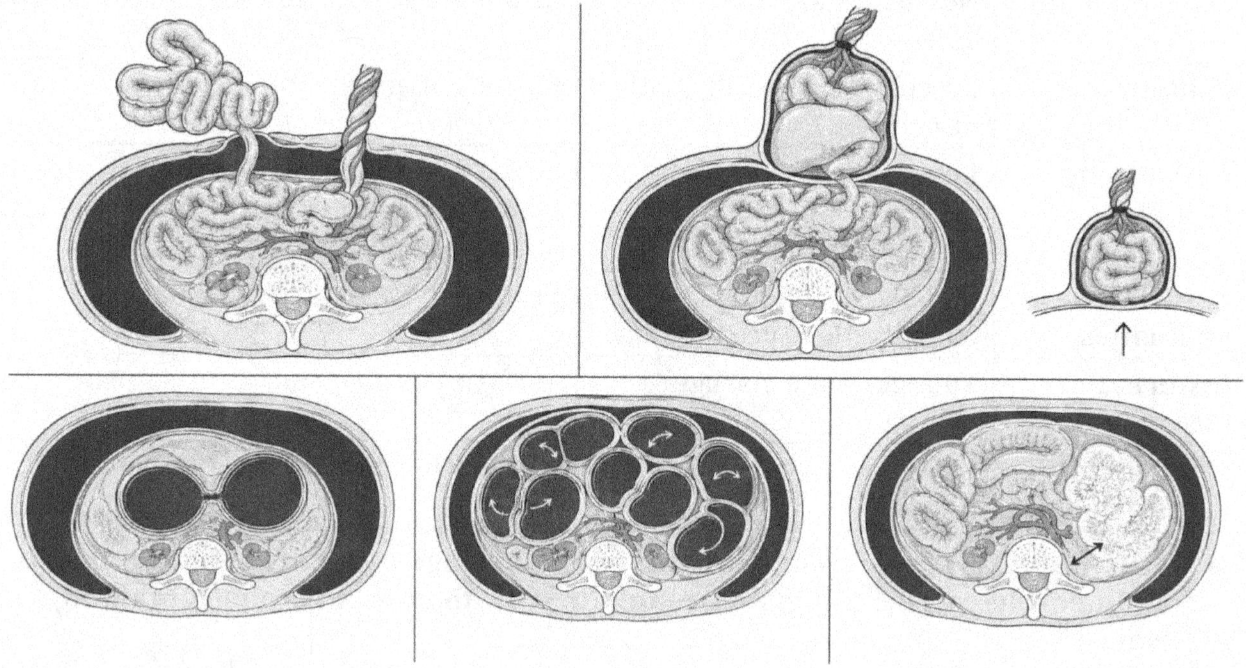

20.7 The Fetal Abdomen and Gastrointestinal Tract

Normal appearances

The stomach lies on the left (Chapter 14 §14.1 — establish situs first). The liver occupies the right upper abdomen, the gallbladder is visible as a small anechoic structure, and **normal bowel is less echogenic than bone**.

The stomach should be visible from early in the second trimester. When it is not, do not conclude on a single observation — **re-look after an interval**, since transient emptying is common.

Absent or small stomach

A persistently absent stomach bubble has a defined differential:

- **Oesophageal atresia** — with **polyhydramnios**
- **Congenital diaphragmatic hernia** — the stomach is in the chest (§20.5)
- **Impaired swallowing** — neurological or neuromuscular conditions, or a neck mass (§20.4)
- **Severe oligohydramnios** — there is no fluid to swallow

Oesophageal atresia: the combination of a **small or absent stomach with polyhydramnios** is the classic presentation, sometimes with a transient **upper pouch** visible in the neck.

> **Most cases have a coexisting tracheo-oesophageal fistula, which allows the stomach to fill — so a visible stomach does not exclude oesophageal atresia.** Detection rates are consequently modest.

Associations: **trisomy 18 and 21**, and the **VACTERL** group (§20.3).

Obstruction

Duodenal atresia — the **"double bubble"**: the fluid-filled stomach and the dilated duodenal bulb.

> **Demonstrate continuity between the two fluid collections**, which distinguishes duodenal atresia from an unrelated abdominal cyst. Turning the fetus or angling the probe usually shows the connecting channel.

Accompanied by **polyhydramnios**, and — the association that must drive management — **a substantial proportion have trisomy 21. Genetic testing and fetal echocardiography must be offered whenever a double bubble is found.**

Jejunoileal atresia and distal obstruction — multiple dilated fluid-filled loops with visible peristalsis, with polyhydramnios in proximal obstruction and less fluid disturbance distally. **Complications to watch for on serial scans are perforation and meconium peritonitis.**

Meconium peritonitis — the sequel to intrauterine bowel perforation: **intra-abdominal calcification**, ascites, and sometimes a walled pseudocyst. It carries an association with **cystic fibrosis**, which should be raised.

Anorectal malformation is rarely diagnosed prenatally, though a dilated distal bowel loop with intraluminal calcification is suggestive, and it may appear within a VACTERL or cloacal pattern.

Echogenic bowel

Defined as bowel echogenicity equal to or greater than adjacent bone, assessed at a moderate gain setting and with harmonics off, since both settings alter the impression.

It is a non-specific finding with a specific workup, because its causes are diverse and several are important:

Cause	Implication
Aneuploidy — particularly trisomy 21	Genetic testing
Cystic fibrosis	Parental carrier screening and fetal testing
Congenital infection — cytomegalovirus especially	Maternal serology
Intra-amniotic bleeding — swallowed blood	Usually benign
Fetal growth restriction / placental insufficiency	Growth and Doppler surveillance
Normal variant	Common

The standard workup is therefore: genetic testing, cystic fibrosis screening, infection serology, and growth surveillance — and reporting the finding without initiating it leaves the work undone. [VERIFY: current grading of echogenic bowel and the recommended investigation pathway]

Abdominal cysts

Ovarian cyst — in a female fetus, a lower abdominal or pelvic cyst, usually simple. **Large cysts carry a risk of torsion**, and a change to a complex appearance with a fluid–debris level suggests it has occurred.

Other cysts: mesenteric, enteric duplication, choledochal (Chapter 12 §12.6), urachal, and hepatic. **Localise the cyst and identify its relationship to normal organs**, since origin determines the differential.

Ascites — either part of hydrops (Chapter 19 §19.11) or urinary in origin from a ruptured obstructed urinary tract (§20.8).

20.8 The Fetal Urogenital System

Normal appearances

The kidneys become reliably visible in the early second trimester as paraspinal structures with a hypoechoic cortex and a slightly echogenic sinus. **The bladder** should be visible and should be seen to fill and empty across the examination.

> **A visible bladder confirms that at least one kidney is producing urine and that the outflow tract is patent.** A persistently absent bladder is a significant finding requiring an explanation, and it should prompt re-examination after an interval rather than a single conclusion.

The two umbilical arteries are identified alongside the bladder (Chapter 19 §19.9).

Renal agenesis

Bilateral renal agenesis — the **empty renal fossae**, **anhydramnios**, and a **persistently absent bladder**. The **"lying-down adrenal" sign** — a flattened, elongated adrenal occupying the empty fossa — supports it.

The consequence is lethal: anhydramnios from early gestation produces **pulmonary hypoplasia** and the associated deformation sequence. **Colour Doppler demonstrating absent renal arteries** confirms the diagnosis and is a useful confirmatory step, since bowel can mimic renal tissue in an anhydramniotic uterus.

Unilateral agenesis — an absent kidney with **compensatory hypertrophy** of the other. **Search the pelvis for an ectopic kidney before concluding absence** (Chapter 7 §7.1), and examine the remaining kidney carefully, since associated anomalies are common.

Cystic and dysplastic kidneys

Multicystic dysplastic kidney — multiple non-communicating cysts of varying size, with no identifiable renal pelvis and no recognisable normal parenchyma (Chapter 12 §12.8). **Examine the contralateral kidney carefully**, since that is where all future function resides and associated anomalies are frequent.

Autosomal recessive polycystic kidney disease — bilaterally enlarged, uniformly and markedly echogenic kidneys with loss of corticomedullary differentiation, the individual cysts being below resolution. Accompanied by **oligohydramnios** and by **congenital hepatic fibrosis.**

Obstructive renal dysplasia — a small echogenic kidney with **cortical cysts**, indicating that obstruction has damaged the parenchyma irreversibly. **The presence of cortical cysts is a prognostic finding, not merely a descriptive one.**

Urinary tract dilatation

Measured as the **anteroposterior renal pelvic diameter** in a transverse plane, and graded using the classification adopted (Chapter 12 §12.8). [VERIFY: current antenatal urinary tract dilatation classification and thresholds]

Determine the level, as in Chapter 7 §7.3: pelvicalyceal dilatation alone suggests **pelviureteric junction obstruction**; dilatation extending down a ureter to the bladder suggests **vesicoureteric junction obstruction or reflux**; and **bilateral dilatation with a distended bladder** indicates **bladder outlet obstruction**.

Lower urinary tract obstruction

> **The pattern: a male fetus, bilateral hydroureteronephrosis, a thick-walled distended bladder, a dilated posterior urethra producing the "keyhole" sign, and reduced amniotic fluid.**

Posterior urethral valves is the commonest cause. **Prognosis is determined by two things**: the **amniotic fluid volume**, since oligohydramnios early in gestation causes pulmonary hypoplasia, and the **renal parenchymal appearance**, since echogenic cortex with cysts indicates established dysplasia.

Urinary ascites or a urinoma may follow forniceal rupture, and paradoxically indicates decompression.

Vesicoamniotic shunting is offered in carefully selected cases (§20.11) — those with preserved renal function and progressive oligohydramnios — and case selection is the difficult part.

Genitalia

Sex determination is subject to the disclosure policies discussed in Chapter 18 §18.2.

Ambiguous genitalia — an important finding requiring genetic and endocrine assessment, with **congenital adrenal hyperplasia** the condition that must not be missed, since it is treatable and potentially life-threatening in the neonate.

> **Discordance between the sonographic appearance of the genitalia and a known fetal sex — from cell-free DNA screening or karyotype — requires investigation rather than assumption of error.**

Hypospadias — a blunt or ventrally curved penile contour with an abnormal urinary stream. **Ovarian cyst** in a female fetus is covered in §20.7.

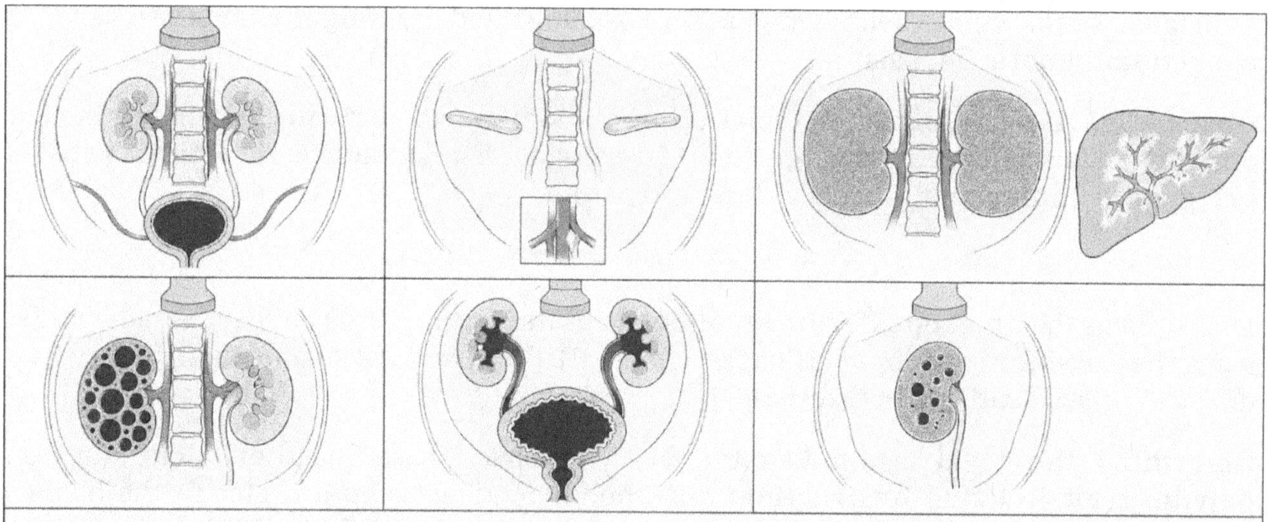

- **Normal kidneys and bladder with the umbilical arteries.** Both kidneys show normal cortical appearance and central sinus. The bladder is present inferiorly, and the umbilical arteries course on each side.
- **Bilateral renal agenesis — empty fossae, lying-down adrenal, anhydramnios, absent renal arteries.** No kidneys or bladder are seen. Flattened adrenals lie in the renal fossae. The uterine space lacks fluid. Colour Doppler shows the aorta without lateral branches.
- **Autosomal recessive polycystic disease with hepatic fibrosis.** Both kidneys are enlarged with uniform microcystic (echogenic) parenchyma and no internal architecture. The liver shows echogenic bands around branching channels.
- **Multicystic dysplastic kidney — examine the other side.** One kidney is replaced by multiple non-communicating cysts of varying sizes and lacks a central sinus. The opposite kidney appears normal but enlarged.
- **Lower urinary tract obstruction with keyhole urethra and thick-walled bladder.** Dilated renal collecting systems, wide ureters, a thick irregular bladder wall, and a short funnel-shaped urethra (keyhole) indicate outflow obstruction.
- **Cortical cysts indicating established dysplasia.** The kidney is small with a densely echogenic cortex containing multiple small cortical cysts within the rim, consistent with established dysplastic change.

20.9 The Fetal Skeleton and Skeletal Dysplasias

The measurements

Femur length is part of routine biometry (Chapter 19 §19.2). Where a dysplasia is suspected, **measure all long bones** — humerus, radius, ulna, tibia, fibula — and assess the hands, feet, spine, skull and thorax.

A systematic approach to short long bones

Short bones are a common referral, and most are not dysplasias. Work through the following in order:

1. Is it early or late in onset? Marked shortening detected in the mid-trimester suggests a **dysplasia**. Shortening that appears only in the third trimester more often reflects **growth restriction or constitutional smallness**, and **achondroplasia characteristically declares itself late**.

2. How severe is the shortening? Mild shortening has a broad and largely benign differential; **severe shortening well below the reference range** points strongly to a dysplasia.

3. Which segments are affected? Rhizomelic (proximal), **mesomelic** (middle), **acromelic** (distal), or **micromelic** (all) — the pattern narrows the differential.

4. What is the thoracic circumference?

> **This is the measurement that predicts survival.** A **narrow thorax** — assessed by thoracic circumference and by the thoracic-to-abdominal or cardiothoracic ratio — indicates **pulmonary hypoplasia**, and it is pulmonary hypoplasia, not the limb shortening, that determines whether a skeletal dysplasia is lethal. **Report it in every suspected dysplasia.**

5. Is mineralisation normal? Poor mineralisation produces a poorly ossified skull that is **abnormally compressible under probe pressure**, unusually clear visualisation of the brain, and reduced acoustic shadowing from bone. It suggests **osteogenesis imperfecta** or **hypophosphatasia**.

6. Are there fractures? Angulation, callus formation and irregular contours indicate fractures, and with poor mineralisation suggest osteogenesis imperfecta.

7. What is the skull shape? A **cloverleaf skull** occurs in thanatophoric dysplasia; frontal bossing in achondroplasia.

8. What do the hands, feet and spine show? Polydactyly, clenched or abnormally postured hands, **talipes**, and **platyspondyly** (flattened vertebral bodies) all narrow the diagnosis.

The principal dysplasias

Dysplasia	Features	Outcome
Thanatophoric dysplasia	Severe micromelia, curved "telephone receiver" femora, **markedly narrow thorax**, cloverleaf skull in one subtype	**Lethal**
Osteogenesis imperfecta type II	**Poor mineralisation**, multiple fractures with angulation, beaded ribs, compressible skull	**Lethal**
Achondrogenesis	Severe micromelia, absent or minimal vertebral ossification, narrow thorax	**Lethal**
Hypophosphatasia (perinatal)	Profoundly deficient mineralisation	**Lethal**
Achondroplasia	**Rhizomelic** shortening declaring in the third trimester, frontal bossing, normal thorax, trident hand	**Non-lethal**
Campomelic dysplasia	Bowed long bones, hypoplastic scapulae, sex reversal in some	Usually lethal

Genetic testing, and particularly exome sequencing, has substantially improved the precision of prenatal dysplasia diagnosis, and it should be offered rather than relying on morphology alone.

Isolated limb and joint anomalies

Radial ray anomalies — absent or hypoplastic radius with a deviated hand — occur in **VACTERL**, **Fanconi anaemia**, and **thrombocytopenia–absent radius syndrome**, and require a full survey and genetic assessment.

Amelia and phocomelia — absent or severely shortened limbs.

Talipes equinovarus (clubfoot) — the foot fixed in a persistently abnormal relationship to the tibia in a coronal plane. **Isolated talipes is common and usually correctable**, but it is associated with **neural tube defects, arthrogryposis, oligohydramnios and aneuploidy**, so a complete survey is required before calling it isolated.

Arthrogryposis — multiple fixed joint contractures with **markedly reduced or absent fetal movement**, which is a real-time observation and cannot be made from still images. Where movement is reduced, observe for an extended period and document it.

Amniotic band sequence — asymmetric, non-anatomical amputations and constriction rings (Chapter 19 §19.11).

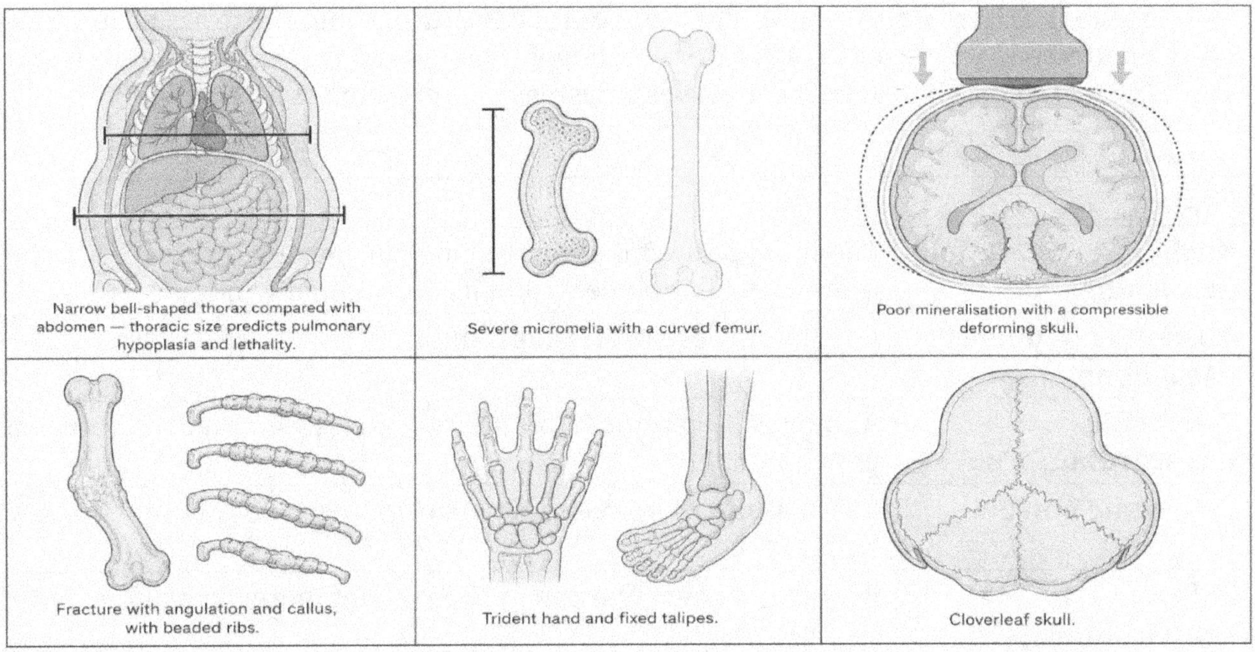

The thorax predicts survival, not the femur.

20.10 Aneuploidy Markers and Syndromic Patterns

What a soft marker is

A soft marker is a normal variant that occurs more frequently in aneuploid fetuses than in euploid ones. It is not a structural anomaly, and in isolation it usually indicates nothing.

Its function is to modify a prior risk — the risk generated by maternal age and by whatever screening has already been performed. A marker multiplies that prior risk by a likelihood ratio, and **the resulting posterior risk depends heavily on what the prior risk was.**

The change that cell-free DNA screening has made

This is the most important shift in this section, and much older teaching predates it:

> **In a woman with a normal cell-free DNA screening result, the prior risk of the common trisomies is already very low. An isolated soft marker in that setting shifts it very little, and reporting it generates anxiety and invasive testing without corresponding benefit.**

Consequently, **many protocols no longer report isolated soft markers in low-risk women**, or report a restricted subset. **A department must adopt a policy and apply it consistently**, rather than leaving each operator to decide. [VERIFY: the current policy on soft marker reporting to be adopted, and which markers remain reportable in isolation]

Two things do remain true:

- **Markers found with a structural anomaly, or in clusters, retain their significance** — the non-isolated principle of §20.1

- **Some markers point to non-chromosomal conditions**, and those associations are unaffected by cell-free DNA results — echogenic bowel and cystic fibrosis or infection (§20.7), and a short femur and skeletal dysplasia or growth restriction (§20.9)

The markers

Marker	Note
Nuchal fold thickening	The most powerful second-trimester marker; measured in the transcerebellar plane within its gestational window
Absent or hypoplastic nasal bone	Population variation is substantial
Echogenic intracardiac focus	A normal variant; frequency varies markedly between populations
Echogenic bowel	Has a **non-chromosomal workup** regardless of aneuploidy risk (§20.7)
Mild ventriculomegaly	Requires its own workup (§20.2) — not merely a marker
Mild pyelectasis	Postnatal follow-up rather than genetic significance in isolation
Short femur or humerus	Consider growth restriction and dysplasia (§20.9)
Aberrant right subclavian artery	Associated with trisomy 21 and with 22q11 deletion
Single umbilical artery	Growth surveillance regardless (Chapter 19 §19.9)
Choroid plexus cyst	Associated with trisomy 18 — but **trisomy 18 almost always has other detectable anomalies**, so an isolated cyst with otherwise normal anatomy is of very limited significance

Syndromic patterns

Recognising a pattern is more useful than recognising any single finding:

Trisomy 21 — atrioventricular septal defect, duodenal atresia, nuchal fold thickening, absent nasal bone, short femur and humerus, echogenic bowel, echogenic intracardiac focus, sandal gap, clinodactyly.

Trisomy 18 — clenched hands with overlapping digits, choroid plexus cysts, rocker-bottom feet, congenital diaphragmatic hernia, omphalocele, cardiac defects, **early-onset growth restriction**, single umbilical artery, and a strawberry-shaped head.

Trisomy 13 — holoprosencephaly with midline facial anomalies, polydactyly, cardiac defects, enlarged echogenic kidneys, growth restriction.

Turner syndrome — cystic hygroma, hydrops, left-sided cardiac lesions including coarctation, horseshoe kidney.

Triploidy — severe early growth restriction with relative head sparing, and an enlarged cystic placenta in the partial molar form (Chapter 18 §18.10).

22q11 deletion — conotruncal cardiac lesions, thymic hypoplasia, cleft palate.

Beckwith-Wiedemann syndrome — macroglossia, omphalocele, macrosomia and organomegaly.

Noonan syndrome — increased nuchal translucency, cystic hygroma, pulmonary stenosis, hydrops.

Meckel-Gruber syndrome — occipital encephalocele, enlarged cystic kidneys, polydactyly.

VACTERL is an **association, not a syndrome** — a non-random co-occurrence without a single genetic cause — and finding one component should prompt a search for the others.

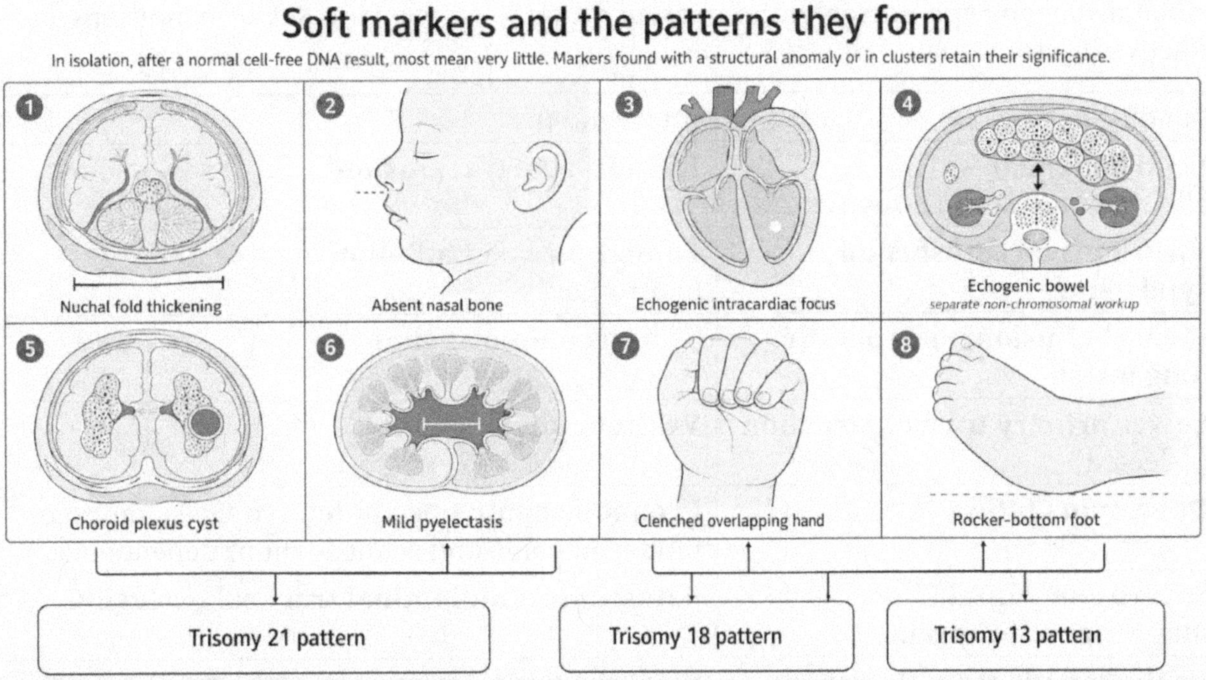

20.11 Counselling, Referral, and Fetal Intervention

The pathway after a diagnosis

A structural anomaly initiates a defined process, and the sonographer's part in it is the first step.

The multidisciplinary team typically includes a **fetal medicine specialist**, the relevant **paediatric surgical or medical subspecialist**, a **clinical geneticist**, a **neonatologist**, a **specialist midwife or nurse**, and access to **psychological support**.

The counselling covers:

- **The diagnosis and its certainty** — including what remains uncertain

- **Whether the finding is isolated**, and what further assessment is planned
- **Genetic testing options** and what each can and cannot exclude
- **The natural history**, and the range of outcomes
- **The treatment pathway**, including any surgery and its staging
- **Delivery planning** — place, mode and timing
- **The options available**, including continuation with active neonatal care, continuation with a palliative care plan, and, where lawful, termination of pregnancy
- **Written information, a second opinion, and support organisations**

Time matters in both directions: decisions have gestational deadlines, but parents also need space to absorb information, and a single consultation is rarely sufficient.

Established fetal interventions

Prenatal diagnosis is not only about preparation — a growing set of conditions has an effective in-utero treatment:

Condition	Intervention
Fetal anaemia — alloimmunisation, parvovirus	**Intrauterine transfusion**
Twin-to-twin transfusion syndrome	**Fetoscopic laser ablation** of placental anastomoses
Pleural effusion; macrocystic lung lesion	**Thoracoamniotic shunt**
Lower urinary tract obstruction (selected)	**Vesicoamniotic shunt**
Open spina bifida	**Prenatal repair**, open or fetoscopic — improves motor outcome and reduces shunt dependence
Severe congenital diaphragmatic hernia	**Fetoscopic endoluminal tracheal occlusion**
Critical aortic stenosis, other selected cardiac lesions	**Fetal cardiac intervention** in specialist centres
Airway obstruction — neck mass, CHAOS	**EXIT procedure** — securing the airway while placental circulation continues
Fetal tachyarrhythmia	**Maternal antiarrhythmic therapy**

All are performed in specialist centres, with careful case selection, and several within trial or registry frameworks. The role of the referring service is to **identify the candidate and refer promptly**, because most of these interventions have a gestational window.

The sonographer's role and boundary

Restating what has appeared throughout this book, because it applies with the greatest force here:

Within scope: performing a technically complete examination; recognising abnormality; **searching deliberately for associated findings**; documenting fully; and **escalating promptly and directly** to the appropriate specialist.

Outside scope: communicating a diagnosis or a prognosis to the parents.

What is required is not silence but a manner of escalation (Chapter 1 §1.3, Chapter 18 §18.2): explain that a colleague needs to review the images, that this is a normal part of the process, and that a specialist will speak with them — without confirming or denying a finding you are not in a position to interpret.

After the pregnancy

Postnatal confirmation of the prenatal findings closes the loop and is how a service learns its own accuracy.

Where a pregnancy is lost or terminated, post-mortem examination or post-mortem imaging, with genetic testing, frequently changes the recurrence risk given to the family — and is therefore offered as part of care rather than as research.

Recurrence counselling and pre-pregnancy care follow: folic acid supplementation for neural tube defects, glycaemic optimisation in diabetes, aspirin prophylaxis where indicated for pre-eclampsia, and specific genetic counselling where a cause has been identified.

A Closing Note

This is the last section of the book, and it is a fitting place to restate what the first chapter argued.

Ultrasound is operator-dependent in acquisition as well as interpretation. A structure that was not insonated does not exist in the record. Everything in the nineteen chapters between — the physics, the protocols, the measurement conventions, the artifact catalogue, the classification systems, the escalation pathways — exists to reduce the distance between what is present in the patient and what appears in the report.

The sonographer's judgement is the instrument. The machine only records what that judgement chose to look at.

Key Points

1. Finding an anomaly is the beginning of the examination. Whether it is isolated determines the aneuploidy risk, the prognosis and the counselling.
2. A normal cell-free DNA result does not reassure in the presence of a structural anomaly — it screens for a limited set of conditions.
3. Describe findings; do not assign a syndrome. A named syndrome in a report becomes the working diagnosis regardless of subsequent testing.
4. An absent cavum septi pellucidi should prompt a deliberate midline assessment for corpus callosum agenesis.

5. The face predicts the brain — midline facial anomalies and holoprosencephaly accompany each other, and finding either obliges a search for the other.
6. Screen the head for open spina bifida. The lemon and banana signs are more sensitive than the spinal defect, and an obliterated cisterna magna should trigger a detailed spinal examination.
7. Closed dysraphism has no Chiari II signs, so a normal posterior fossa does not exclude it.
8. Isolated cleft palate without cleft lip is frequently undetectable — a normal lip does not exclude it.
9. Any large fetal neck mass raises the question of neonatal airway obstruction and changes the delivery plan.
10. In diaphragmatic hernia, the diagnostic observation is abdominal contents at the same axial level as the heart. Liver herniated into the chest worsens the prognosis substantially.
11. Every echogenic lung lesion needs colour Doppler — a systemic feeding vessel from the aorta identifies a sequestration.
12. Gastroschisis is paraumbilical, uncovered and carries low aneuploidy risk; omphalocele is central, covered and carries high risk — higher still when the liver is not herniated.
13. In gastroschisis the surveillance is directed at growth and bowel; in omphalocele it is directed at genetics and the heart.
14. A visible stomach does not exclude oesophageal atresia, because most cases have a fistula that allows the stomach to fill.
15. Demonstrate continuity between the two collections before calling a double bubble, and offer genetic testing and echocardiography whenever you find one.
16. Echogenic bowel has a defined workup — genetic testing, cystic fibrosis screening, infection serology and growth surveillance. Reporting it without initiating that leaves the work undone.
17. A persistently absent bladder requires an explanation. Re-look before concluding.
18. In lower urinary tract obstruction, the prognosis lies in the amniotic fluid volume and the renal cortical appearance, not the degree of dilatation.
19. In suspected skeletal dysplasia, the thoracic circumference predicts survival — not the femur length.
20. A poorly mineralised skull deforms under probe pressure; that compressibility is a finding, not an artifact.
21. Isolated talipes is usually correctable, but a complete survey is required before calling it isolated.
22. Reduced fetal movement in suspected arthrogryposis is a real-time observation that still images cannot capture.
23. After a normal cell-free DNA result, an isolated soft marker shifts risk very little — and reporting it generates anxiety and invasive testing without benefit.
24. Markers found with a structural anomaly or in clusters retain their significance, and some point to non-chromosomal conditions unaffected by cell-free DNA.

25. Identify candidates for fetal intervention and refer promptly — most of these treatments have a gestational window.
26. Escalate promptly; do not diagnose or prognosticate. The alternative to disclosure is an explanation of the process, not silence.

Registry Check

1. A fetus has an isolated omphalocele containing bowel but no liver. Compared with a large omphalocele containing liver, the aneuploidy risk is:

A. Lower **B.** Higher **C.** The same **D.** Absent

> **Answer: B.** Counterintuitively, a smaller omphalocele containing only bowel carries a higher risk of aneuploidy than a larger one containing liver. Genetic testing and fetal echocardiography are indicated in all omphaloceles, and the associated anomalies frequently determine outcome more than the defect itself.

2. During the transcerebellar view, the cisterna magna cannot be identified and the cerebellum appears curved anteriorly around the brainstem. The next step is:

A. Repeat the measurement in a different plane **B.** Perform a detailed examination of the fetal spine **C.** Report an isolated posterior fossa abnormality **D.** Arrange fetal echocardiography

> **Answer: B.** The banana sign with an obliterated cisterna magna is the cranial manifestation of the Chiari II deformity, which accompanies open spina bifida. The cranial signs are more sensitive than direct visualisation of the spinal defect, and their presence should always trigger a detailed spinal examination.

3. An echogenic mass is seen in the fetal thorax. Colour Doppler demonstrates a feeding vessel arising from the descending aorta. This indicates:

A. Congenital pulmonary airway malformation **B.** Bronchopulmonary sequestration **C.** Congenital diaphragmatic hernia **D.** Congenital high airway obstruction sequence

> **Answer: B.** A microcystic pulmonary airway malformation and a sequestration can appear identical on greyscale. The discriminator is vascular: a sequestration has a systemic arterial supply from the aorta, and colour Doppler should be applied to every echogenic lung lesion for this reason.

4. A "double bubble" is seen in the fetal abdomen with polyhydramnios. Which additional step is essential?

A. Serial growth scans only **B.** Demonstrating continuity between the two fluid collections, and offering genetic testing and fetal echocardiography **C.** Assessment of the fetal spine **D.** Amniotic fluid index measurement alone

> **Answer: B.** Continuity between the stomach and the dilated duodenal bulb distinguishes duodenal atresia from an unrelated abdominal cyst. A substantial proportion of cases have trisomy 21, so genetic testing and echocardiography must be offered whenever the finding is made.

5. Bilateral hydroureteronephrosis, a thick-walled bladder and a dilated posterior urethra are seen in a male fetus. Prognosis is best predicted by:

A. The degree of pelvicalyceal dilatation **B.** The bladder wall thickness **C.** The amniotic fluid volume and the renal cortical appearance **D.** The size of the keyhole

> **Answer: C.** In lower urinary tract obstruction, oligohydramnios early in gestation causes pulmonary hypoplasia, and an echogenic renal cortex with cortical cysts indicates established dysplasia. Neither the degree of dilatation nor the bladder wall thickness predicts outcome as reliably.

6. In a fetus with markedly short long bones, which measurement most reliably predicts lethality?

A. Femur length **B.** Femur length to abdominal circumference ratio **C.** Thoracic circumference **D.** Biparietal diameter

> **Answer: C.** Lethality in skeletal dysplasia is determined by pulmonary hypoplasia, which follows from a narrow thorax. Thoracic circumference and the thoracic-to-abdominal ratio should be reported in every suspected dysplasia, since the degree of limb shortening itself does not predict survival.

7. An isolated echogenic intracardiac focus is found in a woman with a normal cell-free DNA screening result and otherwise normal anatomy. The appropriate response is:

A. Offer amniocentesis **B.** Recognise that the finding shifts an already very low risk very little, and follow the departmental policy on soft marker reporting **C.** Arrange serial fetal echocardiography **D.** Report it as a cardiac abnormality

> **Answer: B.** An echogenic intracardiac focus is a normal variant. With a normal cell-free DNA result the prior risk of the common trisomies is already very low, and an isolated marker changes it minimally. Many protocols no longer report isolated markers in this setting, and a consistent departmental policy is required.

8. Which of the following has an established in-utero treatment that improves outcome?

A. Gastroschisis **B.** Trisomy 21 **C.** Open spina bifida **D.** Renal agenesis

> **Answer: C.** Prenatal repair of open spina bifida, whether open or fetoscopic, improves motor outcome and reduces shunt dependence compared with postnatal repair in appropriately selected cases. Identifying candidates and referring promptly matters because the intervention has a gestational window.

Chapter Notes for the Editorial Pass

Verification queue. In priority order: **the soft marker reporting policy to be adopted** (§20.10) — this is the chapter's most consequential editorial decision, because practice has changed substantially since cell-free DNA screening became widely available and much published material predates it; **genetic testing recommendations by indication and their diagnostic yields** (§20.1); **normal ranges for atrial diameter, cisterna magna,**

transcerebellar diameter and nuchal fold, and the ventriculomegaly grading bands (§20.2); **lung-to-head ratio methodology and prognostic thresholds** and **the volume ratio for pulmonary airway malformation** (§20.5); **the echogenic bowel investigation pathway** (§20.7); **the antenatal urinary tract dilatation classification** (§20.8, consistent with the decision taken for Chapter 12); **sacrococcygeal teratoma classification** (§20.3); and the **current status and case selection criteria for each fetal intervention** (§20.11), which is an actively developing area.

Consistency check across the book. Three classification decisions taken elsewhere reappear here and must match: **urinary tract dilatation** (Chapter 12 §12.8), **the adnexal and cardiac descriptive systems**, and the **soft marker policy**, which interacts with the first-trimester screening material in Chapter 18 §18.7. The five-system editorial session flagged in the Chapter 17 notes should be extended to include the soft marker policy, making six.

Figure count: 7 Lane A, 1 Lane B. The Lane B request is deliberately modest — a normal reference set — because this chapter's material is overwhelmingly pattern-based and the schematics carry it. If the digital edition supports video, the highest-value clip for this chapter is **observed fetal movement in suspected arthrogryposis**, which cannot be conveyed by any still image.

Cross-reference targets to fix at layout: §20.1 screening versus diagnosis → Chapter 18 §18.7; §20.2 corpus callosum and posterior fossa → Chapter 13 §13.6; §20.5 cardiac assessment → Chapter 15 §15.7; §20.6 physiological herniation → Chapter 18 §18.5; §20.7 choledochal cyst → Chapter 12 §12.6; §20.8 urinary tract dilatation and multicystic dysplastic kidney → Chapter 12 §12.8; §20.8 ectopic kidney → Chapter 7 §7.1; §20.9 amniotic band sequence → Chapter 19 §19.11; §20.10 first-trimester screening → Chapter 18 §18.7; §20.11 ethical framework and disclosure → Chapter 18 §18.2 and Chapter 1 §1.2–1.3; §20.11 counselling after cardiac diagnosis → Chapter 15 §15.10.

Word count: approximately 10,400 excluding image prompt blocks, learning objectives, registry questions, and these notes.